Innovative Approaches
in Drug Discovery

Innovative Approaches in Drug Discovery

Ethnopharmacology, Systems Biology, and Holistic Targeting

Bhushan Patwardhan, PhD, FAMS
Professor, Interdisciplinary School of Health Sciences and
Director, Center for Complementary and Integrative Health
Savitribai Phule Pune University
Pune, India

Rathnam Chaguturu, PhD
Founder and CEO, iDDPartners
Princeton Junction, NJ, United States

AMSTERDAM • BOSTON • HEIDELBERG • LONDON
NEW YORK • OXFORD • PARIS • SAN DIEGO
SAN FRANCISCO • SINGAPORE • SYDNEY • TOKYO
Academic Press is an imprint of Elsevier

Academic Press is an imprint of Elsevier
125 London Wall, London EC2Y 5AS, United Kingdom
525 B Street, Suite 1800, San Diego, CA 92101-4495, United States
50 Hampshire Street, 5th Floor, Cambridge, MA 02139, United States
The Boulevard, Langford Lane, Kidlington, Oxford OX5 1GB, United Kingdom

British Library Cataloguing-in-Publication Data
A catalogue record for this book is available from the British Library

Library of Congress Cataloging-in-Publication Data
A catalog record for this book is available from the Library of Congress

ISBN: 978-0-12-801814-9

For Information on all Academic Press publications
visit our website at https://www.elsevier.com

  Working together
to grow libraries in
ELSEVIER Book Aid developing countries
International

www.elsevier.com • www.bookaid.org

Acquisition Editor: Kristine Jones
Editorial Project Manager: Tracy Tufaga
Production Project Manager: Lucía Pérez
Designer: Vicky Pearson

Typeset by MPS Limited, Chennai, India

Contents

About the Editors   xiii
About the Authors   xv
Foreword   xxv
Preface   xxix
Dedication   xxxvii

1. Drug Discovery Impasse: Pharmacognosy Holds the Key   1

Rathnam Chaguturu and Bhushan Patwardhan

Historical Perspectives   2
Synthetic Drugs   3
Ethnopharmacology and Natural Products   3
Emergence of Biotechnology   5
Drug Discovery Process   6
Drug Discovery Impasse   8
New Drug Approvals   9
Drug Recalls and Withdrawals   10
Why Drugs Fail?   12
Need for Novel Approaches   13
Chemical Approaches   14
Pharmacology Approaches   16
Biological Approaches   16
Formulation Discovery   18
Concluding Remarks   19
References   19

2. Why and How Drugs Fail   23

Dada Patil, Bhushan Patwardhan and Kalyani Kumbhare

Introduction   23
Drug Withdrawals: Analysis of Six Decades   23
Case Study 1: Statins   25
Discovery and Development of Statins   25
Statin-Induced Diabetes   29
Case Study 2: Example of Troglitazone   31
Mechanism   32
Evidence of Toxicity   34

TGZ Withdrawals: European and USFDA Responses 37
Cytotoxic Response to Liver Cells: Probable Role
of Mitochondrial Injury 38
Inhibition of Bile Salt Export Pump (BSEP) 39
Formation of Electrophilic Reactive Intermediates 41
Role of Host-Related Factors 41
Case Study 3: Example of Rofecoxib 41
Development of Vioxx 42
The Downfall of Vioxx 46
Withdrawal of Vioxx: The "Blockbuster" Drug 47
Rofecoxib and Cardiovascular Toxicity: Role of On-Target,
Off-Target, and Intrinsic Chemical Properties 48
Case Study 4: Example of Thalidomide 49
Conclusions and Future Perspectives 51
References 56

3. **Holistic Drug Targeting** 65
Anuradha Roy and Rathnam Chaguturu

Introduction 65
Single-Target Specificity Approach 67
Target Identification and Validation 67
Chemical Genetics 68
High-Throughput Screening (HTS) of Druggable Targets 69
Rational Drug Design 71
Pharmacognosy 72
Target to Lead Bottleneck 73
Biological Redundancy and the Holistic Advantage 73
Approaches for Holistic Drug Targeting 75
Drug Repositioning 78
Combination Therapy 81
Multitarget Drug Discovery 83
Concluding Remarks 85
References 86

4. **Reverse Pharmacology** 89
*Ashwinikumar A. Raut, Mukund S. Chorghade and
Ashok D.B. Vaidya*

Introduction and Background 89
Introduction 89
Background of Reverse Pharmacology 90
The Roots of Modern Drugs in Traditional Remedies/Poisons 91
The Definition of Reverse Pharmacology and Its Different Origins 94
Ayurvedic Pharmacoepidemiology and Observational Therapeutics 95
Ayurvedic Pharmacoepidemiology 96
Observational Therapeutics 97

Clinical Study Designs and Para-Clinical Models in Reverse
  Pharmacology 98
Ayurveda-Inspired Hits and Leads for New Drug Discoveries 100
Discovery of Natural Products-Based New Chemical Entities via
  Chemistry and Chemical Biology Technologies 102
Introduction and Background 102
Isolation of Natural Products From Plant Species with Established
  Indian Folk Medicine Properties 105
Design and Synthesis of Natural Product Analogs 106
Reverse Pharmacology and New Domains in Life Sciences 108
Automated Oxidation Chemistry for Diversified Analogues 108
Reverse Pharmacology Approach to GPCR-Focused Drug
  Discovery 110
Reverse Pharmacology and Novel Biodynamic Actions 111
Unique Dimensions of Ayurveda Therapeutics 112
Organization for Academic Development of Reverse Pharmacology 115
Challenges and Opportunities in Reverse Pharmacology 117
Future Direction and Scope of Differentiation in Reverse
  Pharmacology 118
References 120

5. Network Pharmacology 127

Uma Chandran, Neelay Mehendale, Saniya Patil,
Rathnam Chaguturu and Bhushan Patwardhan

Introduction 127
Network Pharmacology 128
Network Biology to Network Pharmacology 129
Network Ethnopharmacology 131
Traditional Medicine Inspired Ethnopharmacological Networks 138
Knowledge Bases for Network Ethnopharmacology 142
Network Construction 144
Ayurveda and Network Ethnopharmacology 146
Network Ethnopharmacology of Triphala 146
Triphala Bioactives 147
Human Proteome and Diseasome Targeting Network of Triphala 147
Microbial Proteome Targeting Network of Triphala 151
Applications of Network Pharmacology 154
Limitations and Solutions 154
Conclusion 157
References 157

6. Genomics-Driven Drug Discovery Process 165

Rathnam Chaguturu

Historical Perspective 165
Basic Research Drives Innovation 166

Drug Discovery: Soup to Nuts   167
Target Identification   170
Lead Identification   172
Lead Optimization Strategies   175
Preclinical Studies   179
Preclinical and Clinical Development of Drug Candidates   182
Clinical Development   182
Designing Clinical Trials   183
Clinical Research Phase Studies   183
FDA Review: Registration and Regulatory Approval   184
Phase IV (Life Cycle Management)   184
INDs for Marketed Drugs   184
Concluding Remarks   185
Acknowledgments   185
Appendix 4   189
Forward Chemical Genetics   189
References   191

7. Pharmacogenomics   195
Yogita A. Ghodke-Puranik and Jatinder K. Lamba

Introduction   195
Absorption, Distribution, Metabolism, and Excretion
   (ADME) of Drugs   196
Role of ADME Genes in Drug Response and Adverse Drug Reactions   197
Pharmacogenetics in Drug Response   198
Pharmacogenomics of Phase I Drug Metabolizing Enzymes   198
Pharmacogenomics of Phase II Drug Metabolizing Enzymes   207
Pharmacogenomics of Drug Transporters   209
Pharmacogenomics of Drug Targets   212
Genetic Variability Affecting Adverse Drug Reactions   214
Drug-Induced Liver Injury   214
Drug Hypersensitivity   215
Irinotecan-Induced Myelosuppression   216
Clinical Implementation of Pharmacogenomics   216
Pharmacogenomics in Drug Development   220
Concept of Personalized Medicine in Traditional Indian
   Medical System: Ayurveda   221
Traditional Medicine to Modern Pharmacogenomics: AyuGenomics   222
Ayugenomics a Tool for Classifying Human Population   223
Ayurveda Prakriti Type Associated With the Metabolic Variability   223
Other Studies on Traditional Medicine   224
Perspectives and Conclusions   225
References   226

8.   Transcriptomics and Epigenomics   235
        Preeti Chavan-Gautam, Tejas Shah and Kalpana Joshi

        Introduction   235
        Transcriptomics   236
        The Interrogation of the Transcriptome   237
        Small Interfering RNAs (siRNA), as Therapeutic Agents   237
        Challenges   238
        The Role of RNAi in Identification and Validation of Drug Targets   240
        Applications of RNAi in Various Diseases   241
        Applications of Transcriptomics in Drug Discovery   248
        Transcriptomics in Herbal Drug Discovery   249
        Transcriptomics for Lead Optimization   251
        Transcriptomics for Avoiding Toxicity Pathways   252
        Transcriptomics in Toxicogenomics   252
        Limitations and Further Scope   253
        Epigenomics   254
        DNA methylation   255
        Histone Modifications   255
        Epigenomics Methodologies   256
        Epigenetic Modifications in Infectious Diseases   257
        Epigenetic Modifications in Lifestyle Diseases   258
        Epigenetic Modifications in Degenerative Diseases   259
        Epigenetic Modifications in Cancer   259
        Epigenetic Machinery as Therapeutic Target   260
        Epigenomics and Ethnopharmacology   261
        Limitations and Scope   262
        References   262

9.   Proteomics   273
        Kalpana Joshi and Dada Patil

        Introduction   273
        Recent Advances in Proteomics Technologies   274
        Two-Dimensional Gel Electrophoresis   274
        Electrospray Ionization   275
        Matrix-Assisted Laser Desorption/Ionization   275
        Surface-Enhanced Laser Desorption/Ionization   275
        Protein Microarray Technology   276
        Applications of Proteomics in Drug Discovery   276
        **Biomarker Discovery and Identification of Potential
            Therapeutic Targets**   278
        Some Key Examples   278
        Understanding Disease Mechanisms—MOA (Mode of Action)   279
        Proteomics in Lead Optimization   281
        Proteomics for Evaluating Drug Toxicity   282
        Proteomics in Ethnopharmacology Research   284
        Investigating MOA Botanical Drugs   284

Quality Control and Standardization	286
Toxicokinetics and Herb–Drug Interactions	287
Limitations and Future Prospective	288
References	289

10. Chemical Informatics — 295

Gerald H. Lushington and Rathnam Chaguturu

Key Informatics Challenges in Drug Discovery	297
Efficient Screen Focusing	298
Target Identification	302
Mechanism of Action Perception	303
Reliable Structure-Activity Relationship (SAR) Elaboration	303
Reliable Structure-Based Design	305
Achieving Target Specificity	308
Accurate Toxicity Prediction	308
Pharmacognosy	310
Conclusions	312
References	313

11. Vaccines and Immunodrugs Discovery — 315

Manish Gautam, Bhushan Patwardhan, Sunil Gairola and Suresh Jadhav

Introduction	315
Discovery Approaches for Vaccines	316
Empirical Approaches	316
Rational Approach to Discovery	317
Genomic Approaches for Discovery of Antigens	317
Proteomics-Based Approaches	318
Other Technologies	318
Vaccines Against Complex Pathogens	320
Case Study 1: HIV/AIDS Vaccine	320
Why HIV Virus is Challenging	321
Current Approaches for HIV Vaccine	324
Case Study 2: Malaria Vaccine	325
First Successful Malaria Vaccine	326
Challenges to Developing Malaria Vaccines	327
Systems Approach to Vaccinology	327
Examples of Systems Approach	328
Vaccine Adjuvants	329
Immune Targets for Adjuvant Discovery	330
Trends in Adjuvants and Immunomodulators	332
Small-Molecule Immunodrugs	333
Botanicals for Vaccine Adjuvants	334
Saponins as Vaccine Adjuvants	334
Botanically Derived Polysaccharides as Vaccine Adjuvants	335
Discovery Approaches	337

Summary and Conclusion   339
References   340

12. Curcumin, the Holistic Avant-Garde   343
Subash C. Gupta, Ajaikumar B. Kunnumakkara and Bharat B. Aggarwal

References   347

13. Safety of Traditional Medicines   351
Dnyaneshwar Warude

Introduction   351
Conventional Approaches of Quality Control   352
Newer Approaches for Quality   352
Hyphenated Techniques   352
Phyto-Equivalence Studies   355
DNA Markers   355
Approaches in Safety   358
Pharmacogenomics   359
Pharmacovigilance   360
Herb—Drug Interactions   361
Conclusion   362
References   362

14. Holistic Lifestyle   367
Girish Tillu and Bhushan Patwardhan

Lifestyle and Behavioral Interventions   369
Emerging Evidence From Research   373
Ayurveda and Yoga   375
Medication to Meditation   378
References   382

15. Collaborative Strategies for Future Drug Discovery   387
Rathnam Chaguturu and Bhushan Patwardhan

Prologe   387
The Need   388
Biomedical Ecosystem   389
The New Academia   390
A Roadmap for Successful Drug Discovery in Academia   391
Clinical Models   392
Open Source and Open Science   393
Coordinated, Collaborative Innovation   394
Key Examples   394
Promising Governmental Partnerships   395
Government—Academia—Industry Collaboration: Case From India   396

NMITLI Herbal Drug Project 396
Open Source Drug Discovery 397
Department of Science and Technology 397
Department of Biotechnology 398
SIBRI and BIRAC 398
Indian Council of Medical Research 398
AYUSH 399
Drugs and Biotech Parks 399
Pharma Courting Academia 400
Open Innovations 402
Risk Versus Reward 402
Philanthropic Investments 402
Protection of Intellectual Property 403
Finding the Common Ground 404
It Takes a Village 406
Final Thoughts 408
Further Reading 409

16. Righting the Ship: The Data Reproducibility Conundrum 411

Gerald H. Lushington and Rathnam Chaguturu

Navigating Innovation 411
Here Be Monsters: Reducing the Risks 412
Shipwrecks on the Reproducibility Seas 414
Avast Ye Swabs! 415
Shipworms in the Hull: Animal Anomalies, Corrupt Cells, and Reckless RNAi 416
Headstrong Helm: Cognitive Bias 417
Rigging the Sails With Bad Statistics 421
Toward Calmer Waters: Resources and Conclusions 424
Shame on Us! 425
References 426

Index 429

About the Editors

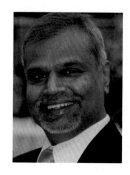

Bhushan Patwardhan, Professor and Director of the Interdisciplinary School of Health Sciences, Savitribai Phule Pune University in Pune, India, is an internationally recognized expert on ethnopharmacology and integrative health. He brings a unique blend of industry/academia executive culture in advancing evidence-based Ayurveda. He is also Chairman of the Academic Planning and Development Committee at the National Institute of Pharmaceutical Education and Research in Mohali, India. He served as advisor for several policy-making bodies, including the Task Forces of the National Knowledge Commission and the Planning Commission, and Commission on Intellectual Property Rights, Innovation and Public Health (CIPIH) of the World Health Organization. Prof Patwardhan is a Fellow of the National Academy of Medical Sciences in India, and the founder and Editor-in-Chief of the *Journal of Ayurveda and Integrative Medicine*, as well as member of the editorial boards of several other journals. He is the recipient of many awards and orations including Parkhe Award for industrial excellence, Dewang Mehta Award for educational excellence, and Sir Ram Nath Chopra Oration. He has guided 18 PhD students, holds eight Indian patents, two US patents, and has written more than 120 research publications. He received his PhD in Biochemistry from the Haffkine Institute in Mumbai, and University of Pune in Pune, India.

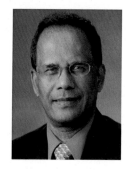

Rathnam Chaguturu is the Founder and CEO of iDDPartners, a nonprofit think-tank focused on pharmaceutical innovation. He has more than 35 years of experience in academia and industry, managing new lead discovery projects and forging collaborative partnerships with academia, disease foundations, nonprofits, and government agencies. He is the Founding President of the International Chemical Biology Society, one of the a founding members of the Society for Biomolecular Sciences, and Editor-in-Chief of the journal *Combinatorial Chemistry and High Throughput Screening*, and he serves on several editorial and scientific advisory boards. Dr Chaguturu has edited the widely received, first-of-its-kind book, *Collaborative Innovation in Drug Discovery: Strategies for Public and Private Partnerships*. And he is also a sought-after speaker at major national and international conferences, where he passionately discusses the need for the reemergence of pharmacognosy, the threat of scientific misconduct in bio-medical sciences, and advocates for the virtues of collaborative partnerships in addressing the pharmaceutical innovation crisis. He received his PhD with an award-winning thesis from Sri Venkateswara University, Tirupati, India.

About the Authors

Ashok D.B. Vaidya, MD (Medicine), PhD (Clinical Pharmacology), is currently Research Director and the Advanced Centre of Reverse Pharmacology, Kasturba Health Society in Mumbai, India. He has a long family lineage of medicine and Ayurveda. Formerly at the helm of affairs at CIBA-GEIGY with an expertise in clinical phases of several new drug molecules, Prof Vaidya has remained engaged in pioneering the development of clinical pharmacology at KEM Hospital, a modern medical institute 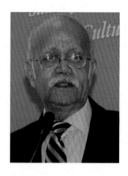 devoted to drug discovery and development from natural products at RAPMC, an Ayurvedic institution. Prof Vaidya has been an expert consultant to government agencies, industries, and research institutes receiving several honors and awards, and has traveled extensively, being a much-sought speaker at scientific conferences and meetings.

Ashwinikumar A. Raut, MD (Ayurveda) is a consultant and researcher blessed with a family tradition of Ayurveda. At present, he is the Director if Clinical Research and Integrative Medicine at Kasturba Health Society's Medical Research Centre in Mumbai, India. Dr. Raut has successfully completed research projects related to Ayurveda formulations and arthritis sponsored by DBT, CSIR, and ICMR Government of India. He received an excellence-in-research award from the Central Drug Research Institute (CDRI) for his work in Ayurveda and rheumatology. Dr. Raut is a 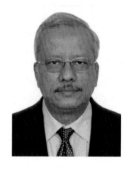 member of the faculty at ARC, KEM Hospital and Seth G S Medical College. He chairs an expert committee at Maharashtra University of Health Sciences, where he prepares the postdoctoral fellowship programs in Reverse Pharmacology.

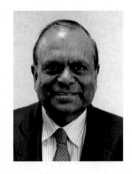

Mukund S. Chorghade, PhD (Organic Chemistry) is an entrepreneur, President and CSO of THINQ Pharma/Discovery. Dr. Chorghade, an adjunct research professor at Harvard, MIT, and Princeton, provides synthetic chemistry and drug development expertise to academia and biopharmaceuticals. He completed his postdoctoral appointments at Universities of Virginia and Harvard. He has also been visiting scientist at the University of British Columbia, the College de France/Université Louis Pasteur, Cambridge, and Caltech, and has directed research at Dow Chemicals, Abbott Laboratories, CytoMed, and Genzyme. Dr. Chorghade, recipient of three Scientist of the Year Awards, and Fellow of the ACS, AAAS, and RSC, has been a featured speaker in several national and international symposia. He serves on several scientific advisory boards at many corporations and foundations.

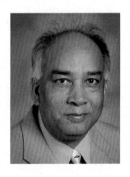

Bharat B. Aggarwal is founding Director of the Anti-inflammation Research Institute in San Diego, CA, United States, and former Professor of Experimental Therapeutics, Cancer Medicine and Immunology, at the University of Texas MD Anderson Cancer Center in Houston, TX, United States. He has been investigating the role of inflammatory pathways mediated through TNFs, NF-kappaB and STAT3, for the prevention and therapy of chronic diseases. While searching for safe antiinflammatory agents, his group has identified more than 50 novel compounds from natural sources that interrupt these cell-signaling pathways. He has published more than 600 papers, edited more than a dozen books, and has been cited by ISI since 2001 as one of the most well-regarded scientists in the world.

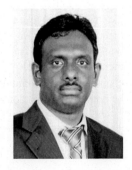

Ajaikumar B. Kunnumakkara is currently working as an Associate Professor in the Department of Biotechnology at the Indian Institute of Technology Guwahati in Assam, India. He obtained his PhD in Biochemistry in 2006 from Amala Cancer Research Center, Thrissur, affiliated with the University of Calicut, Kerala, India. Dr. Kunnumakkara did his first postdoctoral work at the University of Texas MD Anderson Cancer Center in Houston,

TX, United States, (2005−08) and his second postdoctoral work at the National Cancer Institute of National Institutes of Health (NCI/NIH), Bethesda, MD, where he was subsequently employed as a NIH scientist. His research interests include the role of inflammatory pathways in cancer development, anti-inflammatory agents in cancer prevention and treatment, chemosensitization of cancer by natural products, and identification of novel biomarkers for cancer diagnosis and prognosis. He is credited with the publication of more than 80 research articles, and he has more than 11,000 citations with an h-index of >37; his work is cited more than 1700 times in the literature annually. Dr. Kunnumakkara has also edited two monographs entitled *Molecular Targets and Therapeutic Uses of Spices: Modern Uses for Ancient Medicine* and *Anticancer Properties of Fruits and Vegetables: A Scientific Review.*

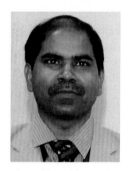

Subash Chandra Gupta, is an Assistant Professor at the Department of Biochemistry, Institute of Science in Banaras Hindu University, India. Dr. Gupta did his postdoctoral training at the Ohio State University and the University of Texas MD Anderson Cancer Center in Houston, TX, and was instructor at the University of Mississippi Medical Center, Jackson, MS, United States. His current research is focused on uncovering the mechanism by which an acidic microenvironment promotes cancer growth. Dr Gupta is also working on cancer chemoprevention and on projects to elucidate the role of inflammatory pathways, cancer stem cells, exosomal microRNAs, and long noncoding RNAs in regulating tumor development. He has published more than 50 peer-reviewed articles in highly prestigious journals and has written several books as well as coedited special issues of scientific journals. He has been honored with prestigious national and international awards, and is member of the editorial board in two reputed scientific journals.

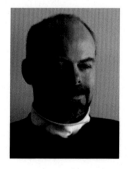

Gerald H. Lushington, brings a wealth of experience in simulations, data mining, and visualization to a diverse range of pharmaceutical and biotechnology research challenges. In addition to skilled application of numerous existing molecular modeling and chemical informatics software tools (including an avid interest in open source initiatives), he is an experienced programmer who has developed and published computational methods. With more than 150 peer-reviewed scientific publications, Lushington is an adjunct faculty member of the Department of Foods, Nutrition, Dietetics and Health at Kansas State University, Manhattan, KS, and the Department of Medicinal Chemistry at the University of Kansas, Lawrence, KS, United States.

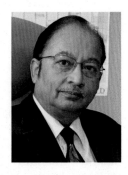

Suresh Jadhav, PhD, M.Pharm., is the Executive Director of Serum Institute of India Pvt. Ltd in Pune, India. His 45 years of technical expertise includes QC/QA/cGMP/GLP/GCP techniques, inspections of laboratories and validation of various production and quality control processes, pharma/ toxicological screening of various drugs, toxins and venoms, and drugs pricing. He successfully led the project of development and introduction of Meningococcal A conjugate vaccine in the sub-Saharan African belt, the development of seasonal and pandemic influenza vaccines, and has also played a major role in the acquisition of Bilthoven Biologicals in The Netherlands. Being associated with DCVMN since its inception, Dr. Jadhav was its President for 5 years. He has been on the board at the GAVI Programme and Policy Committee, and is also member of the European Vaccine Initiative, FastVac, and the Health Innovation in Practice Board, etc. He is closely associated with various advisory committees, like the Task Force of Sabin Vaccine Institute, WHO IVR-IVAC, and Decades of Vaccines (DoV), and is also affiliated with several Indian universities, AICTE, UGC, and the State Directorate of Technical Education. He is the Chairman of Expert Committee on Vaccines and other Biologicals and a member on the Scientific Body of Indian Pharmacopoeia Commission.

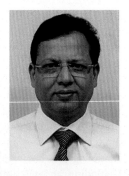

Sunil Gairola is a microbiologist, who graduated from the Department of Microbiology, Himachal Pradesh University in Shimla, India. He worked at the National Control Laboratory, Central Research Institute in Kasauli, and the Serum Institute of India Ltd., where he has been the Director of Quality Control since 2005. He has 30 years of technical experience in quality control of vaccines, adjuvant development, and managing quality control-related activities, and has significantly contributed towards the development and calibration of National Reference Standards for Vaccines and Antisera. Gairola has been a collaborator on many international initiatives of WHO, NVI, NIBSC, EDQM, and PATH, aimed at the harmonization of regulatory requirements, the establishment of international standards, and the development of quality control release assays for immunobiologicals. He is a member of, and a panelist on, the Indian Pharmacopoeia Commision, and the United States Pharmacopeia.

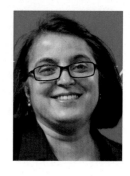

Anuradha Roy, PhD, has been the director of the High Throughput Screening (HTS) Laboratory at the University of Kansas, Lawrence, KS, United States, since 2013. She has 23 years of academic and biotech experience, and has managed development, optimization and execution of early drug discovery projects from target identification, and assay development for high-throughput screening campaigns. As director of the HTS core, her professional responsibilities include helping academic investigators across state universities through the process of developing their target ideas into screenable assays for probe identification. She received her doctoral as well as her MD in Life Sciences from Jawaharlal Nehru University in New Delhi, India.

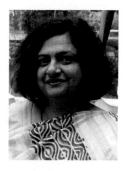

Kalpana Joshi, received her PhD in Microbiology from the Biochemical Science Division of National Chemical Laboratory (CSIR-NCL), and has worked at Lupin R&D as drug discovery manager. At present, she is Professor and Head of the Department of Biotechnology at Sinhgad College of Engineering, SP Pune University, in Pune, India. She has taught for more than 20 years and has lead several prestigious projects funded by DST, ICMR, the Office of the Principal Scientific Adviser (Government of India), and several private companies like Intel, and Glenmark. Her research specialization is molecular and cell biology, pharmacogenomics, biochemistry, immunology, and network pharmacology, whereas the main focus of her research are maternal health and nutrition, pharmacogenomics and ayurvedic biology are her research interests.

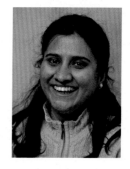

Yogita A. Ghodke-Puranik received her PhD in Health Sciences (Human Genetics and Pharmacogenomics) in 2010 from the Interdisciplinary School of Health Sciences, University of Pune in Pune, India, before going to the University of Minnesota in Twin Cities, MN, United States, for her Postdoctoral training. During her PhD program, she has received several fellowships from the Government of India. She has more than 7 years of experience in the field of human genetics and has worked in broad areas of drug metabolism pharmacogenetics of anticancer, anti-retroviral, antiepileptic, and antirheumatic agents, epigenetic regulation of drug response in cancer patients, as well as and explored the role of mRNAs and miRNAs in transcriptional regulation in human liver. As a research associate at the Mayo Clinic, Rochester, MN, her current research is focused on the genetics of type I interferon pathway in systemic lupus erythematosus patients. She serves as an expert reviewer for journals such as *Clinical and Developmental Immunology, Cytokine, Journal of Proteomics, International Journal of Rheumatic Diseases*, and the *Journal of Ayurveda and Integrative Medicine*. She has authored 19 peer-reviewed research articles and has received several highly cited reviews.

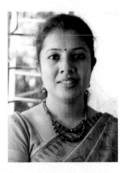

Preeti Chavan-Gautam is Assistant Professor at the Interactive Research School for Health Affairs (IRSHA), Bharati Vidyapeeth University (BVU) in Pune, India. She received her PhD in Health Sciences from the Interdisciplinary School of Health Sciences at the University of Pune in Pune, India, where she worked on applications of DNA markers in the standardization of herbal drugs. She then joined the Interactive Research School for Health Affairs (IRSHA) at Bharati Vidyapeeth Deemed University in Pune, India, as sponsored Research Associate for the Indian Council of Medical Research, where she worked on epigenetic changes in the preterm placenta. At present, Dr Chavan-Gautam is Assistant Professor at the Mother and Child Health Program at IRSHA, where she is interested in understanding placental biology in adverse pregnancy outcomes.

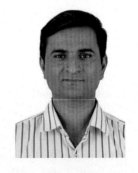

Dnyaneshwar Warude is a drug discovery scientist at Takeda Ltd. Japan, one of the top 10 global pharmaceutical companies, where he is responsible for the repositioning of the company's small molecule asset to fulfill medical needs. His areas of interest include drug discovery and development, ethnopharmacology, and molecular biology. In 2003, he completed an MD in Pharmaceutical Science at the Bharati Vidyapeeth University in Pune, India, and earned his PhD in 2007 at the Savitribai Phule Pune University under the able guidance of Prof Patwardhan. After a short stint as research associate at CSIR, he joined the Lupin Research Center at Pune. As a team leader, he was instrumental in preclinical drug discovery and development for inflammatory and neurological disorders. He has more than 10 publications in peer-reviewed journals to his credit (scopus h-index 8) travels frequently to participate in scientific conferences and deliver lectures.

Manish Gautam has a PhD in Pharmaceutical Sciences from the University of Pune in Pune, India, and currently works as team leader for analytics at Serum Institute of India Pvt Ltd. He is part of the vaccine development group and responsible for assay development, quality control activities, process characterization, and CMC activities for translation of multivalent vaccines from early phase to licensure. His expertise and research interests include immunopharmacology, adjuvant development, ethnopharnacology, glycobiology, and analytics of polysaccharide protein conjugate vaccines.

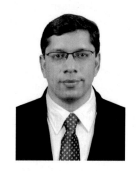

Dada Patil is an analytical scientist at Serum Institute of India Pvt. Ltd. in Pune, India. In his work, he is involved with phyto-metabolomics, pharmacokinetics of small molecules, and an in-depth characterization of vaccine preparations using mass spectrometric platforms. He has published more than 10 research publications in international journals, and was Postdoctoral Research Fellow, at the Interdisciplinary School of Health Sciences, Savitribai Phule Pune University in Pune, India, where he worked on botanical drug development and pharmacokinetics.

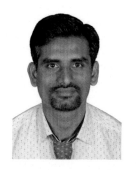

Vaidya Girish Tillu is an Ayurveda physician and researcher at the Interdisciplinary School of Health Sciences at the Savitribai Phule Pune University, in Pune, India. He contributed to AyuSoft, a knowledge-base and decision support system of Ayurveda promoted by the Center for Development in Advanced Computing (C-DAC). He is involved in the study of Ayurveda through interdisciplinary approaches, including clinical and community research, health-seeking behavior, pharmacoepidemiology, lifestyle, and gut health. He is working on observational studies on clinical practice

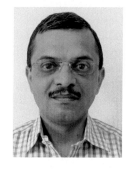

data at the Transdisciplinary University in Bangalore, India. Girish Tillu is associate editor of the *Journal of Ayurveda and Integrative Medicine (J-AIM)* and has received a Hinduja Merit Scholarship, a Vaidya-Scientist Fellowship, and an Arogya Deep Award for his work in the field.

Uma Chandran, PhD, is a Dr. D.S. Kothari post-doctoral fellow at Savitribai Phule Pune University in Pune, India, under the mentorship of Prof Patwardhan. She graduated in Biotechnology from the Rajiv Gandhi Centre for Biotechnology (RGCB) in Kerala, a national research centre of the Government of India. Her research focuses on exploring the Ayurvedic system of medicine using a network pharmacology approach.

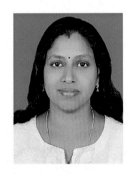

Tejas Shah holds an MD in Biomedical Sciences, with a specialization in Drug Discovery and Development, and is pursuing a PhD. He has worked on a number of prestigious projects funded by different government agencies such as DST, ICMR, and the Department of AYUSH, and is Senior Research Fellow at the Sinhagad College of Engineering. He has acquired expertise in developing animal models for diseases such as diabetes and GDM. His areas of interest are molecular and cell biology, molecular pharmacology, and pharmacogenomics.

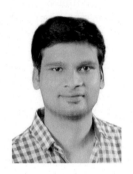

Ms. Kalyani Kumbhare has a BA in Microbiology (Industrial Microbiology) and an MD in Health Sciences from the Interdisciplinary School of Health Sciences, Savitribai Phule Pune University in Pune, India. She has experience in animal handling and has worked in transdisciplinary projects involving herb-drug interactions of antidiabetic drugs, pharmacoepidemiology, and macrofungal diversity. She was awarded a scholarship in the Naturalist Scholarship Program, 2011, organized by the Research and Action in Natural Wealth Administration (RANWA) and has also presented a poster at the National Conference on Biodiversity Assessment, Conservation and Utilization in Pune, India.

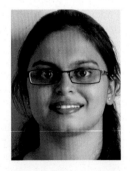

Neelay Mehendale is a graduate of the Savitribai Phule Pune University in Pune, India. He has completed his Integrated MSc in Biotechnology from the Institute of Bioinformatics and Biotechnology, and has carried out his dissertation under the guidance of Prof Patwardhan. His research interest lay in the areas of biochemistry, biophysics, and computational biology. He is also an accomplished Indian classical vocalist.

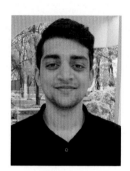

Saniya Patil is currently in her fourth year of studies at the Institute of Bioinformatics and Biotechnology, Savitribai Phule Pune University in Pune, India, where she is pursuing her Integrated M.Sc. in Biotechnology. She has worked on projects involving network pharmacology to study the antimicrobial effect of Ayurvedic formulations, and the cytotoxic effect of gold nanoparticles on cancer cells.

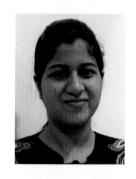

Jatinder K. Lamba has around 20 years of expertise in the field of pharmacogenomics and is currently Associate Professor and Graduate Program Coordinator in the College of Pharmacy at the University of Florida in Gainesville, FL, United States; she has served as a grant reviewer for numerous NIH study sections and is currently a regular member of XNDA study section. Her research is focused on identification, characterization, and clinical validation of genomic/epigenomic markers predictive of therapeutic outcome in cancer

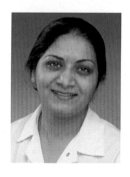

patients, and it spans from preclinical basic research utilizing cell line model systems to translational/clinical phase in patient populations from multiinstitute clinical trials. Research in her laboratory on pharmacogenomics/epigenomics in pediatric AML is focused on identification, characterization, and clinical validation of predictive genetic markers of response to multiple anticancer agents used in AML treatment, and has been funded by NCI since 2008. Dr. Lamba's group is working on developing algorithms to incorporate pharmacogenomics/epigenomic markers with other prognostic factors to advance precision medicine in oncology; identification of such patients upfront will provide opportunity to tailor the initial chemotherapy to achieve maximum benefit.

Foreword

NATURAL PRODUCTS ARE DEAD—LONG LIVE NATURAL PRODUCTS!

We are pleased to write this Foreword for *Innovative Approaches in Drug Discovery: Ethnopharmacology, Systems Biology and Holistic Targeting*, by Bhushan Patwardhan and Rathnam Chaguturu. Both editors are experts in their fields, but more importantly they are original thinkers. Given that innovation may be the only way to survive "creative destruction," as described by McKinsey's Foster and Kaplan, it is important for readers to know that Drs. Patwardhan and Chaguturu understand this need fully. As the editors propose, the present book shows the ongoing revolution in biomedical research and development (R&D), reaching from yesterday's disease- and target-centric mindsets to the more person- and phenotype-centric therapeutic solutions of tomorrow. The book thus paints a "precision medicine" approach that builds on today's growing foundation of scientific insights, but realizes that "good enough never is." At its zenith, what is covered herein elucidates the perspective required to leverage the latest multitarget systems-based mindsets to achieve a better, more holistic, health care outcome. The final installment of the revolution we foresee in medicine will be counted in lives saved, every one of them a miracle made possible by the vision and creativity of people like the editors and authors of this book.

At a core level, the present book is about "pharmacognosy," and the possibility that its reintroduction into the fundamentals and modern practice of biomedical R&D may provide the necessary insights that catapult the next generation of drugs to success. What is pharmacognosy? If you look in a dictionary, you will first see that pharmacognosy is pronounced [färmə'kägnəsē]. You will next see that it is a noun meaning a "branch of knowledge dealing with medicinal drugs that are obtained from plants or other natural sources." Indeed, the word's origin is said to trace back to the mid-1800s, from "pharmaco," which means "of drugs," and "gnosis," which means "knowledge." From this definition, readers will rightly conclude that, in many cases, pharmacognosy involves the study of natural products. As long-time students and practitioners of biotechnology and pharmaceutical R&D, we know about pharmacognosy, but many of today's educators and researchers have forgotten about its importance. The present book is thus even more important in correcting such a significant lapse in institutional memory.

Why are natural products so important? Natural products have always been an integral part of an almost infinite molecular diversity that accesses interesting biology, and during our careers we have been front and center in characterizing and filling this chemical space. Recent estimates suggest that natural products account for a large proportion of drugs on the market today. For example, Newman and Cragg in their analysis on sources of new drugs for the period of the 1940s through 2014 concluded that roughly 50% of the anticancer drugs approved in that timeframe were either natural products or drugs derived directly from natural products. Numerous examples of natural products and drugs derived therefrom can be found throughout major treatises on medicinal chemistry. In sum, this certainly sounds like an important area!

Noteworthy leadership in natural products discovery and development was evident at many longstanding pharmaceutical leaders a few decades ago. Roche, e.g., was particularly invested in marine natural products. Their Australian Research Institute of Marine Pharmacology discovered a number of interesting and unusual but still drug-like molecules, including nucleosides such 1-methylisoguanosine, also known as doridosine. Doridosine bound to adenosine receptors, an important pharmaceutical target at the time, and a class of targets that are still the subject of ongoing R&D today. Many of us were fascinated by the creativity of nature in devising these novel chemical structures.

As cell and molecular biology, genomics, high-throughput screening, and structure-based design technologies advanced through the 1980s, 1990s, and 2000s, progressively only those drugs with a selective activity against an isolated molecular target were in favor in the pharmaceutical industry. While new approaches to discovering natural products continued to be developed during this same period of time using technologies such as proteomics, natural products, as the basis for drug discovery in large pharmaceutical companies ("Big Pharma"), fell out of favor. Among other factors, high-throughput screening of natural product extracts proved difficult, which contributed to Big Pharma's move away from natural products. In fact, we personally witnessed the closure of natural products efforts during our careers at a large pharmaceutical company in the 1990s.

Another reason for the exit of Big Pharma from natural products R&D was the difficulty of synthesizing large quantities of complicated organic molecules cost effectively. Discodermolide, an anticancer polyketide lactone with 13 stereogenic centers isolated from a Caribbean sponge, proved to be a rare example of at least a chemical if not a human safety and efficacy success on the latter front. Novartis required a more than 30-step synthesis to produce just a few tens of grams of material for clinical trials, and also required the use of fragments prepared by fermentation. The other example that comes readily to mind is the anticancer agent, paclitaxel (Taxol). It took nearly 25 years to realize commercial success from the original discovery to total synthesis and scaleup, even with a number of the best academic minds hard at work on the problem.

Other questions have been raised about natural products in recent years, such as invalid bioactives possibly undermining drug discovery. This concern stems from the recent elucidation of pan-assay interference compounds, so-called PAINs, which can give rise to false positives in drug screening campaigns. But the same issues with promiscuous compounds have been known for a long time to present themselves for nonnatural product leads, and if one isn't careful, good leads can be discarded by being too worried about PAINs. Recent natural products-based efforts have even run into problems of possible misidentification of chemical structures. If the chemical structure is correct, then perhaps the biology or purity of the active pharmaceutical ingredient are in question. Consider, e.g., the controversy with antroquinonol A, a fungal-derived anticancer compound being developed by Golden Biotechnology. However, this type of issue isn't only a problem for natural products, as another finding outside the natural products arena uncovered a chemical structure error in an Oncoceutics drug. Thus, there are complexities to worry about with natural products, but they are often no different than with any source of chemical diversity being explored in drug discovery and development.

Can a small biotechnology company succeed where Big Pharma has chosen not to go? Kosan is one example of a biotech venture that worked successfully on complex natural products and derivatives, especially polyketides. It was founded in 1995 and ultimately acquired by Bristol-Myers Squibb in 2008, which, interestingly, had substantially reduced its natural products programs in the late 1990s. Thus, in this case, Big Pharma chose to buy rather than (re)build its own natural products pipeline. Nereus is another example of a meaningfully successful natural products venture, founded in 1998 to exploit new therapeutics derived from marine microbial sources. Nereus had founder ties to the Scripps Institution of Oceanography, part of the University of California San Diego, which may have helped to extend its lifetime as an independent company. However, while Nereus discoveries reached clinical trials, it was ultimately acquired too, in 2012, by Triphase. With these and a few other rare historical exceptions, natural products-based biotech and pharma efforts have been hard to find lately.

It is important to note that challenges remain to find therapies for malaria and drug-resistant tuberculosis, among many other chronic ailments. Nonetheless, the future awaits exactly what is discussed in this book. Powerful new technologies should over time help to reignite natural products R&D in biotech and pharma concerns. For example, Amyris was founded in 2003 to exploit biotechnology and chemical engineering in a number of industries, ranging from petroleum products to pharmaceuticals. Early work on the chemical biology-assisted semi-synthetic approaches to the antimalarial drug, artemisinin, led by University of California Berkeley's Keasling, garnered much attention. These techniques will increasingly buttress work on drugs with structures even more complicated than the artemisinin, discodermolide, and Taxol examples noted above. Novel application of natural molecules may offer an avenue to revisit old ailments with old cures!

No doubt there are many lessons left for us to ponder as we revisit natural molecules. New approaches to integrate high-content screening with the latest omics technologies are appearing in the literature regularly. For sure, new ways to connect chemotypes with phenotypes in natural products are more and more evident, providing yet one more tool to accelerate the essential work of drug hunters. Can a powerful reemergence of natural products in all their glory be far away?

Hopefully you, the reader, will get a sense of the excitement of these times through this book.

Enjoy!

K. Kodukula[1] and W.H. Moos[2]
[1]Bridgewater College, Bridgewater, VA, United States
[2]University of California San Francisco, San Francisco, CA, United States

Preface

Imagine a world free of diseases!

What a wonderful thought and sight. A pinnacle of unimaginable human achievement, a defining hallmark of excellence in human endeavor, and a lofty goal from times immemorial, but *not* yet achieved. The utopian thought is nowhere near our sightline. On the other hand, *is* it ever achievable?

According to the US Center for Disease Control and Prevention, people tend to die of 113 causes, categorized in to 20 categories. Cancer is the most prevalent for the age group in its 60s, and for children it is infectious diseases. Keeping the disparity among rural and urban populations aside, almost 90% of deaths in the developed nations were caused by noncommunicable, lifestyle, chronic diseases; in low-income countries (Asia, Africa, and the Americas), people predominantly die of communicable (infectious and parasitic) diseases. A majority of the anticancer and antibacterial drugs have originated with natural products; yet natural product-based drug discovery efforts were deemphasized about two decades ago because of the issues of gaining intellectual property (IP) rights with regard to composition of matter, material sourcing, complex chemistry, total synthesis and scaleup, and the advent of combinatorial chemistry.

New drugs entering the market are, for the most part, new and improved old wine in new bottles! New derivatives, new targets, new analogues, new scaffolds, but no real breakthroughs. The heat of innovation deficit intensified during the global financial crisis that we witnessed during the last decade. The pharmaceutical industry's response mainly was around business strategy, consolidation, cost cutting, layoffs, and such measures. The era has also witnessed an increased incidence of drug recalls and withdrawals due to untoward effects and drug toxicity. The industry experienced several closures and acquisitions. During the last two decades we also witnessed rapid growth in biologicals.

Any pragmatic discussion on pharmaceutical innovation almost always brings up the topic of rare and neglected diseases. Rare diseases are those that affect a smaller population, while neglected diseases are, in general, infectious diseases that are endemic or prevalent in developing countries. Because of the affected population size (rare) or the affordability (neglected) constraints, pharmaceutical companies have traditionally shied away in developing drugs against these health concerns. But in recent years the mind-set has changed, if nothing else, because of improved public relations. Given the promiscuity of leading drugs and the very limited capital expenditure expected/involved, finding new uses for old (and new) drugs (drug repurposing/repositioning) has taken on a new dimension in recent years for their curative potential against risky, rare, and neglected disease targets, but the path for commercialization seems not quite thought through or bumpy.

Medicines are the greatest gift to humanity, by way of pharmacognosy and ethnopharmacology, the bedrock foundation for modern medicine. Yet, we have forgotten this monumental truth that has saved millions of lives over the last several decades. For the last quarter century, we succeeded in sequencing the human genome. We have developed high-throughput infrastructures that encompass robust assay formats, robotics, and signal-detection technologies. We conquered the ensuing Big Data (volume, velocity, variety, and veracity) with the aid of crowdsourcing and chemo/bio informatics. Combinatorial chemistry has come of age to fill the chemistry space more than ever. Open innovation, collaborative or otherwise, has become the mantra to reenergize pharmaceutical innovation. Personalized/precision medicine, making the treatment as individualized and customized as the disease, and immune-therapeutics have become the emerging paradigms for combating hard-to-treat diseases. Yet, the past two decades have become an era of "high throughput and low output." Could it be that the consequence of a one protein-one drug-one disease paradigm, an otherwise blind-sided, singular focus on developing highly selective drug leads to acting on individual therapeutic protein targets, aka, target-site–based, bench-to-bedside endeavors? Simply put, we are paying the price for pursuing the modern reductionist approach, in place of the yesteryear, proven, holistic reverse pharmacology endeavors.

We now have come to realize that any disease we encounter is almost certainly the tip of an iceberg, with a "disease syndrome" lurking underneath. Instead of a holistic approach, the current health care system focuses on a "reactive response" to a specific disease with a specific drug, while the disease syndrome culprits go unchecked. We face unique challenges in the diagnosis and treatment of each and every disease indication, which goes on to manifest from a simple disease to a more complex, multifactorial risk factors (syndrome), warranting a unified approach from several fronts. This calls for a new paradigm in how we deliver health care to the patient. Think about diabetes, for example. It is no longer a case of simple elevation of blood glucose levels. Prediabetic conditions eventually lead, according to Yensen and Naylor, to type 1, type 2 or gestational diabetes, with several associated risk factors: abdominal obesity, elevated blood triglyceride levels, low HDL cholesterol, high blood pressure, and high-fasting blood sugar. Diabetic complications, if unchecked, lead to retinopathy, coronary heart disease, nephropathy, peripheral vascular disease of the lower limbs, cerebrovascular disease, pregnancy complications, peripheral vascular neuropathy (CNS, diabetic foot), etc. Hence, diseases may initially manifest symptoms that outwardly look simplistic, but masquerade underneath with octopus-like tentacles affecting and invading many physiological processes. The holistic approach of treating the underlying causes of the symptoms, the principle way of ethnopharmacology, begs for serious reconsideration.

We have a translational gap. The public sector has stepped in a big way to understand disease biology and to find new and improved drugs, exemplified by the billions of dollars poured in by the governmental agencies in to the public sector. Venture-backed biopharmaceutical companies are sprouting across the globe to fill niche needs. Philanthropic disease foundations are making their mark against rare diseases—diseases with a personal family connection, and affecting few. Contract research organizations are here to augment preclinical proof of concept endeavors. Collaborative public–private partnerships are all around us, with some success at least in Europe. This dynamic landscape, call it a sort of a business model, while much desired and cherished, has very little in return to show for because of the uncoordinated translational gap. Pharmaceutical precompetitive collaborations should make note of the superb advances made by the automotive and computer (semiconductor and IT) industries in this respect and come up with effective models that accelerate the discovery and development of therapeutics. The pharmaceutical industry's vast experience in developing drugs has not effectively transcended to the academic corridors. The academic drug hunter is pursuing risky targets, largely defined and mandated by the funding agencies' directive. Because of the inherently limited perspective of the academic scientist, the therapeutic relevance of the target, in the context of the complex disease biology/physiology, is not always closely interconnected. The hits identified in academic high-throughput screening centers are riddled with Pan-Assay Interference Compounds, those that show activity across a range of assay platforms and against a range of proteins. The biology-centric academic drug hunters have no way of knowing this promiscuity due to their siloed approach and from not being the beneficiaries of comprehensive knowledge that comes from running screens against multiple targets. The drug hunters also are largely unaware of the compensating cellular mechanisms available when a protein therapeutic target is singularly cornered. This is where a comprehensive, multifactorial knowledge of systems biology/pharmacology or physiopathology (pathophysiology) comes to rescue an otherwise stellar therapeutic, target-driven drug discovery effort. It is therefore all too important to consider designing multitarget compounds or drug cocktails that would not only interact with the key therapeutic target but also with the allied, compensatory pathways, akin to the polypharmacology of plant extracts that are enriched toward achieving the desired biological effect. In the absence of an industry-trained medicinal chemist connected with the project, the drug leads identified through academic high-throughput screening endeavors find no real value, and with no knowledge of translating the discoveries beyond target site efficacy. This is the new "valley of death" for academic discoveries. Clinical efficiency, and what is needed to navigate this valley of death, is a strength endemic to pharma, but is largely unknown to the academic scientist. Things would be different if he/she were to understand the principles of reverse pharmacology, the bedside-to-bench principle.

Monetization of IP, unlike the case with the highly profitable IT industry, drives the pharmaceutical sector. This promotes monopoly and kills innovation, and in turn deprives the discovery and development of life-saving medicines and making patients' lives better. The security of IP is essential, but the incentive model is simply outdated and needs to change; better yet, it should cease to exist. The pharmaceutical innovation model for the third millennium calls for outside-the-box thinking. Think of Uber, the world's largest taxi company that owns no cars; Facebook, the world's most popular social media site, creates no content; Alibaba, the world's most valuable retailer, owns no inventory, Airbnb, the world's largest hotelier, owns no real estate, etc. (Tom Goodwin, WetPaint). These are disruptive innovation models unlike any others.

There are about 7000 diseases that afflict mankind, but we only have treatments available for fewer than 2–3% of these diseases. The most curious thing is that we know the genetic basis for most of these diseases. There are about 25,500 protein-coding genes in the human genome, and a gazillion number of possible small molecules with 30 or fewer heavy atoms. Within the human genome, there are about 4500 genes that are disease relevant, and ~ 3000 are druggable by small molecules. About 12,000 of these are prime targets for protein therapeutics. However, FDA-approved drugs target less than 0.5% of the entire human genome. This means that there is plenty of opportunity to mine the human genome and identify new and novel therapeutic targets. Pharma and academia routinely screen large compound libraries, virtual compound collections, vendor's databases, etc., but with a very limited knowledge of what to look for, not exactly knowing the size or shape of the so called needle (in a haystack) or even if it is there. If we do find a hit, optimization of it to become a bona fide drug lead is a herculean task. There are about 143 well-defined substituents reported in the literature. If we use all of them in just three positions, we would have 143^3 or 2,924,207 possible compounds. This just hints at the fact that we can never be certain. An experienced medicinal chemist might consider making a drastic structural change, based on (1) historical perspective, (2) prior hands-on knowledge, and (3) chemoinformatic input.

It is all too common to see that most targets/assets fail in phase II. Poor understanding of human disease, inadequate biomarkers, and poorly predictive preclinical assays are some of the key contributing factors. It may come as a big surprise that nearly all novel targets, resulting from the mining of the genomic data, fail at clinical proof of concept. This failure is repeated many times within each company and across the industry, a result of the non-sharing, secretive business model of the pharmaceutical industry. We tend to work under the lamp post (e.g., Kinome), and the animal models do not necessarily help prioritize therapeutic targets. How much does it cost to develop a drug? How long does it take? What is the attrition rate between phase I, II, III, and IV? Too many questions without any answers, exacerbated by the modus operandi of lack of public disclosure of key facts, thus enabling a "reinvent the wheel" syndrome over and over by each company, thus wasting precious resources and time and money countless times.

Even though there has been an uptick in the number of drugs approved by the FDA over the last 2 years, the pharmaceutical productivity defined by the number of diseases for which we have effective therapies remains almost unchanged despite huge investments in biomedical research infrastructure. The business model is a game of attrition, takes too long, costs too much, and with no guarantee of ensuring success. The origin of most modern medicines could be traced to an enlightened awareness and pursuit of anecdotal evidence from reverse pharmacology and bedside-to-bench observations. The rich potential of holistic ethnopharmacology and pharmacognosy has largely been forgotten, partly due to the difficulty in gaining rights to the associated IP, ambiguous claims, the advent of combinatorial chemistry, total reliance on bench-to-bedside strategies, and unproven clinical relevance of the therapeutic targets pursued. Pharma's innovation crisis is perhaps tied to its neglect of natural product-based drug discovery. This reminds us of the now famous quote by the late George Allen, Sr., "Forget the past, the future will give you plenty to worry about."

Both academia and pharma are now engaged in screening large compound libraries to identify lead drug candidates. Since the chemical diversity of these libraries is not always relevant to biological function, this approach has not been as successful as was hoped. With increased emphasis on high-throughput screening and combinatorial chemistry, and the clarity that target-based research provides with regard to the site of action as well as IP, there has been a deemphasis on natural product-based drug discovery programs over the last 20 years. The wealth of chemical diversity that has evolved with biological diversity is underrepresented in the commercial chemical library offerings, but needs to be expanded to strategically cover available chemical space and include drug-like compounds with improved pharmacologic, pharmacodynamic, and pharmacokinetic properties as compared to their current nitrogen-rich counterparts.

More than 80% of the world's population relies mainly on traditional medicines for its primary health care. The origins of many drugs that are currently in use could be traced to pharmacognosy and the fruits of reverse pharmacology. Natural products are "designed" to interact with enzymes and/or receptors. Natural products occupy an important part of small molecule space because they are recognized by at least two proteins: (1) the one at the end of their biosynthetic pathway and (2) their evolutionary biological target. Natural products are the products of an organism's evolutionary path, successfully navigating the selective forces toward survival. Of the 325,000 plant species (compared to existing 1.6 million life forms) known to man, we have some knowledge of only about 1500 plants, and the therapeutic relevance of the rest of the plant species yet to be explored. The 1992 Rio convention on biodiversity laid the groundwork toward sustainable use of biodiversity, conservation and benefit sharing, and the legal framework in place to allow for bioprospection.

The authors vigorously argue that any drug, whether New Chemical Entity (NCE) or New Molecular Entity (NME), botanical or biologic, will have an inherent limitation due to a single-target approach in a multitarget and complex biological system. This book critically reviews the drug discovery strategies during the last five decades and analyzes reasons as to why drugs fail. Starting from thalidomide to rofecoxib, the contributing authors collectively analyze physiological reasons from systems biology perspective with chemistry, metabolic pathways, interactions, and cascading effects of one-target modulation on other metabolic processes. This argues for a reconsideration of the present one-target-one drug approach for a given disease. The genomic approach to personalized/precision medicine will be a long, expensive, and risky haul, whereas traditional, knowledge-inspired integrative personalized approaches will be the future of therapeutics. A clear distinction between drug discovery, medicine discovery, and treatment discovery is all too necessary at this critical juncture.

Several thematic concepts are articulated in this book. First, as editors, we emphasize the need for innovative, integrated, interdisciplinary approaches and include knowledge gained from natural product-based, traditional and alternative medicines to drive future drug discovery efforts. Natural products offer an almost infinite structural diversity that accesses interesting, therapeutically relevant biology. As such, systematic, genome-wide, bioinformatics-based, disease-centered, chemotype-to-phenotype systems biology approaches are required to take advantage of the recent advances in omics technologies and to identify novel therapeutic targets. A process is presented for the seamless use of bioinformatics, chemical biology, proteomics, structural biology, and medicinal chemistry−based approaches along with high-throughput, cell-free and cell-based assays to identify novel, druggable protein targets and novel "drug-like" chemical probes. New techniques and resources, grounded in sound scientific reasoning and rational, well-validated approaches that exploit a growing volume of publically available data, stand to become cornerstones of the new pharmaceutics arena (see Chapter 6: Genomics-Driven Drug Discovery Process). A compelling case is then presented by Anu Roy for holistic drug targeting. While preferential drug specificity toward a target is effective against diseases that are monogenic, a majority of the diseases are complex and multifactorial, and are modulated by genetics, environment, age, and sometimes, gender. Successful outcomes may rely on polypharmacology of a given drug or drug cocktails, a new emerging paradigm for targeting multifactorial complex diseases. Patil et al. boils down the causative factors involved in the failure of drugs leading to their eventual recall. Drug toxicity, the primary cause for a drug recall, is primarily due to a cumulative effect of target modulation and intrinsic property of drugs, widely known as "toxicity triangle effect" or "butterfly effect."

Ethnopharmacology, natural products, and traditional medicine systems are considered by Chandran et al. (see Chapter 5: Network Pharmacology) as attractive options to overcome the drug discovery impasse. Network ethnopharmacology of botanical bioactives can serve as a valuable tool for evidence-based Ayurveda and Traditional Chinese Medicine to understand the medicines' putative actions, indications, and mechanisms. We also caution that consumers find it very frustrating to sort through a lot of ambiguous information put out by natural product manufacturers who cannot legally label their goods with condition-specificity. Warude (see Chapter 5: Network Pharmacology) lays out a path for assuring the quality and safety of the herbal products. A cost-effective and time-effective approach to drug discovery could effectively come from reverse pharmacology, a trans-discipline that strikes a balance between relevant pharmacology/toxicity sciences and clinic-centric approaches (see Chapter 9: Proteomics). Proteomics, pharmacogenomics, epigenetics, and transcriptomics are integral to a comprehensive understanding of systems biology of disease pathophysiology, thus leading a desired shift from target-centric approach to disease-centric approach. Collaborative public—private partnerships are integral to the paradigm shift espoused in the new pharma business models, but to be successful, the public must be allowed to share in profits that result from federally financed research. The concluding chapter brings forth the point that there is no use in attempting revolutionary new paradigms unless we also devote our attention to how irreproducibility has pervaded our discipline, and what resources and strategies exist to counteract the problems.

Finally, a greater acceptance of natural product extracts as a key (if complex) source of novel chemistries as well as increased appreciation for holistic approaches in therapeutic optimization, offers critical avenues for growing the pipeline of new candidate prospects, and achieving more systematic guidance regarding the most important optimization criteria for safe, effective medicines (see Chapter 6: Genomics-Driven Drug Discovery Process). Finally, the drug discovery efforts need not be limited to a pharmacology approach with "drug" as a chemical or biological entity. The new discovery paradigm should also include physiological interventions where meditation, diet, exercise, and behavioral changes play an important role, especially in the management of chronic conditions and lifestyle diseases. The authors critically explore these seemingly divergent, albeit fundamental principles, and lay a path for reigniting pharmaceutical innovation through a disciplined reemergence of pharmacognosy, embracing open innovation models and collaborative, trusted public—private partnerships. With unprecedented advances made in the development of biomedically relevant tools and technologies, *the need is great and the time is now* for a renewed commitment toward expanding the repertoire of medicines, the greatest gift to humanity.

Having led drug discovery efforts, both in academia and in industry in the arena of random and focused chemical library screens, drug repurposing and bio-prospection, being beneficiaries of local health traditions, and having first-hand knowledge of reviewing project funding proposals to NIH and other governmental agencies, we have used our unique perspectives to bring together an eclectic group of thought leaders to offer their ideas in reenergizing pharmaceutical innovation, especially from a holistic, pharmacognosy vista. The book in your hands could not have been what it is without the time and energy of these original thinkers. We thank the contributing authors for their distinct, scholarly and personal perspectives, and Ms. Kristine Jones, Ms. Tracy Tufaga, and others at Elsevier for their valuable guidance and support. We sincerely hope that the concepts articulated here resonate with our colleagues in the public and private sectors in bringing effective, timely therapies to the patients' bedside.

Again, the yardstick for pharmaceutical innovation is not the number of blockbuster drugs introduced in to the market place (business-centric), but the number of patients' lives saved and life-threatening diseases eradicated (patient-centric). As Drs. Kodukula and Moos, well-seasoned experts with unparalleled experience in driving pharmaceutical drug discovery efforts so eloquently declare in the Foreword, "Innovation may be the only way to survive creative destruction"—and to achieve a better, more holistic, health care outcome!

Bhushan Patwardhan
and
Rathnam Chaguturu

Dedication

New Drug Discovery and Therapy is like a space odyssey, where no human has ever gone before. It is in this spirit, we dedicate this humble effort with immense gratitude...

...to those who helped pave the way for traditional and contemporary approaches which marked an epoch in drug discovery and therapy;

...to those who find inspiration to uncover new insights from this narrative;

...to our mentors and colleagues, for shaping our ideas;

...to our families, for their unconditional support and love;

and

...to our grandchildren, Chitra, Arjun, Rohan, and Mira...

...we might be traversing the heavenly bodies seeking the meaning of life by the time you get to comprehend all that is discussed.

Chapter 1

Drug Discovery Impasse: Pharmacognosy Holds the Key

Rathnam Chaguturu[1] and Bhushan Patwardhan[2]

[1]*iDDPartners, Princeton Junction, NJ, United States* [2]*Savitribai Phule Pune University, Pune, Maharashtra, India*

The biomedical enterprise spans discovery, development and delivery of drugs in highly complex ways from bench to the bedside. The current therapeutics landscape benefits from public and private sectors and includes knowledge gained from traditional to alternative medicines. The pharmaceutical/biotechnology industry spends over $140 billion on research and development in introducing 25−35 *new* drugs annually, but still experiences a steep innovation crisis. It takes almost 15 years, and $3−$10 billion, including the cost of failures, to find and bring a drug to patients. The cost is too high, the time is long, and both are unsustainable. Clearly, we need a better way to discover and deliver effective treatments.

It is estimated that over 7000 drugs are in development around the world, with three-fourths being first-in-class. Cancer death rates keep falling, thanks to new treatment options and medicines. Cancer immunotherapy, exemplified by Bristol-Myers Squibb's Opdivo and Merck's Keytruda, is now a reality. The HIV/AIDS death rate has fallen by 80−90% in the last two decades. Though we now have a near 90% cure, the cost to develop the drugs is still in excess of US $3 billion, with only 20% of the marketed drugs yielding revenues that either match or exceed the R&D costs incurred. It takes more than 15 years to develop a drug, with less than 10−12% of drugs entering clinical trials ever getting FDA approvals. The current failure rate of >80% is unsustainable and we need to find better ways to shepherd clinical candidates towards a successful outcome.

In the drug discovery arena, big strides are being made in the use of biomarkers and stem cells. The promise of embryonic stem cells discovered back in 1998 with the much-heralded potential for self-renewal has not yielded any major clinical advancements or treatments. With more than 300 trials on human mesenchymal stem cells currently underway for a variety of diseases, the promise of stem cell therapy or made-to-order organs is still a

Innovative Approaches in Drug Discovery. DOI: http://dx.doi.org/10.1016/B978-0-12-801814-9.00001-5
1

distant dream. It is indeed important to keep a reality check on the real-world status of the development and application of any science.

The need is greater than ever for the creation of smarter chemical libraries to improve the chances of new drug lead discovery. Highly intelligent, automated organic synthesis schemes have recently been introduced for producing large amounts of complex, biologically relevant or drug-like compounds. The renaissance in ethnopharmacology and natural products research over the last few years appears to be a response towards creating innovative approaches, giving due recognition to traditional knowledge that was once the foundation of modern medicine. Holistic targeting and disease biology in the context of systems biology are seriously explored as innovative approaches in drug discovery. While we witness these technological breakthroughs, biomedical research has now become hyper-specialized into subdisciplines (Chaguturu, 2015).

Scientific advances over the last 25 years, especially in omics, high throughput screening (HTS) technologies, combinatorial chemistry, instrumentation and informatics, have opened exciting avenues for the discovery of new drug candidates. Nevertheless, major challenges remain and are constantly evolving. The rate of *new* discoveries is falling and many drugs approved by regulators are being withdrawn due to toxicity and safety concerns. The drug discovery process is facing severe innovation deficit, which is putting the pharmaceutical industry under severe pressure. Chemical biology and genomic approaches, primarily monogenic, based on one target-one gene-one disease are not offering desired results.

HISTORICAL PERSPECTIVES

Drugs and pharmaceuticals have played significant roles in the prevention and treatment of several diseases. The history of using drugs in some form or other for treating diseases and alleviating symptoms dates back to ancient times. Most of the early discoveries resulted from natural sources, traditional knowledge, community experiences and a great deal of serendipity. Some of the early-discovered drugs like morphine, cocaine, tubocurarine, codeine, quinine, colchicine, belladonna and many others actually originated from potentially poisonous plants. It is so much easier to identify poisonous characteristics of substances than it is to recognize therapeutic, medicinal properties (Patwardhan and Vaidya, 2010).

The Greek physician, Galen (129−200 AD) devised the first modern pharmacopoeia, describing the appearance, properties and uses of many plants of his time. The foundations of the modern pharmaceutical industry were laid when techniques to produce synthetic replacements for many of the natural medicines were developed. Natural products chemistry, as a branch, seems to have begun in 1804 when a German pharmacist, Frederik Serturner, isolated morphine from opium. He was the first chemist to isolate an alkaloid from a botanical source. Morphine was obtained from *Papaver somniferum*, the poppy plant, properties of which were known for over 5000 years.

SYNTHETIC DRUGS

The seeds of synthetic drugs were sown in 1874, when salicylic acid was isolated from willow bark. This is the precursor of the synthetic drug popularly known as aspirin. Pharmaceutical research took a major leap when organic synthetic chemistry was developed. During that time, pharmacologists, microbiologists and biochemists began to unravel the chemistry of natural processes in humans, animals, plants and microorganisms. This led to the identification of many key chemical molecules and provided more opportunities to develop novel compounds. Many new drugs emerged to treat infections, infestations, cancers, ulcers, and heart and blood pressure conditions. Many drugs were developed through random screening of thousands of synthetic chemicals. Many also came about through serendipity, discovered as a result of the sharp-eyed observations of physicians and scientists. Examples of such drugs include sulfonamides, isoniazid, antipsychotic drugs, antihistamines and penicillin.

The pharmaceutical industry started taking stronger roots after World War II. High competencies were acquired during the war by developing more efficient processes for the mass production of penicillin. Chemists at the pharmaceutical giants synthesized a large number of antibacterial drugs and other compounds creating a prosperous market. The world witnessed growing expenditure for drugs in a free market. During these times, the pharmaceutical sector was confronted with several factors including loose regulations regarding drug safety, patent protection in the country of origin, and access to capital and know-how. The success of random screening drug discovery tools began to decline, and the industry underwent a crisis due to increasing R&D costs coupled with decreasing revenues. This led to a renaissance in ethnopharmacology and pharmacognosy.

ETHNOPHARMACOLOGY AND NATURAL PRODUCTS

The investigation of ethnopharmacology and natural products as a source of novel human therapeutics became popular in the Western pharmaceutical industry during the 1960s, resulting in a pharmaceutical landscape heavily influenced by natural and synthetic molecules like reserpine. It is now estimated that out of 877 small-molecule new chemical entities (NCEs) introduced between 1981 and 2002, roughly half were from compounds based on natural products (Koehn, 2005). It was estimated in 1991 that 121 drugs in use in the United States were derived from plants. It is reported that 25% of all prescriptions dispensed from community pharmacies in the United States between 1959 and 1973 contained one or more ingredients derived from higher plants. A study of the top 150 proprietary drugs used in the United States in 1993 found that 57% of all prescriptions contained at least one major active compound derived from natural sources.

Financially, the retail sales of pharmaceutical products reached a milestone of US$1 trillion, and is forecast to reach $1.8 trillion by 2018 (http://thomsonreuters.com/en/articles/2015/global-pharma-sales-reach-above-1-trillion.html), with drugs derived from medicinal plant origins contributing significantly. A study of the 25 best-selling pharmaceutical drugs in 1997 found that 11 of them (42%) were biological, natural products or entities derived from natural products, with a total value of US$17.5 billion. The world market for herbal remedies will reach $107 billion by 2017 (http://www.nutraceuticalsworld.com/contents/view_breaking-news/2012-03-07/global-herbal-supplement-market-to-reach-107-billion-by-2017) with Europe in the lead (US$6.7 billion), followed by Asia (US$5.1 billion), North America (US$4.0 billion), Japan (US$2.2 billion) and then the rest of the world (US$1.4 billion). The total sales value of Taxol, derived from just one plant species (*Taxus baccata*) was US$3 billion since its introduction.

Among prominent successes of natural product-based drug discovery include the antimalarial drug, artemisinin and the anticancer drug, Taxol. The discovery of Taxol is an important milestone in natural product-based drug discovery. This came out of a program initiated in the late 1950s at the National Cancer Institute in the United States, which involved examination of 35,000 plant species with the goal of finding an ingredient that could later be developed to target cancer cell growth. Of all the samples examined, the bark of the pacific yew tree showed exemplary properties that led to the discovery of the anticancer agent Taxol, which was approved by the FDA in 1990s for the treatment of both ovarian and breast cancers. Substantial clinical evidence is available as well to support the use of Taxol in the treatment of advanced breast cancer where previous standard treatments have failed. Taxol is therapeutically effective and well tolerated, enabling patients to survive significantly longer than those treated with standard combination therapy (Bishop et al., 1999; Jassem et al., 2001). It has demonstrated positive response rates of over 60% in advanced breast cancer in clinical trials (Seidman et al., 1995) compared to previous standard therapy.

Evidence suggests that Taxol prolongs the survival in advanced lung cancer as compared to standard chemotherapy with cisplatin and etoposide (Bonomi et al., 2000). Taxol binds to the beta tubulin of microtubules and stabilizes the assembly, preventing the detachment of subunits. This proves beneficial in proliferative diseases like cancer. Prolonging the state of frozen tubulin assembly prompts dividing cells to undergo apoptosis or revert to the G phase of the cell cycle. This property of Taxol has helped scientists develop it into a potent anticancer drug. And it remains one of the best-selling cancer drugs ever manufactured.

Today, pharmaceutical scientists are experiencing difficulty in identifying new lead structures, templates and scaffolds in the finite world of chemical diversity. A number of synthetic drugs have adverse and unacceptable side effects. There have been impressive successes with eth-nopharmacology and botanical medicines, most notably, *quinghaosu*, an artemisinin from traditional Chinese medicine. Considerable research on pharmacognosy, chemistry, pharmacology and clinical therapeutics has been carried out on medicinal plants. Numerous molecules have come out of the traditional knowledge, examples include rauwolfia alkaloids for treating hypertension, psoralens for vitiligo, holarrhena alkaloids for amebi-asis, guggulsterons as hypolipidemic agents, mucunapruriens for Parkinson's disease, piperidines as bioavailability enhancers, baccosides in mental retention, picrosides for hepatic protection, phyllanthins as antivir-als, curcumines for inflammation, ginsenoids, withanolides and many others as immunomodulators (Patwardhan, 2000).

Many ethnopharmacology-based natural product leads have not been sys-tematically followed except a few, like ginsenoids and curcumin. Although fairly extensive research has been carried out on these leads, none has reached the level of an approved drug. The spectacular successes in medici-nal chemistry, and the development of synthetic drugs, has resulted in natural product-based chemistry becoming less popular; it has been virtually aban-doned by major drug companies. While drug discovery was becoming more specific and commercially lucrative, efforts to develop new drugs for the treatment of communicable diseases particularly affecting poor communities like malaria, trypanosomiasis, filariasis, tuberculosis, schistosomiasis, leshma-niasis and amebiasis came to a near standstill. Although botanical medicines were produced in many countries, the clinical efficacy of these medicines was systematically left unevaluated. The composition of these complex herbal mixtures was only crudely analyzed. Thus, herbal medicines came to be asso-ciated with anecdotes or "old wives tales," quack medicine or snake oil, and was believed to exploitat the sick, the desperate and the gullible. Sadly, herbal medicines continue to be poor in quality control, both in material and clinical efficacy.

EMERGENCE OF BIOTECHNOLOGY

Drug discovery moved away from serendipity to rational drug design when Hitchings and Elion worked on DNA-based antimetabolites, leading to ana-logues of purines as anticancer agents. Watson and Crick's discovery of DNA structure, and a better understanding of the processes of replication, transcription and translation helped in the discovery of antiviral drugs. Recombinant DNA technology, molecular cloning and other developments in molecular biology helped advance the progression of biologicals as new ther-apeutic agents. The chemical dominance of biologicals and vaccines began to evolve. The discovery of polymerase chain reaction (PCR), combinatorial chemistry, HTS, molecular modeling and bioinformatics has substantially contributed to the new era of genomic-based drug discovery.

The emergence of the modern pharmaceutical industry is the outcome of different activities that developed potent, single molecules with highly selective activity for different pathological conditions. In many cases, synthetic drugs improved upon nature. For example, a new range of local anesthetics derived from cocaine avoided its dangerous effects on blood pressure. Chloroquine is much less toxic than naturally occurring quinine. The pharmaceutical sector witnessed stricter regulations that resulted in increased costs, the lengthening of clinical trials leading to longer time-to-market and thus shorter patent cover during commercialization. During this period many new pharmaceutical companies developed and the dominance of the Swiss-German firms began to dwindle.

After the 1980s, new technological paradigms in biotechnology and informatics started to emerge. Advances in bio- and chemo informatics made it possible to mine data generated from HTS, biochips and combinatorial chemistry, resulting in a several-fold increase in the number of compounds tested per year. The Bayh–Dole Act in 1980 facilitated commercialization of publicly funded research and encouraged entrepreneurial entities. Substantial investments through government and private equities were made in the biotech sector.

The US pharmaceutical market rapidly expanded into the European sector, representing today almost half of the total world's total sales. This dramatic change forced European companies to increase competitiveness through decentralization, mergers, acquisitions and specialization. Many large European chemical industries like Hoechst and the Swiss Imperial Chemical Industry (ICI) de-merged their pharmaceutical subsidiaries from their bulk chemical activities. Alliances and mergers came into vogue—Glaxo and Welcome merged in 1995 forming Glaxo-Welcome; Sandoz and Ciba-Geigy formed Novartis in 1996; Astra and Zeneca merged in 1998; Hoechst and Rhone-Poulenc formed Aventis in 1999. Finally, many of these firms started specializing in a particular area of pharmaceutical research, such as cardiovascular or neural-system drugs, and developed strong collaboration in world regions that exceled in these areas.

DRUG DISCOVERY PROCESS

Modern drug discovery has significantly contributed to improving our quality of life, and has been responsible for curing, eradicating and controlling several diseases and disorders. While many drugs may have untoward effects, the benefits from drugs are far-reaching. The undesirable effects occur, to a large extent, due to the misuse of painkillers, tranquilizers, opioids and such other drugs (Harmon, 2010).

Drugs and pharmaceuticals are essentially chemical or biological materials. The process of identifying potential substances, and converting them into drugs and pharmaceuticals is a long, investment-intensive and complex process. However, to identify the missing links in the discovery process, a brief summary is provided here. The discovery and development pipeline involves many steps — basic research, discovery of therapeutic targets, target validation, hit identification and lead candidate development, safety and efficacy assessment, drug manufacturing and distribution.

The first step is exploratory, which involves several years of scientific research to understand the biochemical and pathophysiological processes of a specific, medical condition for which a drug is required. The exploratory steps involve basic research, which can give indications of specific gene/protein targets to be modulated. Once the targets are identified, the next step is to find promising lead compounds, which can bind and interact with the target receptors. This binding and interaction is quite similar to any enzyme action, where there is a high degree of specificity—like a lock and key arrangement. The challenging task is to find the most appropriate key as the lead compound, or candidate drug that can modulate the target in the desired direction.

This discovery of candidate drug molecules leads to the next step of screening potential compounds, using suitable assay systems. Currently, various powerful and rapid technologies are available. In the past, various closely related analogues of lead molecules were synthesized manually, which took months to years to accomplish. With the advent of combinatorial chemistry, hundreds of close congeners can be generated within a short time. The high throughput assays can rapidly test activities of these compounds, by the thousands, in an automated fashion. This helps in identifying the best potential candidates, which may have high degree of specificity, and affinity to the target. Many times these studies can also be done in silico, using suitable software and bio/chemo-informatics tools.

Selected lead compounds follow a rigorous path through in silico, in vitro and in vivo assays in the process of optimization. Out of hundreds of selected leads, only a few may emerge as potential drug candidates. This is followed by the preclinical phase, which involves cell-based and small animal-based assays to screen the safety and efficacy of drug candidates. At this stage a lot of pharmaceutical development work also happens involving the formulation of dosage form, delivery system, stability, pharmacokinetics, bioavailability, pharmacodynamics and dosing studies. Here the industry may decide whether the candidate drug merits further study. If the decision is positive, the industry has to file an investigational new drug (IND) application with a regulatory authority, such as the FDA. Once the safety and efficacy is established, and the regulatory compliances are made, the candidate drugs may become eligible for clinical studies involving phase I to phase IV clinical trials. It is generally estimated that out of hundreds of thousands of compounds screened, only about 250 may enter into the preclinical phase, about two to five may enter the clinical phase and, if lucky, one drug molecule may get approval from the regulatory authority. This is a very long, drawn-out, investment-intensive process involving commitments of 10 to 15 years and around $3 billion.

In addition to the complexity of the discovery process, the discovery space size has become too large for efficient data mining. It is becoming exceedingly difficult to explore and validate new targets, leads and candidate drugs. According to theoretical estimations, about 10^{60} small molecules exist in the world of which about 21 million have been studied for commercial uses. Over 10,000 ligand-binding domains are known. The therapeutic target database of the National University of Singapore contains about 2015 targets of which only 286 are in clinical trials. Out of about 18,000 drug candidate molecules, only about 1540 are approved.

DRUG DISCOVERY IMPASSE

Drug discovery and development has undergone several transitions during the last 25 years. The advances in biomedical sciences, biotechnology, vaccinology, computer-aided drug design, genomics and molecular technologies have brought mind-boggling changes, leading to a broader spectrum of more powerful drugs for many diseases. The chemical drugs are rapidly being replaced with biological drugs. With the advent of pharmacogenomics and systems biology concepts, pharmaceutical medicine is becoming more personalized. The ever-increasing cost of prescription drugs makes them out of reach for a majority of the global population. The new business model embraced by the industry is mainly through reducing R&D costs, cutting jobs and increasing prices to astronomical levels. This is not a smart strategy nor is it in the best interest of the pharmaceutical industry.

It was hoped that with the use of high throughput technologies, supported by genomics, computational sciences and bioinformatics, the drug discovery process would be faster, more economic and safer. Unfortunately, this hope has not become a reality. In fact, the number of new drugs entering the market through these technologies has actually been substantially low. Moreover, the number of drugs withdrawn after market launch is increasing as well. There is certainly something fundamentally wrong in the present approaches used for drug discovery. The pharmaceutical sector seems to be going in circles—doing more of the same, with the determined, but irrational hope that this will disrupt the current impasse (Patwardhan, 2014b).

With the pharmaceutical sector facing a severe innovation deficit, industry leaders and scientists from the pharmaceutical and biomedical sectors are desperately looking for novel approaches, new ideas and innovations to disrupt this discovery bottleneck. Several strategies have been discussed and practiced, including strategic alliances and mergers, open-innovations, industry-academia and industry-industry collaborations, and many other recent initiatives intended to expedite lead generation. These efforts are indicative of both the desperation and aspirations of the industry (Simpson and Reichman, 2013), but strategies of the past may not guarantee success in the future (Schmid and Smith, 2004).

Many new approaches have been explored during the last few years. For instance, RNAi screening remained the fastest growing field during the last decade with the promise to better understand gene function at the genome level. It was hyped as the second genomics wave, which in combination with the human genome-sequencing projects would revolutionize modern drug discovery. However, despite substantial efforts, trials and tribulations, not much success has been realized. Today, RNAi remains surrounded more by controversy, questioning breakthrough discoveries of genes allegedly identified through this random process. There is a critical need for novel gene targets to fight disease but no two RNAi screens show any commonality in the outcome, thus questioning the promise of such new technologies (Bhinder and Djaballah, 2013).

The pharmaceutical industry has historically seen an incredible growth of blockbuster drugs, however, recent trends indicate that present model may not be sustainable in the future. The average cost and time of discovering, developing and launching new drugs is steadily increasing, but without a commensurate increase in the number of newer, safer and better drugs. The situation is quickly deteriorating and the worst is yet to come.

The increased competitiveness of the pharmaceutical marketplace was likely fueled by changes over time on both the supply and demand sides. The development histories of entrants to new drug classes suggest that development races better characterize new drug development than does a model of *post hoc* imitation. Thus, the usual distinctions drawn between breakthrough and "me-too" drugs may not be very meaningful. The pharmaceutical industry has not been as innovative as it claims to be and the regulatory processes are adding more risk and years for pharmaceutical companies and the future does not look promising. Most of the big pharmaceutical manufacturers spend more on marketing than on research and development.

NEW DRUG APPROVALS

The USFDA's Center for Drug Evaluation and Research (CDER) ensures that all approved drugs are safe and effective. Industries submit IND followed by a new drug application to introduce new drugs into the market along with evidence regarding their safety and efficacy. The USFDA has defined novel drugs as "innovative products that serve previously unmet medical needs or otherwise significantly help to advance patient care and public health" (USFDA, 2015). The USFDA publishes a year-wise list of approved drugs. With 45 novel drugs gaining approval from the CDER, year 2015 recorded the highest number in the last 10 years. In 2014, 41 novel drugs were approved by the CDER as compared to 18 in 2007. In the 2015 list of approved novel drugs, 16 out of 45 (36%)

were classified as first-in-class drugs with different mechanisms of action from existing drugs. These could be taken as trends towards overcoming the discovery impasse.

The following figure depicts novel drug approvals over the past decade:

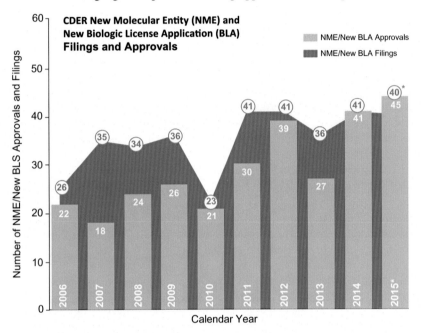

*The 2015 filed numbers include those filed in CY 2015 plus those currently pending filing (i.e., within their 60 day filing period) in CY 2015.

- Receipts that received a "Refuse to File" (RTF) or "Withdrawn before filing" (WF) identifier are excluded.

- Multiple submissions (multiple or split originals) pertaining to a single new molecular/biologic entity are only counted once.

- The filed number is not indicative of workload in the PDUFA V Program.

(USFDA: Novel Drugs Summary, 2015).

DRUG RECALLS AND WITHDRAWALS

Although the rate of new drug discovery seems to have picked up pace, it may not completely address the discovery impasse because the rate of drug recalls and withdrawals are alarmingly increasing. According to the FDA, "a drug is removed from the market when its risks outweigh its benefits. A drug is usually taken off the market because of safety issues with the drug that cannot be corrected, such as when it is discovered that the drug can cause serious side effects that were not known at the time of approval." Usually this is triggered by unexpected adverse effects that were not detected during Phase III clinical trials and were only apparent from postmarketing surveillance data from the wider patient community. The FDA has further defined "recalls" as actions taken by a firm to remove a product from the market due to the firm's own initiative, by the request of the FDA or by FDA order under statutory authority (USFDA. Drug Recalls). A product may be recalled from the market for correction because the product is either defective or potentially harmful; the recalls are classified as Class I, Class II and Class III. The FDA has defined "market withdrawals" as removal of a product from the market due to a minor violation that is not subject to FDA legal action (USFDA. Drug Recalls). A firm may remove the product from the market or correct the violation. The FDA publishes a weekly Enforcement Report which contains all recalls, even those which are not announced in the media or on the FDA's press release page (USFDA. Recalls, Market Withdrawals, & Safety Alerts). In December 2015, the FDA recalled a total of 142 drugs. Drug recalls and withdrawals may be due to various reasons such as contamination, wrong dose or release mechanism, adverse events, product mix-up, and/or wrong labeling (Wang et al., 2012).

A critical retrospection of the whole drug discovery process indicates that it is becoming more complex with drugs failing at the end of the pipeline even in Phase III or Phase IV, exemplified by postapproval or postmarketing withdrawal cases like anticoagulant Ximelagatran of AstraZeneca or Cox II inhibitor Vioxx of Merck. Vioxx (Rofecoxib) a "blockbuster drug" introduced by Merck was approved by the FDA in 1999. Why rofecoxib failed and was recalled is discussed in more details in Chapter 2, Why and How Drugs Fail. However, a short description is given here in order to provide context.

Rofecoxib is used for the treatment of osteoarthritis, rheumatoid arthritis, acute pain, primary dysmenorrheal and as an acute treatment for migraine attacks (PubChem). The approval of Rofecoxib was based on the data available from several short-term trials with traditional nonsteroidal antiinflammatory drug (tNSAIDs). This data suggested that Rofecoxib demonstrated equal efficacy and fewer gastrointestinal side effects as compared to tNSAIDs (Cairns, 2007). Rofecoxib is a selective cyclooxygenase 2 (COX-2) inhibitor and is classified as a NSAID (Fitzgerald, 2004). It is the only drug, when introduced to the market, that had established superiority over tNSAIDs in terms of gastrointestinal outcomes (Brunton et al., 2006). However, Merck voluntarily withdrew it from the market in 2004, just five years after its launch. This decision was a result of data obtained from two major studies funded by Merck, namely Vioxx Gastrointestinal Outcomes Research (VIGOR) and Adenomatous Polyp Prevention on Vioxx (APPROVe), both published in the New England Journal of Medicine. The VIGOR study was a comparative study between Vioxx and Naproxen with a study population of 8076 participants. It proved that Vioxx had lesser gastrointestinal side effects than Naproxen in patients with rheumatoid arthritis. However, this study also reported that Vioxx carried four-times higher risk of myocardial infarction compared to Naproxen (Ferraz et al., 2000). It favored the gastrointestinal effects of Vioxx and understated its cardiovascular risk.

In a study population of 2586 patients, the APPROVe trial began enrollment in 2000 to evaluate the effect of three years of treatment with Vioxx on risk of recurrent adenomatous polps in patients with a history of colorectal cancer. The trial was monitored by an external independent data safety monitoring board. Increased cardiovascular risk was seen in the Vioxx group when compared with the placebo after 18 months of treatment. The study was terminated 2 months before its planned completion due to the recommendation of the external data safety monitoring board (Bresalier et al., 2005). Subsequently, Merck withdrew Vioxx from the worldwide market. Over this background it will be interesting to understand why and how drugs fail. Such end-of-the-pipeline failures are becoming nightmares for pharmaceutical companies. New drug discovery approaches must effectively address and overcome such problems and become more dynamic, focused and predictive where safety and efficacy issues are addressed alongside the developmental costs.

WHY DRUGS FAIL?

While this question has been discussed more in Chapter 2, Why and How Drugs Fail, few pointers are provided here to better understand the context. Any drug, whether chemical, botanical or biological, will have inherent limitations if it is focused only on a single-target. The high specificity to a particular target can actually turn out to be a limitation. Like enzyme action, the drug-receptor relation is considered to be highly specific—like a lock and key. However, just as one master key can open many locks, many drugs may modulate multiple proteins rather than act upon single-targets. As compared with multitarget drugs, highly selective, single-target compounds may actually have less clinical efficacy. When the single-target-based drug discovery approach was evolving, knowledge of biology and pathophysiology was limited. Diseases were looked at more in terms of symptoms and therapeutics were targeted mainly to relieve symptoms. This triggered discovery efforts towards identifying specific targets and receptors. Modulating these receptors either by blocking or stimulating the respective biological pathways with specific chemical entities was the predominant discovery strategy employed by the pharmaceutical industry, as well as in academia and biotechnology start-ups. The drugs discovered from such "specificity-targeted" efforts have been highly successful in relieving "specific" symptoms. For example, hypertension can be controlled by beta-blockers, calcium channel blockers and angiotensin-converting enzyme inhibitors. Hyperglycemia can be treated with drugs stimulating insulin secretion; hypercholesteromia can be treated with drugs inhibiting cholesterol synthesis; pain and inflammation can be treated with prostaglandin inhibitors, and so on. Many drugs may fail, especially in the treatment of chronic diseases, because they modulate only one target and are not able to address complex metabolic system in a systems biology context. Contemporary relevance and importance of holistic drug targeting is discussed in Chapter 3, Holistic Drug Targeting.

Well over 185 drugs have been recalled from the market, either in the United States, Europe or both, since the 1970s, some that had been in use since the 1930s (List of withdrawn drugs). Very few exceptional drugs, such as aspirin, have been able to sustain for reasonably long durations of time. Drugs fail and are withdrawn from the market for several reasons (Patwardhan, 2014a). Drugs fail most of the time because of undesirable off-target effects, toxicity and other serious safety-related issues. Drugs like antibiotics also fail, either because of microbes developing resistance, or simply because the target in which the drug is acting is modulated, making that drug redundant. Drugs acting on single-targets as agonists or antagonists are likely to produce direct and/or indirect cascading effects in the whole physiological system; because the body actually constitutes a meta-network of targets, interacting with each other to regulate complex, biological, metabolic processes (Pujol et al., 2010). Systems biology principles indicate that a seemingly simple drug acting on a specific target can actually trigger a complex sequence of reactions quite distant from the site of action, quite similar to the butterfly effect. Also, drugs fail if they are ineffective. Interestingly, drugs are also withdrawn by pharmaceutical companies for business reasons. When new generation drugs are developed, older ones are withdrawn. As a principle, drug discovery scientists would like to "kill" a drug lead candidate as early as possible in the pipeline, because carrying a bad drug to the end of the pipeline increases the risks and costs.

Regulatory authorities such as the FDA terminate many drugs—even after they are approved. This is worrying, especially because the regulatory process to approve any drug is indeed a very stringent, drawn-out process in which the safety and efficacy of any new drug is assured by a series of chemical, biological and clinical investigations. Still, starting with thalidomide in 1950s and continuing today, hundreds of drugs have been killed by regulators and were withdrawn from markets (List of withdrawn drugs). This massacre of drugs has resulted in significant financial loss, sending the whole sector into a traumatic, panic situation. Clearly, market-driven approaches to drug discovery have not been successful or sustainable. Moreover, there seems to be a substantial decline in pharmaceutical ethics. We need novel approaches to address issues related to drug discovery impasse, innovation deficit and bottlenecks to improve the efficiency.

NEED FOR NOVEL APPROACHES

In the sequence of their appearance, the scientific disciplines involved in drug discovery were: chemistry, pharmacology, physiology, microbiology, biochemistry and molecular biology. Most of the new therapeutic classes of drugs like muscle relaxants; diuretics, L-dopa, antibiotics, recombinant proteins, monoclonal antibodies and others were generated on the basis of scientific opportunities rather than therapeutic need. As seen from the earlier sections, new drug discovery is presently facing many challenges of safety, efficacy and sustainability.

Novel approaches in drug discovery are required as they may reduce costs of R&D, improve safety and efficiency and hence, reduce the chances of market withdrawal of drugs postlaunch. To add to these challenges already discussed, regulatory processes are becoming more stringent and many new drugs are being recalled from postmarketing or postapproval stages (Patwardhan and Mashelkar, 2009). In the past, the industry has witnessed serious challenges regarding drug safety that led, e.g., to withdrawal of Merck's Vioxx and the lawsuit involving GlaxoSmithKline (GSK's) Avandia. Social scrutiny about drug safety and efficacy has greatly increased as well. Since the safety of new drugs may not be known with certainty until they have been in the market for many years, a critical re-evaluation of existing process of drug regulation is needed (Patwardhan and Mashelkar, 2009). Pharmaceutical companies are interested in developing new drugs or maximizing sales from current block-buster drugs in order to maintain high profits. They have to sustain in challenging environments with increasing costs of R&D, marketing costs and loss due to patent expiration (Malik, 2008; Cuatrecasas, 2006).

CHEMICAL APPROACHES

Drug researchers desperately need more new scaffolds and diverse structural analogues. Small organic molecules from natural products and biological systems have in-built substantial structural diversity. It has been very difficult to create such huge structural diversity even with routine combinatorial methods. To effectively address this limitation − highly intelligent, automated organic synthesis schemes were recently introduced by Burke et al. that are capable of efficiently producing and simultaneously purifying large amounts of complex biologically relevant or drug-like compounds.

Of the drugs that are chiral, nearly 90% of the ones marketed close to 2006 were racemic, consisting of an equimolar mixture of the enantiomers. In spite of having the same chemical structure, most isomers of chiral drugs display stark differences in biological activities such as pharmacology, toxicology, pharmacokinetics, metabolism, etc. Some of the isomers may have no biological activity, or a different one, or totally undesirable effects. In a racemic mixture with only one isomer being the drug of choice, the purity of the drug drops to just 50%. Hence, chiral separation and analysis of racemic drugs are absolutely essential to eliminate the unwanted isomer from exhibiting undesirable effects, and to provide an effective means of therapy to patients (Nguyen et al., 2006).

The term "chiral switch" was coined to refer to the substitution in the marketplace of a racemic drug with a single-enantiomer version. It is a procedure used to transform an old racemic drug into its single active enantiomer. One prominent example of a chiral switch occurred in 2001 when the FDA approved AstraZeneca's esomeprazole (Nexium), a proton pump inhibitor used to treat gastroesophageal reflux disease and erosive esophagitis. Omeprazole was marketed by AstraZeneca as "the purple pill." The S-omeprazole enantiomer was responsible for the drug's clinical properties while the R-omeprazole enantiomer was inactive. After FDA approval, esomeprazole was marketed as "the new purple pill" to be used in place of generic omeprazole (Gellad et al., 2014).

Drug repurposing or repositioning is another strategic chemical approach to drug development. It evolved in the early 1990s and has now caught the interest of academia. Drug repurposing extracts added value from prior research and development investments. Drugs with good candidature for repurposing are those that have not succeeded in previous advanced clinical trials for reasons other than safety. A search can also be directed towards exploring new therapeutic applications of existing compounds. Identifying alternative potential disease areas for an approved drug enables the drug to be repurposed for a new market at a fraction of the cost it takes to get a new drug to market.

The drug's known pharmacological mechanism can be applied to a new therapeutic indication. It could also be for an altogether different clinical application. The repurposing of a drug can also involve exploring the pharmacological mechanisms of the drugs, which have not yet been described for the molecule. The avenue opens up new possibilities for drugs that are on the market as well as those that have been on the market, as failure is not a criterion.

The case of thalidomide exemplifies drug repurposing, as is seen in its success as an anticancer agent in recent years. It was used in the late 1950s to treat morning sickness. Its teratogenic effects earned it great notoriety as it was responsible for severe skeletal birth defects (Fletcher, 1980; Knobloch and Rüther, 2008). In spite of this debacle, the potentially therapeutic properties of thalidomide are being re-explored. More than 700 thalidomide clinical trials are currently registered in almost every cancer type and is currently approved for the treatment of multiple myeloma (Breitkreutz and Anderson, 2008; Palumbo et al., 2008). Although the exact mechanism of action for thalidomide is unknown, possible mechanisms include antiangiogenic and oxidative stress-inducing effects as it inhibits NF-κB and COX-2 activity (Kim and Scialli, 2011). Thalidomide is off-patent, cheap and relatively well evaluated, making it the choice of repurposing studies. Thus, with the large amount of pharmacological and biological knowledge available in literature, it has become increasingly feasible to find novel drug indications for existing drugs, aiding the drug repurposing movement.

Many natural product scaffolds can be used for discovering new lines of chemical structures, which can be synthesized, redesigned and repurposed. Many of the natural products especially obtained from traditional medicine sources have evidence of use and safety over many years. Therefore, they can be very good sources for new drug discovery. In such cases, the discovery pipeline can flow in a reverse direction—from clinics to laboratories. This approach known as "reverse pharmacology" is discussed in Chapter 4, Reverse Pharmacology.

PHARMACOLOGY APPROACHES

Ethnopharmacology has already re-emerged as an innovative approach for drug discovery. Most of the ethnopharmacology research is on botanicals, which offer natural libraries of diverse chemical scaffolds and structures. Every botanical contains hundreds of molecules and bioactive compounds. Each of the bioactives may have the capability to modulate one or more targets. Each target may have an effect on one or more genes and metabolic pathways, which can be involved in one or more diseases. This becomes a very complex biological system with interactive networks of bioactives—targets—genes—pathways—diseases. A new branch that attempts to study these complex bioactive interactions with multiple targets is known as polypharmacology or network pharmacology. Network pharmacology uses computational power and supercomputer-based virtual HTS for docking studies to improve efficiency of discovery process. Network pharmacology also attempts repurposing existing drug molecules for different therapeutic conditions.

Network pharmacology is an integration of chemo-informatics and bioinformatics that helps us build a network-centric view of drug action. It is an emerging paradigm, which integrates systems biology and computational biology to study multicomponent and multitargeted drugs and formulations. It uses computational power and computer-based virtual HTS for docking studies to improve efficiency of discovery process. Studying complex relationships between the bioactives, targets, diseases and genes is now possible with the help of network pharmacology. Implementing network pharmacology with the help of the large amount of biological and pharmacological information available in literature is a promising means for drug repurposing as well (Hopkins, 2007; Ellingson et al., 2014). Network pharmacology and its use in drug discovery and drug repurposing have been further explained in Chapter 5, Network Pharmacology.

BIOLOGICAL APPROACHES

After the Human Genome Project (HGP) was launched in the year 1990, applications of genomics in drug discovery became more main-stream. Soon after the first draft of HGP was completed, simultaneously the first Biotechnology Company Genentech celebrated 25 years with a number of new biotechnology products. The USFDA has granted approvals to many biotechnology based products, including: Novartis: Gleevec—for the treatment of chronic myeloid leukemia; Genezyme: Carticel-cartilage regeneration; Immunex: Enbrel—for rheumatoid arthritis; Genenentech: Herceptin—for Brest cancer; CDR Therapeutics: Integrilin - for heart diseases; Organogenesis: Apligraft - a skin substitute. Over 300 drugs are in Phase III and over 200 are expected to be in the market in the near future.

There are many alliances, collaborations, mergers and acquisitions that have become part of the new trend in drug discovery and development. A business cooperation of US$1.5 billion between Bayer and CuraGen for genetic targets of small-molecule drugs; and a Novartis and Vertex Pharma deal of $800 million for rational drug design technology and a strategic alliance between GSK and Ranbaxy for new discovery leads set the standards. This strategy is primarily coming from the pressing need to increase productivity and the success rate of new drug discoveries. The expected growth rate cannot be maintained if the present 0.5 new drug registered/annum/industry is not increased to a minimum of three new drugs registrations/annum/industry.

The drug discovery process is becoming more and more complex and capital intensive and has remain "Target rich" — "Lead poor" with lead discovery as a greater bottleneck. Although HTS and combinatorial chemical synthesis are explored with great hope, general experience tells that in most companies the investments in HTS and combinatorial chemistry have not reaped the rewards in new lead discovery as expected. There is a need for a systematic and critical review of methods and mindset involved in drug discovery, and there is a need to rediscover the drug discovery process afresh.

The chemical biology approach helped to bring more specificity in drug discovery. Understanding of precise targets and their role in pathophysiology of diseases has led to many new drugs. However, single-target single molecule based drug discovery also faced many drawbacks. Development of biotechnology as a new discipline also resulted in an increasing shift from chemical to biological products.

Many advances in biotechnology and omics technologies, especially pharmacogenomics, proteomics, metabolomics, transcriptomics and epigenomics, are emerging as new approaches to innovate drug discovery process. The newly invented genome editing technology platform of clustered regularly interspaced short palindromic repeats or CRISPR-Cas system might open new innovative pathways for biomedical research and help engineer any organism one chooses by modifying its own genome (Doudna and Charpentier, 2014). We discuss these innovative approaches including genomic, pharmacogenomics, transcriptomics, proteomics and chemical informatics approaches in Chapter 6, Genomics-driven Drug Discovery Process;

Chapter 7, Pharmacogenomics; Chapter 8, Transcriptomics and Epigenomics; Chapter 9, Proteomics; and Chapter 10, Chemical Informatics, respectively.

In addition to therapeutic biologic products, vaccine discovery has also benefited significantly through biological approaches. Development of therapeutic adjuvants and vaccines is discussed in Chapter 11, Vaccines and Immunodrugs Discovery.

FORMULATION DISCOVERY

The magic bullet approach was relevant in the 20th century when infectious diseases were predominant. This single-target single molecule approach dominated discovery science for several years. It exists even now and may still be valid for infectious diseases and treatment of specific symptoms like pain, inflammation and edema. But in the 21st century, the world is facing major epidemics of lifestyle diseases like obesity, diabetes, asthma and metabolic syndromes where multiple genes and multiple targets are involved. Many metabolic networks are collectively responsible for pathogenesis of complex syndromes and clusters of diseases. Lifestyle disorders require a multitargeted approach. Chapter 12, Cucurmin, the Holistic Avant-Garde gives an interesting example of curcumin as a holistic targeting agent. Curcumin is a bioactive from the medicinal plant turmeric that has shown efficacy in various diseases including cancer, diabetes, acid peptic, musculo-skeletal, gastrointestinal as well as in wound healing.

There are clear trends that show the main-stream pharmaceutical research is moving away from single molecule or single-target approaches in favor of combinations and multiple target approaches. A shift in mindset from NCE based "drug discovery" to rational "formulation discovery" seem to be an emerging approach. Here, ethnopharmacology and traditional knowledge can play major roles. Most traditional medical products contain natural resources like medicinal plants and minerals where quality control remains the most crucial for safety and efficacy. Chapter 13, Safety of Traditional Medicines, discusses some of the approaches in quality control of traditional medical products.

Opportunities for multidisciplinary research that joins the forces of natural products chemistry, molecular and cellular biology, synthetic and analytical chemistry, biochemistry and pharmacology to exploit the vast diversity of chemical structures and biological activities of natural products have the capability of multitargeting. The exploration of structural chemical databases comprising a wide variety of chemotypes, in conjunction with databases on target genes and proteins, will facilitate the creation of NCE through computational molecular modeling for pharmacological evaluation. The conventional pharmacology routes to drug discovery involving testing analogues of active drugs or mass screenings in chemical libraries are not enough. In this book we portray the past, present and future of drug discovery and highlight novel approaches that might help in overcoming the present impasse.

CONCLUDING REMARKS

Discovery efforts need not be limited only to material pharmaceutical drugs. We bring in point that in the present era of lifestyle epidemics, it is important to consider physiological approaches as well. Physiological interventions can be done through body-mind medicine, lifestyle and behavioral modifications. For many lifestyle diseases "meditation" may be better than "medication". Chapter 14, Holistic Lifestyle, discusses physiological approaches as therapeutic ways based on lifestyle and behavioral medicine.

Drug discovery requires seemingly diverse, but connected, expertise to develop effective therapeutics. Coordinated collaborative partnerships, as illustrated in Chapter 15, Collaborative Strategies for Future Drug Discovery, are mandatory to pave the path and eventually lead to effective innovations in drug discovery. The much-heralded "open source/science" presents new avenues to foster biomedical innovations through *precompetitive* strategies that can develop targeted therapeutics for all diseases. Changing the culture the partners are involved in is challenging, but new models will build teamwork, clear boundaries for competition and reward innovators who embrace these changes (Collyar and Chaguturu, 2015). Currently, the discovery sector is facing a serious problem regarding data reproducibility. Desperate attempts based on compromised ethics and scientific misconduct are unlikely to give sustained solutions to discovery impasse. Chapter 16, Righting the Ship: The Data Reproducibility Conundrum, discusses problems and the context related to these important issues.

The 18 year-high of new drug introductions in 2014 made the rock-bottom approvals experienced over the past decade a distant memory, but it is the changed mindset of the pharmaceutical industry that embraced coordinated, collaborative innovation that made it all possible. While we preach for effective collaborations between pharmaceuticals and academia, it is equally critical that pharmaceutical players engaged in therapeutics for a given disease join hands together for better outcomes (Collyar and Chaguturu, 2015).

It takes a village to raise a child. The same is certainly true for discovering drugs that are efficacious, safe and patient-centric. The need for new approaches to combat the next healthcare crisis is greater than ever.

REFERENCES

Berenson, A., 2007. Merck Agrees to Pay $4.85 Billion in Vioxx Claims. The New York Times [cited 2016 Mar 15] Available from: http://www.nytimes.com/2007/11/09/business/09cndmerck.html?_r=1.

Bhinder, B., Djaballah, H., 2013. A decade of RNAi screening: too much hay and very few needles. Drug Discov. World 14, 31–41.

Bishop, J.F., Dewar, J., Toner, G.C., Smith, J., Tattersall, M.H., Olver, I.N., et al., 1999. Initial paclitaxel improves outcome compared with CMFP combination chemotherapy as front-line therapy in untreated metastatic breast cancer. J. Clin. Oncol. 17, 2355–2364.

Bonomi, P., Kim, K., Fairclough, D., Cella, D., Kugler, J., Rowinsky, E., et al., 2000. Comparison of survival and quality of life in advanced non–small-cell lung cancer patients treated with two dose levels of paclitaxel combined with cisplatin versus etoposide with cisplatin: results of an eastern cooperative oncology group trial. J. Clin. Oncol. 18, 623.

Breitkreutz, I., Anderson, K.C., 2008. Thalidomide in multiple myeloma--clinical trials and aspects of drug metabolism and toxicity. Expert Opin. Drug. Metab. Toxicol. 4, 973–985.

Bresalier, R.S., Sandler, R.S., Quan, H., Bolognese, J.A., Oxenius, B., Horgan, K., et al., 2005. Cardiovascular events associated with rofecoxib in a colorectal adenoma chemoprevention trial. N. Engl. J. Med. 352, 1092–1102.

Brunton, L.L., Lazo, J.S., Parker, K.L. (Eds.), 2006. Autacoids: drug therapy of inflamation. In: Goodman and Gilman's The Pharmacological Basis of Therapeutics, eleventh ed. McGraw-Hill, New York.

Cairns, J.A., 2007. The coxibs and traditional nonsteroidal anti-inflammatory drugs: a current perspective on cardiovascular risks. Can. J. Cardiol. 23, 125–131.

Chaguturu, R., 2015. A look back at 2015: hope, hype and hypocrisy. Comb. Chem. High Throughput Screen. 19, 2–3.

Collyar, D., Chaguturu, R., 2015. Renaissance in biomedical innovation: global villages raise effective therapies. Future Med. Chem. 7 (8), 971–974.

Cuatrecasas, P., 2006. Drug discovery in jeopardy. J. Clin. Invest. 116, 2837–2842.

Doudna, J.A., Charpentier, E., 2014. The new frontier of genome engineering with CRISPR-Cas9. Science 346, 1258096.

Ellingson, S.R., Smith, J.C., Baudry, J., 2014. Polypharmacology and supercomputer-based docking: opportunities and challenges. Mol. Simul. 40, 848–854.

Ferraz, M.B., Bombardier, C., Day, R., Hawkey, C.J., Laine, L., Shapiro, D., et al., 2000. Comparison of upper gastrointestinal toxicity of rofecoxib and naproxen in patients with rheumatoid arthritis. VIGOR Study Group. N. Engl. J. Med. 343, 1520–1528, 2 p following 1528.

Fitzgerald, G.A., 2004. Coxibs and cardiovascular disease. N. Engl. J. Med. 351, 1709–1711.

Fletcher, I., 1980. Review of the treatment of thalidomide children with limb defeciency in Great Britain. Clin. Orthop. Relat. Res. 18–25.

Gellad, W.F., Choi, P., Mizah, M., Good, C.B., Kesselheim, A.S., 2014. Assessing the chiral switch: approval and use of single-enantiomer drugs, 2001 to 2011. Am. J. Manag. Care 20, e90–e97.

Harmon, K., 2010. Prescription drug deaths increase dramatically. Sci. Am.

Hopkins, A., 2007. Network pharmacology. Nat. Biotechnol. 25, 1110.

Jassem, J., Pienkowski, T., Pluzanska, A., Jelic, S., Gorbunova, V., Mrsic-Krmpotic, Z., et al., 2001. Doxorubicin and paclitaxel versus fluorouracil, doxorubicin, and cyclophosphamide as first-line therapy for women with metastatic breast cancer: final results of a randomized phase III multicenter trial. J. Clin. Oncol. 19, 1707–1715.

Kim, J.H., Scialli, A.R., 2011. Thalidomide: the tragedy of birth defects and the effective treatment of disease. Toxicol. Sci. 122, 1–6.

Koehn, F.E., Carter, G.T., 2005. The evolving role of natural products in drug discovery. Nature reviews Drug discovery 4 (3), 206–220.

Knobloch, J., Rüther, U., 2008. Shedding light on an old mystery: thalidomide suppresses survival pathways to induce limb defects. Cell Cycle 7, 1121−1127.

List of withdrawn drugs [Internet]. Available from: <https://en.wikipedia.org/wiki/List_of_withdrawn_drugs>.

Malik, N.N., 2008. Drug discovery: past, present and future. Drug Discov. Today 13, 909−912, 21−22.

Medicines and Healthcare Product Regulatory Agency. Drug safety updates Statins: Risk of hyperglycemia and diabetes.2012. Available from https://www.gov.uk/drug-safety-update/statins-risk-of-hyperglycaemiaand-diabetes.

MERCK & CO., Inc. Patient Information about VIOXXÒ (rofecoxib tablets and oral suspension) for Osteoarthritis, Rheumatoid Arthritis, Juvenile Rheumatoid Arthritis, Pain and Migraine Attacks. Whitehouse Station,NJ, USA.2004. Available at https://www.merck.com/product/usa/pi_circulars/v/vioxx/vioxx_ppi.pdf.

Matheson, A.J., Figgitt, D.P., 2001. Rofecoxib: a review of its use in the management of osteoarthritis, acute pain and rheumatoid arthritis. Drugs 61 (6), 833−865.

National Clinical Guideline Centre (UK). Lipid Modification: Cardiovascular Risk Assessment and the Modification of Blood Lipids for the Primary and Secondary Prevention of Cardiovascular Disease. London:National Institute for Health and Care Excellence (UK); 2014 Jul. (NICE Clinical Guidelines, No. 181.) 2, Development of the guideline. Available from: http://www.ncbi.nlm.nih.gov/books/NBK268937/.

Nguyen, L.A., He, H., Pham-Huy, C., 2006. Chiral drugs: an overview. Int. J. Biomed. Sci. 2, 85−100.

Palumbo, A., Facon, T., Sonneveld, P., Bladè, J., Offidani, M., Gay, F., et al., 2008. Thalidomide for treatment of multiple myeloma: 10 years later. Blood 111, 3968−3977.

Patwardhan, B., 2000. Ayurveda: the "Designer" medicine: a review of ethnopharmacology and bioprospecting research. Indian Drugs 213−227.

Patwardhan, B., 2014a. Death of drugs and rebirth of health care: Indian response to discovery impasse. Collaborative Innovation in Drug Discovery. John Wiley & Sons, Inc., pp. 173−194.

Patwardhan, B., 2014b. The new pharmacognosy. Comb. Chem. HighThroughput Screen. 17, 97.

Patwardhan, B., Mashelkar, R.A., 2009. Traditional medicine-inspired approaches to drug discovery: can Ayurveda show the way forward? Drug Discov. Today 14, 804−811.

Patwardhan, B., Vaidya, A.D.B., 2010. Natural products drug discovery: accelerating the clinical candidate development using reverse pharmacology approaches. Indian J. Exp. Biol. 48, 220−227.

PubChem, available at https://pubchem.ncbi.nlm.nih.gov/.

Pujol, A., Mosca, R., Farrés, J., Aloy, P., 2010. Unveiling the role of network and systems biology in drug discovery. Trends Pharmacol. Sci. 115−123.

Schmid, E.F., Smith, D.A., 2004. Is pharmaceutical R&D just a game of chance or can strategy make a difference? Drug Discov. Today 18−26.

Seidman, A.D., Tiersten, A., Hudis, C., Gollub, M., Barrett, S., Yao, T.J., et al., 1995. Phase II trial of paclitaxel by 3-hour infusion as initial and salvage chemotherapy for metastatic breast cancer. J. Clin. 13, 2575−2581.

Simpson, P.B., Reichman, M., 2013. Opening the lead generation toolbox. Nat. Rev. Drug Discov. 13, 3−4.

USFDA. Drug Recalls. Available at http://www.fda.gov/drugs/drugsafety/DrugRecalls/.

USFDA. Recalls, Market Withdrawals, & Safety Alerts: Enforcement Reports. Available at http://www.fda.gov/safety/recalls/enforcementreports/.

USFDA. Novel Drugs Summary 2015, available at http://www.fda.gov/drugs/developmentappro-valprocess/druginnovation/ucm474696.htm.

Wang, B., Gagne, J.J., Choudhry, N., 2012. The epidemiology of drug recalls in the United States. Arch. Intern. Med. 172, 1110–1111.

Chapter 2

Why and How Drugs Fail

Dada Patil[1], Bhushan Patwardhan[2] and Kalyani Kumbhare[2]

[1]Serum Institute of India Private Limited, Pune, Maharashtra, India, [2]Savitribai Phule Pune University, Pune, Maharashtra, India

INTRODUCTION

Drug failures, postmarket launch, are more of a norm than an exception. This happens mainly because of toxicity, untoward events and other serious safety related concerns. Drugs also fail because the target microbes or systems become resistant. The pharmaceutical companies for business reasons also withdraw drugs, especially when the company introduces a newer drug with enhanced properties. The regulatory authorities recall many approved drugs. This is more worrisome because substantial investments have been made by the industry to execute safety and efficacy-related clinical investigations to meet the very stringent, long and arduous process of drug approval. Still, starting with thalidomide in the decade of 1950 till today, hundreds of drugs have been recalled by regulators and were withdrawn from markets. This has resulted in significant financial loss to the pharmaceutical industry. A three prong approach—first, discover safer drugs; second, try to repurpose old drugs and third, use adjuvants to counter toxicity and enhance safety of existing drugs—is being actively explored by the industry to remedy the situation. These approaches require an in-depth knowledge of the interconnected and interdependent metrics of metabolic processes and systems biology of the disease target involved.

DRUG WITHDRAWALS: ANALYSIS OF SIX DECADES

Many drugs have been withdrawn from the market since 1950. This is mainly due to reasons of safety, efficacy, quality, and commercial viability. Drug-induced toxicities remain the main cause behind these withdrawals. For instance, among the 59 withdrawals reported from the British market during the years 1972−94, 39% were due to safety concerns and 59% for commercial reasons, while only $\sim 2\%$ were for efficacy concerns. Main reasons for a total of 168 drugs withdrawn from 1950 to 2015; the data was compiled from various agencies including World Health Organization, United States

Innovative Approaches in Drug Discovery. DOI: http://dx.doi.org/10.1016/B978-0-12-801814-9.00002-7
23

Food and Drug Administration (USFDA), European Medicines Evaluation Agency, United Kingdom Medicines Control Agency, Canadian Health Protection Branch, Australian Therapeutic Goods Administration and Wikipedia (Fung et al., 2001; Wysowski and Swartz, 2005; Lasser et al., 2002; Qureshi et al., 2011; List of withdrawn drugs). The decade of 1980–1990 saw the withdrawal of 49 drugs (Fig. 2.1). The withdrawn drugs have association with different organ toxicities such as hepatic (rosiglitazone),

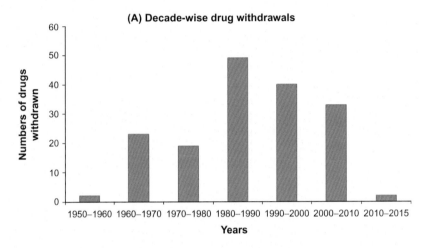

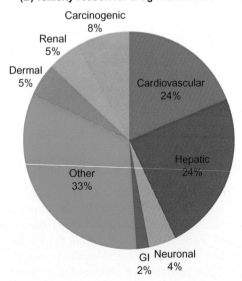

FIGURE 2.1   (A) Worldwide drug withdrawals from 1950 to 2015, (B) Pie chart showing percentages of particular toxicities behind drug withdrawals.

cardiovascular (rofecoxib), neuronal (clioquinol), gastrointestinal (indopro-fen), dermal (sulphacarbamide), renal (thiobutabarbital), genotoxicity and carcinogenicity (ethyl carbamate), and other toxicities (methaqualone) as shown in Fig. 2.1A. The data suggest that hepatic toxicity (24%) and cardio-vascular toxicity (19%) are the main reasons for drug withdrawals. Other reasons (33%) for drug withdrawals include allergies, teratogenicity, psychiatric, hemorrhagic conditions, drug abuse, and overdose (Fig. 2.1B).

An in-depth knowledge of the molecular mechanisms involved is required to understand the underlying reasons of *how* and *why* these drugs failed and had to be recalled or withdrawn from the market. This would also help in any efforts to repurpose these drugs for new indications, to alleviate the asso-ciated toxicities and the revival of withdrawn drugs.

CASE STUDY 1: STATINS

Discovery and Development of Statins

Increased cholesterol levels have widely been attributed to cardiovascular disorders (CVDs). Cholesterol biosynthetic pathway encompasses four major stages: (1) condensation of three acetate units to form a six-carbon interme-diate, mevalonate; (2) conversion of mevalonate to activated isoprene units; (3) polymerization of six 5-carbon isoprene units to form the 30-carbon linear squalene; and (4) cyclization of squalene to form the steroid nucleus, with a further series of changes to produce cholesterol. The reduction of 3-hydroxy-3-methylglutaryl-coenzyme A (HMG-CoA) to mevalonate with HMG-CoA reductase is a rate-limiting step. Therefore, considerable efforts had been directed over the last half a century toward the discovery of HMG-CoA reductase inhibitors as cholesterol-lowering agents. The family of statins has been shown to impair cholesterol production by inhibiting the synthesis of mevalonate, the rate-limiting step in the cholesterol biosynthetic pathway.

Compactin

This first statin, a competitive inhibitor for HMG-CoA reductase, was iso-lated in 1973 by Japanese scientist Akira Endo and his colleagues from the mold *Penicillium citrinum.* Compactin was extensively studied in animal models including rats, hens, dogs, and monkeys for cholesterol lowering effect. These primary findings showing the dramatic effects of compactin in dogs and monkeys, although initially found to be inactive in rat models, had inspired many pharmaceutical companies to begin research programs toward the discovery of statins with more desirable properties. The timeline of statin development is shown in Fig. 2.2. In February 1979, Merck had isolated a statin very similar to compactin, called mevinolin from the fungus *Aspergillus terreus.* In November 1986, Merck submitted a New Drug Application (NDA) to the USFDA for lovastatin, which was approved in

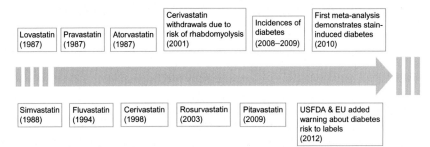

FIGURE 2.2   Timeline: history of statins.

September 1987. Thus lovastatin was the first commercial statin introduced into the market. Currently, there are seven statins available for clinical use: lovastatin (1987), simvastatin (1988), pravastatin (1991), fluvastatin (1994), atorvastatin (1997), rosuvastatin (2003), and pitavastatin (2009). Another drug, cerivastatin, was approved by the USFDA and launched in January 1998, but was subsequently withdrawn from the market in August 2001 because of adverse event reports of rhabdomyolysis.

Guidelines from the American College of Cardiology/American Heart Association and the National Institute for Health and Care Excellence recommend moderate- to high-intensity statin therapy for primary prevention of CVD (Stone et al., 2014; National Institute for Health and Care Excellence, 2014). Statins are generally well tolerated but can produce a variety of skeletal muscle associated, dose-dependent adverse reactions, ranging from muscle pain to muscle cell damage and severe rhabdomyolysis (Thompson et al., 2003). The incidence of rhabdomyolysis is approximately 1 per 10,000; however, fatalities have been reported (Graham et al., 2004). The incidences appear more frequently with cerivastatin especially when used in high doses, in the elderly or when taken along with gemfibrozil, another cholesterol lowering drug. A total of 52 (31 in the United States and 21 worldwide) deaths occurred due to severe rhabdomyolysis associated with the use of cerivastatin; 12 involved concomitant use of gemfibrozil. Additionally, 385 nonfatal cases were reported among 700,000 users in the United States, most of whom required hospitalization (Furberg and Pitt, 2001). Therefore, cerivastatin was voluntarily withdrawn worldwide in August 2001 (USFDA, 2001). An increased risk of Type 2 diabetes associated with statin therapy has been reported when compared with usual care or placebo and also with high dose versus usual dose of statins (Sattar et al., 2010; Preiss et al., 2011). Meta-analyses of large-scale placebo versus standard care controlled trials observed a 9% increased risk for incident diabetes associated with the statin therapy. Systematic review of 17 randomized controlled trials showed an increased risk of the development of diabetes. Other minor adverse events associated with statin treatment include hemorrhagic stroke, cancers, depression, liver enzyme elevation, renal dysfunction and arthritis have been reported. The precise mechanism behind statin-induced myopathy has not been fully understood, but may include on-target modulation contributing to the alteration of muscle cell membrane function, deficits in energy metabolism associated with ubiquinone deficiency and reduction of small GTP-binding proteins involved in myocytes preservation (Nishimoto et al., 2003; Pierno et al., 1995).

Reduced Cholesterol Synthesis and Membrane Excitability

Cholesterol is a key component of the structure and function of cell membranes. Statins seem to alter the membrane cholesterol in different tissues, including skeletal muscle (Nishimoto et al., 2003). The depletion of the cholesterol content of skeletal muscle could lead to changes in membrane stability and fluidity. A change in membrane fluidity may affect muscle membrane excitability through modulation of different ion channels such as sodium, potassium and chloride channels. A dose-dependent reduction of membrane chloride conductance in muscle fibers was seen in simvastatin treated rats (Pierno et al., 1995). However, reduction in cholesterol in human skeletal myotubules using squalene synthetase inhibitors have not shown the association of myotoxicity suggesting this mechanism is less plausible (Flint et al., 1997).

Isoprenoids Depletion

Role of Coenzyme Q10

Isoprenylation is a fundamental element of post-transcriptional lipid modification of proteins and other compounds. It has an important role in the synthesis of ubiquinone (coenzyme Q10), selenoproteins and maintaining cell growth, proliferation and differentiation, and also for calcium homeostasis in the skeletal muscle (Castets et al., 2012). Statin treatment decreases the level of mevalonate, an intermediate product of cholesterol synthesis pathway, which is responsible for donation of isoprenyl unit. The depletion of isoprenylation, especially farnesyl pyrophosphate to geranyl-geranyl pyrophosphate, causes the decrease in the synthesis of coenzyme Q10—a steroid isoprenoid that is involved in the electron transport chain and participates in oxidative phosphorylation in mitochondria. The coenzyme Q10 also serves as an important antioxidant in both mitochondria and lipid membranes (Littarru and Tiano, 2007). Thus, reduction in formation of isoprenoids could cause decrease in synthesis of coenzyme Q10 (Baker and Tarnopolsky, 2001). Several studies have been undertaken to evaluate the correlation of serum and muscle coenzyme Q10 levels with symptoms of myopathy following statin administration. Few studies have shown that the statins have lowered the circulating levels of coenzyme Q10 up to 54%, whereas other studies did not confirm a lowering of coenzyme Q10 levels in muscles during statin therapy (Dasa et al., 2010). Keith et al. showed that supplementation can help in raising the plasma levels of coenzyme Q10 of those taking statins (Keith et al., 2008). Other studies show that supplementation using coenzyme Q10 can improve the symptoms of myopathy (Caso et al., 2007; Langsjoen et al., 2005). However, the few studies which show changes in both plasma and intramuscular coenzyme Q10 concentrations with statin therapy are inconsistent (Joy and Hegele, 2009). Therefore, a direct association between decreased coenzyme Q10 and myopathy has not been conclusively proven (Harper and Jacobson, 2010; Abd and Jacobson, 2011; Littlefield et al., 2014). Furthermore, randomized, double-blind clinical trials have failed to show that coenzyme Q10 supplementation decreases statin-associated myopathy (Young et al., 2007).

Role of Selenoproteins

Selenoproteins have an important role in skeletal muscle regeneration, cell maintenance, oxidative and calcium homeostasis, thyroid hormone metabolism, and immune responses (Castets et al., 2012). Moosmann and Behl have hypothesized that statin-induced myotoxicity could be associated with decrease in selenoprotein synthesis due to depletion in isoprenylation of selenocysteine-tRNA, an essential component of selenoprotein synthesis (Moosmann and Behl, 2004). This hypothesis was tested by Moosmann and his colleagues in human HepG2 hepatic cells, cultivated myoblasts and skeletal muscle cells treated with different statins. HepG2 cells treated with atorvastatin, cerivastatin, and lovastatin at clinically common concentrations lead to differential loss of selenoprotein expression such as glutathione peroxidase (GPx). The mRNA levels were found unchanged after the treatment of statins suggesting posttranscriptional mechanism of selenoprotein suppression (Kromer and Moosmann, 2009). Similarly, cultivated myoblasts and skeletal muscle cells treated with different statins resulted in suppression of biosynthesis of GPx and selenoprotein N (Fuhrmeister et al., 2012). These studies suggest that the statins inhibit the expression of inducible selenoproteins by preventing the mevalonate-dependent maturation of the single human selenocysteine-tRNA and may thereby evoke an increased vulnerability of the liver and skeletal muscles to secondary toxins leading to toxicity.

Role of Apoptosis, Necrosis, and Atrophy

Apoptosis is programmed cell death that is regulated and executed via activation of specific signaling pathways. Statins induce apoptosis in skeletal myoblasts, myotubes and in differentiated primary human skeletal muscle cells, most often in a concentration-dependent manner (Mutoh et al., 1999; Sacher et al., 2005; Sakamoto and Kimura, 2013). The postulated underlying mechanism behind statin-induced apoptosis is largely in part due to the depletion of isoprenoids, which in-turn could decrease protein geranylgeranylation and/or farnesylation (Dirks and Jones, 2006). The isoprenoid depletion leads to the elevated levels of cytosolic calcium and activation of calpain causing release of Bax; a pro-apoptotic protein. Sacher et al. have shown that translocation of Bax to the mitochondria in response to statin treatment may lead to the release of cytochrome c (Sacher et al., 2005). The released cytochrome c increases the activity of caspases-9 and 3 causing skeletal muscle cell apoptosis. These results suggest that the depletion of downstream products of mevalonate synthesis induces apoptosis of skeletal muscle cells in a mitochondrial-mediated manner. This was supported by studies where the addition of mevalonate prevented statin-induced apoptosis and caspase-3 activation (Johnson et al., 2004). The depletion of isoprenoids were also known to cause interference with post-translational modifications of membrane associated with small guanosine triphosphate-binding (GTPase) proteins such as Ras, Rho, and Rab (Laufs and Liao, 2003; Liao, 2002). Among GTPases, Ras acts as an apoptosis suppressor and enhances cell proliferation, Rho modulates cytoskeleton formation and adhesion, and Rab activates intracellular vesicle traffic. Statin-induced apoptosis is linked with depletion of farnesyl Ras (F Ras) protein in L6 rat myoblasts treated with different statins (Matzno et al., 2005). In contrast to the role of apoptosis seen from in vitro studies, several in vivo and clinical studies have demonstrated that statins induced myotoxicity is associated with formation of vacuoles and degenerated organelles followed by necrosis (Nakahara et al., 1998; Westwood et al., 2005). These observations were clearly seen from Sakamoto and his colleagues' studies on single skeletal muscle fibers treated with different statins (Sakamoto et al., 2007, 2011). The underlying mechanism suggested that depletion of geranylgeranlyation of Rab 1 GTPase (GG-Rab) and the subsequent inhibition of ER-to-Golgi traffic involved in statin-induced skeletal myotoxicity (Sakamoto and Kimura, 2013). Recent studies also demonstrated the role of muscular atrophy in biopsied human skeletal muscle tissues exposed to statins (Hanai et al., 2007). It may be that statin-induced depletion in GG-Rab results in increased expression of atrogin-1, an ubiquitin ligase that enhances skeletal muscle weakness (Fig. 2.3) (Cao et al., 2009).

Statin-Induced Diabetes

Although safe and generally well tolerated, emerging data have suggested that statins are associated with an increased risk of new-onset diabetes (NOD) (Medicines and Healthcare Product Regulatory Agency, 2012). Several meta-analyses of clinical trials conducted during the years of 2008−14 showed the association of NOD in the range of 5−27% in patients and about 48% in menopausal woman treated with different statins (Sattar et al., 2010; Preiss et al., 2011; Waters et al., 2011; Culver et al., 2012). All the statins including hydrophilic (e.g., pravastatin and rosuvastatin) as well as hydrophobic (e.g., atorvastatin, lovastatin, pitavastatin, and simvastatin) have been reported for their association for NOD risk in dose-dependent manner. For these reasons,

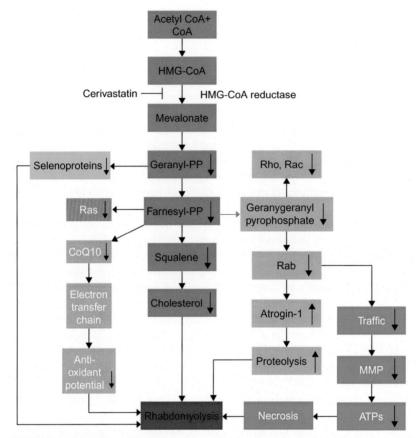

FIGURE 2.3 Plausible molecular mechanism of cerivastatin-induced rhabdomyolysis through modulation of on-target effects mainly on isoprenoids depletion leading to: decrease in coenzyme Q10 synthesis; reduction in biosynthesis of selenoproteins; decline in small guanosine triphosphate-binding (GTPase) proteins such as Ras, Rho, and Rab causing apoptosis and necrosis. The reduction in cholesterol synthesis leads to increase in membrane excitability.

USFDA added a warning about diabetes risk to the labels of all statin agents and similar concern was raised by European drug authorities (USFDA, 2012; [Internet]). A recent Canadian study on 136,966 patients aged ≥ 40 years old showed the use of higher potency statin (e.g., rosuvastatin, atorvastatin, and simvastatin) was associated with a moderate increase in the risk of NOD compared with lower potency statins in patients treated for secondary prevention of cardiovascular disease (Dormuth et al., 2014). Although the precise pathways behind statin-induced NOD is still unknown, there are several postulated mechanisms, categorized into on-target and off-target modulation as schematically shown in Figs. 2.4 and 2.5 (Brault et al., 2014; Sampson et al., 2011; Banach et al., 2013; Eitel et al., 2011; Sattar and Taskinen, 2012).

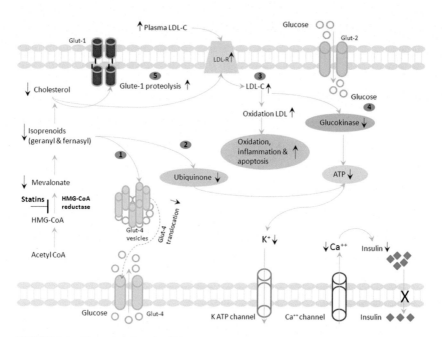

FIGURE 2.4   The underlying plausible mechanism of statin-induced NOD showed role of on-target modulation in cholesterol biosynthesis. The inhibition of HMG-CoA reductase by statins leads to isoprenoids depletion causing an increase in blood glucose through (1) decrease in Glut-4 translocation; (2) decrease in insulin secretion via decrease in ATP-dependent potassium and calcium channel activity mainly due to declined ubiquinone synthesis. The reduced biosynthesis of cholesterol could lead to (3) increased level of low density lipoprotein cholesterol (LDL-C) causing oxidation, inflammation, and apoptosis through increased LDL oxidation; (4) decreased insulin release through a decrease in ATP-dependent potassium and calcium channel activity due to declined glucokinase activity, and (5) increased Glute-1 proteolysis comprising the glucose transport.

Thus, statins are used to prevent cardiovascular diseases by interfering cholesterol biosynthesis. However, a network pharmacology analysis shows its adverse effects, which can induce NOD and specifically cerivastatin-induced rhabdomyolysis (Fig. 2.6).

CASE STUDY 2: EXAMPLE OF TROGLITAZONE

A variety of treatments are available for Type 2 diabetes mellitus. Insulin therapy is used for Type 1 diabetes although it may be used for Type 2 diabetes as well. Oral hypoglycemic agents (OHAs) are predominantly used for the management of Type 2 diabetes mellitus. The OHAs are divided into different classes. Thiazolidinediones (THZs) (Glitazones) is one such class. This class includes Troglitazone, Pioglitazone and Rosiglitazone. Rezulin is a Troglitazone which was the first Glitazone to be discovered. It is a

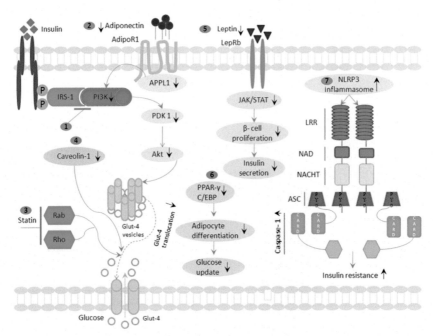

FIGURE 2.5   Off-target modulation by statins could lead to statin-induced NOD. The underlying plausible mechanism showed role of modulation of multiple targets such as (1) IRS-1-PI3PK dislocation; (2) decrease in adiponectin level (3) reduced synthesis of Rab and Rho and (4) decline in Caveolin leading to decreased Glut-4 translocation and thereby increased plasma glucose level. (5) Statin also has leptin inhibitory action leading to decline in insulin secretion through JAK/STAT pathways. (6) Statins have also decreased uptake of glucose mainly through decreased PPAR-γ levels via declined adipocyte differentiation. Statins have also been known to increase the insulin resistance through activation of NLRP3 inflammasome via stimulation of Caspase-1 mechanism.

synthetic drug which mimics natural products (Newman and Cragg, 2007). It was developed by Daichi Sankyo, a Japanese pharmaceutical company. It was later manufactured by Parke-Davis/Warner-Lambert. Rezulin was approved by the USFDA in January 1997 and introduced in the market in March 1997 (Cohen, 2006). Trogliatzone was used as an investigational drug in the Diabetes Prevention Program (DPP) in 1996, a year before it was approved by the USFDA.

Mechanism

THZs reduce insulin resistance. They bind to a nuclear receptor called peroxisome proliferator-activated receptor-γ ($PPAR\gamma$), which is abundantly present in the adipose tissue, liver, heart, and skeletal muscle. After binding to this

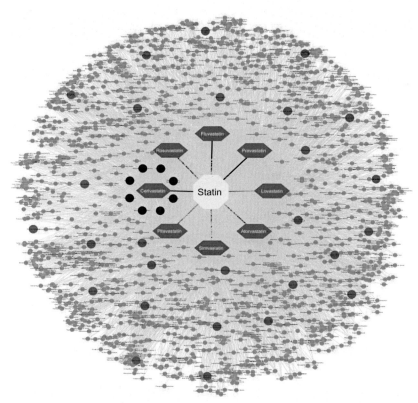

FIGURE 2.6 Brown hexagons indicate statin derivatives. All circles show diseases associated with statins. Pink circles represent statin induced 27 diseases leading to NOD and blue circles around cerivastatin hexagon represent cerivastatin-induced 8 diseases leading to rhabdomyolysis.

receptor, these drugs modulate the gene expression involved in glucose and lipid metabolism, insulin signal transduction and adipocyte differentiation and proliferation. These drugs reduce peripheral resistance to insulin and increase insulin sensitivity of adipose tissue, liver and muscles. They reduce the production of the pro-inflammatory cytokines, increase production of adiponectin by the adipose tissue, increase subcutaneous and small adipocyte mass, lower hepatic fat content, lower hepatic glucose production, increase glucose uptake by skeletal muscle, and preserve and enhance beta cell and vascular function.

The mechanism of THZs is illustrated in Fig. 2.7 (Kahn et al., 2000; Hauner, 2002).

In insulin resistance of Type 2 diabetes, fat cells are larger than normal due to increased production of FFA, TNF-α, and leptin. This leads to insulin resistance that in turn leads to increased peripheral insulin

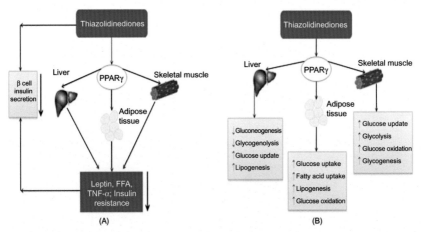

FIGURE 2.7   (A) Mechanism of THZs. (B) THZs have a widespread action.

produced by the pancreatic β cells. THZs, on the other hand, stimulate adipocyte differentiation. These adipocytes are more numerous and smaller as well as more insulin-sensitive. They produce less FFA, TNF-α, and leptin. Hence, insulin is more effectively utilized and there is lesser need to secrete insulin by the pancreatic β cells (Kahn et al., 2000). The effects of THZs on liver, adipose tissue and skeletal muscle is illustrated in Fig. 2.7B (Hauner, 2002).

Troglitazone is primarily an OHA. However, using network pharmacology, it may be observed that Troglitazone also has an effect on other body systems as well. This is illustrated in Figs. 2.8 and 2.9.

Evidence of Toxicity

After the recall of Rezulin, evidence came to light regarding the hepatotoxicity caused by the drug. It was observed that adverse events were present even before the drug was approved. It was also observed that both the manufacturing company and USFDA had knowledge regarding the hepatotoxicity. In spite of this, Rezulin was approved by the USFDA. Dr. John L. Gueriguian, a medical officer at the USFDA had reported the potential of Rezulin to harm the liver during the reviewing process and had recommended against the drug's approval. However, the FDA dismissed Dr. John L. Gueriguian on November 4, 1996, due to a complaint from the manufacturing company (Gale, 2006).

The first sign of hepatotoxicity was observed in 1997–1998. Audrey LaRue Jones, a 55-year-old woman, had taken part in a major trial sponsored by the National Institute of Diabetes and Digestive and Kidney

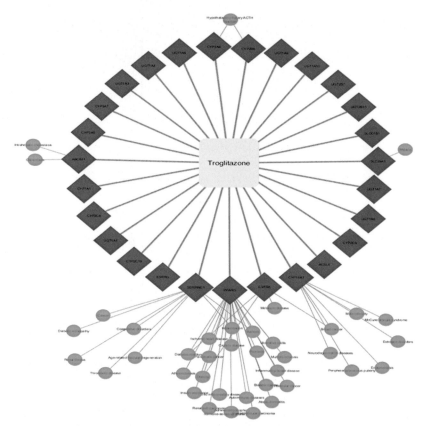

FIGURE 2.8 The red diamonds represent targets of Troglitazone. The green circles represent the diseases targeted by these targets. Using network pharmacology, we also notice the diseases associated with the liver, as Troglitazone is known to cause hepatotoxicity.

Diseases (NIDDK). Audrey had impaired glucose tolerance and was not on medication. Hence, there was a risk of progression of the disease and the trial was designed to prevent this from happening. She was randomized to the Troglitazone group. However, after 7 months of treatment, despite regular monitoring, she underwent liver failure and died on May 17, 1998 after an unsuccessful liver transplant. After this incident, the NIDDK announced that it would be terminating its Troglitazone arm. However, the manufacturers, hushed up this incident and issued a press release stating that Audrey had died due to 'complications unrelated to the study or medication' (Gale, 2006).

The DPP was initiated in order to determine whether Type 2 diabetes could be prevented or delayed by lifestyle modifications or medications in

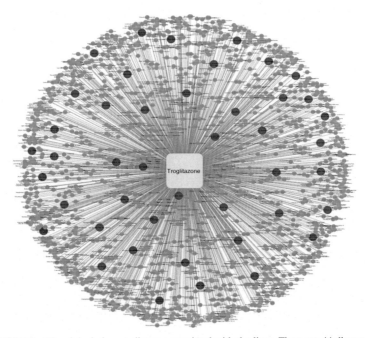

FIGURE 2.9   The pink circles are diseases associated with the liver. There are 44 diseases that are associated with liver and which may occur upon consumption of Troglitazone. The green circles represent diseases associated with other systems/organs.

high-risk populations. Troglitazone was one of the drugs selected for this study even before it had gained approval from the USFDA. This selection was purely based on evidence suggesting that Troglitazone reduced insulin resistance. However, it was withdrawn from the study on June 4, 1998, due to fatal hepatotoxicity which was recognized only after tens of thousands of patients were treated. Also, this decision was taken due to the death of a Troglitazone treated participant. The DPP conducted an analysis of Troglitazone before and after its withdrawal. It was observed that Troglitazone was the most effective treatment for diabetes when compared with other treatments viz. placebo, metformin, or ILS interventions (Knowler et al., 2005).

In March 1998, Watkins and Whitcomb representing Parke-Davis acknowledged that toxicity was observed in the pre-approval clinical trials of Troglitazone. They described that 20 patients had elevated alanine aminotransferase (ALT) which were more than 10 times the upper limit of normal (ULN) and 5 additional patients had developed elevations more than 20 times ULN. However, this information was not entirely true. It later emerged that 5 patients with the highest ALT elevations had levels more than 30 times ULN. This finding indicated more severe adverse hepatic events than those cited by Watkins and Whitcomb (Cohen, 2006).

TGZ Withdrawals: European and USFDA Responses

TGZ was first launched in the United Kingdom by Glaxo Wellcome in October 1997. There were 135 cases of serious hepatotoxicity and six deaths reported from the United States and Japan and therefore, it was voluntarily withdrawn on December 1, 1997, in Europe. In the United States, it was first introduced in January 1997 and August 1997 as combination therapy with insulin and as mono-therapy respectively (Gale, 2001). It seems remarkable that the USFDA took so long to act, although hepatic toxicity signs were clearly seen in conducted clinical trials. The baseline safety review of North American clinical trials included 2510 patients, 48 of whom (1.9%) had ALT 3 times higher than the ULN, as against (0.6%) in the placebo group. Data suggested that out of 20 patients who already showed ALT levels over 10 times the ULN; 5 of those had a 20-fold increase. By March 2000, 60 patients had died as the result of liver damage, a further 10 had received liver transplants (three deaths), 10 had recovered and the outcome of a further 10 was unknown. The incidence of TGZ-induced acute liver failure has been estimated at between 1 in 8000 and 1 in 20,000 patients treated. The delayed act on TGZ withdrawal from the USFDA also received support from physicians who wanted to keep it on the market because of the presence of unconfirmed toxicity, which was not seen by regular liver function tests. It was also argued that the risk of liver failure with TGZ could be related to the risk of hypoglycemia with sulfonylureas and of lactic acidosis with metformin.

Rezulin was recalled by the USFDA in 2000. By that time, Parke-Davis/Warner-Lambert had made billions of dollars. This decision was made based on various studies which showed that Rezulin caused hepatotoxicity. A review of safety data of Rezulin and the other two Glitazones, viz. Avandia (Rosiglitazone) and Actos (Pioglitazone), showed that Rezulin is more toxic to the liver than the other two (USFDA, 2000). However, both Avandia and Actos have been issued a black box warning due to their toxicity. The USFDA was criticized for helping the manufacturers in the approval process of the drug in spite of its known hepatotoxicity. Warner-Lambert had collaborated closely with some senior USFDA members who favored the company and provided inside information in order to speed up the approval process (Gottlieb, 2001). Thus the agency, which took over 25 years to approve Metformin, let Troglitazone through within 6 months. This might be due to fast-track approval by the USFDA because of an increase in political pressure to adopt a less adversarial stance in relation to companies. Pfizer, which acquired Warner-Lambert in 2000, had to resolve all the lawsuits filed against Warner-Lambert and lost millions of dollars.

The delayed act toward withdrawal of TGZ by the USFDA highlighted the crucial role of regulatory decisions and postapproval drug related toxicities (Table 2.1).

A considerable effort has been made to elucidate the mechanism of TGZ-induced hepatotoxicity. A number of hypotheses were brought forward to explain TGZ-induced cell injury.

TABLE 2.1 Time Base Events Toward TGZ Discovery to Withdrawal (Willman, 2000)

Sr. No.	Event	Time
1.	Discovery by Sankyo in Japan	1979
2.	US investigational new drug opened	1989
3.	Approved by regulated in Europe and Japan	Late 1996
4.	Marketed in Europe	October 1997
5.	Marketed in combination with insulin in the US	January 1997
6.	Marketed as monotherapy in the US	August 1997
7.	Withdrawn from Europe	December 1997
8.	First revision of labeling: serum ALT levels should be monitored within first 2 months of TGZ treatment, every 3 months thereafter in its first year and periodically thereafter	October 1997
9.	Second revision of labeling: ALT levels should be checked at the start of the treatment and every 2 months for a period of 1 year and periodically thereafter	December 1997
10.	Advisory committee meeting suggested labeling change, need for more study and to be keep on the market	March 1999
11.	Third revision of labeling: ALT levels at start of therapy, every month for 8 months, every 2 months for remainder of its first year and periodically thereafter	July 1998
12.	Fourth labeling revision: TGZ monotherapy was withdrawn, ALT checks at every months for 12 months. If ALT levels increase 3 times more than the upper normal limits, then discontinue the treatment and patients with liver disease and alcohol abuse TGZ should not be given	June 1999
13.	First public petition to initiate withdrawal action	July 1999
14.	Withdrawn from the US	March 2000

TGZ: Troglitazone; ALT: Alanine transaminase.

Cytotoxic Response to Liver Cells: Probable Role of Mitochondrial Injury

Several cell based mechanistic studies have demonstrated the cytotoxic response of TGZ through mitochondrial apoptosis and necrosis. In 1999, Ramachandran et al. have reported that TGZ increased cytochrome P4503A activity in human hepatocytes at less than 5 μM but became toxic to the cells above 25 μM (Ramachandran et al., 1999). Similar observations were reported by Sahi et al. using rat and human hepatocytes (Sahi et al., 2000). Kostrubsky et al. then reported the effects of TGZ in human and porcine hepatocytes (Kostrubsky et al., 2000). Treatment of human hepatocytes for 2 h with ≥ 25 μM TGZ produced an irreversible inhibition of protein synthesis and cytotoxicity, whereas in porcine hepatocytes 100 μM was lethal. The most likely mechanism by which TGZ is toxic to hepatocytes is via effects on mitochondria, producing the depletion of ATP and release of cytochrome c, which induces apoptosis leading to cell death. Further, molecular mechanism studies by Bae and Song have demonstrated that TGZ leads to activation of JNK, p38 kinase and elevation of pro-apoptotic protein levels (Bax, Bad, release cytochrome c), and cleavage of Bid protein, which resulted in TGZ-induced liver cell apoptosis (Bae and Song, 2003). Another study based on gene and protein expression after TGZ treatment to human hepatocarcinoma (HepG2) cells showed that hepatic injury was associated with the degradation of peroxisome proliferator-activated receptor-γ coactivator-1α (PGC-1 α) protein, leading to reductions in mitochondrial mass and the expression of superoxide dismutase 1 (SOD1) and SOD2, and the induction of ROS that then initiate apoptosis process (Liao et al., 2010). A recent proteomics-based study suggested that TGZ-induced mitochondrial injury was associated with decreased decarboxylation carrier; a glutathione (mGSH) import protein and the specific activation of ASK1-JNK and FOXO3a with prolonged TGZ exposure in knockout Sod2 + / − mice (Lee et al., 2013). Preclinical studies also demonstrated TGZ-induced hepatotoxicity via mitochondrial necrosis using superoxide dismutase 2 gene models (Ong et al., 2007). Ong et al. showed intra peritonial administration of TGZ (30 mg/kg per day, ip, for 4 weeks) at an equivalent bioavailable human oral dose (200 mg) to knockout mice resulted in significant increase in ALT activity associated with varying degrees of hepatocellular necrosis whereas, wild mice did not show any apparent abnormalities in serum ALT and liver histopathology. Interestingly, Fujimoto K et al. showed that the oral administration of TGZ at a higher dose of 300 mg/kg per day resulted in no significant change in hepatocellular necrosis (Fujimoto et al., 2009). These studies demonstrated the mitochondrial damage alone might not be the major cause of the TGZ-induced idiosyncratic liver injury observed in humans. Fig. 2.10 summarizes mechanisms of TZD-induced hepatotoxicity.

Inhibition of Bile Salt Export Pump (BSEP)

Another probable mechanism of TGZ-induced hepatotoxicity suggested that TGZ and/or TGZ sulfate cause inhibition of BSEP, leading to the accumulation of toxic bile salts in liver cells. BSEP has an important role in removing bile salts from liver cells using ATP-dependent active transport (Kullak-Ublick et al., 2000). Retention of bile salts in the liver cells during

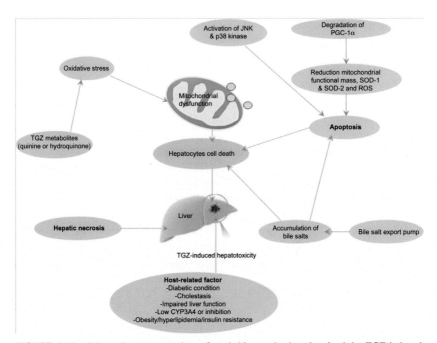

FIGURE 2.10 Schematic representation of probable mechanism involved in TGZ-induced hepatotoxicity through several cellular and molecular events via modulation of off-target effects. TGZ resulted in hepatotoxicity through (1) a direct-acting hepatotoxin producing apoptosis and necrosis of hepatocytes; (2) retention of bile salt due to inhibition of the bile salt export pump (BSEP) leading to apoptosis; (3) formation of metabolites that are capable of covalently binding to key cell macromolecules and enhancing the oxidative stress causing mitochondrial dysfunction; (4) activation of JNK and p38 pathways and degradation of PGC-1α leading to a decrease in mitochondrial mass; (5) host-related factors such as diabetic condition, cholestasis, impaired liver function, low or inhibition of CYP3A4 activity, obesity, hyperlipedemia, and insulin resistance.

cholestasis is associated with hepatocyte apoptosis (Patel et al., 1999). Several in vitro and in vivo studies have shown the role of TGZ and/or TGZ sulfate in inhibition of BSEP, causing accumulation of bile salts in the liver. Preininger et al. reported in 1999 that TGZ declined the bile flow by 67% within 1 h of exposure (3.15 μM) in isolated perfused rat livers (Funk et al., 2001b). Further, Funk et al. observed this cholestatic effect in vivo rat models with IC_{50} values of 3.9 and 0.4 μM for TGZ and TGZ sulfate respectively (Funk et al., 2001a, b). It has been well established that increased levels of bile salts caused cell death and mitochondrial dysfunction because of their intrinsic detergent properties (Gores et al., 1998). Further, molecular mechanisms by which bile salts induce apoptosis in liver cells leading to injury have been studied. Faubion et al. showed involvement of Fas death receptor pathway for apoptosis (Faubion and Gores, 1999). Fas is one of the major death receptors expressed by hepatocytes and liver cells. Bile salts promote the transport of cytoplasmic vesicular Fas to the cell surface and in this manner stimulate Fas aggregation at the cell surface, triggering the caspase cascade and subsequent apoptosis (Faubion et al., 1999).

Formation of Electrophilic Reactive Intermediates

It was hypothesized that TGZ-induced hepatotoxicity, mediated by the formation of electrophilic reactive intermediates including quinones and quinone methides, leading to a classic glutathione depletion/covalent binding or an increase in oxidative stress through redox cycling (Smith, 2003). However, this hypothesis has several limitations due to the following reasons: (1) the quinone metabolite was cytotoxic to human and porcine hepatocytes when compared with TGZ alone, (2) TGZ has potent antioxidant properties similar to vitamin E (Tettey et al., 2001; Yoshioka and Fujita, 1997), thus it was not clear how lipid peroxidation could play much of a role, (3) the onset of TGZ hepatotoxicity is typically delayed and does not usually occur within a day or two as acetaminophen hepatotoxicity does, and (4) finally, high levels of P4503A4 actually protected hepatocytes from cytotoxicity, thus metabolism/metabolic activation are protective in most circumstances (Hewitt et al., 2002).

Role of Host-Related Factors

Along with the above factors, host-related factors could have a role in the TGZ-induced hepatotoxicity. The host-related factors such as (1) the presence of diabetes with ongoing cholestasis; (2) co-administration of other cholestatic drugs; (3) impaired liver function leading to a decrease in TGZ metabolism and clearance; (4) low P4503A4 activity or inhibition of this activity by other drugs or dietary factors; and (5) obesity/hypertriglyceridemia/insulin resistance lead to non-alcoholic steatohepatitis (characterized by inflammation of the liver with concurrent fat accumulation in liver). The systemic evaluation of the mechanisms of TGZ-induced hepatotoxicity suggested the role of hepatic injury due to multiple modulation of cellular and molecular events, through the off-target effect and host-related factors.

CASE STUDY 3: EXAMPLE OF ROFECOXIB

Vioxx (Rofecoxib) was a "blockbuster drug" introduced by Merck and approved by the USFDA in 1999. It is used for the treatment of osteoarthritis, rheumatoid arthritis, acute pain in adults, primary dysmenorrhea and as an acute treatment for migraine attacks (Pubchem). Rofecoxib is a selective cyclooxygenase-2 (COX-2) inhibitor and is classified as a non-steroidal anti-inflammatory drug (NSAID) (Fitzgerald, 2004). NSAIDs are a heterogeneous group of anti-inflammatory, analgesic, and antipyretic compounds, which may often be chemically unrelated but still have similar therapeutic actions and side effects. NSAIDs are classified as non-selective COX inhibitors and selective COX-2 inhibitors. The non-selective NSAIDs are further classified into eight classes while the selective NSAIDs are classified into four classes (Brunton et al., 2006). Some of the prominent examples from this class include aspirin, ibuprofen, naproxen, indomethacin, piroxicam, and diclofenac. Rofecoxib belongs to the diaryl-substituted furanones class of selective NSAIDs. The other Coxibs are Celecoxib, Valdecoxib, Etoricoxib, and Meloxicam (Katzung, 2007). Celebrex is a Celecoxib, which belongs to the diaryl-substituted pyrazoles class of selective NSAIDs. Rofecoxib was manufactured by Merck and was introduced to the market in 1999 under the brand name Vioxx while Celecoxib is manufactured by Pfizer and was introduced in 1998 under the brand name Celebrex. Rofecoxib was the second Coxib to be introduced to the market and the first one to be recalled.

The Vioxx case is one of the most famous recall cases and will always be etched in history, as it was a blockbuster drug. It held the tenth position of the best selling drugs worldwide with an annual turnover of 2.6 billion dollars (Harten and Moosig, 2004).

Development of Vioxx

Discovery of the First NSAID-Aspirin

The bark of willow tree possesses many medicinal properties. The active ingredient present in the willow bark, known as salicin, was crystallized by Leroux in 1829 and salicylic acid was isolated by Pina in 1836. Kolbe synthesized salicylic acid and by 1874 the industrial production was undertaken. Salicylic acid was used for the treatment of rheumatic fever, gout, and as an antipyretic. However, due to the emergence of adverse gastrointestinal effects, it became difficult to tolerate salicylic acid for more than short periods of time. This prompted Hoffman, a chemist at Bayer, to conduct experiments in order to improve the safety profile. He used the earlier work of Gerhardt, a French chemist who had used acetylated salicylic acid to reduce adverse effects. Bayer began testing acetylsalicylic acid in animals by 1899; this was the first time a drug was tested on animals in an industrial setting. Later, it proceeded to clinical studies and then was finally marketed as aspirin (Brunton et al., 2006).

Mechanism of Action

The mechanism of action of aspirin and other anti-inflammatory drugs was discovered by John Vane in the 1970s. Since then, many studies have been carried out to understand and explain the mechanism of NSAIDs, thereby increasing the potential to discover and develop novel therapies for inflammation. One of these therapies was the discovery of selective NSAIDs.

An attempt to inhibit the prostaglandin synthesis induced at sites of inflammation by the COX-2 enzyme without affecting the action of COX-1 enzyme led to the development of Coxibs (Katzung, 2007). Coxibs were originally developed to minimize the adverse effects of the gastrointestinal tract associated with traditional NSAIDs (tNSAIDs).

In order to understand the mechanism of the Coxibs, it is imperative to understand the mechanism of tNSAIDs. tNSAIDs act by inhibiting the function of both COX-1 and COX-2 isoforms of cyclooxygenase (COX) enzyme. The COX-1 enzyme is expressed in most tissue and cell types whereas the COX-2 enzyme is involved in inflammation and carcinogenesis (Cairns, 2007). The COX-2 enzyme was discovered by Daniel Simmons. The function of the COX enzyme is cyclooxygenase activity, as well as conversion of arachidonic acid liberated from the phospholipid membrane by phospholipase to prostaglandin (PG) G_2. This PGG_2 is then converted to PGH_2, which is subsequently converted to prostanoids by tissue-specific isomerases. These prostanoids include thromboxane (TX) A_2 which is present in platelets, PGE_2 and PGI_2 present in gastric mucosa, PGE_2 and PGI_2 in the kidney, PGE_2 in joints, PGI_2 in endothelial cells, and PGE_2 in the central nervous system (Cairns, 2007; Donnelly and Hawkey, 1997). The inhibition of COX-2-mediated formation of PGE_2, which induces inflammation, pain, and fever, decides the therapeutic efficacy of a NSAID. On the other hand, inhibition of COX-1-mediated PGE_2 present in gastric mucosa increases the risk of adverse gastrointestinal events such as mucosal damage and bleeding.

Coxibs, however, inhibit only the COX-2 mediated pathways, thereby reducing inflammation and pain and improving the efficacy of the drug. This is brought about by the blocking of the formation of PGE_2. The coxibs maintain the COX-1 mediated pathways thereby maintaining the gastro-protective effect of COX-1. Both the coxibs and tNSAIDs inhibit renal PGE_2 and PGI_2, which help in sodium and water retention as well as increased blood pressure. This may contribute to cardiovascular events. Also, it has been found that inhibition of PGI_2 due to the inhibitory actions of COX-2 selective drugs may lead to adverse cardiovascular events, as PGI_2 is vascular protective. The mechanism of coxibs is illustrated in Fig. 2.11 [Internet]; (Wolfe et al., 1999; Howard and Delafontaine, 2004).

Using the discovery of coxibs, Pfizer developed and marketed Celebrex (Celecoxib) in 1998. The following year witnessed the appearance of another Coxib, Rofecoxib and was marketed under the brand name Vioxx by Merck, in 1999. The FDA and Merck have published the composition of the Vioxx tablet and oral suspension (USFDA, 2004; Merck & Co., 2004). The active ingredient in both the tablet and suspension is Rofecoxib. Apart from this, the tablet also contains croscarmellose sodium, hydroxypropyl cellulose, lactose, magnesium stearate, microcrystalline cellulose, and yellow ferric oxide. The suspension contains citric acid (monohydrate), sodium citrate

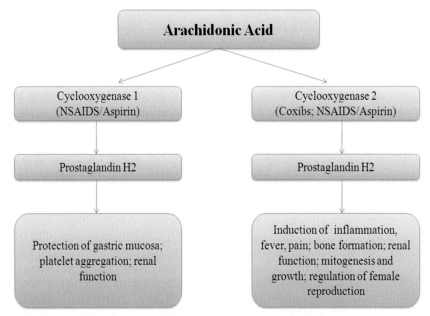

FIGURE 2.11   Mechanism of coxibs.

(dihydrate), sorbitol solution, strawberry flavor, xanthan gum, purified water, and 0.13% sodium methylparaben and 0.02% sodium propylparaben as preservatives.

Rofecoxib primarily acts as an anti-inflammatory drug. However, using network pharmacology, it can be observed that Rofecoxib also has an effect on other systems as well, as illustrated in Fig. 2.12.

Preclinical and Clinical Studies

After the discovery of Rofecoxib, it underwent a series of preclinical and clinical studies in order to assess the safety and efficacy. Several preclinical studies have been performed in order to evaluate the pharmacokinetics of Rofecoxib. Halpin et al. (2000) have reported that the absorption of Rofecoxib was higher in rats as compared to dogs. However, the metabolism of the drug was more complex in dogs. It has also been found that Rofecoxib in rats tends to be more concentrated in the kidneys when compared to Meloxicam (Davies and Jamali, 2004). In mice, it has been observed that a COX-2 blockade causes an increased risk of atherosclerosis in apoE-deficient mice (Verma and Szmitko, 2003). However, Burleigh et al. (2002) have reported that Rofecoxib treatment is associated with reduction in atherosclerosis. Most preclinical data, however, does not report any adverse events associated with the cardiovascular system. It mainly reports a decrease in cardiovascular events on administration of Rofecoxib.

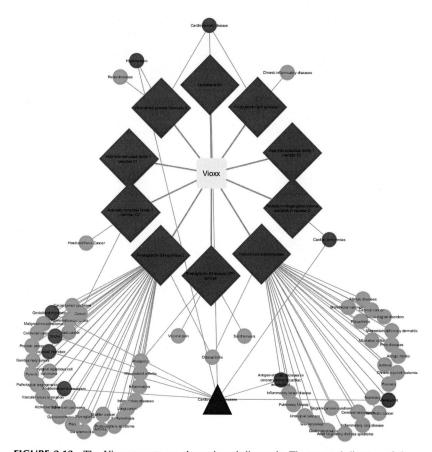

FIGURE 2.12 The Vioxx targets are shown in red diamonds. The targeted diseases of these targets are shown in green and pink circles. Cardiovascular diseases are some of the target diseases of Vioxx and are shown in pink circles. The blue triangles depict cardiovascular diseases. Through this network, it may be observed that Vioxx may have an effect on the cardiovascular system and may contribute to cardiovascular diseases such as myocardial infarction, stroke, hypertension, gestational hypertension, cardiac arrhythmia, vasospasm, antigen-induced decrease in coronary flow and cardiac anaphylaxis and abdominal aortic aneurysm.

In humans, it has been observed that Rofecoxib is extensively absorbed after oral administration and eliminated into the urine through kidneys (Halpin et al., 2002). Early clinical studies involving Vioxx were not designed to evaluate the cardiovascular risk despite suspicions of its effect on the cardiovascular system. In fact, Vioxx was approved based on the results of many short-term, randomized experiments with tNSAIDs. These results demonstrated equal efficacy and fewer adverse gastrointestinal effects when compared to tNSAIDs (Cairns, 2007). Also, the patients enrolled were at low risk of cardiovascular diseases and the studies did not have a standardized procedure to collect and analyze data pertaining to cardiovascular events (Krumholz et al., 2007).

In spite of this, a NDA of Vioxx was submitted to the USFDA in 1998 and was approved in 1999. Henceforth, Vioxx was available on the market.

The Downfall of Vioxx

Major Studies Postapproval

Two major studies were undertaken after the approval of Vioxx. These were the Vioxx Gastrointestinal Outcomes Research (VIGOR) and Adenomatous Polyp Prevention on Vioxx (APPROVe). The VIGOR study was a double-blind, randomized, comparative study between Vioxx and Naproxen with a study population of 8076 and was initiated in 1999. It was the largest study conducted by Merck for Rofecoxib. It was conducted at 301 centers in 22 countries. Vioxx was shown to have lesser gastrointestinal side effects than Naproxen in patients with rheumatoid arthritis. However, this study also reported that Vioxx carried a four-times higher risk of myocardial infarction as compared to Naproxen (Bombardier et al., 2000). It favored the gastrointestinal effects of Vioxx and understated its cardiovascular risk. Concerned with this outcome, Mukherjee et al. (2001) conducted a review in order to analyze the risk of cardiovascular events associated with COX-2 inhibitors. They found that in the VIGOR trial, 111 patients in the Rofecoxib group and 50 patients in the Naproxen group reported serious cardiovascular events, provided these events where termed "serious" by the USFDA medical reviewer. They also found in Study 090, conducted in 2001 with 978 participants given Rofecoxib, Nabumetone, or a placebo, that a total of nine serious cardiovascular events where reported. Of these, six events where reported in the Rofecoxib group, two in the Nabumetone group and one in the placebo group. A search of the Adverse Event Reporting System revealed 159 thrombotic and embolic cases for Rofecoxib.

Rofecoxib was also found to cause 46,783 acute myocardial infarctions and 31,188 hemorrhages in the US population in a study conducted from 1999 to 2004 (Vaithianathan et al., 2012).

On the other hand, Konstam et al. (2001) reported that Rofecoxib was not associated with adverse cardiovascular events. They further stated that the results obtained in the VIGOR study might be due to the cardio-protective effect of Naproxen. This study favored the safety of Rofecoxib as five out of the seven authors were employees at Merck, and two academic authors were hired as consultants by Merck (Krumholz et al., 2007).

The other major trial to be conducted for Vioxx, which ultimately decided its fate, was the APPROVe trial. It was a double-blind, multicenter, randomized, long-term trial. The APPROVe trial began enrollment in 2000 with a study population of 2586 patients. The study was initiated to evaluate the effect of 3 years of treatment with Vioxx on the risk of recurrent adeno-matous polyps in patients with a history of colorectal cancer. It was con-ducted at 108 centers across 29 countries. The trial was monitored by an external independent data safety monitoring board. It was observed that increased cardiovascular risk is seen in the Vioxx group when compared with the placebo. This risk was observed only after 18 months of treatment. The APPROVe trial also reported 10 deaths in each group viz. Rofecoxib and pla-cebo. Of these, deaths due to myocardial infarction were two in the Rofecoxib group and three in the placebo group. Three patients from the Rofecoxib group died due to sudden death arising from cardiac events while one patient died due to ischemic stroke. The study was terminated on September 30, 2004, 2 months before its planned completion, due to the recommendation of the external data safety monitoring board (Bresalier et al., 2005).

A follow-up study was carried out after the discontinuation of the APPROVe trial. This follow-up study, which was termed as the final analysis of the APPROVe trial, was also funded by Merck and the findings were pub-lished in The Lancet (Baron et al., 2008). This post-APPROVe analysis was a yearlong follow-up of all the participants recruited in the APPROVe trial. The participants were recruited from 108 centers worldwide and the study was conducted from August 2005–March 2006. The aim of this trial was to find the cardiovascular risks associated with Rofecoxib even after its discon-tinuation. It was observed that myocardial infarction and stroke were the most common adverse cardiovascular events reported after treatment with Rofecoxib. It cited that COX-2 inhibitors reduce the production of PGI2 by vascular endothelium, which may lead to increased cardiovascular risk. Fluid retention and increased blood pressure, which are side effects of Rofecoxib, may also lead to adverse cardiovascular events.

Withdrawal of Vioxx: The "Blockbuster" Drug

Based on the outcomes of the APPROVe trial, Merck finally decided to vol-untarily withdraw its blockbuster drug, Vioxx. Vioxx was withdrawn from the US market on September 30, 2004, just 5 years after its successful launch. Merck had made billions of dollars by then. After its withdrawal, evidence suggesting that Merck had committed violation of publication ethics came to light. The *New England Journal of Medicine* alleged that Merck had not provided sufficient data regarding adverse cardiovascular events reported during the VIGOR study. Elsevier, a leading publishing house based in Amsterdam, admitted accepting money from Merck in order to publish research articles in one of their journals. These research articles published data regarding the safety of Vioxx and generally favored the drug. These reports were misleading. Lawsuits were filed against Merck and the company agreed to pay 4.85 billion dollars to settle these impending lawsuits (Berenson, 2007).

Rofecoxib and Cardiovascular Toxicity: Role of On-Target, Off-Target, and Intrinsic Chemical Properties

The mechanism behind the cardiovascular toxicity (myocardial infarction and stoke) was not known. Several studies have been directed to understand plausible mechanism using in vitro and in vivo models. These studies speculated the underlying molecular mechanism of Rofecoxib on cardiovascular toxicity mediated through on-target (1), off-target (2) and intrinsic property of Rofecoxib and its metabolites (chemical based). Earlier studies reported that coincidental increases in biosynthesis of PGI2 with TXA_2 reflected a homeostatic response to accelerated platelet−vascular interactions demonstrating that PGI2 modulates the cardiovascular effects of TXA_2 in vivo (FitzGerald et al., 1984; Cheng et al., 2002). Therefore, Rofecoxib could inhibit COX-2 in endometrium leading to an imbalance between COX-1-dependent platelet production of thromboxane (TXA_2) and partly COX-2-dependent endothelial production of prostacyclin (PGI_2) that resulted in cardiovascular events.

Walter et al. reported another mechanism behind cardiovascular events of Rofecoxib to have pro-oxidant activity and to increase the formation of reactive molecules leading to increased oxidative damage to LDL-cholesterol (Walter et al., 2004). His group suggested the role of isoprostanes formation, which act as important mediators of inflammation in the atherosclerotic plaque from membrane lipids containing arachidonic acid. In addition, there could be Rofecoxib-specific events such as the facile formation of a cardiotoxic maleic anhydride derivative from Rofecoxib that may contribute to its adverse effects (Mason et al., 2007). Liu et al. have reported detailed profiling of arachidonic acid metabolites in chronically treated mice with Rofecoxib using metabolomics approach in order to investigate the role of such metabolites behind the cardiovascular toxicity (Liu et al., 2010). This study demonstrated that dramatic increase in 20-hydroxyeicosatetraenoic acid (20-HETE) level after exposure of Rofecoxib could be due inhibition of COX (COX-1 and COX-2). It has been well documented that 20-HETE is a potent vasoconstrictor, thus increasing the risk for Myocardial Infarction (MI) and stroke and inhibition of the production of 20-HETE decreases the infarct size and ablates strokes in several animal models (Miyata et al., 2005; Escalante et al., 1993). This hypothesis suggests 20-HETE as a biomarker for cardiovascular risk from coxibs as well as possible strategies for attenuation of their adverse effects. A recent study demonstrated that combination therapy with Rofecoxib and a potent CYP4a inhibitor (HET0016) resulted in significant reduction in Rofecoxib-induced cerebrovascular damage and stroke outcomes, along with enhanced antitumor efficacy of Rofecoxib (Zhang et al., 2014). Molecular mechanism of cardiotoxicity of Rofecoxib is shown in Fig. 2.13.

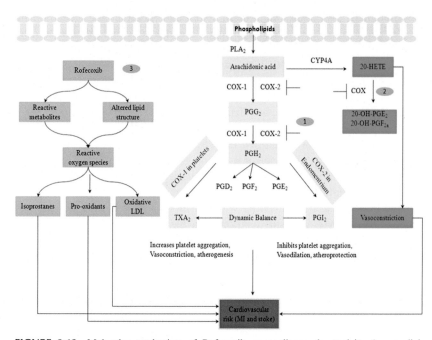

FIGURE 2.13 Molecular mechanism of Rofecoxib on cardiovascular toxicity (myocardial infarction and stoke) mediated through on-target (1) off-target, (2) and intrinsic property of Rofecoxib and (3) its metabolites (chemical based). Rofecoxib inhibits COX-2 in endometrium leading to an imbalance between COX-1-dependent platelet production of thromboxane (TXA_2) and partly COX-2-dependent endothelial production of prostacyclin (PGI_2) that resulted in cardiovascular events. Rofecoxib has been described to have pro-oxidant activity and to increase the formation of reactive molecules leading to increased oxidative damage to LDL-cholesterol. In addition, there could be Rofecoxib-specific events such as the facile formation of a cardiotoxic maleic anhydride derivative from Rofecoxib that may contribute to its adverse effects. Rofecoxib increases formation of (20-HETE) leading to cardiovascular adverse though inhibition of COX (COX-1 and COX-2).

It has been nearly 11 years since Vioxx was recalled. The question that arises here is whether all the Coxibs are associated with adverse cardiovascular events? Or was it just Rofecoxib? Soon after Vioxx was recalled from the market, new evidence emerged saying that cardiovascular events are associated with almost all Coxibs. This was followed by the withdrawal of Valdecoxib for the same reasons.

CASE STUDY 4: EXAMPLE OF THALIDOMIDE

Thalidomide was marketed as a non-addictive, non-barbiturate sedative to treat morning sickness in pregnant women. The drug is a synthetic derivative of glutamic acid, a naturally occurring amino acid involved in important physiological processes, e.g. brain neurotransmission and metabolism. Thalidomide consists of two linked rings, a glutarimide and pthalimide ring. Thalidomide has a chiral carbon, which is unstable and allows two enantiomers to co-exist, which can inter-switch between the two states rapidly in bodily fluids and in water. Teratogenic effects of S-enantiomer of thalidomide have been reported. Within a few years of the widespread use of thalidomide in Europe, Australia, and Japan, approximately 10,000 children were born with phocomelia (condition known as sealed limbs), leading to the ban of thalidomide in most countries in 1961/62. Some countries continued to provide access to thalidomide for a couple of years thereafter. In addition to limb reduction anomalies, other effects later attributed to thalidomide included congenital heart disease, malformations, and ocular abnormalities.

The underlying mechanism by which thalidomide causes a wide range of damage to embryos was still unknown. In the last 50 years (from 1966 to 2003) over 30 separate models/theories for thalidomide embryopathy have been proposed and are reviewed in detail suggesting modulation of multiple targets as well as intrinsic chemical properties of thalidomide (Ito et al., 2011; Vargesson, 2009). It includes (1) acylation of macromolecules, (2) ascorbic acid synthesis, (3) down regulation of adhesion receptors, (4) alteration of cytokine synthesis, (5) folic acid antagonism, (6) inhibition of DNA synthesis, (7) DNA oxidation, (8) interference of glutamate metabolism, and (9) mesonephros-stimulated chondrogenesis. More recently research has focused on hypotheses involving thalidomide's antiangiogenic actions— the drug's ability to induce cell death and generate reactive oxygen species; the thalidomide binding target, Cereblon, a ubiquitin ligase, which if prevented from binding can reduce thalidomide-induced damage in embryos (Vargesson, 2015). Thalidomide toxicity matrix is shown in Fig. 2.14.

Earlier gene expression studies have reported as many as 2000 gene expression profiles after thalidomide exposure. Many of these gene expression profile changes were in vascular-related and cytoskeletal-related genes (Meganathan et al., 2012; Ema et al., 2010). Recent gene expression studies on thalidomide treated mouse embryonic stem cells using microarrays have been reported by Gao et al. (2015). Global gene expression analysis using microarrays revealed hundreds of differentially expressed genes upon thalidomide exposure that were enriched in gene ontology terms and canonical pathways associated with embryonic development and differentiation. In addition, many genes were found to be involved in small GTPases-mediated signal transduction, heart development, and inflammatory responses, which coincide with clinical evidences and may represent critical embryo toxicities of thalidomide.

Primarily, thalidomide is prescribed as sedative or hypnotic drug claimed to cure anxiety, insomnia, gastritis, and tension. It was used against nausea and to alleviate morning sickness in pregnant women. However, using network pharmacology, its adverse effects on fetuses viz. Phocomelia which led to its recall can be observed (Fig. 2.15).

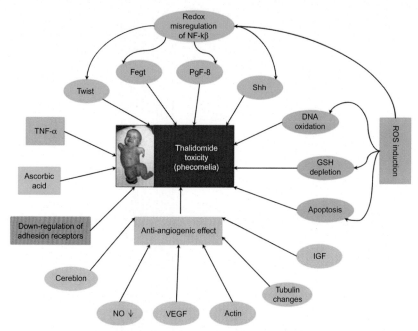

FIGURE 2.14   Thalidomide induced embryopathy (Phocomelia) mediated through modulation of multiple targets involved reactive oxygen substance (ROS), redox misregulation of NF-kβ, TNF-α, ascorbic acid synthesis inhibition, down-regulation of adhesion receptors, and antiangiogenic effects.

Since thalidomide was banned and withdrawn in 1961/62, the drug has been discovered to have antiangiogenic, anti-inflammatory, and antimyeloma roles. In fact, thalidomide was found to be useful in treating leprosy as early as 1965 and is now used to treat complications of the condition around the world. In 1994, thalidomide was demonstrated to possess antiangiogenic actions, which were suggested could be the cause of thalidomide embryopathy. Thalidomide is now used to treat some cancers. Thalidomide has also been demonstrated to be a potent inhibitor of the inflammatory response, through inhibiting the production of TNF-a. Indeed this action has made the drug very successful for treatments for conditions including leprosy and multiple myeloma, Crohn's disease, Behcet's disease, HIV, lupus, and leprosy.

CONCLUSIONS AND FUTURE PERSPECTIVES

Drugs are failing because of safety, efficacy, quality and economic reasons. Our analysis of last six decades (from 1950 to August 2015) shows that failed drugs are recalled or withdrawn mainly due to safety concerns. Major types of toxicities, among others, include hepatic, cardiovascular, neuronal,

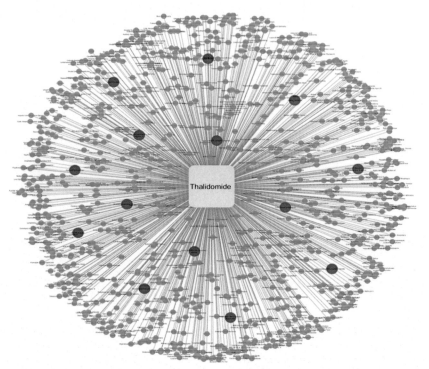

FIGURE 2.15   All circles indicate diseases associated with Thalidomide. The pink circles represent Thalidomide induced 14 diseases leading to Phocomelia.

gastrointestinal, dermal, and renal carcinogenicity. Out of these, hepatic toxicity (24%) and cardiovascular toxicity (19%) are predominantly associated with drug withdrawals. In order to address the question *how* these drugs were withdrawn from the market, molecular mechanisms behind these toxicities were studied on selected case examples of thalidomide, rofecoxib, statins, and troglitazone using systems biology and network pharmacology approach. The case studies clearly demonstrated that these toxicologic effects were associated with on-target, and/or off-target modulation, and/or intrinsic property of drugs (chemical based) or cumulative of these three effects. These are called drug withdrawal "toxicity triangle effect" or "the butterfly effect" (Fig. 2.16).

In order to alleviate these drug-induced toxicities (drug revival approach), the following strategies have been proposed based on intrinsic properties and target modulation:

1. Intrinsic properties modulation:
      Strategy 1: Chemical modulation of the drug.
      Strategy 2: Use of adjuvant (chemical or botanical).

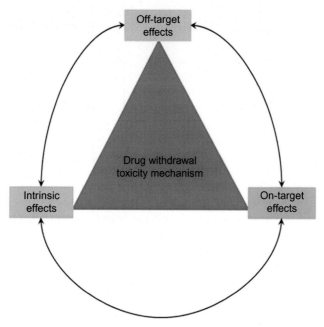

FIGURE 2.16 Drug withdrawal toxicity mechanism called as "toxicity triangle effect."

2. Target modulation (On-target and off-target effects of withdrawal drug):
     Strategy 1: Multitarget modulation.
     Strategy 2: Repurposing for another indications.

Intrinsic properties modulation:
Strategy 1: Chemical modulation of the drug.

It has been well reported that most drugs are transformed into reactive/toxic metabolites in physiological conditions (e.g., R form of Thalidomide into racemic mixture; S form from racemic mixture is known for teratogenic effect) and through metabolism leading to adverse effects. Thiazolidinedione ring (e.g., troglitazone) is responsible for the generation of reactive metabolites after metabolism. Few studies directed toward chemical modification of pyrrolidinedione ring to thiazolidinedione ring suggested improved safety and anti-diabetic effects (Saha et al., 2012).

Strategy 2: Use of adjuvant (chemical or botanical).

Most of the synthetic chemotherapeutic agents available in the market today are immunosuppressants, cytotoxic, and exert variety of side effects that are particularly evident in cancer chemotherapy. Mesna (2-mercaptoethane sulfonate sodium) is an organosulfur compound used as an adjuvant

to alleviate toxicity during cancer chemotherapy involving cyclophosphamide and ifosfamide (Shaw and Graham, 1987). Cyclophosphamide and ifosfamide, an active metabololite of cyclophosphamide, are converted to its
urotoxic metabolite called acrolein in the body. The urotoxicity of acrolein
has been reported mainly through the formation of glutathione adduct
(known as 3-oxopropylglutathione) that stimulate the release of oxygen radi-
cals leading to genotoxic effects (Adams and Klaidman, 1993). Mesna assists
to detoxify these metabolites by reaction of its sulfhydryl group with
α,β-unsaturated carbonyl containing compounds such as acrolein. Botanical
based immunomodulators are often employed as supportive or adjuvant therapy to overcome the undesired effects of cytotoxic chemotherapeutic agents
and to restore normal health. Our earlier studies on traditional ayurvedic
botanicals such as *Withania somnifera* (Linn Dunal), *Tinospora cordifolia*
(Miers), and *Asparagus racemosus* (Willd) have demonstrated protection
toward cyclophosphamide (CP)-induced myelo- and immunoprotection as
evident by significant increase in white cell counts and hemagglutinating and
hemolytic antibody titers (Diwanay et al., 2004). This has suggested the
potential use of these Ayurvedic botanicals as cancer adjuvant during cancer
chemotherapy. Concomitant administration of these botanical adjuvants with
cancer chemotherapeutics such as CP may lead to potential herb-drug interactions. The hepatic enzymes such cytochrome p450 isoenzymes and transporter proteins are considered fugitive targets for such interactions. Our
studies have shown that the effect of these botanicals such as *W. somnifera*,
T. cordifolia, and *A. racemosus* extracts on cytochrome p450 (CYP450)
3A4; a major isoenzyme responsible for metabolism of most of cancer chemotherapeutics, do not have significant inhibition of CYP3A4 even at dose
equivalent to their human dose (Patil et al., 2014). This has suggested that
use of these botanical cancer adjuvants during cancer chemotherapeutics is
safe. This was further evident from animal studies aimed to evaluate pharmacokinetic and pharmacodynamic interactions (Patil et al., 2013). PHY906, a
traditional Chinese formula containing four botanicals such as *Glycyrrhiza
uralensis*, *Paeonia lactiflora*, *Scutellaria baicalensis*, and *Ziziphus jujuba,*
has been demonstrated as potential cancer adjuvant by decreasing gastrointestinal toxicity and enhanced antitumor activities when administered with
Irinotecan and Sorafenib (Lam et al., 2010, 2015). Several traditional botanicals and derived phytochemicals are extensively studied for their potential
adjuvant effect during cancer therapeutics. A list of potential botanical adjuvants used during the chemotherapeutics has been shown in Table 2.2.

Target modulation (On-target and off-target effects):

Strategy 1: Multitarget modulation.

During the past two decades, drug discovery has mainly focused on a
single-target paradigm, which has achieved considerable success and will
continue being pursued in the future. However, the single-target drugs are
limited in the treatment of complex diseases such as cancer, depression, and

TABLE 2.2 The Potential Botanical Adjuvants Used for Alleviating Associated Side Effects During Cancer Chemotherapeutic

Sr. No.	Botanical/ Derived Compounds	Chemotherapeutic Drug	Role in Alleviation in Side Effect	References
1	Silymarin	Ifosfamide and cisplatin	Nephrotoxicity	Kaur and Agarwal (2007), Wu et al. (2009)
2	Propolis	5-fluorouracil	Cytopenia	Kumar (2014)
3	Curcumin	5-fluorouracil	Gastrointestinal dysfunction	Yao et al. (2013)
4	Curcumin	Mitomycin	Nephro and Bone marrow toxicity	Zhou et al. (2009)
5	Ginsenosides	Cyclophosphamide	Bone marrow toxicity	Zhang et al. (2008)
6	Quercetin	Cisplatin	Nephrotoxicity	Kuhlmann et al. (1998)
7	Green tea	Irinotecan	Gastrointestinal toxicity	Wessner et al. (2007)
8	*Astragalus* spp.	Cyclophosphamide and 5-fluorouracil	Nephrotoxicity and hematotoxicity	Zee-Cheng (1992)
9	*Scutellaria baicalensis* and Qing-Shu-Yi-Qi-Tang	5-fluorouracil	Catechexia	Wang et al. (2012)
10	Resveratrol	Cisplatin	Nephrotoxicity	Osman et al. (2015)

Alzheimer's disease, because complex diseases have multiple pathogenic mechanisms and are not likely to result from a single defect. This has suggested the need for more safe and effective drugs for the treatment of such diseases. Recent advances in systems biology and network pharmacology pave the way for designing and development of more comprehensive treatment targeting multiple targets known as a multitarget modulation approach. In this approach, a single drug or multicomponent system could modulate the multiple targets minimizing the on-target or off-target effects with the hope of avoiding unwanted side effects. Traditional Chinese medicine and

Traditional Indian medicines that are usually composed of several medicinal herbs/components can serve as a typical representative of compound medicines promoting efficacy and reducing toxicity.

Strategy 2: Repurposing for another indications.

Repurposing, also called repositioning, reprofiling or rediscovering, refers to the concept or process of taking a drug developed for one indication and applying it to another. Similar risk factors and biological pathways can underlie seemingly unrelated diseases, opening the door for novel hypothesis-driven and data-driven repurposing strategies (Dudley et al., 2011; Sirota et al., 2011). For example, Thalidomide has been repurposed for new conditions such as leprosy and multiple myeloma, Crohns disease, Behcets disease, HIV for its on-target as well off-target effects through antiangiogenic and TNF-α inhibition and anti-inflammatory effects (Hicks et al., 2008). Earlier, these effects were considered for their teratogenic effects. Another well-known example of drug repositioning is the use of sildenafil (Viagra) in erectile dysfunctions. Sildenafil is an inhibitor of cyclic guanosine monophosphate (cGMP)-specific phosphodiesterase type 5 (PDE5) and was originally developed for the treatment of coronary artery disease by Pfizer in the 1980s. The side effect of Sildenafil, marked induction of penile erections, was serendipitously found during the Phase I clinical trials for the patients with hypertension and angina pectoris (Terrett et al., 1996). After Sildenafil failed in Phase II clinical trials for the treatment of angina, it was redirected to the treatment of erectile dysfunctions. Sildenafil received USFDA approval and it entered the US market in 1998, quickly becoming a blockbuster.

REFERENCES

Abd, T., Jacobson, T., 2011. Statin-induced myopathy: a review and update. Expert. Opin. Drug. Saf. 10 (3), 373–387.

Adams, J., Klaidman, L., 1993. Acrolein-induced oxygen radical formation. Free. Radic. Biol. Med. 15, 187–193.

Bae, M., Song, B., 2003. Critical role of c-Jun N-terminal protein kinase activation in troglitazone-induced apoptosis of human HepG2 hepatoma cells. Mol. Pharmacol. 63 (2), 401–408.

Baker, S., Tarnopolsky, M., 2001. Statin myopathies: pathophysiologic and clinical perspectives. Clin. Invest. Med. 24 (5), 258–272.

Banach, M., Malodobra-Mazur, M., Gluba, A., Katsiki, N., Rysz, J., Dobrzyn, A., 2013. Statin therapy and new-onset diabetes: molecular mechanisms and clinical relevance. Curr. Pharm. Des. 19 (27), 4904–4912.

Baron, J.A., Sandler, R.S., Bresalier, R.S., Lanas, A., Morton, D.G., Riddell, R., et al., 2008. Cardiovascular events associated with rofecoxib: final analysis of the APPROVe trial. Lancet. 372 (9651), 1756–1764.

Berenson, A., 2007. Merck Agrees to Pay $4.85 Billion in Vioxx Claims. The New York Times [cited 2016 Mar 15] Available from: http://www.nytimes.com/2007/11/09/business/09cndmerck.html?_r=1.

Bombardier, C., Loren, L., Reicin, A., Shapiro, D., Burgos-Vargas, R., Davis, B., et al., 2000. Comparison of upper gastrointestinal toxicity of rofecoxib and naproxen in patients with rheumatoid arthritis. N. Engl. J. Med. 343, 1520–1528.

Brault, M., Ray, J., Gomez, Y.H., Mantzoros, C.S., Daskalopoulou, S.S., 2014. Statin treatment and new-onset diabetes: a review of proposed mechanisms. Metabolism. 63 (6), 735–745.

Bresalier, R.S., Sandler, R.S., Quan, H., Bolognese, J.A., Oxenius, B., Horgan, K., et al., 2005. Cardiovascular events associated with rofecoxib in a colorectal adenoma chemoprevention trial. N. Engl. J. Med. 352, 1092–1102.

Brunton, L.L., Lazo, J.S., Parker, K.L., 2006. Autacoids drug therapy of inflamation, Goodman and Gilman's The Pharmacological Basis of Therapeutics, eleventh ed. McGraw-Hill medical, United States of America.

Burleigh, M.E., 2002. Cyclooxygenase-2 promotes early atherosclerotic lesion formation in LDL receptor-deficient mice. Circulation. 105 (15), 1816–1823.

Cairns, J.A., 2007. The coxibs and traditional nonsteroidal anti-inflammatory drugs: a current perspective on cardiovascular risks. Can. J. Cardiol. 23 (2), 125–131.

Cao, P., Hanai, J., Tanksale, P., Imamura, S., Sukhatme, V., Lecker, S., 2009. Statin-induced muscle damage and atrogin-1 induction is the result of a geranylgeranylation defect. FASEB J. 23 (9), 2844–2854.

Caso, G., Kelly, P., McNurlan, M., Lawson, W., 2007. Effect of coenzyme Q10 on myopathic symptoms in patients treated with statins. Am. J. Cardiol. 99 (10), 1409–1412.

Castets, P., Lescure, A., Guicheney, P., Allamand, V., 2012. Selenoprotein N in skeletal muscle: from diseases to function. J. Mol. Med. 90 (10), 1095–1107.

Cheng, Y., Austin, S.C., Rocca, B., Koller, B.H., Coffman, T.M., Grosser, T., et al., 2002. Role of prostacyclin in the cardiovascular response to thromboxane A2. Science 296 (5567), 539–541.

Cohen, J.S., 2006. Risks of troglitazone apparent before approval in USA. Diabetologia 49 (6), 1454–1455.

Culver, A.L., Ockene, I.S., Balasubramanian, R., Olendzki, B.C., Sepavich, D.M., Wactawski-Wende, J., et al., 2012. Statin use and risk of diabetes mellitus in postmenopausal women in the Women's Health Initiative. Arch. Intern. Med. 172 (2), 144–152.

Dasa, S., Pella, D., Kozlikova, K., Rybar, R., 2010. Is there is need for Ubiquinone (CoQ10) supplementation in statin- associated myopathy? Open Nutraceuticals J. 3, 242–247.

Davies, N.M., Jamali, F., 2004. COX-2 selective inhibitors cardiac toxicity: getting to the heart of the matter. J. Pharm. Pharm. Sci. 7 (3), 332–336.

Dirks, A., Jones, K., 2006. Statin-induced apoptosis and skeletal myopathy. Am. J. Physiol. Cell. Physiol. 291 (6), C1208–C1212.

Diwanay, S., Chitre, D., Patwardhan, B., 2004. Immunoprotection by botanical drugs in cancer chemotherapy. J. Ethnopharmacol. 90, 49–55.

Donnelly, M., Hawkey, C.J., 1997. COX-II inhibitors—a new generation of safer NSAIDs? Aliment. Pharmacol. Ther. 11, 227–236.

Dormuth, C., Filion, K., Paterson, J., James, M., Teare, G., Raymond, C., et al., 2014. Higher potency statins and the risk of new diabetes: multicentre, observational study of administrative databases. BMJ. 348, g3244.

Dudley, J., Sirota, M., Shenoy, M., et al., 2011. Computational repositioning of the anticonvulsant topiramate for inflammatory bowel disease.. Sci. Transl. Med. 3, 96ra76.

Eitel, J., Suttorp, N., Opitz, B., 2011. Innate immune recognition and inflammasome activation in Listeria monocytogenes infection. Front Microbiol. 1, 149.

Ema, M., Ise, R., Kato, H., et al., 2010. Fetal malformations and early embryonic gene expression response in cynomolgus monkeys maternally exposed to thalidomide. Reprod. Toxicol. 29, 49–56.

Escalante, B., Omata, K., Sessa, W., Lee, S., Falck, J., Schwartzmann, M., 1993. 20-hydroxyeicosatetraenoic acid is an endothelium-dependent vasoconstrictor in rabbit arteries. Eur. J. Pharmacol. 235, 1–7.

Faubion, W., Gores, G., 1999. Death receptors in liver biology and pathobiology. Hepatology 29 (1), 1–4.

Faubion, W., Guicciardi, M., Miyoshi, H., Bronk, S., Roberts, P., Svingen, P., et al., 1999. Toxic bile salts induce rodent hepatocyte apoptosis via direct activation of Fas. J. Clin. Invest. 103 (1), 137–145.

Fitzgerald, G.A., 2004. Coxibs and cardiovascular disease. N. Engl. J. Med. 351 (17), 1709–1711.

FitzGerald, G.A., Smith, B., Pedersen, A.K., Brash, A.R., 1984. Increased prostacyclin biosynthesis in patients with severe atherosclerosis and platelet activation. N. Engl. J. Med. 310, 1065–1068.

Flint, O., Masters, B., Gregg, R., Durham, S., 1997. Inhibition of cholesterol synthesis by squalene synthase inhibitors does not induce myotoxicity in vitro. Toxicol. Appl. Pharmacol. 145 (1), 91–98.

Fuhrmeister, J., Tews, M., Kromer, A., Moosmann, B., 2012. Prooxidative toxicity and selenoprotein suppression by cerivastatin in muscle cells. Toxicol. Lett. 215 (3), 219–227.

Fujimoto, K., Kumagai, K., Ito, K., Arakawa, S., Ando, Y., Oda, S., et al., 2009. Sensitivity of liver injury in heterozygous Sod2 knockout mice treated with troglitazone or acetaminophen. Toxicol. Pathol. 37 (2), 193–200.

Fung, M., Thornton, A., Mybeck, K., Wu, J.H., Hornbuckle, K., Munit, E., 2001. Evaluation of the characteristics of safety withdrawal of prescription drugs from worldwide pharmaceutical markets-1960 to 1999. Drugs Inf. J. 35 (1), 293–317.

Funk, C., Pantze, M., Jehle, L., Ponelle, C., Scheuermann, G., Lazendic, M., et al., 2001a. Troglitazone-induced intrahepatic cholestasis by an interference with the hepatobiliary export of bile acids in male and female rats. Correlation with the gender difference in troglitazone sulfate formation and the inhibition of the canalicular bile salt. Toxicology. 167 (1), 83–98.

Funk, C., Ponelle, C., Scheuermann, G., Pantze, M., 2001b. Cholestatic potential of troglitazone as a possible factor contributing to troglitazone-induced hepatotoxicity: in vivo and in vitro interaction at the canalicular bile salt export pump (Bsep) in the rat. Mol. Pharmacol. 59 (3), 627–635.

Furberg, C., Pitt, B., 2001. Withdrawal of cerivastatin from the world market. Curr. Control. Trials. Cardiovasc. Med. 2 (5), 205–207.

Gale, E., 2001. Lessons from the glitazones: a story of drug development. Lancet 357 (9271), 1870–1875.

Gale, E.A.M., 2006. Troglitazone: the lesson that nobody learned? Diabetologia. 49 (1), 1–6.

Gao, X., Sprando, R., Yourick, J., 2015. Thalidomide induced early gene expression perturbations indicative of human embryopathy in mouse embryonic stem cells. Toxicol. Appl. Pharmacol. 287 (1), 43–51.

Gores, G., Miyoshi, H., Botla, R., Aguilar, H., Bronk, S., 1998. Induction of the mitochondrial permeability transition as a mechanism of liver injury during cholestasis: a potential role for mitochondrial proteases. Biochim. Biophys. Acta 1366 (1–2), 167–175.

Gottlieb, S., 2001. Company played down drug's risks, report says. Br. Med. J. 322 (7288), 696.

Graham, D.J., Staffa, J.A., Shatin, D., Andrade, S.E., Schech, S.D., La Grenade, L., et al., 2004. Incidence of hospitalized rhabdomyolysis in patients treated with lipid-lowering drugs. JAMA 292 (21), 2585−2590.

Halpin, R.A., Geer, L.A., Zhang, K.E., Marks, T.M., Dean, D.C., Jones, A.N., et al., 2000. The absorption, distribution, metabolism and excretion of rofecoxib, a potent and selective cyclooxygenase-2 inhibitor, in rats and dogs. Drug. Metab. Dispos. 28 (10), 1244−1254.

Halpin, R.A., Porras, A.G., Geer, L.A., Davis, M.R., Cui, D., Doss, G.A., et al., 2002. The disposition and metabolism of rofecoxib, a potent and selective cyclooxygenase-2 inhibitor, in human subjects. Drug. Metab. Dispos. 30 (6), 684−693.

Hanai, J., Cao, P., Tanksale, P., Imamura, S., Koshimizu, E., Zhao, J., et al., 2007. The muscle-specific ubiquitin ligase atrogin-1/MAFbx mediates statin-induced muscle toxicity. J. Clin. Invest. 117 (12), 3940−3951.

Harper, C., Jacobson, T., 2010. Evidence-based management of statin myopathy. Curr. Atheroscler. Rep. 12 (5), 322−330.

Harten, P., Moosig, F., 2004. The rofecoxib scandal. Br. Med. J. 329, 816.

Hauner, H., 2002. The mode of action of thiazolidinediones. Diabetes Metab. Res. Rev. 18, S10−S15.

Hewitt, N., Lloyd, S., Hayden, M., Butler, R., Sakai, Y., Springer, R., et al., 2002. Correlation between troglitazone cytotoxicity and drug metabolic enzyme activities in cryopreserved human hepatocytes. Chem. Biol. Interact. 142 (1−2), 73−82.

Hicks, L., Haynes, A., Reece, D., Walker, I., Herst, J., Meyer, R., et al., 2008. A meta-analysis and systematic review of thalidomide for patients with previously untreated multiple myeloma. Cancer Treat. Rev. 34 (5), 442−452.

Howard, P., Delafontaine, P., 2004. Nonsteroidal anti-inflammatory drugs and cardiovascular risk. J. Am. Coll. Cardiol. 43 (4), 519−525.

Ito, T., Ando, H., Handa, H., 2011. Teratogenic effects of thalidomide: molecular mechanisms. Cell. Mol. Life Sci. 68, 1569−1579.

Johnson, T., Zhang, X., Bleicher, K., Dysart, G., Loughlin, A., Schaefer, W., et al., 2004. Statins induce apoptosis in rat and human myotube cultures by inhibiting protein geranylgeranylation but not ubiquinone. Toxicol. Appl. Pharmacol. 200 (3), 237−250.

Joy, T., Hegele, R., 2009. Narrative review: statin-related myopathy. Ann. Intern. Med. 150 (12), 858−868.

Kahn, C.R., Chen, L., Cohen, S.E., 2000. Unraveling the mechanism of action of thiazolidinediones. J. Clin. Invest. 106 (11), 1305−1307.

Katzung, B.G., 2007. Nonsteroidal Anti-Inflammatory Drugs, Disease-Modifying Antirheumatic Drugs, Nonopioid Analgesics, & Drugs Used in Gout, Basic & clinical pharmacology, tenth ed. McGraw-Hill Medical, United States of America.

Kaur, M., Agarwal, R., 2007. Silymarin and epithelial cancer chemoprevention: how close we are to bedside? Toxicol. Appl. Pharmacol. 224 (3), 350−359.

Keith, M., Mazer, C., Mikhail, P., Jeejeebhoy, F., Briet, F., Errett, L., 2008. Coenzyme Q10 in patients undergoing CABG: effect of statins and nutritional supplementation. Nutr. Metab. Cardiovasc. Dis. 18 (2), 105−111.

Knowler, W.C., Hamman, R.F., Edelstein, S.L., Barrett-Connor, E., Ehrmann, D.A., Walker, E. A., et al., 2005. Prevention of type 2 diabetes with troglitazone in the diabetes prevention program. Diabetes 54, 1150−1156.

Konstam, M.A., Weir, M.R., Reicin, A., Shapiro, D., Sperling, R.S., Barr, E., et al., 2001. Cardiovascular thrombotic events in controlled, clinical trials of rofecoxib. Circulation 104 (19), 2280−2288.

Kostrubsky, V., Sinclair, J., Ramachandran, V., Venkataramanan, R., Wen, Y., Kindt, E., et al., 2000. The role of conjugation in hepatotoxicity of troglitazone in human and porcine hepatocyte cultures. Drug. Metab. Dispos. 28 (10), 1192−1197.

Kromer, A., Moosmann, B., 2009. Statin-induced liver injury involves cross-talk between cholesterol and selenoprotein biosynthetic pathways. Mol. Pharmacol. 75 (6), 1421−1429.

Krumholz, H.M., Ross, J.S., Presler, A.H., Egilman, D.S., 2007. What have we learnt from vioxx? Br. Med. J. 334 (7585), 120−123.

Kuhlmann, M.K., Horsch, E., Burkhardt, G., Wagner, M., Köhler, H., 1998. Reduction of cisplatin toxicity in cultured renal tubular cells by the bioflavonoid quercetin. Arch. Toxicol. 72 (8), 536−540.

Kullak-Ublick, G., Beuers, U., Paumgartner, G., 2000. Hepatobiliary transport. J. Hepatol. 32 (1 Suppl.), 3−18.

Kumar, V.L.S., 2014. Propolis in dentistry and oral cancer management. N. Am. J. Med. Sci. 6 (6), 250−259.

Lam, W., Bussom, S., Guan, F., Jiang, Z., Zhang, W., Gullen, E., et al., 2010. The four-herb Chinese medicine PHY906 reduces chemotherapy-induced gastrointestinal toxicity. Sci. Transl. Med. 2, 45ra59.

Lam, W., Jiang, Z., Guan, F., Huang, X., Hu, R., Wang, J., et al., 2015. PHY906(KD018), an adjuvant based on a 1800-year-old Chinese medicine, enhanced the anti-tumor activity of Sorafenib by changing the tumor microenvironment. Sci. Rep. 5, 9384.

Langsjoen, P., Langsjoen, J., Langsjoen, A., Lucas, L., 2005. Treatment of statin adverse effects with supplemental Coenzyme Q10 and statin drug discontinuation. Biofactors 25 (1−4), 147−152.

Lasser, K., Allen, P., Woolhandler, S., Himmelstein, D., Wolfe, S., Bor, D., 2002. Timing of new black box warnings and withdrawals for prescription medications. JAMA 287 (17), 2215−2220.

Laufs, U., Liao, J., 2003. Isoprenoid metabolism and the pleiotropic effects of statins. Curr. Atheroscler Rep. 5, 372−378.

Lee, Y., Goh, W., Ng, C., Raida, M., Wong, L., Lin, Q., et al., 2013. Integrative toxicoproteomics implicates impaired mitochondrial glutathione import as an off-target effect of troglitazone. J. Proteome. Res. 12 (6), 2933−2945.

Liao, J., 2002. Isoprenoids as mediators of the biological effects of statins. J. Clin. Invest. 110, 285−288.

Liao, X., Wang, Y., Wong, C., 2010. Troglitazone induces cytotoxicity in part by promoting the degradation of peroxisome proliferator-activated receptor γ co-activator-1α protein. Br. J. Pharmacol. 161 (4), 771−781.

List of withdrawn drugs [Internet]. Available from: <https://en.wikipedia.org/wiki/List_of_withdrawn_drugs>.

Littarru, G., Tiano, L., 2007. Bioenergetic and antioxidant properties of coenzyme Q10: recent developments. Mol. Biotechnol. 37 (1), 31−37.

Littlefield, N., Beckstrand, R., Luthy, K., 2014. Statins' effect on plasma levels of Coenzyme Q10 and improvement in myopathy with supplementation. J. Am. Assoc. Nurse Pr. 26 (2), 85−90.

Liu, J., Li, N., Yang, J., Li, N., Qiu, H., Ai, D., et al., 2010. Metabolic profiling of murine plasma reveals an unexpected biomarker in rofecoxib-mediated cardiovascular events. Proc. Natl. Acad. Sci. U. S. A. 107 (39), 17017−17022.

Mason, R., Walter, M., Day, C., Jacob, R., 2007. A biological rationale for the cardiotoxic effects of rofecoxib: comparative analysis with other COX-2 selective agents and NSAids. Subcell. Biochem. 42, 175−190.

Matzno, S., Yasuda, S., Juman, S., Yamamoto, Y., Nagareya-Ishida, N., Tazuya-Murayama, K., et al., 2005. Statin-induced apoptosis linked with membrane farnesylated Ras small G protein depletion, rather than geranylated Rho protein. J. Pharm. Pharmacol. 57 (11), 1475−1484.

Meganathan, K., Jagtap, S., Wagh, V., et al., 2012. Identification of thalidomide-specific tran-scriptomics and proteomics signatures during differentiation of human embryonic stem cells. PLoS ONE 7, e44228.

Medicines and Healthcare Product Regulatory Agency, 2012. Statins: Risk of hyperglycemia and diabetes. In: Drug Safety Update. Available from https://www.gov.uk/drug-safety-update/sta-tins-risk-of-hyperglycaemiaand-diabetes.

Merck & Co., 2004. Patient Information about VIOXX® (rofecoxib tablets and oral suspension) for Osteoarthritis, Rheumatoid Arthritis, Juvenile Rheumatoid Arthritis, Pain and Migraine Attacks. Merck & Co., Inc.: Kenilworth, NJ, United States. Available from <https://www.merck.com/product/usa/pi_circulars/v/vioxx/vioxx_ppi.pdf>.

Miyata, N., Seki, T., Tanaka, Y., Omura, T., Taniguchi, K., Doi, M., et al., 2005. Beneficial effects of a new 20-hydroxyeicosatetraenoic acid synthesis inhibitor, TS-011 [N-(3-chloro-4-morpholin-4-yl) phenyl-N'-hydroxyimido formamide], on hemorrhagic and ischemic stroke. J. Pharmacol. Exp. Ther. 314 (1), 77−85.

Moosmann, B., Behl, C., 2004. Selenoprotein synthesis and side-effects of statins. Lancet 363 (9412), 892−894.

Mukherjee, D., Nissen, S.E., Topol, E.J., 2001. Risk of cardiovascular events associated with selective COX-2 inhibitors. JAMA 286 (8), 954−959.

Mutoh, T., Kumano, T., Nakagawa, H., Kuriyama, M., 1999. Involvement of tyrosine phosphor-ylation in HMG-CoA reductase inhibitor-induced cell death in L6 myoblasts. FEBS Lett. 444 (1), 85−89.

Nakahara, K., Kuriyama, M., Sonoda, Y., Yoshidome, H., Nakagawa, H., Fujiyama, J., et al., 1998. Myopathy induced by HMG-CoA reductase inhibitors in rabbits: a pathological, electrophysiological, and biochemical study. Toxicol. Appl. Pharmacol. 152 (1), 99−106.

National Institute for Health and Care Excellence, 2014. Cardiovascular disease: risk assessment and reduction, including lipid modification. NICE Guidelines [CG181]. National Institute for Health and Care Excellence: London, UK. Available from <https://www.nice.org.uk/guidance/cg181>.

Newman, D.J., Cragg, G.M., 2007. Natural products as sources of new drugs over the last 25 years. J. Nat. Prod. 70 (3), 461−477.

Nishimoto, T., Tozawa, R., Amano, Y., Wada, T., Imura, Y., Sugiyama, Y., 2003. Comparing myotoxic effects of squalene synthase inhibitor, T-91485, and 3-hydroxy-3-methylglutaryl coenzyme A (HMG-CoA) reductase inhibitors in human myocytes. Biochem. Pharmacol. 66 (11), 2133−2139.

Ong, M., Latchoumycandane, C., Boelsterli, U., 2007. Troglitazone-induced hepatic necrosis in an animal model of silent genetic mitochondrial abnormalities. Toxicol. Sci. 97 (1), 205−213.

Osman, A., Telity, S., Damanhouri, Z., Al-Harthy, S., Al-Kreathy, H., Ramadan, W., et al., 2015. Chemosensitizing and nephroprotective effect of resveratrol in cisplatin -treated ani-mals. Cancer Cell. Int. 15, 6.

Patel, T., Steer, C., Gores, G., 1999. Apoptosis and the liver: a mechanism of disease, growth regulation, and carcinogenesis. Hepatology 30 (3), 811–815.

Patil, D., Jadhav, S., Patwardhan, B., 2013. Botanical Drug Interactions Case Studies From Traditional Medicines. Lambert Academic Publishing, Germany.

Patil, D., Gautam, M., Gairola, S., Jadhav, S., Patwardhan, B., 2014. Effect of botanical immunomodulators on human CYP3A4 inhibition: implications for concurrent use as adjuvants in cancer therapy. Integr. Cancer Ther. 13 (2), 167–175.

Pierno, S., De Luca, A., Tricarico, D., Roselli, A., Natuzzi, F., Ferrannini, E., et al., 1995. Potential risk of myopathy by HMG-CoA reductase inhibitors: a comparison of pravastatin and simvastatin effects on membrane electrical properties of rat skeletal muscle fibers. J. Pharmacol. Exp. Ther. 275 (3), 1490–1496.

Preiss, D., Seshasai, S., Welsh, P., Murphy, S., Ho, J., Waters, D., et al., 2011. Risk of incident diabetes with intensive-dose compared with moderate-dose statin therapy: a meta-analysis. JAMA 305 (24), 2556–2564.

Qureshi, Z., Seoane-Vazquez, E., Rodriguez-Monguio, R., Stevenson, K., Szeinbach, S., 2011. Market withdrawal of new molecular entities approved in the United States from 1980 to 2009. Pharmacoepidemiol. Drug Saf. 20 (7), 772–777.

Ramachandran, V., Kostrubsky, V., Komoroski, B., Zhang, S., Dorko, K., Esplen, J., et al., 1999. Troglitazone increases cytochrome P-450 3A protein and activity in primary cultures of human hepatocytes. Drug Metab. Dispos. 27 (10), 1194–1199.

Sacher, J., Weigl, L., Werner, M., Szegedi, C., Hohenegger, M., 2005. Delineation of myotoxicity induced by 3-hydroxy-3-methylglutaryl CoA reductase inhibitors in human skeletal muscle cells. J. Pharmacol. Exp. Ther. 314 (3), 1032–1041.

Saha, S., Chan, D., Lee, C., Wong, W., New, L., Chui, W., et al., 2012. Pyrrolidinediones reduce the toxicity of thiazolidinediones and modify their anti-diabetic and anti-cancer properties. Eur. J. Pharmacol. 697 (1–3), 13–23.

Sahi, J., Hamilton, G., Sinz, M., Barros, S., Huang, S., Lesko, L., et al., 2000. Effect of troglitazone on cytochrome P450 enzymes in primary cultures of human and rat hepatocytes. Xenobiotica 30 (3), 273–284.

Sakamoto, K., Kimura, J., 2013. Mechanism of statin-induced rhabdomyolysis. J. Pharmacol. Sci. 123 (4), 289–294.

Sakamoto, K., Honda, T., Yokoya, S., Waguri, S., Kimura, J., 2007. Rab-small GTPases are involved in fluvastatin and pravastatin-induced vacuolation in rat skeletal myofibers. FASEB J. 21 (14), 4087–4094.

Sakamoto, K., Wada, I., Kimura, J., 2011. Inhibition of Rab1 GTPase and endoplasmic reticulum-to-Golgi trafficking underlies statin's toxicity in rat skeletal myofibers. J. Pharmacol. Exp. Ther. 338 (1), 62–69.

Sampson, U.K., Linton, M.F., Fazio, S., 2011. Are statins diabetogenic? Curr. Opin. Cardiol. 26 (4), 342–347.

Sattar, N., Taskinen, M.-R., 2012. Statins are diabetogenic--myth or reality? Atheroscler. Suppl. 13 (1), 1–10.

Sattar, N., Preiss, D., Murray, H., Welsh, P., Buckley, B., de Craen, A., et al., 2010. Statins and risk of incident diabetes: a collaborative meta-analysis of randomised statin trials. Lancet 375 (9716), 735–742.

Shaw, I., Graham, M., 1987. Mesna—a short review. Cancer Treat. Rev. 14 (2), 67–86.

Sirota, M., Dudley, J., Kim, J., et al., 2011. Discovery and preclinical validation of drug indications using compendia of public gene expression data.. Sci. Transl. Med. 3, 96ra77.

Smith, M., 2003. Mechanisms of troglitazone hepatotoxicity. Chem. Res. Toxicol. 16 (6), 679–687.

Stone, N.J., Robinson, J.G., Lichtenstein, A.H., Bairey Merz, C.N., Blum, C.B., Eckel, R.H., et al., 2014. 2013 ACC/AHA guideline on the treatment of blood cholesterol to reduce atherosclerotic cardiovascular risk in adults: a report of the american college of cardiology/american heart association task force on practice guidelines. Circulation 129 (25 Suppl. 2), S1–45.

Terrett, N.K., Bell, A.S., Brown, D., Ellis, P., 1996. Sildenafil (VIAGRATM), a potent and selective inhibitor of type 5 cGMP phosphodiesterase with utility for the treatment of male erectile dysfunction. Bioorg. Med. Chem. Lett. 6 (15), 1819–1824.

Tettey, J., Maggs, J., Rapeport, W., Pirmohamed, M., Park, B., 2001. Enzyme-induction dependent bioactivation of troglitazone and troglitazone quinone in vivo. Chem. Res. Toxicol. 14 (8), 965–974.

Thompson, P.D., Clarkson, P., Karas, R.H., 2003. Statin-associated myopathy. JAMA 289, 1681–1690.

USFDA, 2000. Rezulin (troglitazone). In: Safety Alerts for Human Medical Products - MedWatch. <http://www.fda.gov/Safety/MedWatch/SafetyInformation/SafetyAlertsforHumanMedical Products/ucm173081.htm>.

USFDA, 2001. Bayer voluntarily withdraws Baycol. FDA Talk Paper, T01-34. Available from <www.bl2.info/pdf/bios_life_fda_talk_papers.pdf>.

USFDA, 2004. VIOXX® (rofecoxib tablets and oral suspension). Available from: <http://www. fda.gov/ohrms/dockets/ac/05/briefing/2005-4090B1_14_OFDA-Tab-I-1.htm>.

USFDA, 2012. FDA Drug Safety Communication: Important safety label changes to cholesterol-lowering statin drugs. In: Drug Safety and Availability. <http://www.fda.gov/Drugs/ DrugSafety/ucm293101.htm>.

Vaithianathan, R., Hockey, P.M., Moore, T.J., Bates, D.W., 2012. Iatrogenic effects of COX-2 inhibitors in the US population. Drug. Saf. 32 (4), 335–343.

Vargesson, N., 2009. Thalidomide-induced limb defects: resolving a 50-year-old puzzle. Bioessays 31, 1327–1336.

Vargesson, N., 2015. Thalidomide-induced teratogenesis: history and mechanisms. Birth. Defects Res. C Embryo. Today 105 (2), 140–156.

Verma, S., Szmitko, P.E., 2003. Coxibs and the endothelium. J. Am. Coll. Cardiol. 42 (10), 1754–1756.

Walter, M., Jacob, R., Day, C., Dahlborg, R., Weng, Y., Mason, R., 2004. Sulfone COX-2 inhibitors increase susceptibility of human LDL and plasma to oxidative modification: comparison to sulfonamide COX-2 inhibitors and NSAIDs. Atherosclerosis 177 (2), 235–243.

Wang, H., Chan, Y., Li, T., Wu, C., 2012. Improving cachectic symptoms and immune strength of tumour-bearing mice in chemotherapy by a combinationof Scutellaria baicalensis and Qing-Shu-Yi-Qi-Tang. Eur. J. Cancer 48 (7), 1074–1084.

Waters, D., Ho, J., DeMicco, D., Breazna, A., Arsenault, B., Wun, C., et al., 2011. Predictors of new-onset diabetes in patients treated with atorvastatin: results from 3 large randomized clinical trials. J. Am. Coll. Cardiol. 57 (14), 1535–1545.

Wessner, B., Strasser, E., Koitz, N., Schmuckenschlager, C., Unger-Manhart, N., Roth, E., 2007. Green tea polyphenol administration partly ameliorates chemotherapy-induced side effects in the small intestine of mice. J. Nutr. 137 (3), 634–640.

Westwood, F., Bigley, A., Randall, K., Marsden, A., Scott, R., 2005. Statin-induced muscle necrosis in the rat: distribution, development, and fibre selectivity. Toxicol. Pathol. 33 (2), 246–257.

Willman, D., 2000. The Rise and Fall of the Killer Drug Rezulin. The Los Angeles Times 4, . Available from http://articles.latimes.com/2000/jun/04/news/mn-37375.

Wolfe, M., Lichtenstein, D., Singh, G., 1999. Gastrointestinal toxicity of nonsteroidal antiinflammatory drugs. N. Engl. J. Med. 340 (24), 1888−1899.

Wu, J., Lin, L., Tsai, T., 2009. Drug-drug interactions of silymarin on the perspective of pharmacokinetics. J. Ethnopharmacol. 121 (2), 185−193.

Wysowski, D., Swartz, L., 2005. Adverse drug event surveillance and drug withdrawals in the United States, 1969−2002: the importance of reporting suspected reactions. Arch. Intern. Med. 165 (12), 1363−1369.

Yao, Q., Ye, X., Wang, L., Gu, J., Fu, T., Wang, Y., et al., 2013. Protective effect of curcumin on chemotherapy-induced intestinal dysfunction. Int. J. Clin. Exp. Pathol. 6 (11), 2342−2349.

Yoshioka, T., Fujita, T., 1997. Studies on compounds with antioxidant activity--development of hypoglycemic agents, troglitazone (CS-045). Yakugaku Zasshi 117 (9), 597−610.

Young, J., Florkowski, C., Molyneux, S., McEwan, R., Frampton, C., George, P., et al., 2007. Effect of coenzyme Q(10) supplementation on simvastatin-induced myalgia. Am. J. Cardiol. 100 (9), 1400−1403.

Zee-Cheng, R., 1992. Shi-quan-da-bu-tang (ten significant tonic decoction), SQT. A potent Chinese biological response modifier in cancer immunotherapy, potentiation and detoxification of anticancer drugs. Methods Find. Exp. Clin. Pharmacol. 14 (9), 725−736.

Zhang, Q.H., Wu, C.F., Duan, L., Yang, J.Y., 2008. Protective effects of total saponins from stem and leaf of Panax ginseng against cyclophosphamide-induced genotoxicity and apoptosis in mouse bone marrow cells and peripheral lymphocyte cells. Food. Chem. Toxicol. 46 (1), 293−302.

Zhang, Y., Hoda, M., Zheng, X., Li, W., Luo, P., Maddipati, K., et al., 2014. Combined therapy with COX-2 inhibitor and 20-HETE inhibitor reduces colon tumor growth and the adverse effects of ischemic stroke associated with COX-2 inhibition. Am. J. Physiol. Regul. Integr. Comp. Physiol. 307 (6), R693−R703.

Zhou, Q., Zhang, H., Lu, Y., Wang, X., Su, S., 2009. Curcumin reduced the side effects of mitomycin C by inhibiting GRP58-mediated DNA cross-linking in MCF-7 breast cancer xenografts. Cancer Sci. 100 (11), 2040−2045.

Chapter 3

Holistic Drug Targeting

Anuradha Roy[1] and Rathnam Chaguturu[2]

[1]University of Kansas, Lawrence, KS, United States, [2]iDDPartners, Princeton Junction, NJ, United States

INTRODUCTION

Unlike Mendelian diseases that are caused by inheritance of single traits, complex diseases are multifactorial and are shaped by interplay of diverse genetic variations, age, gender, environmental factors, and lifestyle choices. Complex diseases include cancers, neurological disorders, metabolic syndromes, and infectious diseases, all of which are characterized by a wide spectrum of biological complexity and are considered to be polygenic syndromes (Kaplan and Junien, 2000; Loktionov, 2003). Treatment of complex diseases with single or small combination therapies, while effective in the short term or at the early stages of a disease, is found to be insufficient in mitigating advanced or recurrent disease progression. Loss of responsiveness due to long-term administration of single agents has been attributed to the robustness of the redundant molecular functions within biological networks. Although the majority of the marketed drugs are approved based on experimental data supporting single-target selectivity against a specific disease, further clinical and basic studies have shown that many marketed drugs lack absolute selectivity (Lounkine et al., 2012). Many such drugs are now increasingly being adopted for treatment of new indications in off-label uses as well as drug repositioning strategies for disease management. Many clinical regimens utilize combination therapies that involve prescribing more than one active ingredient for treatment of polygenic diseases. For example, developing drugs targeting redundant functions like the pan-kinase inhibitors has been proposed to improve effectiveness of treatment regimens against pathological conditions that are kinase-dependent. There has been a recent shift in the drug discovery paradigm from single-target single-drug to a multitarget drug discovery approach (MTDD). Targeting several disease-contributing factors is a more holistic approach to drug management wherein the drug development strategies are guided by integrating all available information from diverse perspectives, such as disease etiology and systems biology. The approach serves to identify underlying molecular mechanisms and define interaction of genetics, environment and/or

Innovative Approaches in Drug Discovery. DOI: http://dx.doi.org/10.1016/B978-0-12-801814-9.00003-9

65

behavioral patterns in disease development and progression. The efficacy of treatment of complex diseases is considered to improve significantly with drug development against biological networks or multiple target proteins. Such holistic approaches will help in further tailoring of personalized care, e.g., utilizing drug cocktails to target multiple individual specific factors involved in pathogenesis or in the development of resistance, and in utilizing alternative medicines or lifestyle choices for disease management. Despite an increasing realization of the multifaceted nature of disease progression, holistic approaches are still underutilized and most drug discovery projects are still focused on finding drugs selective for just one therapeutic target of interest. Further improvement in computational data mining and data integration approaches as well as development of multitarget drug screens have the potential of developing more effective drugs in the future (Fig. 3.1).

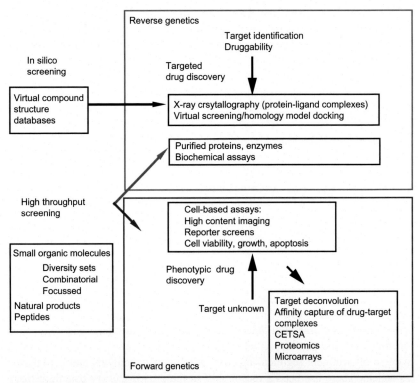

FIGURE 3.1   Schematic depicting the forward and reverse genetics screening approaches in drug discovery. In absence of target information, forward genetics screens are facilitated by phenotypic cell screens, identification of hits followed by target deconvolution. Reverse genetics starts with identification of a specific target via basic/clinical studies. Once the druggability of target is established, biochemical or cell-based assays are set up to screen for hits by high throughput screening. In silico drug discovery is an alternative approach to ligand identification on specific targets. The in silico screening can probe much larger sets of virtually available scaffolds in contrast to high throughput screening where the physically available compounds define the screening sets.

SINGLE-TARGET SPECIFICITY APPROACH

Targeted therapies are based on identifying drugs that are directed against single causative agents like dysregulated protein expression or activity in a diseased state. In a recent systematic analysis of the DrugBank database, 435 drug targets in the human genome are modulated by 989 unique drugs through 2242 drug target interactions (Rask-Andersen et al., 2011). Current approved drugs show activity against a small number of human proteins which include receptors (ligand-gated ion channels, receptor tyrosine kinases, and GPCRs), enzymes, transporter proteins and ligands, or some interacting proteins. Targeted therapies include hormones, signal transduction inhibitors, gene expression modulators, apoptosis inducers, angiogenesis inhibitors, cancer vaccines, immunotherapies, and humanized monoclonal antibodies.

TARGET IDENTIFICATION AND VALIDATION

Establishing that a target plays a pivotal role in development, progression and maintenance of a pathological event is an essential first step in drug discovery, and requires providing evidence at various levels (Bunnage et al., 2015). The development of primary and secondary screens in a drug development program are strongly dependent upon (1) how well a target has been characterized for its role in homeostasis or disease, (2) any homology to known functional domain families, (3) alternatively spliced isoforms, subcellular localization, species/tissue/cell expression patterns and distribution, (4) its interactions with other proteins or nucleic acids, (5) potential for posttranscriptional or posttranslational regulation, (6) its half-life, and (7) constitutive or inducible expression (Bunnage et al., 2015). The target involvement in a disease may result from an increase or decrease in the activity of a protein or association of mutant proteins in gain-of-function through association with new protein partners or new nucleic acid binding sites as seen with p53 conformational or p53 DNA domain mutants. The target may also act by being overexpressed due to gene amplification, or silenced due to epigenetic events. Transcriptional or posttranscriptional expression modulated by noncoding microRNAs or siRNAs can further modulate the physiological state of a cell. Availability of small molecules (chemical genetics) or availability of phenotypic mutants by deleting or amplifying a target can accelerate understanding of target(s) in normal homeostasis or in disease. Numerous approaches as well as databases are currently available to define druggability of targets which have been summarized in (Schenone et al., 2013). The tool boxes available to translational scientists have expanded exponentially over that last two decades and include, among other technologies, protein microarrays (probed with antibodies), RNA microarrays, bioinformatics analysis of protein interaction maps, pathway analysis, phenotypic changes by functional studies using genetic-based technologies (RNA interference, knockdowns, genomic mutations using clustered regularly interspaced short palindromic repeats (CRISPR-Cas), mouse or zebrafish models), overexpression of target protein to mimic the effect of agonist function. Once a reasonable supporting data for target involvement in a disease is made available, the next step in single-target drug discovery is to screen large chemical libraries to identify compounds that can serve as chemical tools to dissect the pathways of interest (Fig. 3.1).

CHEMICAL GENETICS

As in classical genetics, forward chemical genetics involves the screening of randomized collection of chemicals with whole cells like mammalian, bacterial, fungal, Saccharomyces cerevisiae, and organisms such as zebrafish embryos, drosophila, and *Caenorhabditis elegans*. Whole cell organism screens are evaluated by changes in phenotypes (growth rates, morphology, growth media requirements) of cells (wild-type, cancerous, or mutants with that of parental wild-type organisms), followed by characterization of the genes involved. Since the screen is based on an observable and quantifiable change and not on any preselected target, the hits from the screen have the potential to act against multiple targets. Identification of specific targets from forward genetics screens is challenging. Diverse approaches like immobilizing lead compound on solid phase resin for affinity chromatography, pull-down experiments, cell-based thermal stability of proteins, protein arrays in combination with mass spectrometry and other proteomics approaches are employed to fish out some or all of the targets that directly bind to the molecule of interest. The phenotypic drug discovery also forms the basis for forward pharmacology.

In reverse chemical genetics, known purified proteins/enzymes are used to set up biochemical assays (enzymatic end point, kinetic assays, protein-protein or protein-nucleic acid interactions) to identify ligands, substrates, or modulators by screening large chemical libraries. The ligands are then tested for their ability to modulate the target in relevant cells/models. The reverse chemical genetics is also referred to as "target-based" drug discovery and is the basis for reverse pharmacology.

Both the forward and reverse genetics/pharmacology approaches can be used to identify chemical tools via experimental high throughput screening (HTS) or by in silico screening of large chemical collections or natural ligand-like molecules. The chemicals that show specificity to the target or to the cell (cancer vs normal) are used as chemical probes for dissecting the pathway involved or for defining mechanism of action. While the starting points for forward and reverse genetics screens may differ, at defining stages of hit to lead optimization the boundaries between the two approaches get blurred when it comes to defining specificity, selectivity, and direct binding to known or unknown targets. The hits from biochemical screens are tested for their activity in relevant cellular phenotypes or physiological states. The hits from phenotypic screens are used to fish out all possible targets they associate with using affinity matrices, protein arrays, etc. Likewise, the ability of hits from reverse genetics screens may also be taken through fishing approaches to study their pleiotropic effects in cell-based systems. The techniques used in target validation are used again at this stage to define target site activity of the available chemical molecules or natural ligands and to validate functionality of targets in experimental disease models (Fig. 3.3).

HIGH THROUGHPUT SCREENING (HTS) OF DRUGGABLE TARGETS

Since the early 1990s, the HTS campaigns became an integral part of drug discovery in industry and a decade later in academia. Highly optimized and controlled assay protocols are developed in HTS labs that enable routine screening of large compound libraries, peptide libraries, virtual compound collections, and vendor databases for identification of chemical probes and leads (Roy et al., 2009). The target site characterization from basic or clinical research ultimately helps to select assay parameters such as relevant cell types, phenotypes, and activity type to develop assays that faithfully reflect the biology of molecular targets. The assays are developed using biochemical methods utilizing purified assay components (enzyme assays, protein-protein interactions, direct binding of compounds to proteins, protein-nucleic acid interactions) or are phenotypic cell-based (reporter screens, stable cell lines expressing mutant proteins, in cell enzymatic activity assays, high content imaging for changes in morphology, localization, internalization, etc.). The commonly used assay detection platforms include fluorescence (fluorescence intensity, polarization, FRET, TR-FRET), absorbance, luminescence, and Alphascreen assays. The phenotypic imaging-based screens (high content screening) is an example of forward genetics approach where images are captured in microwell format to quantify the number and morphology of nuclei, cells, cell membrane blebbing, nuclear-cytoplasmic localization changes, neuronal growths, EMT transitions, cell differentiation, etc.

Chemical diversity is critical to identification of hits against novel target families. A recent study of a small molecule universe was estimated to contain over 10^{60} synthetically feasible drug-like molecules. The predicted chemical space is impossible to cover and only a very small fraction of the available chemical space has been explored so far. This highlights the fact that it would be impractical to make all the compounds available to identify the best lead compounds. Therefore, knowledge-based methodologies are utilized to identify compound collections for screening campaigns. Compound libraries available from various chemical vendors include around 12 million compounds with considerable overlap (Roy et al., 2009). The cost of acquiring all available compounds as well as the costs associated with their storage, maintenance and screening costs are financially prohibitive for academia and for large pharmaceutical companies as well. Internal compound collections range from a few thousand in academia to several million in large pharmaceutical companies. Knowledge-based selection of scaffolds is employed to select compound collections, but are limited to few target classes like kinases. Chemical library collections are also compiled using computational selection tools guided by Lipinski's rule of five (drug-like and bioavailable) as well as utilization of pan-assay interference compounds (PAINS) filters (Baell and Holloway, 2010) to deprioritize promiscuous hits, or compounds with chemical reactivity, denaturing agents, mercaptans, oxidizing/reducing agents, heavy metals, and chemically undesirable and synthetically challenging scaffolds. Compound libraries include diverse small organic molecules or may be a collection of bioactives, compounds that have been shown to have activity against molecular targets or may have been approved by the United States Federal Drug Administration (USFDA) and are marketed drugs. Natural product collections may contain purified larger molecular species and may be only partially purified fractions. The library diversity is also expanded by recent open innovation trends in compound-sharing across institutes and companies. For example, a compound-sharing partnership was set up in 2015 between the United Kingdom Medical Research Council (MRC) and seven drug companies including AstraZeneca, GlaxoSmithKline, Johnson & Johnson, Eli Lilly, Pfizer, Takeda, and UCB. The compound collections being shared with academics are the compounds that were identified as actives but were triaged during development, for off-target activities, lack of potencies, etc. but may show useful activity against another disease (Rees et al., 2016). In another form of compound collaboration, the Eli Lilly-PD2/TD2 Initiatives (https://pd2.lilly.com, https://td2.lilly.com) seek to test molecules and promising compounds originating from academic research in the Eli Lilly phenotypic/target discovery platform. The profiling data and the secondary assay information are shared with the academic researchers. All compounds with significant and selective biological activity are identified and future collaborations are established for furthering drug discovery efforts. All such collaborations hold promise to expand utility of in-house compound collections.

The assays used for screening compound collections are designed to address the biological function of a target. The assays, both cell based and biochemical, are miniaturized for precision, robustness and reproducibility in multiwell microplates, generally 384 or 1536 well plates. The assay development as well as screening data is subjected to rigorous quality control statistical analysis methods as Z' scores, plate uniformity assays, positive and negative control behavior, and signal windows. The robotic liquid handling is calibrated extensively to ensure homogeneity in compound and reagent transfers. Once a miniaturized assay passes statistical acceptance criterion, the assay is used to screen a small collection of upto 10,000 compounds (validation library) to study assay performance and hit rates. Screening a larger compound collection of hundreds of thousands of compounds at a single or multiple concentrations usually follows a successful completion of a small screen. The primary hits are selected several standard deviations from the plate median. Concentration response curves are generated in reconfirmation assays using compounds cherry-picked from stock library. Medicinal chemists further evaluate the hits that are dose-responsive and clusters of structure-activity series are identified via cheminformatics. Representative compounds from several series are repurchased as fresh powders (>95% pure) and tested in the primary assay as well as few downstream secondary assays. Secondary assays should be distinct from the primary assay platform and preferably be more representative of the physiology of the system being studied. The compound activity using selectivity assays helps to define compound specificity for the target being studied. These initial studies help provide proof of concept for the HTS assay. The hits from these studies form the basis for analoging by catalog or by synthesis. Numerous iterative rounds of analoging are performed to improve the potency and selectivity of primary hits and establish putative quantitative structure-activity relationships. The success of HTS is dependent upon quality and diversity of chemical libraries used as well as by the type of assay technologies employed. While the majority of screens were performed on purified recombinant proteins as well as engineered cell lines, the recent shift to stem cells or primary cells or in 3D spheroids or cocultures of multiple cell lines is believed to make a screen more disease-relevant.

RATIONAL DRUG DESIGN

In silico rational drug design or virtual HTS (vHTS) or protein structure-based docking screen can be employed at all stages of hit to lead compound selection and design and can also directly be used in lieu of experimental HTS to identify chemical scaffolds that can dock directly to the binding pockets in protein structures (Bajorath, 2002). When the target protein or its functional domains are crystallized alone or in the presence of a ligand, computer-based in silico docking and scoring studies can be performed to identify chemical scaffolds that can occupy the target binding sites. When the crystal structures are unavailable, the amino acid sequence of a target protein is used to construct a homology model based on an experimental 3D structure of a related homologous protein. Molecular docking is used to dock molecules and select the most appropriate ligand conformation. Virtual screening uses computational algorithms to evaluate for their potential to bind specific sites on target proteins, for which a 3D structure is known or can be established. The bound conformations are used to obtain the binding energy or related affinity of all compounds that bind to the protein. Virtual HTS allows exploration of a larger chemical space, but in general, limitations in computer hardware allows for only small sample handling and often results in high false negatives. Fragment-based drug discovery (FBDD) is a viable alternative to HTS or virtual screening and can be used to identify compounds with weak affinities. The follow-up strategies involve intense medicinal chemistry efforts to build up and connect the small fragments as starting points and to arrive at molecules with higher affinities.

PHARMACOGNOSY

Pharmacognosy focuses on the study of medicinally active ingredients (secondary metabolites, extracts, etc.) that have their origin in nature or living systems like plants, fungi, and bacteria. Herbal and other preparations involving minerals and metals have been described for the medical treatment of ailments. Folk medicines across ancient civilizations and world cultures (Patwardhan, 2012) have provided historical records of treatment of certain diseases used from animals, animal parts, plants, plant-parts, bacteria, fungi, etc. Many anticancer drugs (cardiac glycosides), two-thirds of antibacterial compounds, antiinflammatory compounds, etc. are natural products. The extensive biodiversity of nature is a largely untapped resource of compounds that may have potent medicinal activities and are evolutionarily selected for their intrinsic cell permeability, scaffold diversity as well as target specificity (Barnes et al., 2016). The natural product-based screens are generally more labor intensive with low turn around because of the need to identify active extracts guided by bioactivity guided fractionation, isolate pure compounds from a mixture in which the active ingredient may be represented in much lower amounts compared with more abundant inactive molecules. Technological advances are being employed to override the commonly encountered barriers in natural product-based discovery. The naturally occurring metabolites from marine invertebrates and their endosymbiotic bacteria are believed to hold promise for unraveling unique scaffolds that are underrepresented in currently available compound collections. A metabolomics and cheminformatics approach was reported recently to establish chemical fingerprinting of marine bacterial extracts in order to identify compounds with MW < 1000 Da that offer chemical diversity (Macintyre et al., 2014). In another study, molecular docking-based virtual screening of 40,000 natural product molecules was used to identify new classes of compounds that inhibit both the wild-type c-KIT (KIT Proto-Oncogene Receptor Tyrosine Kinase), which is deregulated in many cancers, as well as its constitutively active gain-of-function mutant form, D816V. The two sets of virtual hits identified 37 dual dockers, of which four were found to inhibit kinase activity of both the forms of c-KIT (Park et al., 2016). Of these, one structure was selected as a scaffold for further analoging to improve potency against the two c-Kit proteins.

Target to Lead Bottleneck

Any experimental or virtual screen results in identification of a large subset of hits which may be true actives (along with some false positives or false negatives), depend on the target, the scaffold composition of the library, and the assay platform. The early compound triage workflows include parallel approaches to define potency, selectivity, specificity, lipophilicity, molecular mass, and early ADME (absorption, distribution, metabolism, and excretion) characterization to identify a relatively small number of compounds with lead potential. Experimental or computationally predicted ADME data are indicators of compound activity in vivo. The high attrition rates at the lead development phase have been attributed to toxicity, target selectivity or efficacy or some combination of all the three parameters. In an effort to provide correlations between compound properties and attrition rates, data analysis was performed on the attrition of drug candidates from AstraZeneca, Eli Lilly and Company, GlaxoSmithKline, and Pfizer. Although the study indicated a statistical significance between the physicochemical properties of compounds and safety failure rates in clinical trials (Waring et al., 2015), no major trends emerged in rational evaluation of compounds that will be successful in clinical trials. Lead compounds share properties of high efficacy and potency against a specific target, for their ability to bind the target directly, at the same cellular site where the target is expressed, low off-target effects and acceptable toxicity profiles. The majority of compounds in the hit to lead phase fail due to lack of efficacy or toxicity issues (Waring et al., 2015). Preclinical drug development that can accurately predict clinical response of drugs can influence the success rate of lead compounds in late stage drug discovery programs. In a recent report, around 1000 mouse patient-derived xenograft (PDX) models were set up using primary tumor derived patient cells (Gao et al., 2015), with a diverse set of driver mutations. Using approved drugs as well as investigational agents, the reproducibility and clinical translatability of their approach was validated by monitoring the response rate of PDX with BRAF V600 mutations to treatment with encorafenib, a rapidly accelerated fibrosarcoma (RAF) inhibitor. As observed with melanoma resistant tumors, continuous drug treatment of the PDX model showed the same mechanism of encorafenib resistance involving amplification of BRAF as well as MEK1&2 genes. In many complex diseases, the mouse models may not correctly represent the human disease due to differences in the pathways between the murine and humans.

BIOLOGICAL REDUNDANCY AND THE HOLISTIC ADVANTAGE

Whole-genome sequencing offers the potential to identify genetic variations that can influence diagnostics and ultimately lead to the development of therapeutics. The genome wide association studies (GWAS) are an important tool to study the role of molecular pathways in complex diseases, and in identifying gene loci predisposing an individual to a disease. DNA variations have been reported for many diseases reproducibly for Crohn's disease, Type 2 diabetes, prostate cancer, serum lipid levels, age-related macular degeneration, obesity, and several other human diseases. In a recent study, whole-genomes from 500 patients with at least 34 distinct genetic disorders including 18 complex diseases were sequenced (Taylor et al., 2015). Large-scale data sets for defined experimental conditions are available from DNA sequencing, transcriptome analysis, proteomics, and metabolomics. The large data sets can theoretically be integrated to create working models of roles of individual genes, pathways and networks that contribute to disease development and manifest complex phenotypes. The models can then be integrated with the chemical/drug database to identify all USFDA-approved drugs that are available for various targets or pathways and a treatment model can then be envisaged. There are limitations in defining protein-protein or protein-nucleic acid interactions as well as establishing a direct and specific causal relationship between the data sets and disease. The interpretation is also affected by lack of meaningful computational algorithms and deep machine learning protocols, which can help interpret the databases. Systems biology includes integrating large data sets to provide an overall model of multiple factors involved in disease development. Systems biology analysis can provide models for targeting multiple factors for disease progression.

Analysis of human genome sequencing data helped in the identification of around 19,000 human protein-coding genes (Ezkurdia et al., 2014), of which only 10% are deemed druggable by in silico analysis. Nearly half of the proteins expressed by the genome are functionally unclassified, and several may be modified posttranslationally (Hopkins and Groom, 2002). The challenge lies in developing high throughput analysis tools to identify targets that are druggable, i.e., play a role in modulating a disease by siRNA or by chemical perturbation in a disease setting. Systems biology approaches have also revealed functional and physical inter-connectedness between molecular components in the same or other signaling pathways. Proteins with five or more interactions with other proteins are referred as "hub" proteins. The hub proteins like p53, p27, BRCA1, ubiquitin and calmodulin may exhibit single transient interaction at a time or may participate in several interactions simultaneously. Such complex networks provide a great degree of robustness since perturbations at few random nodes does not disrupt the functioning of interaction network. Recent advances in network analysis have shown the interdependence of biological networks in modulating responses to treatments with chemicals, biologics as well as other factors. Thus, inhibition of proteins upstream of a signaling pathway will have more impact in reducing activity of several downstream effectors and phenotypes. Targeting redundant activities in the cell will ensure significant improvement in efficiency of cellular response.

A long-standing paradigm for drug discovery and development has focused on identification and development of drugs that act against a specific target with high potency and selectivity. As a result, the mechanism-based reductionist approach to drug screening has utilized a very small tractable target space. The single-target single-drug approach over-simplifies a pathological state and also disregards evolutionary complexity, relationships between biological networks and pathway redundancy. The single-targeted therapy approaches cannot be used to design treatment regimens in the context of the clinical reality of polygenic, complex diseases. Continuous treatments with targeted therapies frequently show limited efficacy, poor safety and development of resistance. The network robustness, redundancy, crosstalk between signaling pathways (Peng et al., 2006), compensatory signaling (Sergina et al., 2007) and counter-target activities or neutralizing actions (Overall and Kleifeld, 2006), have all been defined as causes underlying the development of drug resistance and efficacy reduction. In targeted drug discovery, the drugs that exhibited large spectrum of biological activities were always deprioritized based on their potential for adverse responses or off-target toxicity, which are the key factors associated with safety issues and high failure rates in clinical studies. The multitarget drug discovery aims to focus on compounds that show functional or binding activity against several targets while at the same time not causing undesirable events like hERG inhibitions. A drug targeting multiple factors or redundant activities may be more efficacious synergistically than a single-target drug, and may also delay or eliminate the development of disease resistance mutations.

APPROACHES FOR HOLISTIC DRUG TARGETING

A drug that acts on multiple targets will be more efficacious than a single active agent in controlling a multifactorial disease at its early onset and also in the treatment of recurrent, chronic advanced stage complex diseases. The rational drug design can help identify compounds with desirable effectiveness against multiple targets while at the same time not being associated with "promiscuity" and high toxicity events, e.g., cardiac side effects due to hERG inhibition (Fig. 3.2). The techniques involved in identification of a wide spectrum of targets against a known bioactive are an extension of the techniques used in initial target validation or defining the mechanism of action of drugs. The techniques include immobilizing the approved drug on a solid matrix for use in affinity chromatography as a bait to trap all cellular targets. The technology uses direct high affinity binding of an organic molecule to putative target proteins (Terstappen et al., 2007). The compounds immobilized to a solid support are incubated with protein extracts from selected cell lines. The specifically bound proteins remaining after extensive washes to remove the unbound components are eluted and analyzed by mass spectrometry. Using unbound matrix, or matrix with inactive structural

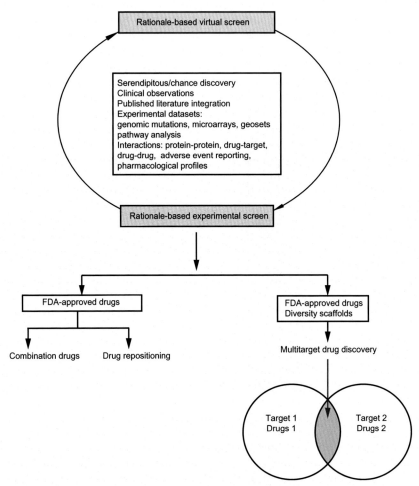

FIGURE 3.2   Holistic drug discovery. Identification of drugs or compounds with multiple functions against targets can involve chance findings (especially prevalent in drug repositioning and combination drugs) or may involve a systematic analysis and mining of all available literature and data bases of several repositories (protein interactions, drug-drug or drug target interactions, safety profiles, etc). The approaches of virtual screening and experimental screenings of FDA-approved drugs, bioactives as well as diversity scaffolds can be used in lieu of each other for validating hits from each screen. Combination drug regimens, combination matrix studies as well as drug repositioning utilizes the activities of FDA-approved drugs. New designs of multi-drug discovery approaches may utilize marketed drugs, bioactives as well as diversity scaffolds, with the goal of identifying hits with multiple activities.

analogs of compounds, or using extracts from a control cell line can further contribute to the specificity of binding. The low affinity binding targets may not be detected by the affinity chromatography approach. Another approach to identifying targets binding to drugs of interest is cellular thermal shift

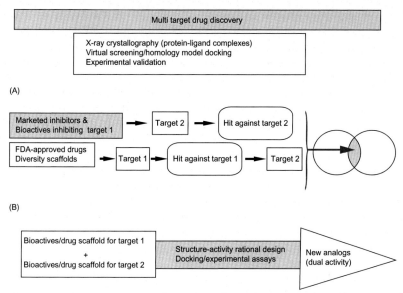

FIGURE 3.3 Approaches to multitarget drug discovery. (A) Using a focused panel of available marketed drugs or bioactives against target 1, in silico screenings or biochemical assays are developed for target 2 to identify the molecules against target 1 that also bind to target 2. Alternatively, all FDA-approved drugs and bioactives, as well as all available diversity scaffolds are screened for actives against target 1. The subset of hits from the first screen is y = used to screen for actives against target 2. The compounds that hit both target 1 and target 2 are prioritized. In (B), the chemical synthesis is performed on a known scaffold active against target 1 and another active against target 2. The structural analogs based on desirable characteristics are developed to identify new analogs with dual target activities.

assay (CETSA). This approach is based on the ability of proteins to tolerate higher temperatures when directly bound to drugs compared with unbound proteins. Technically, CETSA involves treating cells with candidate compounds, heating to denature and precipitate unbound proteins, removal of cell debris and aggregates from soluble protein fraction. The soluble proteins are then detected by Western blotting or mass spectrometric analysis (Jafari et al., 2014), as shown for a cyclin-dependent kinase (CDK) inhibitor that selectively engaged with CDK4 and CDK6, but did not bind to CDK2 or CDK9, confirming results from activity assays. CETSA has greater utility in evaluating effectiveness of engagement of target protein, which is a function of local drug concentration and its binding efficiency. CETSA may have a potential role in quantifying drug efficacy in diverse disease backgrounds, since target engagement can vary between patients and also contribute to designing personalized care regimens. In addition to the basic research to explore additional targets that approved drugs or known bioactives engage with, alternate approaches to holistic treatment strategies have involved drug repositioning and off-label treatments, combination of distinct active ingredients as well as high throughput or in silico screening protocols to identify compounds showing activity against two or more distinct targets.

DRUG REPOSITIONING

Drug repositioning or drug repurposing is a widely used strategy that seeks to identify new targets for drugs that are already approved for the treatment of a disease (Table 3.1). Repurposing is supported by observations that most drugs have pleiotropic effects and most diseases are multifactorial. Utilization of marketed approved drugs is both time and cost effective since the pharmacology, formulation, safety and toxicity profiles are already established (Huang et al., 2011). Drug repositioning may also use as starting points, compounds shown to be safe in the late stage clinical trials but which were shelved due to their failure to meet the required endpoints in a clinical trial. Drug repositioning also helps in giving a new lease on life of an expired patent. The rare and neglected diseases due to single gene mutations (http://rarediseases.info.nih.gov), that affect small patient populations previously neglected by big pharma due to low returns on investment, are proposed to benefit the most by drug repurposing projects. A detailed analysis of all available drugs, a total of 8969 unique molecular entities (approved or registered drugs) were reported to be available for repurposing projects (Huang et al., 2011).

Anecdotal drug repurposing is generally based on clinical observations and chance findings when approved drug use data accumulates from large population groups and shows effects that were not reported at the time of USFDA approval. The chlorpromazine derivative of the antihistamine promethazine was to have both antihistaminic and antiemetic barbiturate enhancing effects. In 1952 Henri Laborit, a French neurosurgeon, used chlorpromazine as a surgical anesthetic, based on which the drug was later repurposed for controlling schizophrenic patients. This was the first antipsychotic drug that blocked D2 dopamine receptors in the brain. In another serendipitous discovery, diphenoxylates used for the treatment of diarrhea were also found to be useful for the treatment of psoriasis. The most successful, serendipitous-based repurposing was reported for sildenafil, a selective phosphodiesterase 5 inhibitor developed as an antihypertensive (Ghofrani et al., 2006) and was repurposed successfully for the treatment of erectile dysfunction based on its effect on different organ. Thalidomide, an antiemetic drug recalled for teratogenicity and embryonic limb deformities, was later approved for the treatment of leprosy and multiple myeloma for its ability to inhibit tumor necrosis factor alpha and angiogenesis (Jacobson, 2000).

The increasing interest and focus on drug repositioning has helped streamline strategies for a more systematic analysis of available data on network data and computational methods to shortlist new indications. One simple strategy for finding new indications for a known drug is direct

TABLE 3.1 Examples of Some Repurposed Drugs

Drug	Original Disease	New Disease
Amphotericin	Antifungal	Leishmaniasis
Amantidine	Influenza	Parkinson's
Arsenic	TB & syphilis	Promyelocytic lukemia
Aspirin	Pain or fever	Antiplatelet
Allopurinol	Cancer	Gout
Azathioprene	Rheumatoid arthritis	Renal transplant
Atomoxetine	Antidepressant	Attention deficit disorder
Bleomycin	Cancer	Pleural effusion
Bromocriptine	Parkinson's	Diabetes mellitus
Bupropion	Depression	Antismoking
Ceftriaxone	Antibiotic	Amyotrophic lateral sclerosis
Colchicine	Gout	Mediterranean fever
Cycloserine	Urinary tract infection	Tuberculosis
Dapsone	Leprosy	Malaria
DB289	Pneumocystis	Malaria & trypanosomiasis
Eflornithine	Cancer	African trypanosomiasis
Everolimus	Renal cancer	Renal transplant
Finasteride	Prostate hyperplasia	Male pattern blindness
Fosmidomycin	Urinary tract infections	Antimalarial
Fumagillin	Antiamoebic	Cancers (angiogenesis)
Gemcitabine	Antiviral	Cancers
IFN alpha	Hepatitis B&C	Cancers
Itraconazole	Antifungal	Cancers
Isoniazid	Tuberculosis	Multiple sclerosis
Miltefosine	Cancer	Visceral leishmaniasis
Minocycline	Antibiotic	Amyotrophic lateral sclerosis
Minoxidil	Hypertension	Hair loss
Nelfiavir	HIV antiprotease	Cancers
Naltrexone	Opioid addiction	Alcohol withdrawal
Nonsteroidal	Antiinflammatory	Alzheimer's disease
Orlistat	Obesity	Cancers
Paromomycin	Amebicide	Visceral leishmaniasis

(Continued)

TABLE 3.1 (Continued)

Drug	Original Disease	New Disease
Pentamidine	Pneumonia	Trypanosomiasis & leishmaniasis
Quinacrine	Antimalarial	Prion diseases
Raloxifene	Osteoporosis	Postmenopausal breast cancer
Retinoic acid	Acne	Promyelocytic leukemia
Ritumaxib	Rheumatoid arthritis	Cancer
Serotonin antagonists	Antipsychotic	Multifocal leukoencephalopathy
Sildenafil	Angina & hypertension	Erectile dysfunction
Thalidomide	Morning sickness	Leprosy, multiple myeloma
Tamoxifen	Antiinflammatory	Parkinson's

phenotypic screening, which is not driven by any underlying hypothesis (Mullard, 2015). The USFDA- approved drug collections are screened in 384 or 1536 well plates to identify drugs that show activity against whole cells. The phenotypic screens are performed in a panel of patient derived cell lines or cell lines representing various stages of a disease with control cells lacking disease-relevant changes, e.g., primary cells. The read-out for phenotypic screens include cell viability, cell migration, caspase activity, physiologically relevant muscle cell contractions, electrophysiology, etc. The activity of drugs is often compared across a panel of cell lines representative of various stages of a disease or across cells derived from various cancers. Any differences or similarities across the panel are utilized to identify drugs that are cytotoxic to subsets of all of the cell lines representing different stages of diseases. The drugs active in a selective cell or with pan-panel activity is further optimized for activity by running combination screens against a set of standard of care drugs used in clinical settings. The synergistic pair is tested in animal models before it is advanced for further clinical investigation. Sorafenib, a marketed C-Raf kinase specific inhibitor, prescribed for the treatment of Raf dependent melanomas, is an example of drug that was also found to inhibit several receptor tyrosine kinases (e.g., VEGFR, PDGFR). The drug is now used for the treatment of renal cell carcinoma, thyroid cancer, and primary hepatocellular carcinoma.

In silico drug repositioning uses bioinformatics tools to define relationships between drugs, their side effects and literature mining public databases, and to systematically identify interaction networks between drugs and protein targets based on literature mining and also include direct experimental screenings (Sirota et al., 2011; Gottlieb et al., 2011; Shameer et al., 2015;

Kuhn et al., 2016). Computational and connectivity map strategies have been reported for comparing publicly available gene expression data from diseased and healthy individuals, from biological samples from drug-treated or control untreated biological samples, and microarray data. A recent report compared gene expression profiles from 164 drug compounds and compared them with gene expression signature of inflammatory bowel syndrome (IBD). By identifying drugs with gene expression signature that is opposite of a disease signature, the group inferred that the epilepsy drug topiramate was a good candidate for the treatment of IBD or Crohn's disease (Dudley et al., 2011). Positive effects of topiramate in rodent model of IBD also supported the computational predictions.

Biovista (Charlottesville, VA, USA), a drug repurposing biopharma, developed a repurposing platform based on a systematic literature-based discovery (LBD) approach which seeks to define connections across biomedical resources like genomic, pathway, drug to target and drug to disease databases. The approach is based on associating biomedical terms in free-text using information extraction (IE) methods. As a proof of concept, Biovista repositioned Pirlindol, a monoamine oxidase A (MAO) inhibitor, approved by the USFDA for the treatment of neurological disorders (psychosis, depression). Pirlindol, with its good safety profile, was selected as a candidate for repositioning based on its ability to reduce oxidative stress and inhibiting lipid peroxidation, processes widely prevalent in multiple sclerosis (MS) (Lekka et al., 2011). The drug was also found to have neuroprotective effects in animal model of MS.

Increase in partnerships across academia and industry can maximize repurposing efforts for new indications. The MRC (UK) works collaboratively with AstraZeneca to fund grants under mechanisms of disease initiative in which AstraZeneca provides academic researchers access to compounds that are not in development (Wadman, 2012). The researchers can use the compounds as probes to study mechanisms of diseases, validate targets and unravel new therapeutic opportunities. Drug repositioning is still in early stages and is mitigated by legal and patenting issues when new safety and efficacy data is made publicly available. While some molecules may serve simply as starting scaffolds, with patents filed on compounds derived from them or protected through method-of-use patents.

COMBINATION THERAPY

One of most prevalent approaches to targeting multiple pathways in clinical medicine is the use of multiple active ingredients in combination therapy. Specific drug combinations can block disease-relevant targets in a given patient population. Studies exposing crosstalk between pathways can for instance support design of appropriate drug combinations for better disease control. For example, a crosstalk between the epidermal growth factor receptor (EGFR) signaling pathway and hypoxia-inducible factor (HIF-1) pathways mediated development of apoptosis resistance preferentially in breast cancer cells compared with normal mammary epithelium. The EGF treated cancer cells activated the phosphoinositide 3-kinase/AKT pathway, subsequently increasing the level of HIF-1alpha under normoxic conditions which activated survivin gene transcription through direct binding to the survivin promoter. The increased expression of survivin (inhibitor of apoptosis) suppressed apoptosis in breast cancer cells (Peng et al., 2006).

Coadministration of two or more drugs may be efficacious but the question of side effects as well as drug-drug interactions may also develop when two distinct drugs are used in combination. The combinations aim to use drugs at much lower doses than when used as single agents, with the goal of minimizing side effects, toxicity and delaying resistance. Phenotypic or targeted screens are performed using combination matrices between two drugs of interest or against a standard of care and a USFDA-approved drug collection. In such studies, drugs interacting with a given therapeutic target or that modulating distinct targets can be combined at concentrations well below their 50% inhibitory concentrations (IC50) to study efficacy. The synergistically or antagonistically active drugs are further characterized in the in vitro and in animal models. Synergetic, additive or antagonistic drug combinations are subjected to mathematical analysis to generate fractional effect analysis, combination index, median drug effect analysis and response surface approaches (Chou, 2006; Greco et al., 1995). A large number of drug combinations curated from 140,000 clinical studies have been compiled into a Drug Combination Database (DCDB), which is a good resource for systems-based drug discovery (Liu et al., 2014). As with other approaches, drug activity and side effects profiling, network crosstalk, and modulation are useful in developing new drug combinations.

A rational design of approved USFDA drug mixture for the treatment of recurrent glioblastoma (GBM) was published recently (Kast et al., 2013, 2014). The Comprehensive Undermining of Survival Paths (CUSP9) study is an attempt to address limited effectiveness of single agents like temozolomide in glioblastoma treatment. Based on an overall analysis of published research, the team identified at least 17 distinct signaling systems or targets that promote rapid growth and migration of glioblastoma cells. At least nine known USFDA-approved drugs that are known to block the activity of the targets include artesuanate (PI3 kinase, AKT, TLR2, TNFα), disulfiram (ALDH), captopril (ACE, AT1, MMP), celecoxib (carbonic anhydrases, COX), aprecipitant (NK-1 receptors), auranofin (thioreductase, STAT3, cathepsin B), itraconzole (P-gp efflux pump, BCRP, Hedgehog, 5 Lipooxygease), ritonavir (AKT, mTOR, cyclin D3, proteasome), and sertraline (TCTP, AKT, mTOR). The side effects and concentrations of individual drugs were carefully evaluated to minimize risks of side effects while at the same time targeting multiple effectors of the disease.

A more comprehensive cancer treatment strategy involves designing protocols where the drug candidates for the primary driver kinase as well as its resistant mutant forms are administered from the beginning of the treatment. For example, targeted first generation kinase inhibitors like Tarceva (OSI pharmaceuticals) and Iressa (AstraZeneca) against EGFR resulted in acquisition of escape mutations in EGFR (T790M) in nonsmall cell lung cancer (NSCLC). AZD9291 (AstraZeneca) and Rociletinib (Clovis Oncology) are third generation EGFR tyrosine kinase inhibitors that are active against NSCLC harboring the T790M EGFR mutants. Treatment protocols utilizing both the first generation kinase inhibitors as well as ones inhibiting the gatekeeper mutations will significantly improve survival (Piotrowska et al., 2015). The HAART (Highly Active Antiretroviral Therapy) for HIV-treatment combines two nucleoside reverse transcriptase (RT) inhibitors lamivudine and zidovudine in the presence of a protease inhibitor (Staszewski, 1995). Clinical data showed that lamivudine treatment alone triggered resistance due to Met 184 Val mutation in viral RT. The mutant form M184V was still sensitive to zidovudine and a combination of the two RT inhibitors effectively suppressed the catalytic activity required for HIV replication. The use of combination therapies is most widespread in clinical practice for managing complex diseases.

MULTITARGET DRUG DISCOVERY

Identification of a single compound with activity against two or more targets has its advantages over combination drug therapies requiring administration of multiple drugs. The pharmacokinetics and safety profiles for single multitarget drug are theoretically more defined than the potential for long-term adverse effects developing with combination drugs. The development of resistance to multitarget drugs is probably lower than that of single-target drugs. A multitarget drug is guaranteed to interact with its targets in the same tissue/cell compartment and unlike the combination drugs, will not have drug-drug interactions (synergistic/antagonistic).

Polypharmacology that does not involve toxic promiscuity of drugs is predicted to be beneficial for the treatment of complex diseases and is of great value in multitarget drug discovery. The compounds with adverse side effects should be deprioritized early in drug discovery while identifying those exhibiting potentiation of therapeutic activity by hitting multiple targets followed by characterization of pharmacological profiles.

Several rational-based designs, computational-based docking, and virtual screening approaches have surfaced for identifying drugs with multiple functions (Fig. 3.3). Based on the reports of synergistic effects of HDAC inhibitors with other anticancer agents like EGFR, Hsp90, and topoisomerase inhibitors, a rational design approach was employed to generate a multitarget compound starting with a Chinese herbal compound derivative of evodiamine, a quinazolinocarboline alkaloid (He et al., 2015). The evodiamine derivative with potent anti-Topo-I and II activity was used to design evodiamine/Vorinostat (HDAC inhibitor) hybrids to target topoisomerase I and II as well as histone deacetylase (HDAC) (He et al., 2015). Several compounds were shown to inhibit all three cancer targets. Some of the compounds also show strong antiproliferative and pro-apoptotic effects in cancer lines, MDA-MB-231 (breast cancer), HCT116 (colon cancer) and HLF (liver cancer).

Another virtual screening approach was published recently to identify inhibitors of EGFR kinase as well as BRD4, a Bromo and Extra-Terminal (BET) domain protein. Both EGFR and bromodomain activity is upregulated in various cancers. BET bromodomain proteins regulate gene transcription by recognizing acetylate lysine residues on histones. Transcriptional profiles of EGFR and BRD4 were found to be different using LINCS. Dual EGFR-BRD4 inhibitors were identified by virtual screening that included data mining E-molecules database (>6 million compounds). Of the 908 predicted EGFR inhibitors, 108 were docked to BRD4 cocrystal structures. Of these, eight were experimentally shown to inhibit BRD4 bromodomain −acetylated biotin histone four peptide Alphascreen assay and other counter assays. Finally, one compound that inhibited BRD4 binding also inhibited EGFR kinase activity (Allen et al., 2015). In another study, new compounds were obtained by modulating the structure of COX inhibitor, Lumiracoxib to obtain multitarget NSAID that is inhibitory to not only COX1 and two but also to the thromboxane A2 prostanoid (TP) receptor, which is associated with chronic pain. Another approach helped design compounds that targeted both the fatty acid amide hydrolase (FAAH) as well as cyclooxygenase (COX)-1 and COX-2. The antipain and antiinflammation effects of NSAIDs, normally limited by its adverse gastrointestinal injury, are greatly improved with concomitant inhibition of FAAH due to the accumulation of protective FAAH substrates, such as the endocannabinoid anandamide (Migliore et al., 2015).

Screening clinical kinase inhibitors for their ability to targeting bromodomains using Alphascreen assay identified a dual kinase/bromodomain inhibitor. Of the 628 kinase inhibitors (bioactives and marked drugs), nine were found to inhibit the poly acetylated histone H4 peptide (Ciceri et al., 2014). The hits were shown to bind directly to the bromodomains by thermal shift assay and also formed cocrystal complexes with the BRD4 bromodomain showing pharmacophore relatedness for kinase and bromodomain binding sites. Kinome wide profiling data showed selectivity of BI-2536 for PLK-1 and selectivity for BET bromodomains. Potent nanomolar activity of the kinase inhibitors, BI-2536 and TG-101348 as well as clinical PLK1 and JAK2/FLT3 kinase inhibitors, acting on distinct BRD4 oncogenic pathway helps provide a strong strategy for polypharmacological targeting.

A more in-depth understanding of drug target, target-disease associations will provide stronger leads for targeting complex diseases. The use of experimental HTS screens as well as in silico methods for predicting polypharmacology of known drugs (Reker et al., 2014) and new molecules by means of structure-based (molecular docking, binding-site structural similarity, receptor-based pharmacophore searching), expression-based (expression profile/signature similarity disease-drug and drug-drug networks), ligand-based (similarity searching, side-effect similarity, QSAR, machine learning), and fragment-based approaches have promising potential in facilitating drug repositioning and the discovery of multitarget drugs.

CONCLUDING REMARKS

Drug discovery process is a challenging, labor, and cost-intensive multistep process involving target identification and validation and identification of chemicals by screening large compound collections experimentally (HTS) or by in silico approaches. Drug discovery is driven by medical needs. As a result, target identification and druggability, as well as ultimate direct demonstration of the drug exposure at its site of action, target occupancy, proof of mechanistic pharmacology and use of disease-relevant phenotypic assays are postulated to increase the probability of generating high quality chemical probes or leads. Numerous techniques have been used to study specific and off-target binding of chemical probe, and have led to the development and approval of compounds that show high target specificity. Complex polygenic diseases are characterized with dysregulation of multiple targets and such diseases cannot be managed with targeted single therapies. More effective and improved therapeutic opportunities emerge from targeting redundancy or network complexity of biological systems. A holistic approach to complex disease treatment is focused on identifying a single molecule that works against several targets implicated in specific disease development and progression. Various combination treatments have been designed, tested, and approved by the USFDA for management of late stage or refractory cancers and neurological diseases. The combination therapies have been efficacious but add to the healthcare costs, require strict adherence to regimens and possibility of developing new adverse side effects with time. Regulatory compliance also complicates combination synergistic therapies and drug repurposing especially if two competing pharmaceutical sources are involved. Multidrug targeting is an emerging and rapidly advancing strategy that holds enormous potential in future therapeutics. The selection of right combination of targets for a disease of interest is critical in multitarget drug discovery and requires good understanding of target-disease associations, pathway-target-drug-disease relationships and adverse events profiling. The field requires further advances in large-scale data integration and analysis of target-target, target-drug and drug-drug relationships.

Finally, the holistic approach to resolving global health crisis will be beneficial to addressing issues with the availability and access to the best available medicines and patient care for the treatment and management of chronic, infectious and neglected diseases, as well as controlling regional breakouts of diseases (Zika virus, Ebola, etc.). World healthcare reform requires a strong collaborative commitment from various sectors engaged in drug discovery including the academia, pharma, philanthropy, government, disease foundations, and patient advocacy groups. Such holistic support from all sources engaged in drug discovery as well as patient care will help enforce research and drug development to address unmet patient needs; develop safe, effective, and sustainable preventative approaches to minimize risk factors to complex as well as infectious diseases; and also introduce changes in health insurance practices. The world resources also would need to be applied towards reforming health education, drug production costs, intellectual/regulatory systems, basic science, and innovation.

REFERENCES

Allen, B.K., Mehta, S., Ember, S.W., Schonbrunn, E., Ayad, N., Schurer, S.C., 2015. Large-scale computational screening identifies first in class multitarget inhibitor of EGFR kinase and BRD4. Sci. Rep. 5, 16924.

Baell, J.B., Holloway, G.A., 2010. New substructure filters for removal of pan assay interference compounds (PAINS) from screening libraries and for their exclusion in bioassays. J. Med. Chem. 53 (7), 2719−2740.

Bajorath, J., 2002. Integration of virtual and high-throughput screening. Nat. Rev. Drug. Discov. 1 (11), 882−894.

Barnes, E.C., Kumar, R., Davis, R.A., 2016. The use of isolated natural products as scaffolds for the generation of chemically diverse screening libraries for drug discovery. Nat. Prod. Rep.

Bunnage, M.E., Gilbert, A.M., Jones, L.H., Hett, E.C., 2015. Know your target, know your molecule. Nat. Chem. Biol. 11 (6), 368−372.

Chou, T.C., 2006. Theoretical basis, experimental design, and computerized simulation of synergism and antagonism in drug combination studies. Pharmacol. Rev. 58 (3), 621−681.

Ciceri, P., Müller, S., O'Mahony, A., Fedorov, O., Filippakopoulos, P., Hunt, J.P., et al., 2014. Dual kinase-bromodomain inhibitors for rationally designed polypharmacology. Nat. Chem. Biol. 10 (4), 305−312.

Dudley, J.T., Sirota, M., Shenoy, M., Pai, R.K., Roedder, S., Chiang, A.P., et al., 2011. Computational repositioning of the anticonvulsant topiramate for inflammatory bowel disease. Sci. Transl. Med. 3 (96), 96ra76.

Ezkurdia, I., Juan, D., Rodriguez, J.M., Frankish, A., Diekhans, M., Harrow, J., et al., 2014. Multiple evidence strands suggest that there may be as few as 19 000 human protein-coding genes. Hum. Mol. Genet. 23 (22), 5866−5878.

Gao, H., Korn, J.M., Ferretti, S., Monahan, J.E., Wang, Y., Singh, M., et al., 2015. High-throughput screening using patient-derived tumor xenografts to predict clinical trial drug response. Nat. Med. 21 (11), 1318−1325.

Ghofrani, H.A., Osterloh, I.H., Grimminger, F., 2006. Sildenafil: from angina to erectile dysfunction to pulmonary hypertension and beyond. Nat. Rev. Drug. Discov. 5 (8), 689−702.

Gottlieb, A., Stein, G.Y., Ruppin, E., Sharan, R., 2011. PREDICT: a method for inferring novel drug indications with application to personalized medicine. Mol. Syst. Biol. 7, 496.

Greco, W.R., Bravo, G., Parsons, J.C., 1995. The search for synergy: a critical review from a response surface perspective. Pharmacol. Rev. 47 (2), 331−385.

He, S., Dong, G., Wang, Z., Chen, W., Huang, Y., Li, Z., et al., 2015. Discovery of novel multi-acting topoisomerase I/II and histone deacetylase inhibitors. ACS Med. Chem. Lett. 6 (3), 239−243.

Hopkins, A.L., Groom, C.R., 2002. The druggable genome. Nat. Rev. Drug. Discov. 1 (9), 727−730.

Huang, R., Southall, N., Wang, Y., Yasgar, A., Shinn, P., Jadhav, A., et al., 2011. The NCGC pharmaceutical collection: a comprehensive resource of clinically approved drugs enabling repurposing and chemical genomics. Sci. Transl. Med. 3 (80), 80ps16.

Jacobson, J.M., 2000. Thalidomide: a remarkable comeback. Expert. Opin. Pharmacother. 1 (4), 849−863.

Jafari, R., Almqvist, H., Axelsson, H., Ignatushchenko, M., Lundbäck, T., Nordlund, P., et al., 2014. The cellular thermal shift assay for evaluating drug target interactions in cells. Nat. Protocols 9 (9), 2100−2122.

Kaplan, J.C., Junien, C., 2000. Genomics and medicine: an anticipation. From boolean mendelian genetics to multifactorial molecular medicine. Comptes rendus de l'Academie des sciences Serie III, Sciences de la vie 323 (12), 1167−1174.

Kast, R.E., Boockvar, J.A., Brüning, A., Cappello, F., Chang, W.-W., Cvek, B., et al., 2013. A conceptually new treatment approach for relapsed glioblastoma: coordinated undermining of survival paths with nine repurposed drugs (CUSP9) by the International Initiative for Accelerated Improvement of Glioblastoma Care. Oncotarget 4 (4), 502−530.

Kast, R.E., Karpel-Massler, G., Halatsch, M.-E., 2014. CUSP9* treatment protocol for recurrent glioblastoma: aprepitant, artesunate, auranofin, captopril, celecoxib, disulfiram, itraconazole, ritonavir, sertraline augmenting continuous low dose temozolomide. Oncotarget 5 (18), 8052−8082.

Kuhn, M., Letunic, I., Jensen, L.J., Bork, P., 2016. The SIDER database of drugs and side effects. Nucl. Acids Res. 44 (D1), D1075−D1079.

Lekka, E., Deftereos, S.N., Persidis, A., Persidis, A., Andronis, C., 2011. Literature analysis for systematic drug repurposing: a case study from Biovista. Drug Disc. Today Therap. Strateg. 8 (3−4), 103−108.

Liu, Y., Wei, Q., Yu, G., Gai, W., Li, Y., Chen, X., 2014. DCDB 2.0: a major update of the drug combination database. Database J. Biol. Databases and Curation 2014, bau124.

Loktionov, A., 2003. Common gene polymorphisms and nutrition: emerging links with pathogenesis of multifactorial chronic diseases (review). J. Nutr. Biochem. 14 (8), 426−451.

Lounkine, E., Keiser, M.J., Whitebread, S., Mikhailov, D., Hamon, J., Jenkins, J.L., et al., 2012. Large-scale prediction and testing of drug activity on side-effect targets. Nature 486 (7403), 361−367.

Macintyre, L., Zhang, T., Viegelmann, C., Martinez, I.J., Cheng, C., Dowdells, C., et al., 2014. Metabolomic tools for secondary metabolite discovery from marine microbial symbionts. Mar. Drugs 12 (6), 3416−3448.

Migliore, M., Habrant, D., Sasso, O., Albani, C., Bertozzi, S.M., Armirotti, A., et al., 2015. Potent multitarget FAAH-COX inhibitors: design and structure-activity relationship studies. Eur. J. Med. Chem. 109, 216−237.

Mullard, A., 2015. The phenotypic screening pendulum swings. Nat. Rev. Drug. Discov. 14 (12), 807–809.

Overall, C.M., Kleifeld, O., 2006. Tumour microenvironment - opinion: validating matrix metallopro- teinases as drug targets and anti-targets for cancer therapy. Nat. Rev. Cancer 6 (3), 227–239.

Park, H., Lee, S., Hong, S., 2016. Discovery of dual Inhibitors for wild type and D816V mutant of c-KIT kinase through virtual and biochemical screening of natural products. J. Nat. Prod..

Patwardhan, B., 2012. Health for India: search for appropriate models. J. Ayurveda Integr. Med. 3 (4), 173–174.

Peng, X.H., Karna, P., Cao, Z., Jiang, B.H., Zhou, M., Yang, L., 2006. Cross-talk between epi- dermal growth factor receptor and hypoxia-inducible factor-1alpha signal pathways increases resistance to apoptosis by up-regulating survivin gene expression. J. Biol. Chem. 281 (36), 25903–25914.

Piotrowska, Z., Niederst, M.J., Karlovich, C.A., Wakelee, H.A., Neal, J.W., Mino-Kenudson, M., et al., 2015. Heterogeneity underlies the emergence of EGFRT790 wild-type clones follow- ing treatment of T790M-positive cancers with a third-generation EGFR inhibitor. Cancer Discov. 5 (7), 713–722.

Rask-Andersen, M., Almén, M.S., Schiöth, H.B., 2011. Trends in the exploitation of novel drug targets. Nat. Rev. Drug. Discov. 10 (8), 579–590.

Rees, S., Gribbon, P., Birmingham, K., Janzen, W.P., Pairaudeau, G., 2016. Towards a hit for every target. Nat. Rev. Drug. Discov. 15 (1), 1–2.

Reker, D., Rodrigues, T., Schneider, P., Schneider, G., 2014. Identifying the macromolecular tar- gets of de novo-designed chemical entities through self-organizing map consensus. Proc. Natl. Acad. Sci. U. S. A. 111 (11), 4067–4072.

Roy, A., Taylor, B., McDonald, P.M., Price, A., Chaguturu, R., 2009. Hit-to-probe-to-lead optimization strategies. Handbook of Drug Screening, Second Edition. Drugs and the Pharmaceutical Sciences. CRC Press, pp. 21–55.

Schenone, M., Dancik, V., Wagner, B.K., Clemons, P.A., 2013. Target identification and mecha- nism of action in chemical biology and drug discovery. Nat. Chem. Biol. 9 (4), 232–240.

Sergina, N.V., Rausch, M., Wang, D., Blair, J., Hann, B., Shokat, K.M., et al., 2007. Escape from HER-family tyrosine kinase inhibitor therapy by the kinase-inactive HER3. Nature 445 (7126), 437–441.

Shameer, K., Readhead, B., Dudley, J.T., 2015. Computational and experimental advances in drug repositioning for accelerated therapeutic stratification. Curr. Top. Med. Chem. 15 (1), 5–20.

Sirota, M., Dudley, J.T., Kim, J., Chiang, A.P., Morgan, A.A., Sweet-Cordero, A., et al., 2011. Discovery and preclinical validation of drug indications using compendia of public gene expression data. Sci. Transl. Med. 3 (96), 96ra77.

Staszewski, S., 1995. Zidovudine and lamivudine: results of phase III studies. J. Acquir. Immune Defic. Syndr. Hum. Retrovirol. Off. Publ. Int. Retrovirol. Assoc. 10 (Suppl. 1), S57.

Taylor, J.C., Martin, H.C., Lise, S., Broxholme, J., Cazier, J.-B., Rimmer, A., et al., 2015. Factors influencing success of clinical genome sequencing across a broad spectrum of disor- ders. Nat. Genet. 47 (7), 717–726.

Terstappen, G.C., Schlupen, C., Raggiaschi, R., Gaviraghi, G., 2007. Target deconvolution strat- egies in drug discovery. Nat. Rev. Drug. Discov. 6 (11), 891–903.

Wadman, M., 2012. New cures sought from old drugs. Nature 490 (7418), 15.

Waring, M.J., Arrowsmith, J., Leach, A.R., Leeson, P.D., Mandrell, S., Owen, R.M., et al., 2015. An analysis of the attrition of drug candidates from four major pharmaceutical companies. Nat. Rev. Drug. Discov. 14 (7), 475–486.

Chapter 4

Reverse Pharmacology

Ashwinikumar A. Raut[1], Mukund S. Chorghade[2] and Ashok D.B. Vaidya[1]

[1]*Kasturba Health Society-Medical Research Centre, Mumbai, Maharashtra, India,*
[2]*THINQ, Boston, MA, United States*

INTRODUCTION AND BACKGROUND

I never found it [drug discovery] easy. People say I was lucky twice but I resent that. We stuck with [cimetidine] for 4 years with no progress until we eventually succeeded. It was not luck, it was bloody hard work.

— Sir James Black, Nobel Laureate (Jack, 2009).

Introduction

The aforementioned quote from Sir James Black, the discoverer of β-adrenergic and H_2- blockers, expresses the exasperation so often felt by many scientists who have dedicated their lives to new drug discoveries. Any new drug discovery for an unmet medical need often grabs headlines in the medical and lay press/media. Overenthusiastic science writers, not infrequently, depict the epitome of medical progress in superlative terms. The current drug discovery and development processes depend heavily on reductionist paradigms. The latter involve identification of drug targets, synthesizing many molecules through combinatorial chemistry/monoclonal antibodies, and testing the drug candidates through high throughput or binding to specific macromolecules. Despite the advances in genomics, proteomics, and metabolomics, the new drug development is costly, time-consuming, less productive, and yields low returns on heavy investments. The current statistics indicate a drying up of the drug discovery pipeline (New Drug Discovery: in 1996 (56), 2007 (17), 2013 (03)) (Mishra, 2014). There is also a further aggravation in the drug supply due to some of the marketed blockbuster drugs that have been withdrawn. There are opinions expressed about the need of a paradigm shift in the processes of drug discovery and development. The transdiscipline of reverse pharmacology (RP)

Innovative Approaches in Drug Discovery. DOI: http://dx.doi.org/10.1016/B978-0-12-801814-9.00004-0
89

offers one such opportunity to shift the paradigm, with an eye to saving cost and time—and with greater chances of success in clinical therapeutics.

Background of Reverse Pharmacology

The large number of the world population (about 70%) still relies on traditional systems of medicine (TSM). In India, more than 500 million people turn to various forms of medicine such as Ayurveda, Unani, Siddha, and homeopathy (AYUSH) (Raut, 2013). The major components of the remedies in the TSM pharmacopoeias are medicinal plants. There are increasing global demands of safe herbal products for many intercurrent and chronic illnesses. Quite a number of Ayurvedic and traditional Chinese medicine (TCM) plants sell in the Western markets as dietary supplements (DS), as over-the-counter drugs, with vague claims of structure and function improvement. There is a disclaimer on every bottle that the United States Federal Drug Administration (USFDA) has not approved the DS. This dichotomy of not accepting the systems of health care (Ayurveda or TCM) and permitting the drugs of those systems as DS is hazardous! More than 100 countries have some form of regulations for herbal medicines. The market for herbal supplements and medicine is expected to cost approximately US $100 billion by 2015 (Stephen Daniells, 2011). There is a World Health Organization (WHO) projection of the global herbal market to reach the figure of $5 trillion by 2050 (India Medical Times). The evidence base of the herbal remedies is considered inadequate despite their long use. What these remedies need are different kinds of evidence—and a different approach. When these age-old natural drugs are taken out of their contextual matrix and subjected to significant statistical studies, their "Cochrane review" often pronounces them as "not convincing" statistically. It is interesting to note what Sir Bradford Hill, the pioneer of controlled clinical trials, said,

> When I got on to the subject of statistical tests of significance I started by stating that these were based on the laws of probability over which statisticians quarreled violently. I was entirely ignorant of them but I knew more than the lady who congratulated her friend on the birth of triplets. "It is remarkable," said the mother. "It happens only one in 8000 times." "Good gracious," said her friend. "However did you find time for the housework?
>
> (Chalmers, 2003)

Reverse pharmacology is essentially a transdisciplinary quest for clinical significance, not merely a matter of flipping a coin. The potential of the widely used TSM drugs/plants can be investigated by RP, which is a novel initiative that offers a paradigm shift in the new drug discovery process. The ingenuity of RP is meant for the integration of traditional remedies with the wisdom of robust documentation of safety and efficacy. RP is staged as experiential knowledge/data, exploratory research, and relevant clinical/experimental studies. Unlike conventional drug discovery and development, RP approach is done from "bedsides to benches." It can also be relevant for new uses of old drugs or for following up on a new unseen indication of a drug candidate. The clinically novel biodynamic actions of traditional remedies may open up new vistas in biomedicine and life sciences. The phytoactive molecules can also provide novel chemical scaffolds for the structural modifications with defined drug targets. Hence, RP can play a dual role—it can inspire new drugs from traditional remedies and enrich the chemical repertoire of medicinal chemists for new chemical entities (NCEs).

THE ROOTS OF MODERN DRUGS IN TRADITIONAL REMEDIES/POISONS

Around half a century before Jesus, Aulus Cornelius Celsus made a profound statement, "That medicines were first found out, and then after the reasons and causes were discoursed; and not the causes first found out, and by light from them the medicines and cures discovered." Unlike this view, it has been emphasized in Ayurveda that the disease is first investigated and only later the medicines: "*Rogamadau parikshet tadanantaram aushadham.*" This obvious difference is primarily due to different epistemologies of the genesis of Greek medicine and that of Ayurveda. As a consequence, the renaissance period of medicine, in Europe, reacted to the Greek physician Galen and his centuries-old entrenched therapeutic concoctions.

Liberated from a blind following, questions were then asked by inquisitive minds about how the tribal poisons worked. This habit of asking how led to developments far beyond the then state of technology. Claude Bernard, the father of physiology and pharmacology, solved the mystery of curare arrow

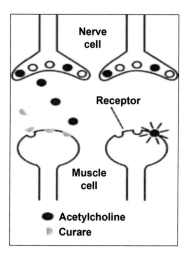
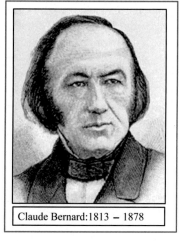

Claude Bernard:1813 – 1878

FIGURE 4.1   From arrow poisoning to drug receptor.

TABLE 4.1 Poisons and Mechanisms of Actions (Vaidya, A.D.B., 2010b)

Medicinal Plant	Clinical Effect	Mechanism
Curare tomentosum	Conscious paralysis & death	Neuromuscular block
Papaver somniferum	Sleep & pain relief	Opioid receptors/endorphins
Physostigma venenosum	Ordeal poison	Anticholineesterase
Claviceps purpurea	Gangrene	α & β adrenergic receptors
Strychnos nux-vomica	Convulsant	Glycinergic receptors
Atropa belladonna	Fatal poisoning	Cholinergic blockade
Melilotus alba	Bleeding disorder	Anti-Vitamin K
Bathraps jaraca	Snake poisoning	ACE inhibition

poison (Fig. 4.1). The victim stays fully conscious but dies of paralysis. Bernard's experiment showed that the curarized muscle can still contract if it is directly stimulated electrically. But if the nerve supplying the muscle is electrically stimulated, then there is no contraction. That was a momentous discovery laying the foundation of the modern pharmacology of drugs binding to targets and receptors. Several poisons and native remedies were studied experimentally, asking *how*?

Table 4.1 lists some of these plants, their clinical effects, and experimental correlates.

The short, 226-page book by Claude Bernard, *An Introduction to the Study of Experimental Medicine*, is considered a classic (Bernard, 1957). L. Bernhard Cohen, in a foreword to its English edition, writes, "The usual definition of a scientific 'classic' is a great work that is venerated, cited, but no longer read. Claude Bernard's book is an exception. . ." The influence of Bernard on modern pharmacology and drug discovery is all pervasive. Mechanistic explanation of the actions of drug molecules is the most dominant reductionist paradigm even in drug discovery, but history has been forgotten! The human and clinical effects of medicinal plants and poisons started the entire enterprise of drug development and the pharmaceutical industry. Bernard himself had said, "The most useful path for physiology and medicine to follow now is to seek to discover new facts instead of trying to reduce to equations the facts which science already possesses." At least in the early decades of the last century, scientists with medical backgrounds pursued the factual activity of plants in man and searched the mechanisms in animals and tissues. They also gave credit to the practitioners of Asian or folk medicine for the current use

TABLE 4.2 Drug Discovery Paradigm (Vaidya, A.D.B., 2010b)

Medicinal Plant	Clinical Facts	Mechanistic Correlates
Nicotiana tabacum	Stimulant	Nicotinic receptors
Cinchona officinalis	Fever cure	Antiplasmodial
Rauwolfia serpentina	Sedative/antihypertensive	Catecholamine reuptake block
Salix alba	Pain & swelling reduction	COX inhibitor
Ephedra sinensis	Antiasthmatic	Sympathomimetic
Thea sinensis	Stimulant	Increase in CAMP
Catharanthus roseus	WBCs reduction	Microtubules
Erythroxylum coca	Stimulant	Local anesthesia

of the many plants they studied. That was a dominant paradigm that provided targets for the drug actions (Table 4.2).

A huge number of drugs during the last century emerged by testing new chemical activities against the targets as per these mechanisms. The ceaseless activity of medicinal chemists, by minor structural variations on the natural actives, led to an eclipse in finding new facts at the bedside. In addition, the advent of molecular biology and immunology led to hype and hubris for the reductionist paradigm. The developed drugs, based on the mechanisms of plant actions (*vide supra*), are as follows: (1) neuromuscular blockade: tubocurarine, pancuronium, galamine, suxamethonium; (2) anticholinergic: scopalamine, cyclopentlate, iratropium; (3) vitamin K antagonist: dicomarol, warfarin; (4) local anesthetic: procaine, lidocaine; and (5) ACE inhibition: captopril, benazapril, and enalapril. Though the list is much longer than given, the point to be made here is that this mechanisms-directed path led to many "me too" drugs. Eventually, there was a need for a shift in the paradigm.

Rauwolfia serpentina was shown to be an antihypertensive and tranquillizer by Indian scientists Sen and Bose and others (Sen and Bose, 1931). Sen also observed side effects of the plant, namely depression, gynecomastia/galactorrhea, Parkinsonian syndrome, hyperacidity, and nasal congestion. As the active principle of reserpine was isolated, its mechanism was proven to be a depletion of catecholamines by inhibition of their reuptake. A watershed in new drugs occurred for hypertension, depression, Parkinson's disease, prolactinoma, and nasal congestion. A paradigm shift had occurred: Ayurvedic drugs and plants can give therapeutic effects, and that there is much to learn and gain about their side effects, if understood mechanistically (Vaidya, 1979). Unfortunately, there was no organized approach to identify and pursue the clinical facts of Ayurvedic drug responses to their logical conclusion. The prejudices against Ayurveda among allopaths and fundamentalists of vaidyas (who practiced Ayurveda) have delayed the exploration of Ayurvedic therapeutics for new world drugs. This situation is now changing with the emergence and development of RP, which has caught the attention of several leaders in drug discovery and development. However, the need of triple competence in RP—Ayurveda/traditional medicine, clinical pharmacology, and drug discovery—is a tall demand. This can be partly resolved by a transsystem and transdisciplinary R&D network (Raut and Chorghade, 2014).

THE DEFINITION OF REVERSE PHARMACOLOGY AND ITS DIFFERENT ORIGINS

The need has been felt to look at medical systems, other than modern medicine, in a different perspective, by the leaders of clinical pharmacology like Louis Lasagna and UK Sheth. Lasagna said, "These systems need different type of evidence" (Lasagna, 1999). Sporadic attempts have been made by many groups to study Ayurvedic plants ethnobotanically, phytochemically, experimentally, and clinically. But in the absence of a clear and defined approach the emergent evidence has often been challenged on quantitative grounds or has remained fragmented and not pursued. Alvan Feinstein, a clinical scientist, epidemiologist, and mathematician, wrote in a visionary paper on the limits of quantitation, "A clinician performs an experiment every time he treats a patient...each treated patient begins in a baseline state, receives an intervention, and has an outcome—exactly as in an experiment ...the 'control' comparison comes from the clinicians awareness of similar patients in the past; and the goal of the 'experiment' is to repeat (or exceed) the best outcomes achieved with those previous patients." (Feinstein, 1994). During a stay at Yale, of one of the authors (ADBV) had several discussions on clinical research with Feinstein, Robert Levine, Arnold Eisenfeld, Mel Van Woert, and Lewis Thomas. A vague sense of direction then emerged, presaging RP. The stress by Feinstein and Levine on starting research from the clinic—a bedside to bench path—made a major impact (Vaidya, 2013).

After much deliberation, an acceptable and pragmatic definition has emerged for RP, which is the science of documenting clinical/experiential hits with basal and postintervention data, and then by relevant trans-system exploratory studies (in vitro and in vivo) of these hits to develop leads. Positive leads are then investigated at different levels of biological organization, experimentally, and clinically as drug candidates.

The scope of RP is immense: (1) to evaluate clinically the evidence of safety, efficacy, and quality of drugs/plants used in the TSM; (2) to discover new drugs from natural products (NPs) already in use by humans; (3) to find new clinical facts and bedside biodynamic phenomena that may lead to new

TABLE 4.3 The Starting Points of Reverse Pharmacology

Systems and Domains	New Approaches	Clinical Research
Ayurveda/siddha	Ayurvedic epidemiology	Anecdotal cases
Traditional Chinese medicine	Observational therapeutics	Case reports
Unani medicine	Systems ayurveda	Case series
Homeopathy	Phytochemistry	Retrospective surveys
Kampo medicine	Golden triangle	Retrolective studies
Tribal medicine	Ayurvedic biology	Prospective Studies
Modern medicine	Phytopharmacolgy	Open clinical trials
Ethnobotany	Ayurgenomics	Controlled trials
Vriksha/prani ayurveda	Molecular botany	Multicentric trials
Nutraceutics	Reverse nutraceutics	Meta-analyses/ Cochrane

insights in human biology; (4) to overcome the current costly, drawn out and attritive process of drug discovery/development; and (5) to complement the extant process by novel phyto-actives as chemical scaffolds for NCEs.

RP need not merely be a linear process or unimodal in its resourcing. The origins of RP can also be from the diverse and rich big data of traditional/modern literature, ethnobotanical, phytochemical, experimental, clinical, and anecdotal cases. Table 4.3 lists systems and domains, new approaches and areas of clinical research. There is a vast scope of exploring RP by a judicious combination of systems of origin, new approaches, and areas of clinical research.

AYURVEDIC PHARMACOEPIDEMIOLOGY AND OBSERVATIONAL THERAPEUTICS

The main domains of RP driven drug discovery are (1) experiential, (2) exploratory, and (3) experimental. These three domains are rather exclusive mutually, not sequential. RP is a circular model with enrichment interconnecting feedbacks. However, experience mostly forms the first platform of RP. The experiential domain of RP would cover Pharmacoepidemiology-resourced information, hints from clinical notes and classical literature, and hits from observational therapeutics as well as from single case studies/case series. Experiential domain would source information coming from unconventional rationales of traditional medicine, from novel clinical observations to serendipitous findings.

Ayurvedic Pharmacoepidemiology

The discipline of pharmacoepidemiology (Strom, 1989) is the outcome of an integrative approach of clinical pharmacology and epidemiology. During the major multiinstitutional national session of the Council for Scientific and Industrial Research sponsored by New Millennium Indian Technology Leadership Initiative (CSIR-NMITLI) in arthritis, diabetes, and hepatitis for developing globally competitive herbal drugs inspired from Ayurvedic heritage, the idea of Ayurvedic pharmacoepidemiology was proposed by Dr. Rama Vaidya (Vaidya et al., 2003). Ayurvedic pharmacoepidemiology would require a collaboration among vaidya scientists, clinical pharmacologists, and epidemiologists.

Ayurvedic pharmacoepidemiology (AyPE) is defined as the "study of the usage, acceptability, efficacy, safety, complementarities, and cost-effectiveness of Ayurvedic drugs in a large number of people." It includes Ayurvedic prescription audits, registration of Ayurvedic drugs utilization, population pharmacodynamics/kinetics, and documentation of untoward or unexpected beneficial effects of Ayurvedic drugs. AyPE aims to study Ayurvedic therapies in various aspects such as the extent of use, level of efficacy, nature of safety, cost-effectiveness, drug interactions, and rationality as per the indications and ingredients of the drugs (Vaidya et al., 2003).

With a global increase in the use of herbal and traditional therapeutics (herbal supplement sales are expected to hit $93.15 billion by 2015: Report [Internet]) the Pharmacoepidemiology of Traditional medicine will become more relevant. In the Indian context, where Ayurveda is deeply rooted in the community at large, Ayurvedic pharmacoepidemiology becomes quite relevant to healthcare. Such an endeavor can be useful in many ways: (1) prevalence and patterns of usage of Ayurvedic drugs; (2) records of field safety for rational therapeutics and precautions; (3) establishing a national drug policy on the pharmaco-economics of Ayurveda; (4) detection of drug interactions due to concomitant intersystem utilization of drugs; and (5) discovery of novel, beneficial effects for developing new drugs.

Two doctoral (PhD) programs were initiated on Ayurvedic pharmacoepidemiology in arthritis and in diabetes. Whereas the program on arthritis has been submitted to the university (Tillu, 2015), the program in diabetes has also progressed well. The review of the literature and current status of indigenous antidiabetic drugs was published in a textbook on diabetes mellitus (Vaidya et al., 2014). A detailed analysis of marketed Ayurvedic antidiabetic formulations for their brand names, dosage forms, ingredients, composition, dosages schedule, and precautions and package insert has provided interesting data on Ayurvedic-marketed products in the Mumbai region of India (Nabar et al., 2013) During a drug utilization study at a healthcare medical camp and at a tertiary care center it became evident that the majority of patients do use indigenous and conventional antidiabetic drugs concomitantly. These can be with or without the information of the treating physician (unpublished data). This raises the question about synergistic or antagonistic activities of drug interactions. The concern for drug interaction got substantiated when in one volunteer the bioavailability of metformin was reduced by Ayurvedic powder (Puranik et al., 2014). The KAP survey (knowledge, attitude, and practice) on the management of diabetes and arthritis is currently in progress on patients as well as for traditional Ayurvedic practitioners.

Observational Therapeutics

Observational therapeutics can be defined as an observational study that carefully documents the therapeutic outcomes and novel biodynamic effects of interventions from conventionally practiced therapy. Several modern drug discoveries have their roots in careful follow-up of chance observations in the field, in patients, or in laboratories. The ancient classical literature of Ayurveda, clinical notes, and observations of Ayurvedic experts and recent clinical use provide a goldmine for further drug research through observational therapeutics (Sen and Bose, 1931; Raut, 2010; Pade, 1973; Aushadhi Baad, 1974; Desai, 1928; Vaidya, 1925). There is an urgent need for a strategic plan to organize observational therapeutics at Ayurvedic teaching hospitals so that the experiential knowledge and wisdom of traditional medicine can help to discover and develop Ayurveda-inspired new drugs or new phytoactive chemical scaffolds.

Dr. Rama Vaidya, in her thought leadership article on *Observational Therapeutics: Scope, Challenges and Organization*, has given key messages relevant to finding new approaches for traditional medicine-inspired new drug discovery (Vaidya, 2011). These are as follows:

- "Exclusive hierarchy of randomized controlled trials, along with evidence-based medicine, has largely eclipsed the significance of even valuable observational studies."
- "Observational studies could be judged on the basis of the validity of causal associations on well-defined criteria such as dose-response relationship, temporal sequence, and biological plausibility."
- "Inspirational impact of new hits and leads has to be shared at the institutional morning reports, grand rounds, continued medical education, and widely read journals."
- "A judicious and economical usage of advanced markers necessitates robust thinking of biological plausibility and rational understanding of *Dravya-Guna-Vidnyan* (Ayurvedic pharmacology)."

Ayurvedic pharmacoepidemiology essentially makes an assessment of the field reality and community practices of Ayurveda therapeutics and principles. Such an endeavor should establish communication with research methodologies to bring scientific credibility to these practices and help correct wherever is needed to rationalize the community practices. Observational therapeutics on the other hand could be more focused to the clinical setups. This has the inbuilt advantage of knowledge and wisdom of practicing physicians. Such an endeavor has the potential to identify emerging hits and leads from clinical practices for new drug discovery and development or even for repurposing traditional drugs for new indications.

CLINICAL STUDY DESIGNS AND PARA-CLINICAL MODELS IN REVERSE PHARMACOLOGY

There are three stages of RP: (1) experiential, (2) exploratory, and (3) experimental. The study designs do not follow the conventional Phases 1−3 that's mandatory for NCEs. This is primarily so because in RP one starts at the bedside first. The physician in charge of the patient carries out the experiential studies in the regular clinical practice settings. The treatment given is a standard practice. The added elements are essentially the records of the baseline clinical and laboratory findings/markers that define the therapeutic or adverse response. A Reverse pharmacologist joins the caretaker physician just to ensure that meticulous attention to the minutest details is a mindful and ceaseless activity. For example, in an experiential study of malaria a remedy was given in a dose and form as per the routine. But the temperature and symptoms profile were meticulously recorded and graded. The malarial parasite (MP) count was carried out basally and followed up. The data suggested early response to the crude plant paste from the leaves of a single tree of *Nyctanthes arbor-tristis* as compared to the natural course of clinical malaria (Karnik et al., 2008). The sample size was large and the Ayurvedic literature too suggested usage and activity against malaria. An experiential stage needs to stress good clinical service practice. Whether these can be called trials is a moot point. In a therapeutic setting, the physician has the patient's trust and he or she knows how to monitor them.

During the exploratory studies—human or in vitro/in vivo models—the choice of methods and design has to be relevant to the earlier observations in Stage 1. The designs can involve $N = 1$ studies, human pharmacology (noninvasive methods) for dynamics, dose-searching/dose-finding/dose-optimizing studies with markers of response, pharmacokinetics (if an assay is available), sequential trial design, and an open comparative or cross-over trials can be scheduled, as per the individual intervention and the indication. The standard clinical pharmacology techniques and design will have to be modified and adopted, without the orthodox Phase 1−3 approaches. For example, the plant studied experientially for malaria was subjected to exploratory studies with more frequent temperature (inner ear) measurements.

Besides the MP counts, a PCR for the plasmodial DNA was conducted for the parasite clearance. The markers of severity—inflammatory cytokines such as TNF-α and ILβ1—were measured basally and serially. A disease modifying activity was observed with a faster amelioration of symptoms (Godse, 2004). The plant was extracted with rigorous protocols and active fractions were identified against *Plasmodium falciparum* strains: resistant and sensitive. The fractions were studied in several other in vitro models. The point to notice is that individualization of the designs and models is a crucial dimension of RP.

The experimental and final clinical stage have the rigor that can match that with any NCEs in terms of the proof of the concept of efficacy, safety, and quality. But again only the relevant science is brought to the fore as the usage safety and therapeutic indications were known to start with. The mechanistic studies can be under taken as paraclinical rather than as preclinical studies. The clinical trial designs have to consider the Ayurvedic *pramanas* (*apta, pratyaksha, anumana, upamana,* and *yukti*), besides the statistical considerations; Ayurvedic statistics are being developed for this purpose (Vaidya, 2007). The clinical trials will have robust markers of efficacy and safety as per the interventions and indications. Instead of double-blind trials, double-vision trials are proposed in RP. The phrase "double vision" implies a conscious consideration of factors that influence drug response. The Ayurvedic modifiers of the therapeutic response are to be factored-in rather than lumped-out as confounding variables to be equally distributed in the control and test groups.

The entire thrust has to develop analogue models of what clinical drug actions have been documented. The bedside-to-bench path has this advantage. The data then can be taken back to the bedside for a drug with much more confidence than we do with NCEs as new drugs. The withdrawal of blockbuster drugs has taught us the lesson to go much earlier in humans (Patwardhan, 2008). Sir John Vane, Nobel Laureate, said,

"[R]egrettably there was ample evidence that the time taken from discovery to marketing was lengthening (8−10 years)...but I was aware of at least one instance where it had taken more than 17 years. Clearly there is a need, to conduct the early evaluation of drugs in humans more effectively and more readily."

RP can provide such a new paradigm. Even a pioneer like Bradford Hill said,

"Such personal observations of a handful of patients, acutely made and accurately recorded by the masters of clinical medicine, have been and will continue to be, fundamental to the progress of medicine...We were to use a new drug upon one proven case of acute leukemia and the patient made an immediate and indisputable recovery, should we not have a result of the most profound importance."

AYURVEDA-INSPIRED HITS AND LEADS FOR NEW DRUG DISCOVERIES

Inspirational elements of Ayurveda are driven from its robust fundamental principles and long-standing social acceptance. The core fundamental principles of *yatha-pinde-tatha-brahmande* (microcosm—macrocosm—continuum) and *sharir-satva-atman* (body-mind-spirit) bespeaks of its holistic and integrative approach. Whereas *panchamahabhuta-tridosha-triguna* (five basic elements-three pathophysiological attributes-three psychological attributes) and *hetu-linga-aushadhi* (cause-manifestations-management) indicate a comprehensive and systems theory approach of Ayurveda. The utility and applicability of this traditional healthcare heritage is evident through its live classical texts with editions and commentaries, several therapeutic compendia, clinical notes of masters, and a large community usage in the Indian and south Asian populace.

Sarpagandha (*Rauwalfia serpentina*) was the first Ayurveda-inspired new drug discovery that made a global impact on modern pharmacotherapeutics of hypertension. It was an early example of antecedent preorganized RP inspired from Ayurvedic therapeutics. A Sarpagandha formulation-called Pagal Buti was popularly used by traditional practitioners of Ayurveda for psychiatric indications. The significance of *R. serpentina* as an antihypertensive was appreciated by Vaidya Kaviraj Gananath Sen along with Kartick Chander Bose in the early 1930s (Sen and Bose, 1931). The study demonstrated a reduction in blood pressure and a tranquilizing effect. This was an experience-driven clinical hit. Subsequent studies by Siddiqui and Siddiqui and others were on the phytochemical analysis (Jain and Murthy, 2009). A historical 1949 paper in the British Heart Journal by Rustom Jal Vakil (Vakil, 1949) summed up his 10 years of study with added opinions of some 50 other physicians with rauwolfia in hypertension. The publication led to the drug finally being brought to Western awareness (Gupta, 2002). CIBA scientists isolated reserpine and a global antihypertensive drug was made available.

Arogyavardhini Vati is one of the popular Ayurvedic formulations classically indicated for diverse clinical conditions. However, it is most commonly used for jaundice, along with Punarnavadi Kwath by Ayurveda practitioners of western India. Inspired from this clinical usage, an open-label clinical study was conducted that showed safety and efficacy of this combination in acute viral hepatitis (Antarkar et al., 1978). Subsequently, a well-designed, double-blind, placebo-controlled clinical study was conducted of only Arogyavardhini Vati in acute viral hepatitis in the mid-1970s. This 14-day clinical study in 38 subjects provided convincing evidence for its efficacy in early reduction of liver transaminases as well as clinical morbidity scores (Antarkar et al., 1980). Further from this complex herbo-mineral formulation of Arogyavardhini; Kutaki (Picrorriza kurroa) a 50% content of it was optimized for the phytoactives; picrocide 1 & 2. Such a standardized Kutaki was subjected to placebo-controlled trial that also demonstrated efficacy in viral hepatitis (Vaidya et al., 1996). These clinical hits and leads were studied further in experimental models of liver injury (Shetty et al., 2010).

Atmagupta (*Mucuna pruriens*) contains formulations that are often used in Ayurveda for improving general vitality and as an aphrodisiac. However, repurposing its use for Parkinson's disease (PD) was based on a phytochemical analogy struck by one of the authors (ADBV). PD is a disease of dopamine deficiency in the corpus striatum. *M. pruriens* contains high levels of L-Dopa (Damodaran and Ramaswamy, 1937). With this literature-driven hit, a clinical study of *M. pruriens* in PD was planned. This exploratory clinical study demonstrated the efficacy of *M. pruriens* in PD with concomitant displays of plasma levels of L-dopa. This single open label, but well-organized study, provided an optimized lead (Vaidya et al., 1978). Recently, in a comparative cross-over clinical study with L-dopa-carbidopa combination, *M. pruriens* has shown better safety and efficacy (Katzenschlager et al., 2004). Compliant formulation with reduced bulk and improved palatability remains the main challenge. There are basic studies showing anti-Parkinson's effects with L-Dopa—free extracts of *M. pruriens*.

Amruta (*Tinospora cordifolia*) is considered a *rasayana* (rejuvenative/ reparative) plant in Ayurveda. Initial investigation of this plant was driven by the hint of a conceptual correlation of rasayana with that of immunomodulation (Dahanukar et al., 1988). This plant has been extensively studied experimentally as well as clinically for diverse pharmacological activities, namely, immunomodulatory, antiinflammatory, antiarthritic, antipyretic, hepatoprotective, antidiabetic, antispasmodic, antioxidant, antiallergic, antistress, antileprotic, antimalarial, and antineoplastic activities (Upadhyay et al., 2010; Panchabhai et al., 2008). Several phytoconstituents have been isolated and characterized including seven immunomodulatory compounds (11-hydroxymustakone, *N*-methyl-2-pyrrolidone, *N*-formylannonain, cordifolioside A, magnoflorine, tinocordiside, syringin) characterized from different parts of this plant (Sharma et al., 2012). However, whole plant extracts are used clinically and are commercially available.

Commiphora wightii (Guggulu) is an illustrious plant medicine from Ayurveda that has gone through all three phases of RP: gaining hits from traditional literature, developing into leads through clinical, animal and laboratory studies and eventually became a natural drug available globally for the specific indication of dyslipidemia. However, in a study published in JAMA in 2003 on Guggulipid for the treatment of hypercholesterolemia (a randomized controlled trial), sponsored by the NIH, the results were negative (Szapary et al., 2003). This single negative paper had an adverse impact on the Guggulipid market and also on the interest of scientists and funding agencies in Guggulu. However, at the same time the molecular mechanism of guggulsterones was demonstrated: Guggulu had lipid-lowering activity through antagonizing Farnesoid X receptor (Urizar et al., 2002). Scientists with clinical conviction continued to work on Guggulu/guggulsterones. Over the last few years guggulsterones/Guggulu components are being experimentally explored for diverse pathological conditions, in particular different cancers, inflammatory colon conditions, ophthalmic and ear inflammatory conditions, synovitis, hepatitis, crystal arthropathy, atherosclerosis, endothelial dysfunction, cardiac dysfunction, insulin resistance, metabolic disorders, bacterial infections, skin aging, and so on. While the current interface of Guggulu with basic sciences is opening windows, the true picture is still eluding scientists (Raut and Mertia, 2012).

Several such Ayurvedic plants/formulations have been investigated, which provide hits and leads with prospective new drug discovery/NPs development. Some of the selected plants/formulations are tabulated (Table 4.4).

A clinical research model taking into account the fundamental principles of traditional medicine would appreciate the therapeutic approach of the traditional medical system. At the same time the application of the methods of relevant drug discovery sciences would be most appropriate. The establishment of such evidence would rationalize traditional medical practices. An RP approach is the most suitable to establish such evidence (Vaidya, 2010a). The untapped potential for the new drug discovery from RP and in traditional medicine is immense.

DISCOVERY OF NATURAL PRODUCTS-BASED NEW CHEMICAL ENTITIES VIA CHEMISTRY AND CHEMICAL BIOLOGY TECHNOLOGIES

Introduction and Background

The natural world is a source for inspiration for chemists and biologists, and NPs have long been a source for novel molecules of broad utility. The exquisite and varied architecture of NPs provides a rich palette for discovery. They can be considered "prevalidated by nature," having been optimized for interaction with biological macromolecules through evolutionary selection processes. Besides being useful in their own right, these compounds represent a diverse source of novel, active agents that can serve as leads/scaffolds for elaboration into NCEs for a multitude of explorations.

Embedded in these NPs are a number of diverse, chiral functional groups that are potential sites for protein interactions. Biologically active NPs generally have frameworks with rigid and complex ring structures and precise stereochemical features. This ensures that derivatives from these starting compounds are likely to yield leads with higher specificity and affinity.

TABLE 4.4 Ayurveda-Inspired and Reverse Pharmacology-Driven Hits and Leads

Plants/ Formulations	Indication/Hit	Activity/Lead	Impact
AmrutBhallatak (Raut et al., 2007; Raut et al., 2013) *Semecarpus anacardium* and *Tinospora cordifolia*	Osteoarthritis	Chondroprotection	Disease modifying antiosteoarthritic
Parijat (Godse, 2004) *Nyctanthes arbor-tristis*	Malaria	Antiparasite	Disease modifying
		Anticytokine	Isolation of bioactive fraction
Mamejawa (Vaidya, 2007) *Enicostema littorale*	Type 2 DM	Lipemic control	Prevention of complications
		Antioxidant	
		DNA protection	
		Glycemic control	
Panchavalkal (Joshi et al., 2007) (five barks)	Wound healing	Vaginal infections	Ayurvedic topical products in market
	Leucorrhoea	Burns wounds	
Ashoka (Shringi, 2000) *Saraca asoca*	Menorrhagia	Ovulatory dysfunctional uterine bleeding	Menorrhagia subset identification
Haridra (Hastak et al., 1997; Joshi et al., 2011) *Curcuma longa*	Oral-submucus fibrosis	Micronuclei reduction in oral smear	Anticancer studies, studies in neurodegenerative disorders
	Cervical precancer	Reduction in persistent cervical precancer	
	Antiaging	Hippocampal neurogenesis	
Shunthi (Altman and Marcussen, 2001; White, 2007) *Zingiber officinalis*	Nausea, vomiting, arthritis	Antiemetic, antiinflammatory, and antiarthritic	High evidence of efficacy levels

Ashok Vaidya et al., in their seminal studies (Patwardhan et al., 2008; Vaidya, 2014), have demonstrated that many modern drugs and agrochemicals have their origin in ethnopharmacology and traditional medicine. Ayurvedic and traditional Chinese systems are living "great traditions." Traditional knowledge and experiential databases can provide new functional leads to reduce time, expense, and toxicity—the three main hurdles. Thus, the normal discovery course of "lab to utility" actually becomes "utility to lab"—a true reversed design approach.

The enthusiasm for NP discovery is dampened by difficult syntheses. A significant disadvantage of NPs, with the exception of those derived from fermentation, is the draconian organic synthesis/medicinal chemistry effort required for commercialization or future functionalization. In many cases, the NP is not available in sufficient quantities for various biological assays, thereby limiting their exploration.

Chemical space must be expanded efficiently. The ability to easily access new chemical space is a major challenge for discovery chemists. Although advances in parallel synthesis/combinatorial chemistry and diversity-oriented synthesis have made great strides towards expanding the accessibility of synthetic compounds that have high levels of diversity (including stereochemical, shape, and bond connectivity), there is room for further improvement. The diversity expansion inherent in transformations that mimic the metabolism of small molecules and NPs can provide a new direction. Simple and well-controlled oxidation, halogenation, and alkylation reactions can afford compounds that have unique physicochemical and biological properties. Indeed, Muller has opined that such biotransformations are the source of remarkable levels of diversity in NPs and investigational agents (Müller, 2004).

Chemists prefer known and reliable chemistry. Despite possessing an enviable armamentarium of techniques and methodologies in organic synthesis, chemists often prefer to focus on the simplest, most robust (and therefore commonly used) transformations. This is driven by premium demands on efficiency and creativity. As a result, much of the emphasis in industrial research involves the study of molecules that can easily be made, rather than on those agents that properly address the question but require significant synthetic innovation, isolation, and synthesis of indigenous NPs and their derivatives. Several plants have been used in traditional Ayurveda and Siddha medicine; the NPs have demonstrated or have been ascribed medicinal value after years of experience. The latest techniques in systems biology and RP can be used to isolate and characterize the bioactive agents and generate key scaffolds with chirality. These architectures have hitherto not been used in discovery chemistry. The need of the hour is to derive inspiration from the wisdom of Mother Nature to reconfigure products into chemical hybrid "molecular legos" and to screen the deck of diverse compounds against targets. Recently, the concept of hybrid molecules has gained currency. Coupling of diverse molecules such as artemisinin and chloroquine with vitamin K3 have generated new molecules with effectiveness in oncology. In addition to diversifying the structure of single molecules, the properties of several NPs can be modulated by such hybrids.

Current chemical investigations center on: (1) expansion of the already known activities of NPs derived from RP by selective functionalization, generation, and derivatization of privileged structures and conducting selective studies; (2) designed organic synthesis of high-recognition libraries focused on specific biological targets; and (3) synthesis of building blocks/scaffolds/high-value intermediates.

We have a repository of molecules that contains:

- Six hundred scaffolds/building blocks derived from purification of extracts from the top 100 medicinally useful plants that have been used in Ayurveda, yoga, Yunani, Siddha, and homeopathy.
- Nearly 1000 pharmaceuticals that are currently available free of patents. These allopathic drugs range from acyclovir to ciprofloxacin to roxithromycin and sidenafil.
- Nearly 2500 intermediates from which the above drugs have been synthesized by nonpatent infringing processes. These molecules are drug-like but, on the whole, have not been tested in the West.

Chemists are actively engaged in the development and streamlining of chemical technologies that enable the transformation of NPs and their derivatives from this repository directly to NP-derived new chemical entities. A collection of existing and novel oxidation approaches that are capable of robustly and predictably converting functionality typically found in the specific classes of NPs are used. These oxidations include metalloporphyrin-mediated oxidations, hepatocyte oxidations, salen-based oxidants, and halogenation reactions. Key automated platform technologies to streamline the application of these oxidation chemistries en masse to NP collections are being deployed. Such technologies include flow chemistry (Ley, Jones), development of new resin-bound reagents (Ley), microwave chemistry (Jones), autopurification (Jones), and automated structure elucidation (Jas and Kirschning, 2003; Sedelmeier et al., 2009; Gedye et al., 1986; Caddick, 1995; Kappe, 2004; Torregrossa et al., 2006; Collins, 2010; de la Hoz et al., 2005; Huber and Jones, 1992; Jones and Chapman, 1993).

Isolation of Natural Products from Plant Species with Established Indian Folk Medicine Properties

Chorghade's discovery approach utilizes biologically active NPs integrated with an established, efficient synthesis toolbox. Our unique access to discovery and development quantities of isolated NPs with known biological activity is an asset. We use a modified bioassay-guided fractionation approach wherein a high throughput separation chemistry approach (using the parallel high-performance liquid chromatography (HPLC) "Sepbox" technology, Sepiatec, Inc.) is coupled with cell-based bioassays to detect and identify putative compounds that offer promise of bioactivity. A significant advantage is that in addition to fast separation and isolation of active fractions, the cell-based phenotypic effects will allow emphasis on bioactive samples.

Some active fractions (possessing other putative biological activities) might be eliminated due to their lack of effect in the assays coupled to fractionation; subsequent testing of these fractions in other phenotypic assays and follow-up of structural identification work will isolate the full spectrum of these bioactive compounds.

Sample Collection

Plant sample collection is an important aspect of NP drug discovery, since the secondary metabolites are formed under certain macro and/or micro environments.

Fractionation

NP drug discovery is always a challenge. The "Sepbox" provides a novel high-throughput approach to support fractionation and subsequent identification of compounds within the fraction. The Sepbox concept is based on a patented combination of HPLC and solid phase extraction (SPE). Using two-dimensional separation, the recovery rate for both polar and nonpolar substances is usually above 90 percent. Using an automated and highly reproducible process, one extract can be completely separated in one day. The pure individual components are solubilized in suitable solvents and collected in microtiter plates or vials. The compounds collected in microtiter plates can be used directly for assaying or can be used as a master plate for making HTS assay plates. Up to 600 fractions with a very high yield of pure compounds can be efficiently obtained to be used in subsequent screenings.

Fractions are evaluated contemporaneously via HPLC/UV/LC-MS and LC-MS-MS detection for chemical composition. The usual spectroscopic tools, FTIR, NMR, CMR, and MALDI-TOF, are used for structure elucidation and characterization. Chiral HPLC ascertains the stereochemical configuration with additional derivatization, as needed.

Design and Synthesis of Natural Product Analogs (McNamara et al., 2002; Sanchez-Martin et al., 2004; Baxendale et al., 2006)

Antimalarial lactones: Secondary metabolites isolated from *Cordeceps militaris* have received attention due to their unique structures and specific biological activities (Fig. 4.2). Compound A was isolated as a white solid from *C. militaris* BCC 2816; the structure was elucidated and the stereochemistry confirmed by spectral data and X-ray crystallographic analysis. Some natural

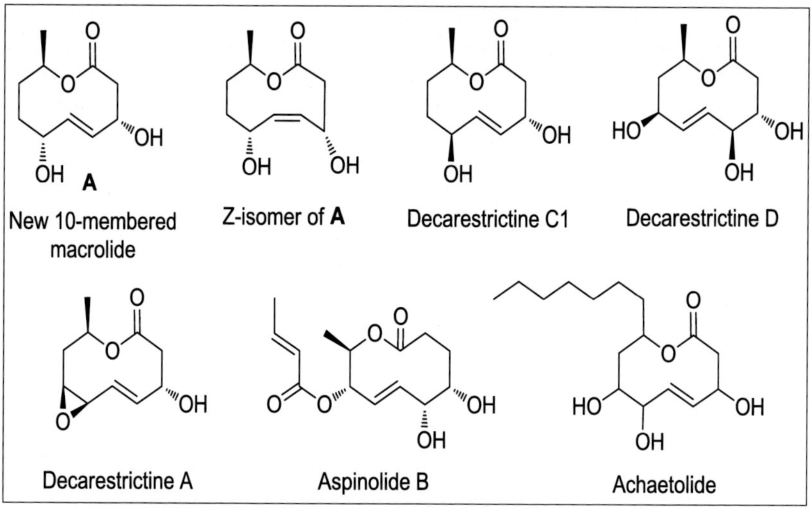

FIGURE 4.2   Natural products derived from *Cordyceps militaris*.

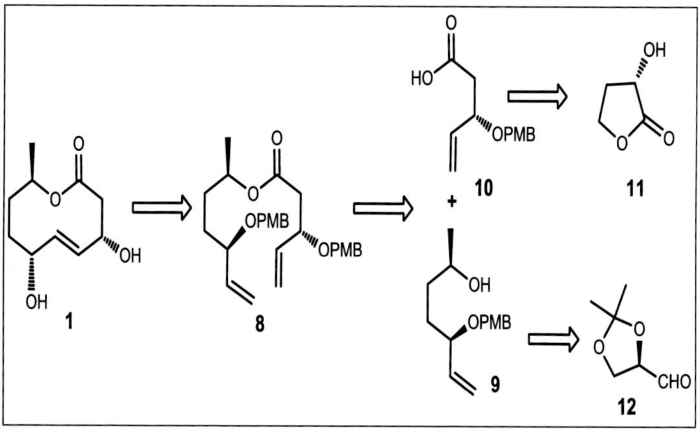

SCHEME 4.1   Retrosynthesis of compound A.

nonenolides possess chiral centers on both sides of a double bond. These have a variety of biological activities ranging from antidiabetic to cholesterol lowering to antileishmanial. The compounds enumerated above could serve as scaffolds that could be elaborated into a variety of applications.

In a collaborative program, with Professors Grubbs and Goddard (California Institute of Technology) on the synthesis of natural lactones that employs ring-closing metathesis (RCM) as key step, Chorghade et al. Mohapatra et al. (2007) devised a stereoselective synthesis of nonenolide (Scheme 4.1). Conventional wisdom held that the stereochemistry of ring-closing metatheses could not be accurately predicted for 8-, 9-, and 10-membered ring lactones. The macrolactonization step relies on a RCM on a diolefinic ester. Strategic bond disconnection in ester 8 leads to chiral, nonracemic fragments 9 and 10 that could be derived from (S)-α-hydroxy-γ-butyrolactone 11 and 1, 2-*O*-isopropylidene (D)-glyceraldehyde 12, respectively. Ester 8 was subjected to RCM reactions in two different sequences: First, the RCM reaction was conducted on the protected species; deprotection yielded a preponderance of the E-isomer. Deprotection, followed by RCM, yielded a preponderance of the Z-isomer. Extensive density functional theory calculations conclusively identified a pivotal role for the protecting groups in directing the stereochemistry of ring closure. The work was instrumental in the elucidation of some specific rules about stereochemical requirements for olefin metathesis.

REVERSE PHARMACOLOGY AND NEW DOMAINS IN LIFE SCIENCES

Once the active NCEs have been isolated from a NP after meticulous RP, many synthetic and analytical techniques can be explored to expand the scope with the naturally available chirality and diversity of these molecules. Extrapolations to pharmaceuticals, agrochemicals, and cosmoceuticals are feasible. Representative new technologies are enumerated below.

Automated Oxidation Chemistry for Diversified Analogues

Chorghade, Dolphin, and colleagues (Andersen et al., 1994; Chorghade et al., 1996a, b; Hill et al., 1996) have developed novel sterically protected and electronically activated porphyrin mediated catalytic oxidation of sophisticated molecular entities and have designed numerous practical and efficacious methods of synthesizing porphyrins with halogens at the ortho-aryl and also the pyrrole positions and central metal atoms such as magnesium, manganese, and ruthenium in the macrocycle. Traditional porphyrins suffer very rapid oxidative degradation and dimerization; the catalytic turnovers and reaction rates are very low. These catalysts have turnover numbers in excess of 100,000 and are extremely stable.

The methodologies have been used to achieve epoxidation, hydroxylation, and *N*-demethylation on numerous targets including functionalized NP substrates; the N and S oxides are also obtained. The oxidation procedure is extremely facile as compared to the biochemical and enzymatic processes. Exogenous cooxidants such as iodosobenzene, cumene hydroperoxide, hydrogen peroxide, or sodium hypochlorite were used; substrates were stirred for one to six hours at ambient temperatures. Products were separated by a combination of HPLC and preparative Thin layer chromatography. A library of compounds, when subjected to porphyrin-mediated oxidation, yield a substantially larger number of compounds. This then provides new compounds that are more polar, water soluble, and contain handles for further derivatization. RP-based new phytoactives can be subjected to the methodologies (*vide supra*) to expand the library of molecules with drug-like activities, as earlier shown, clinically, with parent molecules.

Transformations in this platform have two ultimate outcomes: (1) modification of lipophilicity: small changes in lipophilicity of a lead molecule provide compounds with significantly different physicochemical and biological properties and (2) enabling rapid compound follow-up: a significant consideration is the amenability of the scaffold for rapid evolution. In addition, installation of a functional group easily transformed into a radiolabel provides rapid inroads to crucial imaging experiments. The likely conversion of rolipram into hydroxylated analogs via oxidation chemistry could make these molecules susceptible to a tosylation/fluorination sequence for installation of ^{18}F for PET or ^{123}I for SPECT imaging.

Similar strategies can be applied to NPs with established biological targets to probe pathways and potentially uncover new analogs with refined properties. Consider the antitumor agent alkaloid camptothecin, isolated from *Camptotheca acuminata*. Targets of this storied agent include the regulatory enzyme topoisomerase I and hypoxia inducible factor 1 [HIF-1α]. This compound exists in the hemiaminal form, and Jones (Torregrossa et al., 2006; Collins, 2010; de la Hoz et al., 2005; Huber and Jones, 1992; Jones and Chapman, 1993; Jones and Mathews, 1997; LaBeaume et al., 2010b) has shown that by using microwave-mediated methods, a facile conversion to derivatives of 5-amino CPT can be effected (Jones). A 5-fluoroethyl derivative shows superior HIF-1α inhibition than CPT, warranting an in-depth synthesis and screening program. Additionally, microwave-mediated fluorination methods would seem to be suited to formation of 5-F and, using radiolabeled fluoride, the corresponding ^{18}F derivative to permit PET imaging for distribution studies. DNA repair enzymes are a target of CPT; another option could include conversion to GlcNAc and other carbohydrate derivatives using established glycosylation coupling chemistries (Ma et al., 2009; Dong et al., 2008; Kallmerten and Jones, 2010; Labeaume et al., 2010a) (Scheme 4.2). Myriad other NP platforms are amenable to selective oxidation chemistry (LaBeaume et al., 2009; Peddibhotla et al., 2007). The bicyclic sesquiterpene caryophyllene, recently identified as a ligand for the cannabinoid CB2 receptor, has folk medicinal applications as an analgesic and antiinflammatory agent. Selective allylic oxidation would allow conversion to a number of derivatives of increasing complexity and differing lipophilicity and transport properties. This could include conversion to a PEGylated analogue, fluorination in order to study metabolic profiles and with labeled [^{18}F, ^{123}I] versions, molecular imaging (Scheme 4.3). Jones employed microwave-mediated Johnson-orthoester Claisen rearrangement on the derivative (Jones et al., 1993). The resulting ester, when subjected to

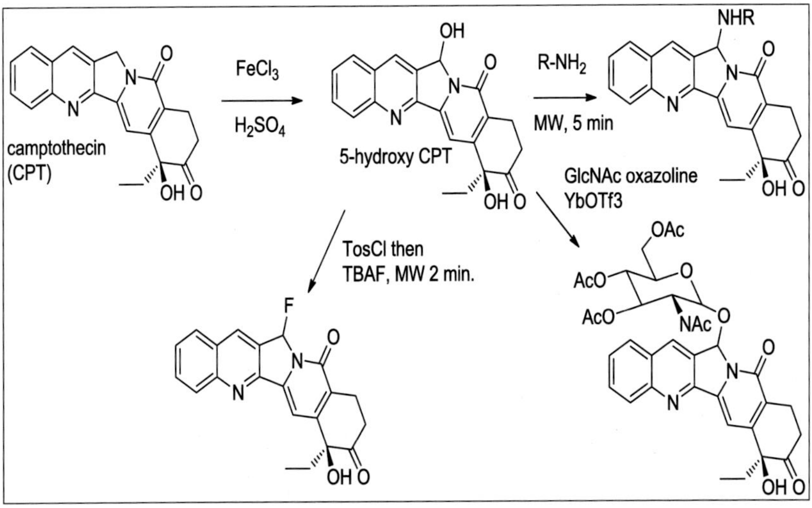

SCHEME 4.2   Hydroxylated CPT derivatives as platforms to substituted analogues and probes of CPT function.

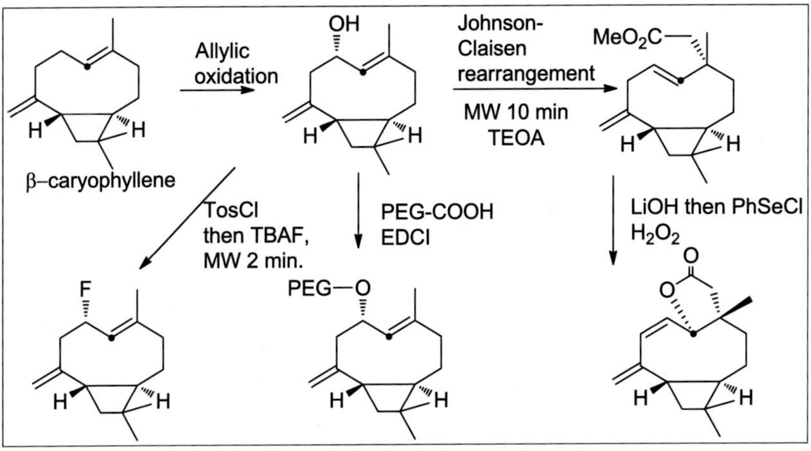

SCHEME 4.3   Selective oxidative strategies en route to beta-caryophyllene derivatives.

selenolactonization, yielded the cyclic lactone derivatives. Given the abundance of cyclic lactones in terpene derived NPs, this could open up new avenues of research in their relevant biochemical pathways and targets.

REVERSE PHARMACOLOGY APPROACH TO GPCR-FOCUSED DRUG DISCOVERY

Bennett et al. (Bennett et al., 2013), in Molecular Pharmacology, describes how RP, enabled by Heptares Therapeutics StaR(R) technology, can be applied to and accelerate GPCR-based drug discovery. The authors studied isolated GPCRs locked in conformations that correspond to agonist or antagonist pharmacology, and elucidated 3D structures. These StaRs and structures were used to select and design compounds with specific pharmacologies such as inverse agonist, partial agonist or full agonist, based on their ability to bind differentially to the agonist and antagonist StaRs.

Finally, new techniques are also used for the standardization and characterization of herbal remedies that are sold as supplements and are contaminated with unlisted ingredients that could pose health risks to consumers. Scientists will now use advanced DNA testing to authenticate all of the plants that are used in its store-brand herbal supplements, and extensively test the products for common allergens like tree nuts, soy, and wheat.

Reverse Pharmacology and Novel Biodynamic Actions

Bedside observations of patients or field observations of people have often identified novel effects of foods, plants, and drugs. The majority of such astute observations are often serendipitous and frequently not followed up scientifically. The organized system of Ayurveda and TCM, as practiced currently, offer unprecedented opportunities for both serendipitous as well as planned records of novel drug effects. Several disciplines of life sciences can be traced back to their roots in novel human biodynamic actions. RP is a multisystem path for a scientific pursuit of such actions. For example, the trichomes of the fruits of *Mucuna pruriens* induces intense itching when in contact with skin. We had studied the scanning electronic microscopic view of the trichome (Fig. 4.3). The trichome was a hollow tube with miniscule reversed hooks on its surface. This structure opened up the field of investigations into the mechanism of pruritus vis-à-vis mast cell degranulation. This would probably enhance the field of mechanistic understanding of allergic urticaria and itching. Another plant, *Gymnema sylvestre*, relieves trichome-induced itching (Vaidya, 1910). RP of this plant would open up the potential for novel phytoactive antipruritic agents.

Ayurveda has given central importance for health on the functional competence of gastrointestinal tract and digestion. Long before the human microbiome revolution occurred, the central attention to Panchakarma (five purifications) was primarily on the digestive tract. The demonstration of the relief in bronchial asthma accompanied by an increase in FEV1 by a Panchakarma—Vamana (medically supervised emesis) was a unique contribution (Dahanukar and Thatte, 1997). Clinically, antiinflammatory plants of Ayurveda like *Boswellia serrata* have shown clinical relief in Crohn's disease (Gerhardt et al., 2001). Chronic smoldering inflammation of the gastrointestinal tract is emerging as a common substratum for diabesity, metabolic syndrome, rheumatoid arthritis, and cancer (Vaidya et al., 2008). RP of

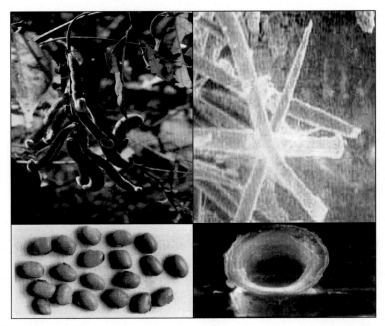

FIGURE 4.3 *Mucuna pruriens* legumes, seeds, and trichomes (under Scanning Electron Microscope).

Panchakarma and Ayurvedic antiinflammatory drugs could open up a novel field for a mechanistic understanding of the aforesaid clinical conditions.

UNIQUE DIMENSIONS OF AYURVEDA THERAPEUTICS

Nanaushadhibhutam Jagati Kinchitdravyam Upalabhyate I
Tam Tam Yuktam Artham Cha Tam Tam Abhipretya II

(Charak Su. 26-12)

"There is no substance in the world which cannot serve as medicine through intelligent application. Ayurveda has always cherished such a broad vision for resourcing medicinal substances for its therapeutics" (Joshi, 2003).

Ayurvedic therapeutics (*chikitsa*) is generally classified as *daivya-vyapashraya* (divine therapies: inclusive of wearing precious stones, reciting prayers, chanting mantras, performing homa-havan, etc.), *yuktivyapashraya* (rational therapies: based on logistics of therapeutic principles), and *satvava-jaya* (mindfulness: yoga and meditation). However, the current mainstream Ayurveda practice primarily adheres to the tenets of *yuktivyapashraya chikitsa*. The therapeutic principles for management logistically involve the reversal of pathogenesis that takes into account *nidana parivarjana* (avoiding causative and precipitating factors), *sanshamana chikitsa* (restoration of

TABLE 4.5 Classical Management Approach in Ayurveda	
Aahara (diet regimen)	*Hitahara* (healthy diet)
	Mitahara (moderate diet)
Vihara (self-efficacy)	*Achara* (behavioral and lifestyle management)
	Vichara (psychological construct)
	Vyayama (physical exercise)
Aushadhi (medical)	*Bheshaja* (pharmacotherapy)
	Yantra-shastra (physical/surgical therapy)

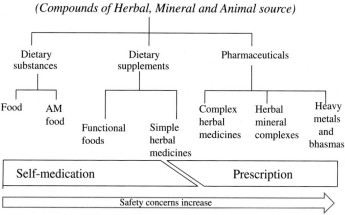

(Compounds of Herbal, Mineral and Animal source)

Plants form important ingredient across the ayurvedic drugs spectrum.
AM food: Ayurvedically modified food, e.g., milk processed with turmeric

FIGURE 4.4   Spectrum of ayurvedic drugs.

physiological homeostasis), *sanshodhana chikitsa* (detoxification procedures for harmonizing human system) and *rasayana chikitsa* (rejuvenative and reparative medicine). The actual clinical management implementation includes *ahar* (diet regimen), *vihar* (self-efficacy), and aushadhi (medical management). Table 4.5 depicts the subclasses of Ayurveda's classical management approach (Raut and Gundeti, 2014).

Pharmacotherapeutics in Ayurveda covers a broad spectrum of drugs: simple kitchen remedies, complex herbo-mineral formulations, preparations of metals, and animal products (Fig. 4.4). However, for this chapter we shall restrict our discussion to herb-based medicines. In Ayurveda, the plant kingdom has been explored for medicinal uses in great depth since ancient times. In the adoptive age, medicines were used in their available natural form; in the cultural period, there was an adaptive age with the art of pharmacy making modifications in the NPs. Thereafter was the creative age, with the analysis and synthesis of the active plant constituents (Parikh, 1992). During this evolutionary progression of Ayurveda, diverse concepts and subbranches were established. The concept of *guna* essentially constitutes the physical/ chemical properties of the material such as density, viscosity, dispersibility, flow properties, etc. (Vaidya, 1992). The concepts of *rasa* (taste), *veerya* (anabolic/catabolic properties), *vipak* (metabolite taste), and *prabhav* (unique efficiency) cover the biodynamic effects of medicinal plant/product. The subbranch of *aushadhi-nirman* and *bhaishajya-kalpana* deals with manufacturing and pharmaceutical developments, whereas the branch of *dravya-guna-karma* deals with Ayurvedic pharmacology.

Much importance is attributed to the habitat, season, and time of collection of medicinal plant material. These factors would influence the concentrations of the phytoconstituents and the methods of collection, preservation, and manufacturing would influence the quality besides the activity of the product (Sharma and Dash, 1985). The aphorism *sanskaro hi gunantaradhanam uchyate* indicates the significance of diverse processes during manufacturing which influences enhancing/modulating of activity and reducing/subduing of toxicity. *Piper longum* is one of the most commonly used ingredients in Ayurvedic formulation. *Chausashti pimpali* is a unique preparation where seed powder of the plant is triturated in its own decoction for specific number of times and duration. This unique preparation is indicated for children for their recurrent respiratory ailments. It has been demonstrated that such a classical method of processing affects the *piperine* content of the product (Raut, 1992).

Besides the aforementioned factors, the product-related attributes such as *ayurvedeeya kalpa* (dosage form), *aushadhi prayoga* (dosage regimen), *aushadhi kala* (dosage schedule), *anupana* (vehicle for administration), and *aharvihar* (concomitant diet and lifestyle regimen) are considered as significant determinants for the therapeutic outcome. Guggulu formulations are very popular amongst Ayurvedic practitioners and used in diverse dosage forms as well as in different combinations with other plants for pertinent clinical conditions (Apte, 1988). *Vardhamanprayoga* is one of the distinctive methods recommended where the drug is initiated with a minimal dose and then gets gradually increased to the maximum tolerable dose; it is then subsequently reduced gradually in a reverse order to the minimum the dose it started with. Such cycles of dosage regimen are repeated a number of times depending on the indications and the formulation used. Different dosage schedules and dose administrations recommended in Ayurveda appear to address the facilitation of absorption, drug-food interactions, and biorhythms. Diverse vehicles are identified along with the drug administration for specific indication. To illustrate: the Bhallatak formulation, when studied for its long-term safety profile, demonstrated no mortality in the group of animals that received milk as a vehicle, whereas other groups had severe toxicity (Dineshkumar and Shashikeran, 2008).

A profound aphorism from Ayurveda states *chikitsa nasti shuddhastu yo anyamanyam udiriyet*, which means the therapy that gives rise to another disease is not a pure and proper one.

ORGANIZATION FOR ACADEMIC DEVELOPMENT OF REVERSE PHARMACOLOGY

RP has emerged as a transdiscipline for more productive drug discovery and cost-effective development. The term underlines two important points: it adheres to the core principles of pharmacology and it provides a different perspective in its approach to drug discovery. This different bedside perspective values a human-centric approach over a techno-centric one. It also proposes therapy-centric attention over pharmaco-centric (Raut et al., 2012). The lack of an organized RP approach has delayed by decades the development of new drugs from existing therapeutic experience. Structural and functional organization, multisystem, and multidisciplinary faculty, and an appropriately placed academic location are essential for the growth and development of the new transdiscipline, RP (Raut and Vaidya, 2011).

The organization of RP will have to maintain dynamism, flexibility, and a progressive approach to adopt and assimilate relevant scientific and technological advancements along with the due cognition of a rich, untapped heritage. The personnel involved would have to have state-of-the art skills and knowledge, but it is more important to have an appropriate attitude. Clinicians would necessarily have to evolve as adepts-physician-scientists/vaidya-scientists (Vaidya, 2010b), and the basic scientists, working in laboratories, would have to be more aware of the clinical relevance and applications of their R&D at patients' bedsides. Optimum product standardization and ethical approvals are the prerequisites for RP studies. The expertise and infrastructure needed are mandatory in RP organization. Other valuable infrastructural setups in RP are multisystem research-based clinics, clinical laboratories with specialty research laboratories, human pharmacology units, Ayur- and pharmaco-informatics, documentation and administrative units. Project-specific and need-based consultations and collaborations with specialists of diverse domains have to be explored and encouraged strongly. Table 4.6 depicts structural and functional elements for the organization of RP.

The path of RP is now internationally pursued (Aggarwal et al., 2011), explored (Willcox et al., 2011), and acknowledged (Raut and Chorghade, 2014). Experiential, exploratory, and experimental domains of RP may have academic locations at different national/international institutions. A robust coordination of team and networking by strong leaders are necessary across institutions. The academic location may even be placed in an individual clinic/laboratory/community setup, provided the individual has internalized and grasped the RP organization and has constant linkages and networking with the advanced center of RP. A larger impact of RP and its long-term

TABLE 4.6 Structural and Functional Elements for Organization of Reverse Pharmacology

Structural Organization	Functional Organization
State of the art integrative research clinics	Effective networking and collaborations
Research laboratories for exploratory studies	Liaison with regulatory agencies
Pharmacy unit for product standardization	Intersystem ethics committee approvals
Human pharmacology unit for dynamic/kinetic studies	Integrative research advisory committee/review board
Animal house essentially for safety pharmacology	Regular interactive scientific sessions for debate & discussions
Major hospital and pharma sector for large scale experiments	Dialogue and interviews of traditional healers
Documentation cell with health care informatics	Visits and excursions to biodiversity spots

sustenance demand well-structured and diligently organized training modules. The Medical Research Center of Kasturba Health Society, which is also an ICMR's Advanced Center for RP had organized a two-week ICMR workshop for training in RP from March 26 to April 9, 2011.

Cognizing of the multisystem-multidisciplinary and integrative nature of the RP training program, and appreciation of the importance and significance of such a program for traditional medical research, inspired Vice Chancellor of Maharashtra University of Health Sciences (MUHS), Dr. Arun Jamkar, to announce a Fellowship Program in RP and Drug Development (FRPDD) under the aegis of MUHS. Two of the authors, AAR and ABDV, spearheaded the preparation of the syllabus. A one-year curriculum was prepared by inviting the inputs from individuals/institutions actively engaged in Ayurveda, natural product-research, and drug development. The curriculum proposed has been approved by board of studies of MUHS. The training module gives more importance to active learning over passive training and is intended to develop appropriate attitude, skills, and knowledge in RP and drug discovery. It is expected that these trainees would eventually devise innovations in healthcare research and in methodology of translational research at the interface of Ayurveda and the basic sciences. The early training of the faculty is already in progress. However, having a suitable and eligible multisystem and multidisciplinary faculty is a challenge. In the absence of standard reference book, an anthology of RP publications is in process and an outline of a textbook on RP is ready.

Finally, regular and periodical training through workshops/postdoctoral fellowship programs in RP and eventual transformation and implementations of RP principles and methodologies by trained participants would determine the futuristic spread, growth and development of RP.

CHALLENGES AND OPPORTUNITIES IN REVERSE PHARMACOLOGY

The fact is that the transdiscipline of RP has grown in the milieu of Ayurveda and that too in India; Ayurveda as an organized system of health-care is neither globally known nor understood. As a consequence, the multinational companies, wedded to the reductionist paradigm of drug discovery, find it difficult to comprehend how RP applied to Ayurveda can be a productive path for new drugs. Ayurveda is not merely an ancient system of health irrelevant to modernity. Ayurveda is still used by 70 percent of 1.25 billion Indians—a vast potential field for novel biodynamic effects. The fundamental principles and practices of Ayurveda are so profound that even its cursory study would convince any open-minded person to mine its wisdom. However, there is no doubt about the stupendous advances that have transformed allopathy into modern medicine. As a result, modern medicine has developed the hubris due to its high-tech success. The humility that allowed Edward Jenner to listen to a milkmaid who said that cowpox prevents smallpox is rare to find (Riedel, 2005). Much hubris prevents a study of the Sanskrit texts of Ayurveda. There is a selective amnesia that most modern drugs owe their success to their origin from NPs. But humility, amidst unprecedented technical progress, is rarely acquired. Dobree puts it well: "It is difficult to be humble. Even if you aim at humility, there is no guarantee that when you have attained the state you will not be proud of the fact." The challenge can be addressed, partly, by some examples of successful products developed through RP for unmet medical needs. The recent Nobel Prize in Medicine received by Professor Tu Youyou is an apt example that illustrates the need for attention to the approach of RP, notwithstanding the long delay from usage in TCM to a global drug (The 2015 Nobel Prize in Physiology or Medicine - Press Release). However, the Nobel committee has stated clearly that the prize is not the recognition for TCM. This is a bit unfortunate because a long usage of a plant in TCM/Ayurveda with clinically proven efficacy and safety is also a major contribution in therapeutics. We observed antimalarial and disease modifying activity with *Nyctanthes arbotristis* at an Ayurvedic hospital with state-of-the art response markers (Godse, 2004). It is suggested that such an interface research in RP would not lead to opportunity loss or long delays in discovering globally relevant natural drugs from ancient systems of medicine.

The irony is that the traditional eminence-based mindset in Ayurveda is late in adopting biomedical advances and technology that are congruent with its basic principles but are badly needed for patient care. This wariness and phobia of advanced technologies also carries over to the relevant science and techniques used by RP. It appears alien to the Ayurvedic faculty with an eminence-based mindset. Among them, there is an element of ancestral vainglory and complacency that prevents them from grasping the opportunities RP offers for evidence-based Ayurveda. This is an even greater challenge than the ones posed by modern medicine. This is primarily so because the experiential robust documentation of hits, at the bedside, is within their domain. In India, a novel initiative has been taken to train and develop vaidya-scientists (Patwardhan et al., 2011). The returns are remarkable, as vaidya-scientists are competent to engage in RP and scientific research with a high motivation.

Another major challenge for RP is its need of a transsystem clinical and basic infrastructure, with a state-of-the art capability to develop a new drug from a clinical hit. Currently, there is a separate Ministry of AYUSH established by the government of India. It is hoped that with this empowerment the public perception of AYUSH will hopefully change, by a judicious adoption of science and technology compatible with fundamentals of Ayurveda (Patwardhan, 2015). There are hardly any integrated medicine departments in India. There is more hope for RP from the universities abroad where many medical colleges do have Departments of Complementary and Alternative Medicine. It is desirable that these departments, in collaboration with their clinical pharmacology units, develop training and research in RP. As most of these colleges do not allow Ayurveda, their chances of getting clinical hits and leads are meager. But there is a vast potential of paraclinical studies for the leads and candidate NPs already discovered in India. Table 4.7 lists some such plants and the relevant experiments for correlates.

The biggest challenge facing a serious enterprise in RP is the mindless marketing of the Ayurvedic and Chinese medicines as over-the-counter DS in the West. These are marketed without any regulatory approvals and with all sorts of claims for health. As a consequence, when scientific evidence generated by RP is presented, the earlier noise in the marketplace affects the credibility of new data. In India, we have taken care of the proper categorization of natural drugs into three groups with their respective standards and regulatory guidelines: (1) Ayurvedic, Siddha, and Unani drugs under AYUSH; (2) phytopharmaceuticals under the drug controllers; and (3) food supplements (ayurceuticals) under Food Safety and Standards Authority of India (FSSAI). This clarity offers unprecedented opportunities to discover and develop, through RP, a remedy under a specific category.

FUTURE DIRECTION AND SCOPE OF DIFFERENTIATION IN REVERSE PHARMACOLOGY

RP, being a very new paradigm, has to face a degree of uncertainty as to its future direction. The analogy of RP to clinical pharmacology would serve as

TABLE 4.7 Opportunities for Reverse Pharmacology Correlates
(Vaidya, A.D.B., 2006; 2010b)

Ayurvedic Drug	Medicinal Plant	Demonstrated Action	Para-Clinical Studies
Arogyawardhani	Picrorhiza kurroa	Hydro-choleretic	Gallstone prevention
Kapikachhupak	Mucuna pruriens	Antiparkinson	Neuroplasticity
Amrutbhallatak	Semicarpus anacardium	Antiarthritic	Chondrocyte stem cells
Asthisandhanak	Cissus quadrangularis	Fracture-healing	Hydroxyapatite laying
Chashashth pippali	Piper longum	Antiasthmatic	LTB-4 antagonist
Ashokarishta	Saraca asoca	Antimenorrhagic	Vascular stability
Ashwagandharishta	Withania somnifera	Anticancer	Immune surveillance
Rasavanti	Berberis aristata	Antiglaucoma	Less intraocular pressure

signpost for an appropriate direction to this new transdiscipline. Clinical pharmacology actually evolved as human pharmacology for studying effects of drugs on human body and what the human organism does to the drugs. Unfortunately, rather than growing as a discovery transdiscipline which would enrich human biology, clinical pharmacology was grabbed and dwarfed by the drug industry. As a consequence, it is sad that it got restricted to Phase I to Phase IV trials. The vast potential of clinical pharmacology was thwarted. For the future direction of RP we have to be cautious that the transdiscipline would be adopted, expanded, and made fruitful by an active collaboration of drug discovery scientists from academia and industry.

The very transdisciplinary nature of RP necessitates its development as an academic endeavor. The initiation of RP being at the bedside, excellent and state-of-the art clinical facilities is at its core of development. The inspirational roots of RP also lie in robust traditions of Ayurveda, TCM, etc.; hence, it is desirable that teaching hospitals of these systems provide a base for observational therapeutics and experiential studies (Vaidya, 2010a; Vaidya and Raut, 2006). Bridges will have to be built with super-specialty clinical research units for relevant human exploratory studies. These units should have linkage with experimental/cellular/biochemical pharmacology for pursuing the clinical hits and leads in appropriate in vitro and in vivo models. Besides the stress on novel clinical pharmacodynamic data providing hits and leads, RP can open up new domains in human biology. Such new generalization at human level could lead to an impact on the cumulative reductionist data from life sciences.

RP has a vast scope for differentiation and emergence of unique specialties. It cannot be overemphasized that clinical and therapeutic freedom and pluralism would provide a rich field for fertile hits and leads of novel biodynamic effects. However, the current undue stress on evidence-based medical practice has often limited the chance of serendipitous discoveries and their follow up. Ayurvedic epistemology has a clarity and simplicity that permits pluralistic therapeutic approaches. The latter are primarily concerned with the reversal of pathogenesis in an individual patient. The training and development of vaidya-scientists, as a specialty, was intended to equip the faculty with a strong foundation in *shastra* and a deep acquaintance in life sciences (Vaidya, 2010b). This would be the front-line differentiated specialty needed in RP. This group would generate hits in experiential stage of RP. For in-depth exploratory studies, objective variables of clinical/laboratory markers are most vital. Noninvasive clinical methods, current biochemical/immune/microbial/molecular markers, and imaging/scopy techniques are essential for the documentation (Hastak et al., 1997; Joshi et al., 2004, 2011; Sheth et al., 2006; Godse et al., 2011). In the future, laboratory medical scientists who focus on RP studies would emerge as investigative reverse pharmacologists. The paraclinical in vitro and in vivo studies in RP demand a unique orientation to novel clinical drug phenomena. For the mechanistic understanding of the drug actions, relevance of pharmacokinetics/metabolism and relevant safety profiles, RP would require experts with a foundation in basic sciences. The specialties which would emerge from the differentiation are reverse pharmacodynamists, reverse pharmacokineticists, safety pharmacologists, and cellular/molecular pharmacologists for NPs. Such a wide scope of super specialties in RP may appear daunting at present. But the vast number of clinically documented hits and leads demand the rigor and expertise to mine the field effectively. The current unmet healthcare needs in communicable and noncommunicable diseases as well as the emergent new challenges could be substantially met with by such a transdisciplinary differentiation of RP.

REFERENCES

Aggarwal, B., Prasad, S., Reuter, S., Kannappan, R., Yadev, V., Park, B., et al., 2011. Identification of novel anti-inflammatory agents from Ayurvedic medicine for prevention of chronic diseases. "reverse pharmacology" and "bedside to bench" approach. Curr. Drug Target 12 (11), 1595–1653.

Altman, R.D., Marcussen, K.C., 2001. Effects of a ginger extract on knee pain in patients with osteoarthritis. Arthritis Rheumatism 44, 2531–2538.

Andersen, J.V., Chorghade, Mukund, S., Dezaro, D.A., Dolphin, D.H., Hill, D.R., et al., 1994. Metalloporphyrins as chemical mimics of cytochrome P-450 systems. Bioorgan. Med. Chem. Lett. 4 (24), 2867.

Antarkar, D., Tathed, P., Vaidya, A., 1978. A pilot phase II trial with arogyavardhini and punarnavadi-kwath in viral hepatitis. Pan Med. 20 (3), 157–160.

Antarkar, D., Vaidya, A., Doshi, J., Athavale, A., Vinchoo, K., Natekar, M., et al., 1980. A double-blind clinical trial of arogyavardhini-an Ayurvedic drug – in acute viral hepatitis. Indian J. Med. Res. 72, 588–593.

Apte, V., 1988. Guggulu ani guggulukalpa sarsangraha. Bharatiya Vidya Bhavan, Mumbai.

Aushadhi Baad, 1974., Compilation of clinical notes of Pade SD, Patil PB, Gadre DV, Padhyegurjar AB. Raghuvanshi Prakashan, Pune.

Baxendale, I., Deeley, J., Griffiths-Jones, C., Ley, S., Saaby, S., Tranmer, G., 2006. A flow process for the multi-step synthesis of the alkaloid natural product oxomaritidine: a new paradigm for molecular assembly. Chem. Commun. 24, 2566–2568.

Bennett, K.A., Tehan, B., Lebon, G., Tate, C.G., Weir, M., Marshall, F.H., et al., 2013. Pharmacology and structure of isolated conformations of the adenosine A2A receptor define ligand efficacy. Mol. Pharmacol. 83 (5), 949–958.

Bernard, C., 1957. An Introduction to the Study of Experimental Medicine. Dover, New York, NY.

Caddick, S., 1995. Microwave assisted organic reactions. Tetrahedron 51 (38), 10403–10432.

Chalmers, I., 2003. Fisher and bradford hill: theory and pragmatism? Int. J. Epidemiol. 32 (6), 922–924.

Chorghade, M.S., Dolphin, D.H., Dupre, D., Hill, D.R., Lee, E.C., Wijesekara, T.P., 1996a. Improved protocols for the synthesis and halogenation of sterically hindered metalloporphyrins. Synthesis (Stuttg).1320.

Chorghade, M.S., Dolphin, D.H., Hill, D.R., Hino, F., Lee, E.C., Zhang, L.-Y., et al., 1996b. Metalloporphyrins as chemical mimics of cytochrome P-450 systems. Pure Appl. Chem. 68 (3), 753.

Collins Jr., M., 2010. Future trends in microwave synthesis. Future Med. Chem 2 (2), 151–155.

Dahanukar, S., Thatte, U., 1997. Current Status of Ayurveda in Phytomedicine, Phytomedicine Vol. 4 (4), 359–368.

Dahanukar, S., Thatte, U., Pai, N., More, P., Karandikar, S., 1988. Immunotherapeutic modification by Tinospora cordifolia of abdominal sepsis induced by caecal ligation in rats. Indian J. Gastroenterol. 7, 21–23.

Damodaran, M., Ramaswamy, R., 1937. Isolation of 1-3:4-dihydroxyphenylalanine from the seeds of Mucuna pruriens. Biochem. J. 31 (12), 2149–2152.

de la Hoz, A., Diaz-Ortiz, A., Moreno, A., 2005. Microwaves in organic synthesis. Thermal and non-thermal microwave effects. Chem. Soc. Rev. 34 (2), 164–178.

Desai, V.G., 1928. Kadu (Picrorhiza kurroa). Aushadhi Sangraha. Gajanan Book Depot, Dadar, Mumbai, p. 542.

Dineshkumar, B. and Shashikeran, B., 2008 Report of acute toxicity study in Swiss albino mice and Sprauge Dawley rats, long-term toxicity study in Sprauge Dawley rats of abfn-02, study no: 03-07. National Institute of Nutrition, Hyderabad, Andra Pradesh, India.

Dong, M., Sitkovsky, M., Kallmerten, A., Jones, G., 2008. Synthesis of 8-substituted xanthines via 5,6-diaminouracils: an efficient route to A2A adenosine receptor antagonists. Tetrahedron. Lett. 49 (31), 4633–4635.

Feinstein, A.R., 1994. Clinical judgment revisited: the distraction of quantitative models. Ann. Intern. Med. 120 (9), 799–805.

Gedye, R., Smith, F., Westaway, K., Ali, H., Baldisera, L., Laberge, L., et al., 1986. The use of microwave ovens for rapid organic synthesis. Tetrahedron. Lett. 27 (3), 279–282.

Gerhardt, H., Seifert, F., Buvari, P., Vogelsang, H., Repges, R., 2001. Therapy of active Crohn disease with *Boswellia serrata* extract H 15. Gastroenterology. 39 (1), 11—17.

Godse, C., 2004. An Exploration and Putative Interventional Effect of Nyctanthes Arbor-Tristis (Parijat) in Malaria: Clinical, Metabolic, Parasite and Immune Changes. University of Mumbai.

Godse, C.S., Nabar, N.S., Raut, A.A., Joshi, J.V., 2011. Reverse pharmacology for antimalarial plants goes global. J. Ayurveda Integr. Med. 2 (4), 163—164.

Gupta, S., 2002. Rustom Jal Vakil (1911—1974) — father of modern cardiology. JIACM 3 (1), 100—104.

Hastak, K., Lubri, N., Jakhi, S., More, C., John, A., Ghaisas, S., et al., 1997. Effect of turmeric oil and turmeric oleoresin on cytogenetic damage in patients suffering from oral submucous fibrosis. Cancer Lett. 116, 265—269.

Hill, D.R., Celebuski, Joseph, E., Pariza, R.J., Chorghade, Mukund, S., et al., 1996. Novel macrolides via meso-tetraarylmetalloporphyrin assisted oxidations. Tetrahedron. Lett. 37 (6), 787.

Huber, R., Jones, G., 1992. Acceleration of the orthoester Claisen rearrangement by clay catalyzed microwave thermolysis: expeditious route to bicyclic lactones. J. Org. Chem. 57 (21), 5778—5780.

India Medical Times. 2013, Global herbal market expected to reach $5 trillion mark by 2050 [Internet], [cited 2015 Jan 12]. Available from: http://www.indiamedicaltimes.com/2013/ 12/ 09/global-herbal-market-expected-to-reach-5-trillion-mark-by-2050/.

Jack, A., 2009. An Acute Talent for Innovation. Financial Times. [Internet] [cited 2016 Aug 6] http://www.ft.com/cms/s/0/29633e10-f0c8-11dd-992c-0000779fd2ac.html#axzz4GX7KJFzW.

Jain, S., Murthy, P., 2009. The other bose: an history of missed opportunities in the history of neurobiology of India. Curr. Sci. 97 (2).

Jas, G., Kirschning, A., 2003. Continuous flow techniques in organic synthesis. Chemistry (Easton). 9 (23), 5708—5723.

Jones, G., Chapman, B., 1993. Decarboxylation of indole-2-carboxylic acids: improved procedures. J. Org. Chem. 58 (20), 5558—5559.

Jones, G., Mathews, J., 1997. Bifunctional antitumor agents. Derivatives of pyrrolo[9, 10-b] phenanthrene--A DNA intercalative delivery template. Tetrahedron 53 (43), 14599—14614.

Jones, G., Huber, R., Chau, S., 1993. The Claisen rearrangement in synthesis: acceleration of the Johnson orthoester protocol en route to bicyclic lactones. Tetrahedron 49 (2), 369—380.

Joshi, J., Rege, V., Bhat, R., Vaidya, R., et al., 2004. Cervical cytology, vaginal pH and colposcopy as adjuncts to clinical evaluation of Panchavalkal, an Ayurvedic preparation, in leucorrhoea. J. Cytol 21, 33—38.

Joshi, J., Paradkar, P., Agashe, S., Vaidya, A.A., et al., 2011. Chemopreventive potential & safety profile of NBFR-03 (supercritical curcuma longa extract) in women with cervical low-grade squammous intraepithelial neoplasia in papanicolaou smears. Asian Pac. J. Cancer Prev. 12, 3305—3311.

Joshi, J.V., Vaidya, R.A., Affandi, M.Z., 2007. Cytology in the Diagnosis of Gardnerella Vaginalis infection. J. Cytology 23, 214.

Joshi, Y.G., 2003. Charak Samhita of Agnivesha, Sutrasthana, Atreyabhadrakappiyaadyaya, first ed. Vaidyamitra Prakashan, Pune, 1(12):318.

Kallmerten, A., Jones, G., 2010. Microwave accelerated synthesis of PET image contrast agents for AD research. Curr. Alzheimer. Res. 7 (3), 251—254.

Kappe, C., 2004. Controlled microwave heating in modern organic synthesis. Angew. Chem. Int. Ed. Engl. 43 (46), 6250—6284.

Karnik, S., Tathed, P., Antarkar, D., Godse, C., Vaidya, R., Vaidya, A., 2008. Antimalarial activity and clinical safety of traditionally used. Indian J. Tradit Knowl. 7 (2), 330–334.

Katzenschlager, A., Evans, A., Manson, P.N., Patsalos, N., Ratnaraj, H., Watt, L., et al., 2004. Mucuna pruriens in Parkinson's disease: a double blind clinical and pharmacological study. J. Neurol. Neurosurg. Psychiatry 75, 1672–1677.

LaBeaume, P., Wager, K., Falcone, D., Li, J., Torchilin, V., Castro, C., et al., 2009. Synthesis, functionalization and photo-Bergman chemistry of enediyne bioconjugates. Bioorg. Med. Chem. 17 (17), 6292–6300.

Labeaume, P., Dong, M., Sitkovsky, M., Jones, E., Thomas, R., Sadler, S., et al., 2010a. An efficient route to xanthine based A(2A) adenosine receptor antagonists and functional derivatives. Org. Biomol. Chem.

LaBeaume, P., Placzek, M., Daniels, M., Kendrick, I., Ng, P., McNeel, M., et al., 2010b. Microwave-accelerated fluorodenitrations and nitrodehalogenations: expeditious routes to labeled PET ligands and fluoropharmaceuticals. Tetrahedron Lett. 51 (14), 1906–1909.

Lasagna, L., 1999. The future of drug development and regulation. Three Steps Forward, One Step Back: Health and Biomedical Issues on the Cusp of a New century. New York Academy of Sciences, USA, pp. 21–27.

Ma, D., Lin, Y., Xiao, Z., Kappen, L., Goldberg, I., Kallmerten, A., et al., 2009. Designed DNA probes from the neocarzinostatin family: impact of glycosyl linkage stereochemistry on bulge base binding. Bioorg. Med. Chem. 17 (6), 2428–2432.

McNamara, C., Dixon, M., Bradley, M., 2002. Recoverable catalysts and reagents using recyclable polystyrene-based supports. Chem. Rev. 102 (10), 3275–3299.

Mishra, V.P., 2014. Keynote address in National Seminar on Concept of Reverse Pharmacology at DMIMS, Wardha, Maharashtra, India.

Mohapatra, D.K., Ramesh, D.K., Gurjar, M.K., Chorghade, M.S., Giardello, M.A., Grubbs, R.H., 2007. First total synthesis of an anti-malarial nonenolide: protecting group directed ring-closing metathesis (RCM). Tetrahedron Lett. 48, 2621–2625.

Müller, M., 2004. Chemical diversity through biotransformations. Curr. Opin. Biotechnol. 15 (6), 591–598.

Nabar, N., Vaidya, R., Narayana, D., Raut, A., Shah, S., Patwadhan, B., et al., 2013. Marketed Ayurvedic antidiabetic formulations: labelling, drug information, and branding. Indian Pract. 66 (10), 631–641.

Noble Prize 2015 in Physiology or Medicine – Press Release, [Internet] [cited 2015 Nov 2]. Available from: http://www.nobelprize.org/nobel_prizes/medicine/laureates/2015/press.html.

Pade, S.D., 1973. Aryabhishak Arthat Hindustancha Vaidyaraj, Shree Gajanan Book Depot, Dadar, Mumbai.

Panchabhai, T.S., Kulkarni, U.P., Rege, N.N., 2008. Validation of therapeutic claims of Tinospora cordifolia: a review. Phytother Res. 22 (4), 425–441.

Parikh, K.M., 1992. Medicinal Preparations and Pharmacy in Ayurveda, in Selected Medicinal Plants of India, a Monograph of Identity, Safety, and Clinical usage, compiled by Bhavan's SPARC. CHEMEXIL371–378.

Patwardhan, B., 2008. Integrated Biomedical Research. Proceedings, ICMR Symposium on Reverse Pharmacology. Medical Research Centre of Kasturba Health Society, Vile Parle (W), Mumbai, pp. 9–18.

Patwardhan, B., 2015. Public perception of AYUSH. J. Ayurveda Integr. Med. 6 (3), 147–149.

Patwardhan, B., Vaidya, A.D.B., Chorghade, M., Joshi, P.S., 2008. Reverse pharmacology and systems approaches for drug discovery and development. Curr. Bioact. Compd. 4 (4), 201–212.

Patwardhan, B., Joglekar, V., Pathak, N., Vaidya, A., 2011. Vaidya-scientists: catalysing ayurveda renaissance. Curr. Sci. 100 (4), 25.

Peddibhotla, S., Dang, Y., Liu, J., Romo, D., 2007. Simultaneous arming and structure/activity studies of natural products employing O-H insertions: an expedient and versatile strategy for natural products-based chemical genetics. J. Am. Chem. Soc. 129 (40), 12222–12231.

Puranik, A., Nabar, N., Joshi, J., Amonkar, A., Shah, S., Menon, S., et al., 2014. Single dose metformin kinetics after co-administration of nisha-amalaki powder or mamejwa ghanavati, Ayurvedic anti-diabetic formulations: a randomized crossover study in healthy volunteers. J. Obes. Metab. Res. 1 (2), 99–104.

Raut, A., 1992. Dissertation for Rasashastra and Bhaishajya-kalpana. Bombay University.

Raut, A., Chorghade, M., 2014. Conference on natural products 2014 held in Chicago 7th To 10th July. J. Ayurveda Integr. Med. 5 (4), 263.

Raut, A., Mertia, P., 2012. Commiphora Wightii (Guggulu): Lessons to be Learned. In: Proceedings of the ICMR Strategic Thrust Symposium on Translational Research and Reverse Pharmacology. The Interface of Basic Sciences with Traditional Medicine. Medical Research Centre-Kasturba Health Society, Vile Parle (W), Mumbai, pp. 107–111.

Raut, A. 2013. Scope and potential of Integrative Medicine in current Healthcare Scenario' in conference Samyukti 2013, an evidence-based approach to Integrating Ayurveda and Allopathy, Organized by MS Ramaiah Academy of Health and Applied Sciences, and Institute of Transdisciplinary Health Sciences and Technology, Bangalore, Karnataka, India. [Internet], [cited 2015 Jan 23]. Available from: http://www.iaim.edu.in/samyukti/resources/ashwini_kumar_raut.pptx.

Raut, A.A., 2010. Vaidya Antarkar Memorial Volume. Antarkar Memorial Forum & Bharatiya Vidya Bhavan, Mumbai.

Raut, A.A., Gundeti, M.S., 2014. Obesity and osteoarthritis comorbidity: insights from ayurveda. J. Obes. Metab. Res. 1, 89–94.

Raut, A., Vaidya, R., 2011. Organization/Faculty/Academic Location for Reverse Pharmacology, Abstracts. ICMR Workshop for Training in Reverse Pharmacology. Medical Research Centre-Kasturba Health Society, Vile-Parle (W), Mumbai, pp. 21–22.

Raut, A., Vaidya, R., Vaidya, A, 2012. Pragmatic Curriculum of Reverse Pharmacology for Integrative Healthcare Research. In: Proceedings of the ICMR strategic thrust symposium on "Translational Research and Reverse Pharmacology: The Interface of Basic Sciences with Traditional Medicine." Medical Research Centre-Kasturba Health Society, Vile-Parle (W), Mumbai, pp. 39–43.

Raut, A.A., Sawant, N.S., Badre, A.S., Amonkar, A.J., Vaidya, A.D.B., 2007. Bhallataka (Semicarpus anacardium Linn)-A Review. Indian Journal of Traditional Knowledge Vol. 6 (4), 653–659.

Raut, A., Bichile, L., Chopra, A., Patwardhan, B., Vaidya, A., 2013. Comparative study of amrutbhallataka and glucosamine sulphate in osteoarthritis: Six months open label randomized controlled clinical trial. J. Ayurveda. Integr. Med. 4, 229–236.

Riedel, S., 2005. Edward Jenner and the history of smallpox and vaccination. Proc. Baylor Univ. Med. Center 18 (1), 21–25.

Sanchez-Martin, R., Mittoo, S., Bradley, M., 2004. The impact of combinatorial methodologies on medicinal chemistry. Curr. Top. Med. Chem. 4 (7), 653–669.

Sedelmeier, J., Ley, S., Lange, H., Baxendale, I., 2009. Pd-EnCatTM TPP30 as a catalyst for the generation of highly functionalized Aryl- and Alkenyl-Substituted acetylenes via microwave-assisted sonogashira type reactions. Eur. J. Org. Chem. 26, 4412–4420.

Sen, G., Bose, K., 1931. Rauwolfia serpentina, a new Indian drug for insanity and high blood pressure. Indian Med. World 21, 194–201.

Sharma, R.K., Dash, B., 1985. Charak Samhita of Agnivesha, Viman sthana, Rogabhishakjitiya, second ed. Chaukhambha Sanskrit Series, Varanasi, p. 256.

Sharma, U., Bala, M., Kumar, N., Singh, B., Munshi, R.K., Bhalerao, S., 2012. Immunomodulatory active compounds from Tinospora cordifolia. J. Ethnopharmacol. 141, 918–926.

Sheth, F.J., Patel, P., Vaidya, A.D.B., Vaidya, R.A., Sheth, J., 2006. Increased frequency of sister chromatid exchanges in patients with type II diabetes. Curr. Sci. 90 (2), 236–240.

Shetty, S.N., Mengi, S., Vaidya, R., Vaidya, A.D.B., 2010. A study of standardized extracts of Picrorhiza kurroa Royle ex Benth in experimental nonalcoholic fatty liver disease. J. Ayurveda Integr. Med. 1 (3), 203–210.

Shringi, M., Galvankar, P., Vaidya, R.A., et al., 2000. Therapeutic profile of an Ayurvedic formulation Ashotone in Dysfunctional Uterine Bleeding (DUB). The Indian Practitioner 53, 193–198.

Stephen Daniells, 2011 Herbal supplement sales to hit $93.15 billion by 2015: Report [Internet], [cited 2015 Jan 12]. Available from: http://www.nutraingredients-usa.com/Markets/Herbal-supplement-sales-tohit-93.15-billion-by-2015-Report.

Strom, B., 1989. Pharmacoepidemiology. Churchil Livingstone, New York, NY.

Szapary, P.O., Wolfe, M.L., Bloedon, L.T., Cucchiara, A.J., DerMarderosian, A.H., Cirigliano, M.D., et al., 2003. Guggulipid for the treatment of hypercholesterolemia: a randomized controlled trial. JAMA 290 (6), 765–772.

Tillu, G., 2015. Pharmacoepidemiology of Ayurveda Medicines. Savitribai Phule Pune University.

Torregrossa, J., Bubley, G., Jones, G., 2006. Microwave expedited synthesis of 5-aminocamptothecin analogs: inhibitors of hypoxia inducible factor HIF-1alpha. Bioorg. Med. Chem. Lett. 16 (23), 6082–6085.

Upadhyay, A.K., Kumar, K., Kumar, A., Mishra, H.S., 2010. Tinospora cordifolia (Willd.) Hook. f. and Thoms. (Guduchi) - validation of the Ayurvedic pharmacology through experimental and clinical studies. Int. J. Ayurveda Res. 1 (2), 112–121.

Urizar, N.L., Liverman, A.B., Dodds, D.T., et al., 2002. A natural product that lowers cholesterol as an antagonist ligand for FXR. Science 296, 1703–1706.

Vaidya, A., 2013. The Splendour of Research Aspirations: From Haffkine Institute to Kasturba Health Society (1961–2013). Seventh Haffkine Oration at The Haffkine Institute for Training, Research and Testing, Parel, Mumbai, India.

Vaidya, A.B., 1979. We can still learn from Indian medicine. CIBA-GEIGY J 4 (17).

Vaidya, A.B., 2007. Ayurvedic statistics—A novel epistemology based discipline. National Seminar on Evidence Based Ayurveda & CME on Biomedical Research Methods. MGIMS Sewagram, Maharashtra, India.

Vaidya, A.B., 2010a. Reverse Pharmacology—A Paradigm Shift for New Drug Discovery Based on Ayurvedic Epistemology. In: Muralidharan, T.S., Raghava, V. (Eds.), Ayurveda in Transition. Arya Vaidya Sala, Kottakkal, Kerala, India, pp. 27–38.

Vaidya, A.B., Antarkar, D., Doshi, J., Bhatt, A., Vijaya, R., Vora, P., et al., 1996. Picrorhiza kurroa (Kutaki) Royle ex Benth as a hepatoprotective agent—experimental and clinical studies. J. Postgrad. Med 42 (4), 105–108.

Vaidya, A.B., Rajgopalan, T.G., Mankodi, N.A., Antarkar, D.S., Tathed, P.S., Purohit, A.V., et al., 1978. Treatment of Parkinson's disease with the cowhage plant-Mukuna pruriens Bak. Neurol. India 26 (4), 171–176.

Vaidya, A.D.B., 1992. Some principles and practices of Ayurveda. In: Selected Medicinal Plants of India: A Monograph of Identity, Safety, and Clinical Usage, Bhavan's SPARC, Mumbai, pp. 365–370.

Vaidya, A.D.B., 2006. Reverse pharmacological correlates of Ayurvedic drug actions. Ind. J. Pharmacol. 38 (5), 311−315.

Vaidya, A.D.B., 2007. Herbal Based formulations in type 2 diabetes mellitus with emphasis on insulin resistance. In: Completion report of CSIR NMITLI Diabetes project 2002−2007. Govt. of India.

Vaidya, A.D.B., 2010b. An advocacy for Vaidya−Scientists in Ayurvedic research. J. Ayurveda Integr. Med 1 (1), 6−8.

Vaidya, A.D.B., 2014. Reverse Pharmacology − A Paradigm Shift for Drug Discovery and Development. Curr. Res. Drug Discov 1 (2), 39−44.

Vaidya, A.D.B., Raut, A.A., 2006. Evidence-based Ayurveda: Sorting fact from fantasy. International Conclave on Traditional Medicine, AYUSH, New Delhi, India, pp. 219−247.

Vaidya, A.D.B., Nabar, N., Vaidya, R., 2014. Current status of indigenous drugs and alternative medicine in the management of diabetes mellitus. In: Tripathy, B., Chandalia, H. (Eds.), RSSDI Textbook of Diabetes, third ed RSSDI, Hyderabad, Andhra Pradesh, India, p. 45.

Vaidya, M.S. 1910. Personal Ayurvedic Notes with the author ADBV.

Vaidya, M.S., 1925. Hadakavana ilajne vadhu pushti (More support for the remedy cited for hydrophobia). Vaidyakalpataru 25, 247−248.

Vaidya, R., 2011. Observational therapeutics: Scope, challenges, and organization. J. Ayurveda Integr. Med. 2 (4), 165−169.

Vaidya, R., Pandey, S., Vaidya, A.D.B., 2008. Polycystic Ovary Syndrome: Is It a Chronic Inflammatory Disease? In: Mukherjee, G.G. (Ed.), Polycystic Ovary Syndrome, ECAB Clinical Update: Obstetrics & Gynecology series. Elsevier, Kalkaji, New Delhi, pp. 42−73.

Vaidya, R.A., Vaidya, A.D.B., Patwardhan, B., Tillu, G., Rao, Y., 2003. Ayurvedic Pharmacoepidemiology: A Proposed New Discipline. J. Assoc. Phys. India 51, 528.

Vakil, R.J., 1949. A clinical trial of Rauwolfia serpentina in essential hypertension. Br. Heart. J. 2, 350−355.

White, B., 2007. Ginger an overview. Am. Fam. Physician 75, 1689−1691.

Willcox, M., Graz, B., Falquet, J., Diakite, C., Giani, S., Diallo, D.A., 2011. "Reverse pharmacology" approach for developing an antimalarial phytomedicine. Malar. J. 10 (Suppl. 1), 1−10.

Chapter 5

Network Pharmacology

Uma Chandran, Neelay Mehendale, Saniya Patil, Rathnam Chaguturu
and Bhushan Patwardhan
Savitribai Phule Pune University, Pune, Maharashtra, India

INTRODUCTION

Drug discovery, the process by which new candidate medications are discovered, initially began with random searching of therapeutic agents from plants, animals, and naturally occurring minerals (Burger, 1964). For this, they depended on the *materia medica* that was established by medicine men and priests from that era. This was followed by the origin of classical pharmacology in which the desirable therapeutic effects of small molecules were tested on intact cells or whole organisms. Later, the advent of human genome sequencing revolutionized the drug discovery process that developed into target–based drug discovery, also known as reverse pharmacology. This relies on the hypothesis that the modulation of the activity of a specific protein will have therapeutic effects. The protein that the drug binds to or interacts with is also referred to as a "target." In this reductionist approach, small molecules from a chemical library are screened for their effect on the target's known or predicted function (Hacker et al., 2009). Once the small molecule is selected for a particular target, further modifications are carried out at the atomic level to ameliorate the lock-and-key interactions. This one-drug/one-target/one-therapeutic approach was followed for the last several decades.

The information technology revolution at the end of 20th century metamorphosed the drug discovery process as well (Clark and Pickett, 2000). Advancements in omics technologies during this time were used to develop strategies for different phases of drug research (Buriani et al., 2012). Computational power was implemented in the discovery process for predicting a drug-likeness of newly designed or discovered compounds and ligand-protein docking for predicting the binding affinity of a small molecule with a protein three-dimensional structure. In silico tools were developed to predict other pharmacological properties of the drug molecules such as absorption, distribution, metabolism, excretion, and toxicity—abbreviated together as ADMET (van de Waterbeemd and Gifford, 2003; Clark and Grootenhuis, 2002). The technological advancements triggered discovery efforts in a

Innovative Approaches in Drug Discovery. DOI: http://dx.doi.org/10.1016/B978-0-12-801814-9.00005-2
127

direction to discover more specific magic bullets that were completely against the holistic approach of traditional medicine. This magic bullet approach is currently in decline phase. The major limitations of this drug discovery approach are side effects and the inability to tackle multifactorial diseases. This is mainly due to the linearity of this approach.

During the peak, historical time of drug discovery and development of natural products—based drugs had played a significant role due to their superior chemical diversity and safety over synthetic compound libraries (Zimmermann et al., 2007). Currently, it is estimated that more than one hundred new, natural product—based leads are in clinical development (Harvey, 2008). Many active compounds (bioactives) from traditional medicine sources could serve as good starting compounds and scaffolds for rational drug design. Natural products normally act through modulation of multiple targets rather than a single, highly specific target. But in drug discovery and development, technology was used to synthesize highly specific mono-targeted molecules that mimic the bioactives from natural compounds rather than understanding the rationale behind their synergistic action and developing methods to isolate the bioactives from natural resources. Researchers understand that most diseases are due to dysfunction of multiple proteins. Thus, it is important to address multiple targets emanating from a syndrome-related, metabolic cascade, so that holistic management can be effectively achieved. Therefore, it is necessary to shift the strategy from one that focuses on a single-target, new chemical entity to one of a multiple-target, synergistic, formulation-discovery approach (Patwardhan et al., 2015). This tempted the research world to go back and extensively explore natural sources, where modern pharmacology had begun. This renewed research focus indicates the need to rediscover the drug discovery process by integrating traditional knowledge with state-of-the-art technologies (Patwardhan, 2014a).

NETWORK PHARMACOLOGY

A new discipline called network pharmacology (NP) has emerged which attempts to understand drug actions and interactions with multiple targets (Hopkins, 2007). It uses computational power to systematically catalogue the molecular interactions of a drug molecule in a living cell. NP appeared as an important tool in understanding the underlying complex relationships between botanical formula and the whole body (Zhang et al., 2013; Berger and Iyengar, 2009). It also attempts to discover new drug leads and targets and to repurpose existing drug molecules for different therapeutic conditions by allowing an unbiased investigation of potential target spaces (Kibble et al., 2015). However, these efforts require some guidance for selecting the right type of targets and new scaffolds of drug molecules. Traditional knowledge can play a vital role in this process of formulation discovery and repurposing existing drugs. By combining advances in systems biology and NP, it might be possible to rationally design the next generation of promiscuous drugs (Cho et al., 2012; Hopkins, 2008; Ellingson et al., 2014). NP analysis not only opens up new therapeutic options, but it also aims to improve the safety and efficacy of existing medications.

NETWORK BIOLOGY TO NETWORK PHARMACOLOGY

The postgenomic era witnessed a rapid development of computational biology techniques to analyze and explore existing biological data. The key aim of the postgenomic biomedical research was to systematically catalogue all molecules and their interactions within a living cell. It is essential to understand how these molecules and the interactions among them determine the function of this immensely complex machinery, both in isolation and when surrounded by other cells. This led to the emergence and advancement of network biology, which indicates that cellular networks are governed by universal laws and offer a new conceptual framework that could potentially revolutionize our view of biology and disease pathologies in the 21st century (Barabási and Oltvai, 2004). During the first decade of the 21st century, several approaches for biological network construction were put forward that used computational methods, and literature mining especially, to understand the relation between disease phenotypes and genotypes. As a consequence, LMMA (literature mining and microarray analysis), a novel approach to reconstructing gene networks by combining literature mining and microarray analysis, was proposed (Li et al., 2006; Huang and Li, 2010). With this, a global network was first derived using the literature−based, cooccurrence method and then refined using microarray data. The LMMA biological network approach enables researchers to keep themselves up to date with relevant literature on specialized biological topics and to make sense of the relevant large-scale microarray dataset. Also, LMMA serves as a useful tool for constructing specific biological network and experimental design. LMMA−like representations enable a systemic recognition for the specific diseases in the context of complex gene interactions and are helpful for studying the regulation of various complex biological, physiological, and pathological systems.

The significance of accumulated-data integration was appreciated by pharmacologists, and they began to look beyond the classic lock-and-key concept as a far more intricate picture of drug action became clear in the postgenomic era. The global mapping of pharmacological space uncovered promiscuity, the specific binding of a chemical to more than one target (Paolini et al., 2006). As there can be multiple keys for a single lock, in the same way, a single key can fit into multiple locks. Similarly, a ligand might interact with many targets and a target may accommodate different types of ligands. This is referred to as "polypharmacology." The concept of network biology was used to integrate data from DrugBank (Re and Valentini, 2013) and OMIM (Hamosh et al., 2005), an online catalog of human genes and genetic disorders to understand the industry trends, the properties of drug targets, and to study how drug targets are related to disease-gene products. In this way, when the first drug-target network was constructed, isolated and bipartite nodes were expected based on the existed one-drug/one-target/one-disease approach. Rather, the authors observed a rich network of polypharmacology interactions between drugs and their targets (Yildirim et al., 2007). An overabundance of "follow-on" drugs that are drugs that target already targeted proteins was observed. This suggested a need to upgrade the single-target single-drug paradigm, as single-protein single-function relations are limited to accurately describing the reality of cellular processes.

Advances in systems biology led to the realization that complex diseases cannot be effectively treated by intervention at single proteins. This made the drug researchers accept the concept of polypharmacology which they previously thought as an undesirable property that needs to be removed or reduced to produce clean drugs acting on single-targets. According to network biology, simultaneous modulation of multiple targets is required for modifying phenotypes. Developing methods to aid polypharmacology can help to improve efficacy and predict unwanted off-target effects.

Hopkins (Hopkins, 2007, 2008) observed that network biology and polypharmacology can illuminate the understanding of drug action. He introduced the term "network pharmacology." This distinctive new approach to drug discovery can enable the paradigm shift from highly specific magic bullet—based drug discovery to multitargeted drug discovery. NP has the potential to provide new treatments to multigenic complex diseases and can lead to the development of e-therapeutics where the ligand formulation can be customized for each complex indication under every disease type. This can be expanded in the future and lead to customized and personalized therapeutics. Integration of network biology and polypharmacology can tackle two major sources of attrition in drug development such as efficacy and toxicity. Also, this integration holds the promise of expanding the current opportunity space for druggable targets. Hopkins proposed NP as the next paradigm in drug discovery.

Polypharmacology expands the space in drug discovery approach. Hopkins had suggested three strategies to the designers of multitarget therapies: the first was to prescribe multiple individual medications as a multidrug combination cocktail. Patient compliance and the danger of drug—drug interactions would be the expected drawbacks of this method. The second proposition was the development of multicomponent drug formulations. The change in metabolism, bioavailability, and pharmacokinetics of formulation as well as safety would be the major concerns of this approach. The third strategy was to design a single compound with selective polypharmacology. According to Hopkins, the third method is advantageous, as it would ease the dosing studies. Also, the regulatory barriers for the single compound are fewer compared to a formulation. An excellent example of this is metformin, the first-line drug for Type II diabetes that has been found to have cancer-inhibiting properties (Leung et al., 2013).

The following years witnessed the application research of NP by integrating network biology and polypharmacology. A computational framework, based on a regression model that integrates human protein—protein interactions, disease phenotype similarities, and known gene—phenotype associations to capture the complex relationships between phenotypes and genotypes, has been proposed. This was based on the assumption that phenotypically similar diseases are caused by functionally related genes. A tool named CIPHER (Correlating protein Interaction network and PHEnotype network to pRedict disease genes) has been developed that predicts and prioritizes disease-causing genes (Wu et al., 2008). CIPHER helps to uncover known disease genes and predict novel susceptibility candidates. Another application of this study is to predict a human disease landscape that can be exploited to study the related genes for related phenotypes that will be clustered together in a molecular interaction network. This will facilitate the discovery of disease genes and help to analyze the cooperativity among genes. Later, CIPHER-HIT, a Hitting-Time-based method to measure global closeness between two nodes of a heterogeneous network, was developed (Yao et al., 2011). A phenotype—genotype network can be explored using this method for detecting the genes related to a particular phenotype. A network—based gene clustering and extension were used to identify responsive gene modules in a condition—specific gene network aimed to provide useful resources to understand physiological responses (Gu et al., 2010).

NP was also used to develop miRNA—based biomarkers (Lu et al., 2011). For this, a network of miRNA and their targets was constructed and further refined to study the data for specific diseases. This process integrated with literature mining was useful to develop potent miRNA markers for diseases. NP was also used to develop a drug gene—disease comodule (Zhao and Li, 2012). Initially, a drug-disease network was constructed by information gathered from databases followed by the integration of gene data. The gene closeness was studied by developing a mathematical model. This network inferred the association of multiple genes for most of the diseases and target sharing of drugs and diseases. These kinds of networks give insight into new drug-disease associations and their molecular connections.

NETWORK ETHNOPHARMACOLOGY

During the progression period of network biology, natural products were gaining importance in the chemical space of drug discovery, as these have been economically designed and synthesized by nature for the benefit of evolution (Wetzel et al., 2011). Researchers began analyzing the logic behind traditional medicine systems and devised computational ways to ease the analysis. A comprehensive herbal medicine information system that was developed integrates information of more than 200 anticancer herbal recipes that have been used for the treatment of different types of cancer in the clinic, 900 individual ingredients, and 8500 small organic molecules isolated from herbal medicines (Fang et al., 2005). This system, which was developed using an Oracle database and Internet technology, facilitates and promotes scientific research in herbal medicine. This was followed by the development of many databases that serve as a source of botanical information and a powerful tool that provides a bridge between traditional medicines and modern molecular biology. These kinds of databases and tools made the researchers conceive the idea of NP of botanicals and their formulations to understand the underlying mechanisms of traditional medicines. We refer to such networks as "ethnopharmacological networks" and the technique as "Network Ethnopharmacology (NEP)" (Patwardhan and Chandran, 2015). Shao Li pioneered this endeavor and proposed this network as a tool to explain the ZHENG (syndrome of traditional Chinese medicine (TCM)) and the multiple-targets' mechanism of TCM (Li, 2007).

Li et al. tried to provide a molecular basis for 1000-year-old concept of ZHENG using a neuro-endocrine-immune (NEI) network (Li et al., 2007). ZHENG is the basic unit and key concept in TCM theory. It is also used as a guideline in disease classification in TCM. The HOT (HANS ZHENG in Mandarin) and COLD (RE ZHENG) are the two statuses of ZHENG which therapeutically directs the use of herbs in TCM. Chinese herbs are classified as HOT−cooling and are used to remedy HOT ZHENG and COLD−warming herbs that are used to remedy COLD ZHENG. According to the authors, hormones may be related to HOT ZHENG, immune factors may be related to COLD ZHENG, and they may be interconnected by neurotransmitters. This study provides a methodical approach to understand TCM within the framework of modern science. Later they reconstructed the NEI network by adding multilayer information including data available on the KEGG database related to signal transduction, metabolic pathways, protein−protein interactions, transcription factor, and micro RNA regulations. They also connected drugs and diseases through multilayered interactions. The study of COLD ZHENG emphasized its relation to energy metabolism, which is tightly correlated with the genes of neurotransmitters, hormones, and cytokines in the NEI interaction network (Zhang et al., 2008; Ma et al., 2010).

Another database, TCMGeneDIT, provides information about TCMs, genes, diseases, TCM effects, and TCM ingredients mined from a vast amount of biomedical literature. This would facilitate clinical research and elucidate the possible therapeutic mechanisms of TCMs and gene regulations (Fang et al., 2008). To study the combination rule of TCM formulae, an herb network was created using 3865 collaterals-related formulae (Li et al., 2010). They developed a distance-based, mutual-information model (DMIM) to uncover the combination rule. DMIM uses mutual-information entropy and "between herb distance" to measure the tendency of two herbs to form an herb pair. They experimentally evaluated the combination of a few herbs for angiogenesis. Understanding the combination rule of herbs in formulae will help the modernization of traditional medicine and also help to develop a new formulae based on the current requirement. A network target–based paradigm was proposed for the first time to understand the synergistic combinations (Li et al., 2011), and an algorithm termed "NIMS" (network target–based identification of a multicomponent synergy) was also developed. This was a step that facilitated the development of multicomponent therapeutics using traditional wisdom. An innovative way to study the molecular mechanism of TCM was proposed during this time by integrating the TCM experimental data with microarray gene expression data (Wen et al., 2011). As a demonstrative example, Si-Wu-Tang's formula was studied. Rather than uncovering the molecular mechanism of action, this method would help to identify new health benefits of TCMs.

The initial years of the second decade of the 21st century witnessed the network ethnopharmacological exploration of TCM formulations. The scope of this new area attracted scientists, and they hoped NEP could provide insight into multicompound drug discoveries that could help overcome the current impasse in drug discovery (Patwardhan, 2014b; Li et al., 2012). NEP was used to study the antiinflammatory mechanism of Qingfei Xiaoyan, a TCM (Cheng et al., 2013). The predicted results were used to design experiments and analyze the data. Experimental confirmation of the predicted results provides an effective strategy for the study of traditional medicines. The potential of TCM formulations as multiple compound drug candidates has been studied using TCM formulations based NP. TCM formulations studied in this way are listed in Table 5.1. Construction of a database containing 19,7201 natural product structures, followed by their docking to 332 target proteins of FDA-approved drugs, shows the amount of space shared in the chemical space between natural products and FDA drugs (Gu et al., 2013a). Molecular-docking technique plays a major role in NP. The interaction of bioactives with molecular targets can be analyzed by this technique. Molecular docking–based NEP can be a useful tool to computationally elucidate the combinatorial effects of traditional medicine to intervene disease networks (Gu et al., 2013c). An approach that combines NP and pharmacokinetics has been proposed to study the material basis of TCM formulations (Pei et al., 2013). This can be extrapolated to study other traditional medicine formulations as well.

In cancer research, numerous natural products have been demonstrated to have anticancer potential. Natural products are gaining attraction in anticancer research, as they show a favorable profile in terms of absorption and metabolism in the body with low toxicity. In a study all of the known bioactives were docked for their property to interact with 104 cancer targets (Luo et al., 2014). It was inferred that many bioactives are targeting multiple

TABLE 5.1 TCM Formulations That Were Explored Using Network Pharmacology

Formulation Name	Observations About Bioactive Compounds	References
QiShenYiQi	Shows antiapoptosis, antiinflammation, antioxidant, anticoagulation, energy utilization facilitation and angiogenesis promotion against myocardial infarction	Li et al. (2014c)
	Useful against acute myocardial ischemia, and it might gain enhanced drug effect by regulating apoptosis and inflammation related pathways together	Wu et al. (2014)
Fufang xueshuantong	Ameliorate the activation of coagulation system in thrombosis	Sheng et al. (2014)
Gansui banxia tang	Modulates Hsp90α, ATP1A1, and STAT3 and combats hepatocellular carcinoma, intestinal tuberculosis, and gastrointestinal inflammation	Zhang et al. (2013)
Bushenhuoxue formula	Useful in chronic kidney disease, as it regulates the coagulation and fibrinolytic balance, expression of inflammatory factors, and inhibits abnormal ECM accumulation	Shi et al. (2014)
Ge-genqin-lian decoction	Useful in Type 2 diabetes, as it increases the insulin secretion in RIN-5F cells and improves insulin resistance	Li et al. (2014b)
Liu-Wei-Di-Huang pill	Deals with Yin deficiency of chen through PPAR signaling, progesterone-mediated oocyte maturation, adipocytokine signaling, and aldosterone-regulated sodium reabsorption	Liang et al. (2014)
Si-Wu-Tang	Useful in primary dysmenorrhea of gynecology blood stasis syndrome, as it regulates lipid metabolism (Shaofu Zhuyu decoction), amino acid metabolism (Xiangfu SWT), carbohydrate metabolism (THSWT), ErbB, and VEGF signal transduction pathway (Qinlian SWT)	Liu et al. (2014)

(Continued)

TABLE 5.1 (Continued)

Formulation Name	Observations About Bioactive Compounds	References
	Useful in climacteric syndrome, blood deficiency, as it regulates TGFβ signaling, pathway, oxidative stress–induced gene expression via Nrf2, and upregulates VEGFα expression	Fang et al. (2013)
	Useful in women's diseases through regulation of Nrf2-mediated oxidative stress response pathways, upregulation of Nrf2-regulated genes, increases an antioxidant-response element activity, phytoestrogenic effect	Wen et al. (2011)
Taohong Siwu decoction	Useful in osteoarthritis, as it inhibits MMP expression, reduces local ILs, ADAMTS-4, TNFα, iNOS, COX, VDR, PPAR-γ, CDK2, HO-1 pathways	Zheng et al. (2013)
Qingfei-Xiaoyan Wan	Useful in inflammation of respiratory system, asthma through reduction in the infiltration of cytokines through ERK1, and five inflammatory pathways	Cheng et al. (2013)
Buchang Naoxintong	Deals with coronary heart disease and stroke by targeting APOB, APOE, APOA1, LPL, LDLR	Chen et al. (2013)
Bushen Zhuanggu formula	Used against metastatic breast cancer, as it regulates OPG/RANKL/RANK system, TGFβ, COX-2, EGFR pathway	Pei et al. (2013)
Qing-Luo-Yin	Used against rheumatoid arthritis, as it regulates angiogenesis, inflammatory responses, and immune response pathways	Zhang et al. (2013)
	Used against rheumatoid arthritis with cold patterns, as it regulates nitrogen metabolism, PXR/RXR activation, linoleic acid metabolism, and metabolism of xenobiotics by CYP	Li et al. (2012)
Zhike Chuanbei Pipa Dropping Pill	Useful in airway inflammation and asthma, as it regulates the Toll-like receptor, TGFβ, MAPK, HSP 90-α pathways, and inhibits NF-κB	Yang et al., (2012)

(Continued)

TABLE 5.1 (Continued)

Formulation Name	Observations About Bioactive Compounds	References
Fufang Danshen formula	Useful in cardiovascular diseases, as it regulates PPARγ, ACE, KCNJ11, KCNQ1, ABCC8 pathways	Li et al. (2011)
Realgar-Indigo naturalis formula	Used against acute promyelocytic leukemia, as it regulates ubiquitination/degradation of promyelocytic leukemia–retinoic acid receptor α oncoprotein, stronger reprogramming of myeloid differentiation regulators, and enhanced G1/G0 arrest in APL cells	Wang et al. (2008)
Panax notoginseng	Useful in cardiovascular disease, as it targets various receptors and transcriptional factors that influence various types of cells in their proliferation, differentiation, migration and secretion, and prevents or inhibits early events of CVDs	Liu et al. (2014)
Xuesaitong injection	Used against myocardial infarction, as it modulates ErbB, MAPK, VEGF, and Wnt pathways	Wang et al. (2013a)
Panax notoginseng/ Salvia miltiorrhiza	Useful in cardiovascular disease	Liu (2013)
Shenmai injection	Used against myocardial ischemia, as it upregulates SPP1, TNC, FST, ITGA11, COMP and downregulates INHBC, ACTN3, PPARα, FGF7, and GP5	Wu et al. (2013)
Da Chuanxiong formula	Useful in migraine and nervous headache, as it dispels wind pathogens and dissipates blood stasis	Wang et al. (2013b)
Danggui/ Chuanxiong	Maintains blood stasis by nourishing and tonifying blood, activates blood circulation and dissolves blood stasis, regulates menstruations, and relieves pain	Li et al. (2012)
Zhi-Zi-Da-Huang decoction	Antioxidant effect helps to treat alcoholic liver disease through regulation of enzymes, cytochrome P450 2E1 (CYP2E1), and xanthine oxidase (XO)	An and Feng (2015)

(Continued)

TABLE 5.1 (Continued)

Formulation Name	Observations About Bioactive Compounds	References
Diesun Miaofang	Used in treatment of traumatic injury and activates blood, removes stasis, promotes qi circulation, and relieves pain	Zheng et al. (2015)
Buyang Huanwu decoction	Qi deficiency and blood-stasis diseases targeted through COX-2 and PPAR-gamma; potentially useful in cancer treatment	Ding et al. (2014)
Modified Simiaowan	Useful in gout diseases and acts through 30 core ingredients in MSW and 25 inflammatory cytokines and uric acid synthetase or transporters	Zhao et al. (2015)
8 formulations for CHD	1588 ingredients from 36 herbs used in 8 core formulae for the treatment of coronary heart disease	Ding et al. (2015)
herb Folium Eriobotryae	Useful in inflammation, and acts through regulation of 43 inflammation-associated proteins, including especially COX2, ALOX5, PPARG, TNF, and RELA	Zhang et al. (2015)
Rhubarb on renal fibrosis	Useful in renal fibrosis through bioactives like rhein, emodin, catechin, and epicatechin	Xiang et al. (2015)
Fructus Schisandrae chinensis	Shows protective activity toward hepatocyte injury by targeting GBA3/SHBGin hepatocytes	Wang et al. (2015)
Ejiao slurry	Regulates cancer cell differentiation, growth, proliferation, and apoptosis, and shows an adjuvant therapeutic effect that enriches the blood and increases immunity	Xu et al. (2014b)
Xiao-Chaihu Decoction and Da Chaihu-Decoction	XCHD treats diseases accompanying symptoms of alternating fever and chills, no desire for food or drink, and dry pharynx, while DCHD treats those with symptoms of fullness, pain in abdomen, and constipation.	Li et al. (2014a)
Dragon's blood	Used in colitis and acts through interaction with 26 putative targets	Xu et al. (2014a)

protein targets and thus are linked to many types of cancers. NP coupled to sophisticated spectroscopical analysis such as ultra-performance liquid chromatography—electrospray, ionization—tandem mass spectroscopy (UPLC-ESI-MS/MS) is a useful approach to study the absolute molecular mechanism of action of botanical formulations based on their constituent bioactives (Xu et al., 2014a). Bioactive—target analysis has shown that some of the botanical formulations are more effective than their corresponding marketed drug—target interactions (Zhang et al., 2014). This indicates the potential of NP to better understand the power of botanical formulations and to develop efficient and economical treatment options. The holistic approach of botanical formulations can be better explained by NP. A study has reported this property by exemplifying a TCM formulation against viral infectious disease (Zhang et al., 2014). Not only does the formulation target the proteins in the viral infection cycle, but it also regulates the proteins of the host defense system; thus, it acts in a very distinctive manner. This unique property of formulations is highly efficient for strengthening the broad and nonspecific antipathogenic actions. Thus, network-based, multitarget drugs can be developed by testing the efficacy of the formulation, identifying, and isolating the major bioactives and redeveloping a multicomponent therapeutic using the major bioactives based on synergism (Leung et al., 2013).

NP also serves to document and analyze the clinical prescriptions of traditional medicine practitioners (Li et al., 2015). A traditional medicine network that links bioactives to clinical symptoms through targets and diseases is a novel way to explore the basic principles of traditional medicines (Luo et al., 2015).

TRADITIONAL MEDICINE INSPIRED ETHNOPHARMACOLOGICAL NETWORKS

The network-based approaches provide a systematic platform for the study of multicomponent traditional medicine and has applications for its beneficial modernization. This platform not only recovers traditional knowledge, but it also provide new findings that can be used for resolving current problems in the drug industry (Zhang et al., 2013). This section explains a handful of ethnopharmacological networks that were developed to understand the scientific rationale of traditional medicine.

Dragon's blood (DB) tablets, which are made of resins from *Dracaena* spp., *Daemonorops* spp., *Croton* spp., and *Pterocarpus* spp., is an effective TCM for the treatment of colitis. In a study, an NP-based approach was adopted to provide new insights relating to the active constituents and molecular mechanisms underlying the effects of DB (Xu et al., 2014a). The constituent chemicals of the formulation were identified using an ultra-performance liquid chromatography-electrospray ionization-tandem mass spectrometry method. The known targets of those identified 48 compounds were mined from literature and putative targets that were predicted with the

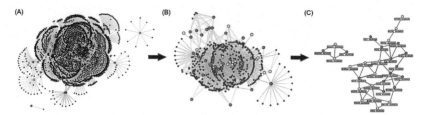

FIGURE 5.1 Putative DB targets-known colitis therapeutic targets protein—protein interaction (PPI) network: (A) The network between all targets and other human proteins. (B) The network of hub proteins in network (A). (C) The network of the major putative DB targets and the major known colitis therapeutic targets in network (B). Yellow spherical nodes indicate the putative targets; pink spherical nodes indicate the known therapeutic targets; purple spherical nodes indicate other human proteins that interact with putative targets or known therapeutic targets. Red edges in (C) indicate the PPIs of targets involved in the NOD—like receptor signaling pathway. *Source: From Xu H, Zhang Y, Lei Y, Gao X, Zhai H, Lin N, et al. A systems biology-based approach to uncovering the molecular mechanisms underlying the effects of dragon's blood tablet in colitis, involving the integration of chemical analysis, ADME prediction, and network pharmacology. PLoS One. 2014;9:e101432.*

help of computational tools. The compounds were further screened for bioavailability followed by the systematic analysis of the known and putative targets for colitis. The network evaluation revealed the mechanism of action of DB bioactives for colitis through the modulation of the proteins of the NOD-like receptor signaling pathway (Fig. 5.1).

The antioxidant mechanism of Zhi-Zi-Da-Huang decoction as an approach to treat alcohol liver disease was elucidated using NP (Li et al., 2011; An and Feng, 2015). An endothelial cell proliferation assay was performed for an antiangiogenic alkaloid, sinomenine, to validate the Network target—based Identification of Multicomponent Synergy (NIMS) predictions. The study was aimed at evaluating the synergistic relationship between different pairs of therapeutics, and sinomenine was found to have a maximum inhibition rate with matrine, both through the network and in vitro studies. The discovery of bioactives and elucidation of the mechanism of action of the herbal formulae, Qing-Luo-Yin and the Liu-Wei-Di-Huang pill, using NP, has given insight to the design validation experiments that accelerated the process of drug discovery (Li and Zhang, 2013). Validation experiments based on the network findings regarding Cold ZHENG and Hot ZHENG on a rat model of collagen—induced arthritis showed that the Cold ZHENG—oriented herbs tend to affect the hub nodes in the Cold ZHENG network, and the Hot ZHENG-oriented herbs tend to affect the hub nodes in the Hot ZHENG network (Li et al., 2007).

NP was used to explain the addition and subtraction theory of TCM. Two decoctions: Xiao Chaihu and Da Chaihu were studied using NP approach to investigate this theory. According to the addition and subtraction theory, the addition or removal of one or more ingredients from a traditional formulation resulted in a modified formula that plays a vital role in individualized

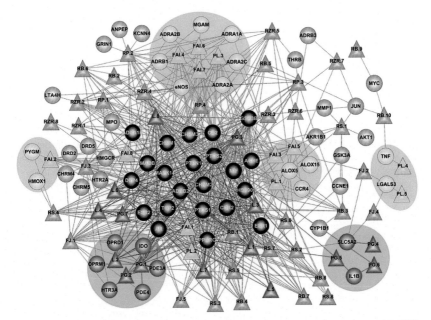

FIGURE 5.2 Drug–target network depicting the addition and subtraction theory of TCM. Drug–target interactions are shown as connecting lines between drugs (compounds, triangles) and targets (circles). The black nodes (circles) represent targets that are targeted by all the herbs of the formulation. Drugs belonging to individual herbs are highlighted in purple and green backgrounds. *Source: From Li B, Tao W, Zheng C, Shar PA, Huang C, Fu Y, et al. Systems pharmacology-based approach for dissecting the addition and subtraction theory of traditional Chinese medicine: An example using Xiao-Chaihu-Decoction and Da-Chaihu-Decoction. Comput. Biol. Med. Elsevier; 2014;53C:19–29.*

medicine. Compounds from additive herbs were observed to be more efficient on disease–associated targets (Fig. 5.2). These additive compounds were found to act on 93 diseases through 65 drug targets (Li et al., 2014a). Experimental verification of the antithrombotic network of Fufang Xueshuantong (FXST) capsule was done through in vivo studies on lipopolysaccharide–induced disseminated intravascular coagulation (DIC) rat model. It was successfully shown that FXST significantly improves the activation of the coagulation system through 41 targets from four herbs (Sheng et al., 2014). NP analysis of the Bushenhuoxue formula showed that six components—Rhein, Tanshinone IIA, Curcumin, Quercetin and Calycosin— Acted through 62 targets for the treatment of chronic kidney disease. These predictions were validated using unilateral ureteral obstruction models, and it was observed that even though the individual botanicals showed a significant decrease in creatinine levels, the combination showed lower blood creatinine and urea nitrogen levels (Shi et al., 2014). The antidiabetic effects of Ge-Gen-Qin-Lian decoction were investigated using an insulin secretion assay, and an insulin−resistance model using 13 of the 19 ingredients showed antidiabetic activity using NP studies (Li et al., 2014b). To confirm the predictions of the network of Liu-Wei-Di-Huang pill, four proteins— PPARG, RARA, CCR2, and ESR1—that denote different functions and are targeted by different groups of ingredients were chosen. The interactions between various bioactives and their effect on the expression of the proteins showed that the NP approach can accurately predict these interactions, giving hints regarding the mechanism of action of the compounds (Liang et al., 2014). Experimental results confirmed that the 30 core ingredients in Modified Simiaowan, obtained through network analysis, significantly increased HUVEC viability and attenuated the expression of ICAM-1 and proved to be effective in gout treatment (Zhao et al., 2015). The role of anthraquinone and flavanols (catechin and epicatechin) in the therapeutic potential of rhubarb in renal interstitial fibrosis was examined using network analysis and by conventional assessment involving serum biochemistry, histopathological, and immunohistochemical assays (Xiang et al., 2015). In silico analysis and experimental validation demonstrated that compound 11/12 of fructus Schisandrae chinensis targets GBA3/SHBG (Wang et al., 2015).

NP is a valuable method to study the synergistic effects of bioactives of traditional medicine formulation. This was experimentally shown on the Sendeng-4 formulation for rheumatoid arthritis (Fig. 5.3). Data and network analysis have shown that the formulation acts synergistically through nine categories of targets (Zi and Yu, 2015). Another network that studied three botanicals, *Salviae miltiorrhizae, Ligusticum chuanxiong*, and *Panax noto-ginseng* for Coronary Artery Disease (CAD), displayed their mode of action through 67 targets, out of which 13 are common among the botanicals (Fig. 5.4). These common targets are associated with thrombosis, dyslipide-mia, vasoconstriction, and inflammation (Zhou and Wang, 2014). This gives insight to how these botanicals are managing CAD.

Another approach using NP is the construction of networks based on experimental data followed by literature mining. This method is very effec-tive for large space data analysis, which will help to derive the mechanism of action of the formulation. A network of QiShenYiQi formulation having cardioprotective effects, constructed based on the microarray data and the published literature, showed that 9 main compounds were found to act through 16 pathways, out of which 9 are immune and inflammation-related (Li et al., 2014c). The mechanism of action for the Bushen Zhuanggu formulation was proposed based on LC-MS/MS standardization, phar-macokinetic analysis, and NP (Pei et al., 2013). The efficacy of Shenmai injection was evaluated using a rat model of myocardial infarction, genome-wide transcriptomic experiment, and then followed by a NP analy-sis. The overall trends in the ejection fraction and fractional shortening were consistent with the network−recovery index (NRI) from the network (Wu et al., 2013).

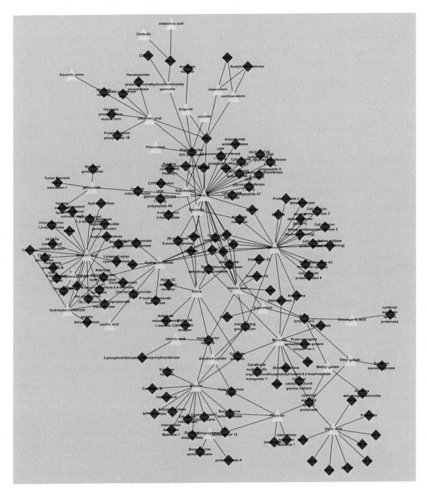

FIGURE 5.3   The chemical composition-target interaction network of Sendeng-4. The yellow nodes represent chemical components and the blue nodes represent targets. The edges represent interactions. *Source: From Zi, T., Yu, D., 2015. A network pharmacology study of Sendeng-4, a Mongolian medicine. Chin. J. Nat. Med. 13, 108–118.*

KNOWLEDGE BASES FOR NETWORK ETHNOPHARMACOLOGY

In order to develop an ethnopharmacological network, exploring the existing databases to gather information regarding bioactives and targets is the first step. Further information such as target-related diseases, tissue distribution and pathways are also to be collected depending on the type of study that is going to be undertaken. The Universal Natural Products Database (UNPD)

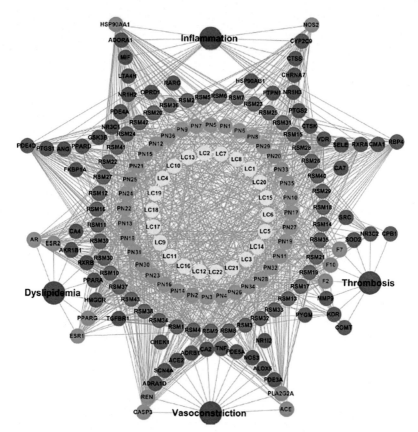

FIGURE 5.4   Network of three botanicals for Coronary Artery Disease (CAD). *Source: From Zhou, W., Wang, Y., 2014. A network-based analysis of the types of coronary artery disease from traditional Chinese medicine perspective: potential for therapeutics and drug discovery. J. Ethnopharmacol. 151, 66—77.*

(Gu et al., 2013a) is one of the major databases that provides bioactives information. Other databases that provide information regarding bioactives include CVDHD (Gu et al., 2013b), TCMSP (Ru et al., 2014), TCM@Taiwan (Sanderson, 2011), SuperNatural (Banerjee et al., 2015), and Dr. Dukes's phytochemical and ethnobotanical database (Duke and Beckstrom-Sternberg, 1994). The molecular structures of bioactives are usually stored as "SD" files and chemical information as smiles and inchkeys in these databases. Any of these file formats can be used as inputs to identify the targets in protein information databases. Binding database or "Binding DB" (Liu et al., 2007) and ChEMBL (Bento et al., 2014) are databases for predicting target proteins. Binding DB searches the exact or similar compounds in the database and retrieves the target information of those compounds. The similarity search gives the structurally similar compounds with respect to the degree of similarity as scores to the queried structure. The information regarding both annotated and predicted targets can be collected in this way. This database is connected to numerous databases, and these connections can be used to extract further information regarding the targets. The important databases linked to binding DB are UniProt (Bairoch et al., 2005), which gives information related to proteins and genes; Reactome, a curated pathway database (Croft et al., 2011); and the Kyoto Encyclopedia of Genes and Genomes (KEGG), a knowledge base for systematic analysis of gene functions and pathways (Ogata et al., 1999).

Therapeutic Targets Database (TTD) (Zhu et al., 2012) gives fully referenced information of targeted diseases of proteins, their pathway information, and the corresponding drug directed to each target. Disease and Gene Annotation (DGA), a database that provides a comprehensive and integrative annotation of human genes in disease networks, is useful in identifying the disease type that each indication belongs to (Peng et al., 2013). The human protein atlas (HPA) database (Pontén et al., 2011) is an open database showing the spatial distribution of proteins in 44 different normal human tissues. The information of the distribution of proteins in tissues can be gathered from HPA. The database also gives information regarding subcellular localization and protein class. An overall review of the methods to implement NP for herbs and herbal formulations is also available, including a systematic review of the databases that one could use for the same (Kibble et al., 2015; Lagunin et al., 2014).

Integration of knowledge bases helps data gathering for network pharmacological studies, and its knowledge base shows the inter-relationships among these databases (Fig. 5.5) (Yang et al., 2013). The counts of entities, such as bioactives, targets, and diseases, can vary based on the knowledge bases that are relied on for data collection. An integration of knowledge bases can overcome this limitation. Another factor that affects the counts of these entities is the time frame for data collection. This change occurs due to the ongoing, periodic updates of the databases.

NETWORK CONSTRUCTION

A network is the schematic representation of the interaction among various entities called nodes. In pharmacological networks, the nodes include bioactives, targets, tissue, tissue types, disease, disease types, and pathways. These nodes are connected by lines termed edges, which represent the relationship between them (Morris et al., 2012). Building a network involves two opposite approaches: a bottom-up approach on the basis of established biological knowledge and a top-down approach starting with the statistical analysis of available data. At a more detailed level, there are several ways to build and illustrate a biological network. Perhaps the most versatile and general way is

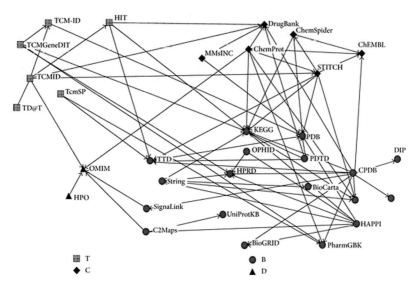

FIGURE 5.5 Database relationship network. *Source: From Yang, M., Chen, J.-L., Xu, L.-W., Ji, G., 2013. Navigating traditional Chinese medicine network pharmacology and computational tools. Evid. Based Complement Alternat. Med. 2013: 731969.*

the *de novo* assembly of a network from direct experimental or computational interactions, e.g., chemical/gene/protein screens. Networks encompassing biologically relevant nodes (genes, proteins, metabolites), their connections (biochemical and regulatory), and modules (pathways and functional units) give an authentic idea of the real biological phenomena (Xu and Qu, 2011).

Cytoscape, a Java-based open source software platform (Shannon et al., 2003), is a useful tool for visualizing molecular interaction networks and integrating them with any type of attribute data. In addition to the basic set of features for data integration, analysis, and visualization, additional features are available in the form of apps, including network and molecular profiling analysis and links with other databases. In addition to Cytoscape, a number of visualization tools are available. Visual network pharmacology (VNP) (Hu et al., 2014), which is specially designed to visualize the complex relationships among diseases, targets, and drugs, mainly contains three functional modules: drug-centric, target-centric, and disease-centric VNP. This disease-target-drug database documents known connections among diseases, targets, and the USFDA-approved drugs. Users can search the database using disease, target, or drug name strings; chemical structures and substructures; or protein sequence similarity, and then obtain an online interactive network view of the retrieved records. In the obtained network view, each node is a disease, target, or drug, and each edge is a known connection between two of them. The Connectivity Map, or the CMap tool, allows the user to compare gene-expression profiles. The similarities or differences in the signature transcriptional expression profile and the small molecule transcriptional response profile may lead to the discovery of the mode of action of the small molecule. The response profile is also compared to response profiles of drugs in the CMap database with respect to the similarity of transcriptional responses. A network is constructed and the drugs that appear closest to the small molecule are selected to have better insight into the mode of action.

Other software, such as Gephi, an exploration platform for networks and complex systems, and Cell Illustrator, a Java-based tool specialized in biological processes and systems, can also be used for building networks (Hu et al., 2014).

AYURVEDA AND NETWORK ETHNOPHARMACOLOGY

Ayurveda, the Indian traditional medicine, offers many sophisticated formulations that have been used for hundreds of years. The Traditional Knowledge Digital Library (TKDL, http://www.tkdl.res.in) contains more than 36,000 classical Ayurveda formulations. Approximately 100 of these are popularly used at the community level and also as over-the-counter products. Some of these drugs continue to be used as home remedies for preventive and primary health care in India. Until recently, no research was carried out to explore Ayurvedic wisdom using NP despite Ayurveda holding a rich knowledge of traditional medicine equal to or greater than TCM. Our group examined the use of NP to study Ayurvedic formulations with the well-known Ayurvedic formulation Triphala as a demonstrable example (Chandran et al., 2015a, b).

In this chapter, we demonstrate the application of NP in understanding and exploring the traditional wisdom with Triphala as a model.

NETWORK ETHNOPHARMACOLOGY OF TRIPHALA

Triphala is one of the most popular and widely used Ayurvedic formulations. Triphala contains fruits of three myrobalans: *Emblica officinalis* (EO; Amalaki) also known as *Phyllanthus emblica*; *Terminalia bellerica* (TB; Vibhitaka); and *Terminalia chebula* (TC; Haritaki).

Triphala is the drug of choice for the treatment of several diseases, especially those of metabolism, dental, and skin conditions, and treatment of cancer (Baliga, 2010). It has a very good effect on the health of heart, skin, eyes, and helps to delay degenerative changes, such as cataracts (Gupta et al., 2010). Triphala can be used as an inexpensive and nontoxic natural product for the prevention and treatment of diseases where vascular endothelial growth factor A—induced angiogenesis is involved (Lu et al., 2012).

The presence of numerous polyphenolic compounds empowers it with a broad antimicrobial spectrum (Sharma, 2015).

Triphala is a constituent of about 1500 Ayurveda formulations and it can be used for several diseases. Triphala combats degenerative and metabolic disorders possibly through lipid peroxide inhibition and free radical scavenging (Sabu and Kuttan, 2002). In a phase I clinical trial on healthy volunteers, immunostimulatory effects of Triphala on cytotoxic T cells and natural killer cells have been reported (Phetkate et al., 2012). Triphala is shown to induce apoptosis in tumor cells of the human pancreas, in both in vitro and in vivo models (Shi et al., 2008). Although the anticancer properties of Triphala have been studied, the exact mechanism of action is still not known. The beneficial role of Triphala in disease management of proliferative vitreoretinopathy has also been reported (Sivasankar et al., 2015). One of the key ingredients of Triphala is Amalaki. Some studies have already shown the beneficial effect of Amalaki Rasayana to suppress neurodegeneration in fly models of Huntington's and Alzheimer's diseases (Dwivedi et al., 2012, 2013). Triphala is an effective medicine to balance all three Dosha. It is considered as a good rejuvenator Rasayana, which facilitates nourishment to all tissues, or Dhatu.

Here we demonstrate the multidimensional properties of Triphala using human proteome, diseasome, and microbial proteome targeting networks.

TRIPHALA BIOACTIVES

The botanicals of Triphala—EO, TB, and TC—contain 114, 25, and 63 bioactives, respectively, according to UNPD data collected during June 2015. Of these, a few bioactives are common among the three botanicals. Thus, Triphala formulation as a whole contains 177 bioactives. Out of these, 36 bioactives were Score-1, based on Binding DB search carried out during June 2015. EO, TB, and TC contain 20, 4, and 20 Score-1 bioactives, respectively (Fig. 5.6). The Score-1 bioactives that are common among three plants are chebulanin, ellagic acid, gallussaeure, 1,6-digalloyl-beta-D-glucopiranoside, methyl gallate, and tannic acid. This bioactive information is the basic step toward constructing human proteome and microbial proteome targeting networks.

HUMAN PROTEOME AND DISEASOME TARGETING NETWORK OF TRIPHALA

Thirty-six Score-1 bioactives of Triphala are shown to interact with 60 human protein targets in 112 combinations (Fig. 5.7). Quercetin, ellagic acid, 1,2,3,4,6-pentagalloylglucose and 1,2,3,6-tetrakis-(O-galloyl)-beta-D-glucose are the four bioactives that interact with the maximum number of targets: 21, 16, and 7, respectively. The other major bioactives that have multitargeting

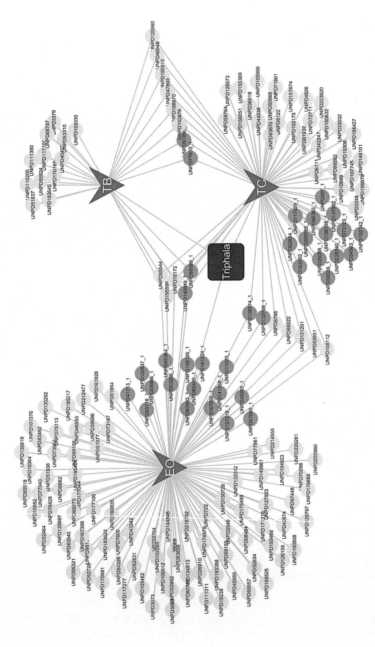

FIGURE 5.6 Bioactive network of Triphala. Dark green versus are the botanicals of Triphala and oval nodes are the bioactives where green represents Score 1 bioactives.

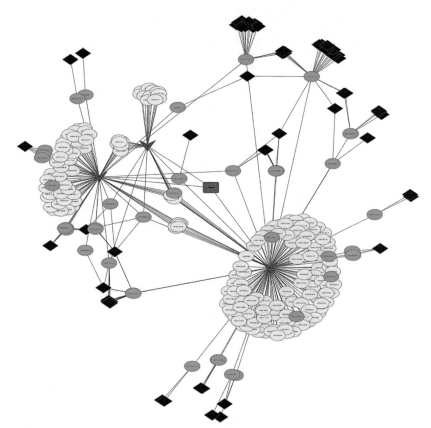

FIGURE 5.7 Bioactive—target network of Triphala. Dark green versus are the botanicals of Triphala and oval nodes are the bioactives where green represents score 1 bioactives. Blue diamonds denote targets.

property include catechin; epicatechin; gallocatechin; kaempferol; and trans-3,3',4',5,7-pentahydroxylflavane. The major protein targets of Triphala include alkaline phosphatase (ALPL); carbonic anhydrase 7 (CA7); coagulation factor X (F10), DNA repair protein RAD51 homolog 1 (RAD51); GSTM1 protein (GSTM1); beta-secretase 1 (BACE1); plasminogen activator inhibitor 1 (SERPINE1), prothrombin (F2); regulator of G-protein signaling (RGS) 4, 7, and 8, tissue-type plasminogen activator (PLAT); and tyrosine-protein phosphatase nonreceptor type 2 (PTPN2).

The 60 targets of Triphala are associated with 24 disease types, which include 130 disease indications (Fig. 5.8). The major disease types in which Triphala targets are associated include cancers, cardiovascular diseases, nervous system diseases, and metabolic diseases. Analysis of existing data indicates that targets of Triphala bioactives are involved in the 40 different types

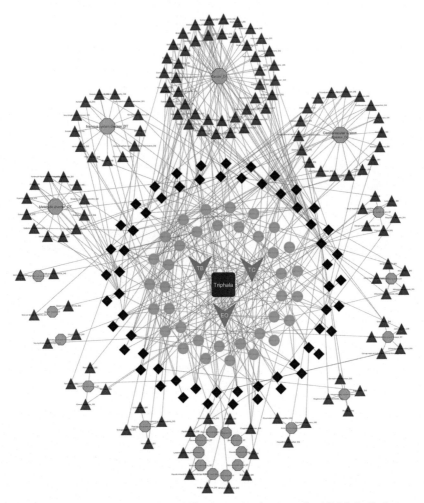

FIGURE 5.8 The human proteome and diseasome targeting network of Triphala. Dark green versus are the botanicals of Triphala and oval green nodes are the score1 bioactives. Targets are represented by blue diamond nodes, red triangle nodes depict diseases, and orange octagons indicate disease types.

of cancers making it the largest group of diseases, involving Triphala targets. This linkage is through the interaction of 25 bioactives and 27 target proteins in 46 different bioactive–target combinations. The types of cancers which are networked by Triphala include pancreatic, prostate, breast, lung, colorectal and gastric cancers, tumors, and more. Quercetin, ellagic acid, prodelphinidin A1, and 1,2,3-benzenetriol are the important bioactives; and RAD51, BACE1, F2, MMP2, IGF1R, and EGFR are the important targets that play a role in cancer.

Triphala shows links to 18 indications of cardiovascular diseases through 12 bioactives and 11 targets. The cardiovascular diseases that are covered in the Triphala network include atherosclerosis, myocardial ischemia, infarction, cerebral vasospasm, thrombosis, and hypertension. The bioactives playing a major role in cardiovascular diseases are quercetin, 1,2,3,4,6-pentagalloyoglucose, 1,2,3,6-tetrakis-(O-galloyl)-beta-D-glucose, bellericagenin A1, and prodelphinidin A1, whereas the targets playing an important role are SERPINE1, F10, F2, and FABP4.

Triphala's network to nervous system disorders contains 13 diseases in which the significant ones are Alzheimer's disease, Parkinson's disease, diabetic neuropathy, and retinopathy. In this subnetwork, 14 bioactives interact with 11 targets through 21 different interactions. Quercetin, 1,2,3,4,6-pentagalloyoglucose, 1,2,3,6-tetrakis-(O-galloyl)-beta-D-glucose, and epigallocatechin-3-gallate are the most networked bioactives whereas the most networked targets are BACE1, SERPINE1, PLAT, ALDR, CA2.

The association of Triphala with metabolic disorders is determined by six bioactives that interact with seven targets. The major metabolic diseases come in this link are obesity, diabetic complications, noninsulin-dependent diabetes, hypercholesterolemia, hyperlipidemia, and more. The bioactives having more interactions with targets are ellagic acid, quercetin, and bellericagenin A1, whereas the highly networked targets are IGF1R, FABP5, ALDR, and AKR1B1. Triphala bioactives are also linked to targets of other diseases comprising autoimmune diseases, ulcerative colitis, McCune–Albright syndrome, psoriasis, gout, osteoarthritis, endometriosis, lung fibrosis, glomerulonephritis, and more.

The proteome-targeting network of Triphala, thus, shows its ability to synergistically modulate 60 targets that are associated with 130 disease indications. This data is generated with the available information that included only one-fifth of the total number of bioactives. Further logical analysis and experimental studies based on the network result are needed to explore the in-depth mechanism of action of Triphala. For researchers in this area, these kind of networks can give an immense amount of information that can be developed further to reveal the real mystery behind the actions of traditional medicine.

MICROBIAL PROTEOME TARGETING NETWORK OF TRIPHALA

Triphala is also referred to as a "tridoshic rasayana," as it balances the three constitutional elements of life. It tonifies the gastrointestinal tract, improves digestion, and is known to exhibit antiviral, antibacterial, antifungal, and antiallergic properties (Sharma, 2015; Amala and Jeyaraj, 2014; Sumathi and Parvathi, 2010). Triphala Mashi (mashi: black ash) was found to have nonspecific antimicrobial activity, as it showed a dose-dependent inhibition of Gram-positive and Gram-negative bacteria (Biradar et al., 2008).

Hydroalcoholic, aqueous, and ether extracts of the three fruits of Triphala were reported to show antibacterial activity against uropathogens with a maximum drug efficacy recorded by the alcoholic extract (Bag et al., 2013; Prasad et al., 2009). The methanolic extract of Triphala showed the presence of 10 active compounds using GC-MS and also showed potent antibacterial and antifungal activity (Amala and Jeyaraj, 2014).

Triphala has been well studied for its antimicrobial activity against Gram-positive bacteria, Gram-negative bacteria, fungal species, and different strains of *Salmonella typhi* (Amala and Jeyaraj, 2014; Sumathi and Parvathi, 2010; Gautam et al., 2012; Srikumar et al., 2007). Triphala showed significant antimicrobial activity against *Enterococcus faecalis* and *Streptococcus mutans* grown on tooth substrate thereby making it a suitable agent for prevention of dental plaque (Prabhakar et al., 2010, 2014). The application of Triphala in commercial antimicrobial agents has been explored. A significant reduction in the colony forming units of oral streptococci was observed after 6% Triphala was incorporated in a mouthwash formulation (Srinagesh et al., 2012). An ointment prepared from Triphala (10% (w/w)) showed significant antibacterial and wound healing activity in rats infected with *Staphylococcus aureus*, *Pseudomonas aeruginosa*, and *Streptococcus pyogenes* (Kumar et al., 2008). The antiinfective network of Triphala sheds light on the efficacy of the formulation in the simultaneous targeting of multiple microorganisms. Also, this network provides information regarding some novel bioactive−target combinations that can be explored to combat the problem of multidrug resistance.

Among the bioactives of Triphala, 24 Score-1 bioactives target microbial proteins of 22 microorganisms. The botanicals of Triphala-EO, TB, and TC-contain 19, 3, and 8 Score1 bioactives respectively which showed interactions with microbial proteins. They act through modulation of 35 targets which are associated with diseases such as Leishmaniasis, malaria, tuberculosis, hepatitis C, acquired immunodeficiency syndrome (AIDS), cervical cancer, candidiasis, luminous vibriosis, yersiniosis, skin and respiratory infections, severe acute respiratory syndrome (SARS), avian viral infection, bacteremia, sleeping sickness, and anthrax (Fig. 5.9). The microorganisms captured in the Triphala antiinfective network includes candida albicans, hepatitis C virus, human immunodeficiency virus 1, human papillomavirus type 16, human SARS coronavirus leishmania amazonensis, *Mycobacterium tuberculosis*, *staphylococcus aureus*, *Plasmodium falciparum*, and *Yersinia enterocolitica*.

In Mycobacterium tuberculosis, dTDP-4-dehydrorhamnose 3,5-epimerase RmlC is one of the four enzymes involved in the synthesis of dTDP-L-rhamnose, a precursor of L-rhamnose (Giraud et al., 2000). The network shows that Triphala has the potential to modulate the protein through four bioactives such as punicalins, terflavin B, 4-*O*-(S)-flavogallonyl-6-*O*-galloyl-beta-D-glucopyranose, and 4,6-*O*-(S,S)-gallagyl-alpha/beta-D-glucopyranose.

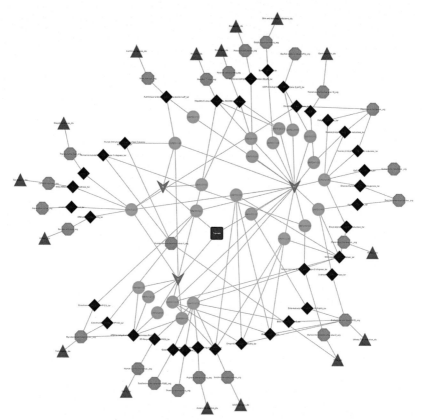

FIGURE 5.9   The microbial proteome—targeting network of Triphala. Dark green verus are the botanicals of Triphala and oval green nodes are the Score1 bioactives. Targets, diseases, and microorganisms are represented by blue diamond nodes, red triangle nodes, and pink octagon nodes, respectively.

Research on new therapeutics that target the mycobacterial cell wall is in progress. Rhamnosyl residues play a structural role in the mycobacterial cell wall by acting as a linker connecting arabinogalactin polymer to peptidoglycan and are not found in humans, which gives them a degree of therapeutic potential (Ma et al., 2001). Triphala can be considered in this line to develop novel antimycobacterial drugs.

The network shows the potential of gallussaeure and 3-galloylgallic acid to modulate human immunodeficiency virus type 1 reverse transcriptase. Inhibition of human immunodeficiency virus at the initial stage itself is crucial and thus, targeting human immunodeficiency virus type 1 reverse transcriptase, at the preinitiation stage is considered to be an effective therapy. Protein E6 of human papillomavirus 16 (HPV16) prevents apoptosis of infected cells by binding to FADD and caspase 8 and hence being targeted for development of antiviral drugs (Yuan et al., 2012). Kaempferol of Triphala is found to target protein E6 of HPV16, which is a potential mechanism to control the replication of the virus.

The network also shows Triphala's potential to act on *Plasmodium falciparum*. Enoyl-acyl carrier protein reductase (ENR) has been investigated as an attractive target due to its important role in membrane construction and energy production in *Plasmodium falciparum* (Nicola et al., 2007) while the parasite interacts with human erythrocyte spectrin and other membrane proteins through protein M18 aspartyl aminopeptidase (Lauterbach and Coetzer, 2008). Trans-3,3',4',5,7-pentahydroxylflavane, epigallocatechin, and epicatechin can modulate both while epigallocatechin 3-gallate can regulate Enoyl-acyl carrier protein reductase and, Quercetin and vanillic acid can act on M18 aspartyl aminopeptidase. Epigallocatechin 3-gallate can also target 3-oxoacyl-acyl-carrier protein reductase which is a potent therapeutic target because of its role in type II fatty acid synthase pathway of *Plasmodium falciparum* (Karmodiya and Surolia, 2006).

Epigallocatechin 3-gallate and Quercetin are the bioactives that have shown maximum antimicrobial targets interaction. While Epigallocatechin 3-gallate shows interaction with 3-oxoacyl-(Acyl-carrier protein) reductase, CpG DNA methylase, Enoyl-acyl-carrier protein reductase, Glucose-6-phosphate 1-dehydrogenase, hepatitis C virus serine protease, NS3/NS4A and YopH of *Plasmodium falciparum, Saccharomyces cerevisiae*, and *Spiroplasma monobiae*; Quercetin acts on 3C-like proteinase (3CL-PRO), arginase, beta-lactamase AmpC, glutathione reductase, M18 aspartyl aminopeptidase, malate dehydrogenase and tyrosine-protein kinase transforming protein FPS of *Escherichia coli*, Fujinami sarcoma virus, human SARS coronavirus (SARS-CoV), *Leishmania amazonensis, Plasmodium falciparum, Saccharomyces cerevisiae*, and *Thermus thermophiles*.

APPLICATIONS OF NETWORK PHARMACOLOGY

NP has gained impetus as a novel paradigm for drug discovery. This approach using in silico data is fast becoming popular due to its cost efficiency and comparably good predictability. Thus, network analysis has various applications and promising future prospects with regard to the process of drug discovery and development. Table 5.2 lists the important applications of NP.

LIMITATIONS AND SOLUTIONS

NP has proven to be a boon for drug research, and that helps in the revival of traditional knowledge. Albeit there are a few limitations of using NP for

TABLE 5.2 Applications of Network Pharmacology

Traditional medicine	• Scientific evidence for use of Ayurvedic medicine • Understanding the rationale of traditional formulations • Understanding the mechanism of action of Ayurvedic medicines • Safety and efficacy of Ayurvedic medicines • Possible substitutes for endangered botanicals • Network-based designing and prescribing of plant formulations • Analysis of multiple bioactives, studying synergistic action • Botanical biomarkers for quality control
Pharmacology	• To develop new leads from natural products • Understanding the mechanism of action of drugs • Determining the possible side effects of drugs • Predicting new indications • Predicting toxicity • Predicting possible drug−drug interactions • Rational design of drugs based on group of interacting proteins • Drug repurposing
Drug research	• Identifying novel drug targets • Reduced cost and time through in silico evaluation • Understanding the signaling pathway of disease types • Designing experiments based on drugs and targets • Therapeutics for multigene-dependent diseases • Discovery of disease-causing genes • Diagnostic biomarkers • Studying drug resistance or antibiotic resistance

studying traditional medicine that would hopefully get resolved in the future. The major limitations and possible solutions are listed:

1. NEP currently relies on various databases for literature and bioactive mining. Databases, though curated, may show discrepancies due to numerous sources of information, theoretical, and experimental data. Moreover, the botanicals that undergo certain preparatory procedures during the formulation of the medicine may have its constituents that have chemically changed due to the procedures; like boiling, acid/ alkali reactions, interactions between the bioactives, etc. A way to navigate around this problem is to make use of modern, high-throughput chemical identification techniques like ultra-performance liquid chromatography−electrospray ionization−tandem mass spectroscopy (UPLC-ESI-MS/MS). This technique will help to identify the exact bioactives or the chemical constituents of the formulation, and will enrich the subsequent

NEP studies. This is because the bioactives form the foundation of any traditional medicine network.

2. Absorption, distribution, metabolism, excretion, and toxic effects (ADMET) parameters associated with the bioactives/formulation when they are administered in the form of the medicine need to be considered in order to extrapolate in silico and cheminformatics data to in vitro and in vivo models. In silico tools that offer the prediction of these parameters can be depended on for this. But traditional medicines are generally accompanied by a vehicle for delivery of the medicine. These vehicles, normally various solvents—water, milk, lemon juice, butter, ghee (clarified butter), honey—that alter the solubility of the bioactives, play a role in regulating ADMET parameters. Experimental validation studies are required to evaluate this principle of traditional medicine.

3. Target identification usually relies on a single or a few databases due to the limited availability of databases with free access. This can occasionally give incomplete results. Also, there may be novel targets waiting to be discovered that could be a part of the mechanism of action of the bioactives. To deal with this discrepancy in the network, multiple databases should be considered for target identification. Integration of databases serving similar functions can also be a solution for this problem. In addition to this, experimental validation of the target molecules using protein–protein interaction studies or gene expression studies will provide concrete testimony to the network predictions.

4. A number of traditional medicines act through multiple bioactives and targets. Synergy in botanical drugs helps to balance out the extreme pharmacological effects that individual bioactives may have. The interactions of bioactives with various target proteins, their absorption into the body after possible enzyme degradation, their transport, and finally their physiological effect are a crucial part of traditional medicine (Gilbert and Alves, 2003). However, in vitro assays or in silico tools are unable to give a clear idea as to the complete and exact interactions in a living organism. NP is only the cardinal step toward understanding the mechanism of bioactives/formulations. But this gives an overview of the action of traditional medicine which can be used to design in vivo experiments and clinical trials. This saves time and cost of research and inventions.

5. It is observed that formulations are working by simultaneous modulation of multiple targets. This modulation includes activation of some targets and inhibition of other. In order to understand this complex synergistic activity of formulation, investigative studies regarding the interactions of ligands with targets are to be carried out. This can be achieved by implementing high-throughput omics studies based on the network data.

CONCLUSION

Network pharmacological analysis presents an immense scope for exploring traditional knowledge to find solutions for the current problems challenging the drug discovery industry. NEP can also play a key role in new drug discovery, drug repurposing, and rational formulation discovery. Many of the bioactive—target combinations have been experimentally studied. The data synthesis using NP provides information regarding the mode of action of traditional medicine formulations, based on their constituent bioactives. This is a kind of reverse approach to deduce the molecular mechanism of action of formulations using modern, integrated technologies. The current network analysis is based on the studies that have been conducted and the literature that is available. Hence, the data is inconclusive as a number of studies are still underway and novel data is being generated continuously. Despite its limitations, this still is a favorable approach, as it gives insight into the hidden knowledge of our ancient traditional medicine wisdom. NP aids the logical analysis of this wisdom that can be utilized to understand the knowledge as well as to invent novel solutions for current pharmacological problems.

REFERENCES

Amala, V.E., Jeyaraj, M., 2014. Determination of antibacterial, antifungal, bioactive constituents of Triphala by FT-IR and GC-MS analysis. Int. J. Pharm. Pharm. Sci. 6, 13—16.

An, L., Feng, F., 2015. Network pharmacology-based antioxidant effect study of Zhi-Zi-Da-Huang decoction for alcoholic liver disease. Evid. Based Complement Alternat. Med. 2015, 1—6.

Bag, A., Bhattacharyya, S.K., Pal, N.K., 2013. Antibacterial potential of hydroalcoholic extracts of Triphala components against multidrug-resistant uropathogenic bacteria--a preliminary report. Ind. J. Exp. Biol. 51, 709—714.

Bairoch, A., Apweiler, R., Wu, C.H., Barker, W.C., Boeckmann, B., Ferro, S., et al., 2005. The universal protein resource (UniProt). Nucl. Acids Res. 33, D154—D159.

Baliga, M.S., 2010. Triphala, ayurvedic formulation for treating and preventing cancer: a review. J. Altern. Compl. Med. 16, 1301—1308.

Banerjee, P., Erehman, J., Gohlke, B.-O., Wilhelm, T., Preissner, R., Dunkel, M., 2015. Super natural II--a database of natural products. Nucl. Acids Res. 43, D935—D939.

Barabási, A.-L., Oltvai, Z.N., 2004. Network biology: understanding the cell's functional organization. Nat. Rev. Genet. 5, 101—113.

Bento, A.P., Gaulton, A., Hersey, A., Bellis, L.J., Chambers, J., Davies, M., et al., 2014. The ChEMBL bioactivity database: an update. Nucl. Acids Res. 42.

Berger, S.I., Iyengar, R., 2009. Network analyses in systems pharmacology. Bioinformatics 25, 2466—2472.

Biradar, Y.S., Jagatap, S., Khandelwal, K.R., Singhania, S.S., 2008. Exploring of antimicrobial activity of Triphala mashi-an ayurvedic formulation. Evidence-based complement. Altern. Med. 5, 107—113.

Burger, A., 1964. Approaches to drug discovery. N Engl. J. Med. 270, 1098—1101.

Buriani, A., Garcia-Bermejo, M.L., Bosisio, E., Xu, Q., Li, H., Dong, X., et al., 2012. Omic techniques in systems biology approaches to traditional Chinese medicine research: present and future. J. Ethnopharmacol. 140, 535−544.

Chandran, U., Mehendale, N., Tillu, G., Patwardhan, B., 2015a. Network pharmacology: an emerging technique for natural product drug discovery and scientific research on ayurveda. Proc. Ind. Natl. Acad. Sci. 81, 561−568.

Chandran, U., Mehendale, N., Tillu, G., Patwardhan, B., 2015b. Network pharmacology of ayurveda formulation Triphala with special reference to anti-cancer property. Comb. Chem. High Throughput Screen 18, 846−854.

Chen, D., Lu, P., Zhang, F.-B., Tang, S.-H., Yang, H.-J., 2013. Molecular mechanism research on simultaneous therapy of brain and heart based on data mining and network analysis. Zhongguo Zhong Yao Za Zhi 38, 91−98.

Cheng, B.F., Hou, Y.Y., Jiang, M., Zhao, Z.Y., Dong, L.Y., Bai, G., 2013. Anti-inflammatory mechanism of qingfei xiaoyan wan studied with network pharmacology. Yao Xue Xue Bao 48, 686−693.

Cho, D.-Y., Kim, Y.-A., Przytycka, T.M., 2012. Chapter 5: network biology approach to complex diseases. PLoS Comput. Biol. 8, e1002820.

Clark, D.E., Grootenhuis, P.D.J., 2002. Progress in computational methods for the prediction of ADMET properties. Curr. Opin. Drug Discov. Devel. 5, 382−390.

Clark, D.E., Pickett, S.D., 2000. Computational methods for the prediction of "drug-likeness.". Drug Discov. Today 5, 49−58.

Croft, D., O'Kelly, G., Wu, G., Haw, R., Gillespie, M., Matthews, L., et al., 2011. Reactome: a database of reactions, pathways and biological processes. Nucl. Acids Res. 39.

Ding, F., Zhang, Q., Hu, Y., Wang, Y., 2014. Mechanism study on preventive and curative effects of buyang huanwu decoction in Qi deficiency and blood stasis diseases based on network analysis. Zhongguo Zhong Yao Za Zhi 39, 4418−4425.

Ding, F., Zhang, Q., Ung, C.O.L., Wang, Y., Han, Y., Hu, Y., et al., 2015. An analysis of chemical ingredients network of Chinese herbal formulae for the treatment of coronary heart disease. PLoS One 10, e0116441.

Duke, J.A., Beckstrom-Sternberg, S.M., 1994. Dr. Duke's phytochemical and ethnobotanical databases. ARS/USDA.

Dwivedi, V., Anandan, E.M., Mony, R.S., Muraleedharan, T.S., Valiathan, M.S., Mutsuddi, M., et al., 2012. In vivo effects of traditional ayurvedic formulations in drosophila melanogaster model relate with therapeutic applications. PLoS One 7, e37113.

Dwivedi, V., Tripathi, B.K., Mutsuddi, M., Lakhotia, S.C., 2013. Ayurvedic Amalaki Rasayana and Rasa-Sindoor suppress neurodegeneration in fly models of Huntington's and Alzheimer's diseases. Curr. Sci. 105 (12), 1711−1723.

Ellingson, S.R., Smith, J.C., Baudry, J., 2014. Polypharmacology and supercomputer-based docking: opportunities and challenges. Mol. Simul. 40, 848−854.

Fang, X., Shao, L., Zhang, H., Wang, S., 2005. CHMIS-C: a comprehensive herbal medicine information system for cancer. J. Med. Chem. 48, 1481−1488.

Fang, Y.-C., Huang, H.-C., Chen, H.-H., Juan, H.-F., 2008. TC;MGeneDIT: a database for associated traditional Chinese medicine, gene and disease information using text mining. BMC Compl. Altern. Med. 8, 58.

Fang, Z., Lu, B., Liu, M., Zhang, M., Yi, Z., Wen, C., et al., 2013. Evaluating the pharmacological mechanism of Chinese medicine Si-Wu-Tang through multi-level data integration. PLoS One 8, 1−8.

Gautam, A.K., Avasthi, S., Sharma, A., Bhadauria, R., 2012. Antifungal potential of Triphala churna ingredients against Aspergillus species associated with them during storage. Pakistan J. Biol. Sci. 15, 244−249.

Gilbert, B., Alves, L.F., 2003. Synergy in plant medicines. Curr. Med. Chem. 10, 13−20.

Giraud, M.F., Leonard, G.A., Field, R.A., Berlind, C., Naismith, J.H., 2000. RmlC, the third enzyme of dTDP-L-rhamnose pathway, is a new class of epimerase. Nat. Struct. Biol. 7, 398−402.

Gu, J., Chen, Y., Li, S., Li, Y., 2010. Identification of responsive gene modules by network-based gene clustering and extending: application to inflammation and angiogenesis. BMC Syst. Biol. 4, 47.

Gu, J., Gui, Y., Chen, L., Yuan, G., Lu, H.Z., Xu, X., 2013a. Use of natural products as chemical library for drug discovery and network pharmacology. PLoS One 8, 1−10.

Gu, J., Gui, Y., Chen, L., Yuan, G., Xu, X., 2013b. CVDHD: a cardiovascular disease herbal database for drug discovery and network pharmacology. J. Cheminform 5, 51.

Gu, S., Yin, N., Pei, J., Lai, L., 2013c. Understanding traditional Chinese medicine anti-inflammatory herbal formulae by simulating their regulatory functions in the human arachidonic acid metabolic network. Mol. Biosyst. 9, 1931−1938.

Gupta, S.K., Kalaiselvan, V., Srivastava, S., Agrawal, S.S., Saxena, R., 2010. Evaluation of anticataract potential of Triphala in selenite-induced cataract: in vitro and in vivo studies. J. Ayurveda Integr. Med. 1, 280−286.

Hacker, M., Messer II, W.S., Bachmann, K.A., 2009. Pharmacology: Principles and Practice. Elsevier/Academic Press.

Hamosh, A., Scott, A.F., Amberger, J.S., Bocchini, C.A., McKusick, V.A., 2005. Online mendelian inheritance in man (OMIM), a knowledgebase of human genes and genetic disorders. Nucl. Acids Res. 33, D514−D517.

Harvey, A.L., 2008. Natural products in drug discovery. Drug Discov. Today 13, 894−901.

Hopkins, A.L., 2007. Network pharmacology. Nat. Biotechnol. 25, 1110−1111.

Hopkins, A.L., 2008. Network pharmacology: the next paradigm in drug discovery. Nat. Chem. Biol. 4, 682−690.

Hu, Q.-N., Deng, Z., Tu, W., Yang, X., Meng, Z.-B., Deng, Z.-X., et al., 2014. VNP: interactive visual network pharmacology of diseases, targets, and drugs. CPT Pharmacometrics Syst. Pharmacol. 3, e105.

Huang, Y., Li, S., 2010. Detection of characteristic sub pathway network for angiogenesis based on the comprehensive pathway network.. BMC Bioinformatics11.

Karmodiya, K., Surolia, N., 2006. Analyses of co-operative transitions in plasmodium falciparum beta-ketoacyl acyl carrier protein reductase upon co-factor and acyl carrier protein binding. FEBS J. 273, 4093−4103.

Kibble, M., Saarinen, N., Tang, J., Wennerberg, K., Mäkelä, S., Aittokallio, T., 2015. Network pharmacology applications to map the unexplored target space and therapeutic potential of natural products. Nat. Prod. Rep. 32, 1249−1266.

Kumar, M.S., Kirubanandan, S., Sripriya, R., Sehgal, P.K., 2008. Triphala promotes healing of infected full-thickness dermal wound. J. Surg. Res. 144, 94−101.

Lagunin, A.A., Goel, R.K., Gawande, D.Y., Pahwa, P., Gloriozova, T.A., Dmitriev, A.V., et al., 2014. Chemo- and bioinformatics resources for in silico drug discovery from medicinal plants beyond their traditional use: a critical review. Nat. Prod. Rep. 31(11), 1585−5611.

Lauterbach, S.B., Coetzer, T.L., 2008. The M18 aspartyl aminopeptidase of plasmodium falciparum binds to human erythrocyte spectrin in vitro. Malar. J. 7, 161.

Leung, E.L., Cao, Z.-W., Jiang, Z.-H., Zhou, H., Liu, L., 2013. Network-based drug discovery by integrating systems biology and computational technologies. Brief. Bioinform. 14, 491—505.

Li, B., Tao, W., Zheng, C., Shar, P.A., Huang, C., Fu, Y., et al., 2014a. Systems pharmacology-based approach for dissecting the addition and subtraction theory of traditional Chinese medicine: an example using xiao-chaihu-decoction and da-chaihu-decoction. Comput. Biol. Med. 53C, 19—29, Elsevier.

Li, H., Zhao, L., Zhang, B., Jiang, Y., Wang, X., Guo, Y., et al., 2014b. A network pharmacology approach to determine active compounds and action mechanisms of Ge-Gen-Qin-Lian decoction for treatment of type 2 diabetes. Evid. Based Complement Altern. Med. 2014.

Li, J., Lu, C., Jiang, M., Niu, X., Guo, H., Li, L., et al., 2012. Traditional Chinese medicine-based network pharmacology could lead to new multicompound drug discovery. Evid. Based. Complement. Alternat. Med. 2012.

Li, S., 2007. Framework and practice of network-based studies for Chinese herbal formula. J. Chinese Integr. Med. 5, 489—493.

Li, S., Zhang, B., 2013. Traditional Chinese medicine network pharmacology: theory, methodology and application. Chin. J. Nat. Med. 11, 110—120.

Li, S., Wu, L., Zhang, Z., 2006. Constructing biological networks through combined literature mining and microarray analysis: a LMMA approach. Bioinformatics 22, 2143—2150.

Li, S., Zhang, Z.Q., Wu, L.J., Zhang, X.G., Li, Y.D., Wang, Y., 2007. Understanding ZHENG in traditional Chinese medicine in the context of neuro-endocrine-immune network. IET Syst. Biol. 1, 51—60.

Li, S., Zhang, B., Jiang, D., Wei, Y., Zhang, N., 2010. Herb network construction and co-module analysis for uncovering the combination rule of traditional Chinese herbal formulae. BMC Bioinformatics 11, BioMed Central Ltd.

Li, S., Zhang, B., Zhang, N., 2011. Network target for screening synergistic drug combinations with application to traditional Chinese medicine. BMC Syst. Biol. 5, BioMed Central Ltd.

Li, W., Tang, Y., Shang, E., Guo, J., Huang, M., Qian, D., et al., 2012. Analysis on correlation between general efficacy and chemical constituents of danggui-chuanxiong herb pair based on artificial neural network. Zhongguo Zhong Yao Za Zhi 37, 2935—2942.

Li, X., Wu, L., Fan, X., Zhang, B., Gao, X., Wang, Y., et al., 2011. Network pharmacology study on major active compounds of fufang danshen formula. Zhongguo Zhong Yao Za Zhi 36, 2911—2915.

Li, X., Wu, L., Liu, W., Jin, Y., Chen, Q., Wang, L., et al., 2014c. A network pharmacology study of Chinese medicine QiShenYiQi to reveal its underlying multi-compound, multi-target, multi-pathway mode of action. PLoS One 9, 1—11.

Li, Y., Li, R., Ouyang, Z., Li, S., 2015. Herb network analysis for a famous TCM doctor' s prescriptions on treatment of rheumatoid arthritis. Evidence-based complement. Altern. Med. 2015.

Liang, X., Li, H., Li, S., 2014. A novel network pharmacology approach to analyse traditional herbal formulae: the Liu-Wei-Di-Huang pill as a case study. Mol. Biosyst. 10, 1014—1022.

Liu, T., Lin, Y., Wen, X., Jorissen, R.N., Gilson, M.K., 2007. BindingDB: a web-accessible database of experimentally determined protein-ligand binding affinities. Nucl. Acids Res. 35, 198—201.

Liu, P., Duan, J.-A., Bai, G., Su, S.-L., 2014. Network pharmacology study on major active compounds of siwu decoction analogous formulae for treating primary dysmenorrhea of gynecology blood stasis syndrome. Zhongguo Zhong Yao Za Zhi 39, 113—120.

Liu, X., 2013. Computational pharmacological comparison of *Salvia miltiorrhiza* and *Panax notoginseng* used in the therapy of cardiovascular diseases. Exp. Ther. Med.1163–1168.

Lu, K., Chakroborty, D., Sarkar, C., Lu, T., Xie, Z., Liu, Z., Basu, S., 2012. Triphala and its active constituent chebulinic acid are natural inhibitors of vascular endothelial growth factor-a mediated angiogenesis. PLoS One 7, e43934.

Lu, L., Li, Y., Li, S., 2011. Computational identification of potential microRNA network biomarkers for the progression stages of gastric cancer. Int. J. Data Min. Bioinform. 5, 519–531.

Luo, F., Gu, J., Chen, L., Xu, X., 2014. Systems pharmacology strategies for anticancer drug discovery based on natural products. Mol. Biosyst. 10, 1912–1917.

Luo, F., Gu, J., Zhang, X., Chen, L., Cao, L., Li, N., et al., 2015. Multiscale modeling of drug-induced effects of ReDuNing injection on human disease: from drug molecules to clinical symptoms of disease. Sci. Rep. 5, 10064.

Ma, Y., Stern, R.J., Scherman, M.S., Vissa, V.D., Yan, W., Jones, V.C., et al., 2001. Drug targeting mycobacterium tuberculosis cell wall synthesis: genetics of dTDP-rhamnose synthetic enzymes and development of a microtiter plate-based screen for inhibitors of conversion of dTDP-glucose to dTDP-rhamnose. Antimicrob. Agents Chemother. 45, 1407–1416.

Ma, T., Tan, C., Zhang, H., Wang, M., Ding, W., Li, S., 2010. Bridging the gap between traditional Chinese medicine and systems biology: the connection of cold syndrome and NEI network. Mol. Biosyst. 6, 613–619.

Morris, J.S., Ph, D., Kuchinsky, A., Pico, A., Institutes, G., 2012. Analysis and Visualization of Biological Networks with Cytoscape. UCSF, p. 65.

Nicola, G., Smith, C.A., Lucumi, E., Kuo, M.R., Karagyozov, L., Fidock, D.A., et al., 2007. Discovery of novel inhibitors targeting enoyl-acyl carrier protein reductase in plasmodium falciparum by structure-based virtual screening. Biochem. Biophys. Res. Commun. 358, 686–691.

Ogata, H., Goto, S., Sato, K., Fujibuchi, W., Bono, H., Kanehisa, M., 1999. KEGG: kyoto encyclopedia of genes and genomes. Nucl. Acids Res. 27, 29–34.

Paolini, G.V., Shapland, R.H.B., van Hoorn, W.P., Mason, J.S., Hopkins, A.L., 2006. Global mapping of pharmacological space. Nat. Biotechnol. 24, 805–815.

Patwardhan, B., 2014a. Rediscovering drug discovery. Comb. Chem. High Throughput Screen 17, 819.

Patwardhan, B., 2014b. The new pharmacognosy. Comb. Chem. High Throughput Screen 17, 97.

Patwardhan, B., Chandran, U., 2015. Network ethnopharmacology approaches for formulation discovery. Ind. J. Tradit. Knowl. 14, 574–580.

Patwardhan, B., Mutalik, G., Tillu, G., 2015. Integrative Approaches For Health: Biomedical Research, Ayurveda and Yoga. Academic Press, Elsevier Inc.

Pei, L., Bao, Y., Liu, S., Zheng, J., Chen, X., 2013. Material basis of Chinese herbal formulas explored by combining pharmacokinetics with network pharmacology. PLoS One 8, e57414.

Peng, K., Xu, W., Zheng, J., Huang, K., Wang, H., Tong, J., et al., 2013. The disease and gene annotations (DGA): an annotation resource for human disease. Nucl. Acids Res. 41, 553–560.

Phetkate, P., Kummalue, T., U-Pratya, Y., Kietinun, S., 2012. Significant increase in cytotoxic T lymphocytes and natural killer cells by Triphala: a clinical phase i study. Evid. Based Complement Alternat. Med. 2012.

Pontén, F.K., Schwenk, J.M., Asplund, A., Edqvist, P.H.D., 2011. The human protein atlas as a proteomic resource for biomarker discovery. J. Intern. Med. 270, 428–446.

Prabhakar, J., Senthilkumar, M., Priya, M.S., Mahalakshmi, K., Sehgal, P.K., Sukumaran, V.G., 2010. Evaluation of antimicrobial efficacy of herbal alternatives (Triphala and green tea polyphenols), MTAD, and 5% sodium hypochlorite against enterococcus faecalis biofilm formed on tooth substrate: an in vitro study. J. Endod. 36, 83–86.

Prabhakar, J., Balagopal, S., Priya, M., Selvi, S., Senthilkumar, M., 2014. Evaluation of antimicrobial efficacy of Triphala (an Indian Ayurvedic herbal formulation) and 0.2% chlorhexidine against Streptococcus mutans biofilm formed on tooth substrate: an in vitro study. Ind. J. Dent. Res. 25, 475.

Prasad, C.P., Rath, G., Mathur, S., Bhatnagar, D., Ralhan, R., 2009. Potent growth suppressive activity of curcumin in human breast cancer cells: modulation of Wnt/beta-catenin signaling. Chem. Biol. Interact. 181, 263–271.

Re, M., Valentini, G., 2013. Network-based drug ranking and repositioning with respect to DrugBank therapeutic categories. IEEE/ACM Trans. Comput. Biol. Bioinform. 10, 1359–1371.

Ru, J., Li, P., Wang, J., Zhou, W., Li, B., Huang, C., et al., 2014. TCMSP: a database of systems pharmacology for drug discovery from herbal medicines. J. Cheminform 6, 13.

Sabu, M.C., Kuttan, R., 2002. Anti-diabetic activity of medicinal plants and its relationship with their antioxidant property. J. Ethnopharmacol. 81, 155–160.

Sanderson, K., 2011. Databases aim to bridge the East-West divide of drug discovery. Nat. Med. 17, 1531, Nature Publishing Group, a division of Macmillan Publishers Limited. All Rights Reserved.

Shannon, P., Markiel, A., Ozier, O., Baliga, N.S., Wang, J.T., Ramage, D., et al., 2003. Cytoscape: a software environment for integrated models of biomolecular interaction networks. Genome Res.2498–2504.

Sharma, S., 2015. Triphala powder: a wonder of ayurveda. Int. J. Recent Res. Asp. 2, 107–111.

Sheng, S., Wang, J., Wang, L., Liu, H., Li, P., Liu, M., et al., 2014. Network pharmacology analyses of the antithrombotic pharmacological mechanism of Fufang Xueshuantong Capsule with experimental support using disseminated intravascular coagulation rats. J. Ethnopharmacol. 154, 735–744.

Shi, S.H., Cai, Y.P., Cai, X.J., Zheng, X.Y., Cao, D.S., Ye, F.Q., et al., 2014. A network pharmacology approach to understanding the mechanisms of action of traditional medicine: bushenhuoxue formula for treatment of chronic kidney disease. PLoS One 9.

Shi, Y., Sahu, R.P., Srivastava, S.K., 2008. Triphala inhibits both in vitro and in vivo xenograft growth of pancreatic tumor cells by inducing apoptosis. BMC Cancer 8, 294.

Sivasankar, S., Lavanya, R., Brindha, P., Angayarkanni, N., 2015. Aqueous and alcoholic extracts of Triphala and their active compounds chebulagic acid and chebulinic acid prevented epithelial to mesenchymal transition in retinal pigment epithelial cells, by inhibiting SMAD-3 phosphorylation. PLoS One 10, e0120512.

Srikumar, R., Parthasarathy, N.J., Shankar, E.M., Manikandan, S., Vijayakumar, R., Thangaraj, R., et al., 2007. Evaluation of the growth inhibitory activities of Triphala against common bacterial isolates from HIV infected patients. Phytother. Res. 21, 476–480.

Srinagesh, J., Krishnappa, P., Somanna, S.N., 2012. Antibacterial efficacy of Triphala against oral streptococci: an in vivo study. Ind. J. Dent. Res. 23, 696.

Sumathi, P., Parvathi, A., 2010. Antibacterial potential of the three medicinal fruits used in Triphala: an ayurvedic formulation. J. Med. Plants 4, 1682–1685.

van de Waterbeemd, H., Gifford, E., 2003. ADMET in silico modelling: towards prediction paradise? Nat. Rev. Drug Discov. 2, 192–204.

Wang, L., Zhou, G.-B., Liu, P., Song, J.-H., Liang, Y., Yan, X.-J., et al., 2008. Dissection of mechanisms of Chinese medicinal formula realgar-indigo naturalis as an effective treatment for promyelocytic leukemia. Proc. Natl. Acad. Sci. U. S. A. 105, 4826−4831.

Wang, L., Li, Z., Zhao, X., Liu, W., Liu, Y., Yang, J., et al., 2013a. A network study of Chinese medicine xuesaitong injection to elucidate a complex mode of action with multicompound, multitarget, and multipathway. Evid. Based Complement Alternat. Med. 2013.

Wang, L., Zhang, J., Hong, Y., Feng, Y., Chen, M., Wang, Y., 2013b. Phytochemical and pharmacological review of da Chuanxiong formula: a famous herb pair composed of chuanxiong rhizoma and gastrodiae rhizoma for headache. Evid. Based Complement Alternat. Med. 2013.

Wang, S.Y., Fu, L.L., Zhang, S.Y., Tian, M., Zhang, L., Zheng, Y.X., et al., 2015. In silico analysis and experimental validation of active compounds from fructus Schisandrae chinensis in protection from hepatic injury. Cell Prolif. 48, 86−94.

Wen, Z., Wang, Z., Wang, S., Ravula, R., Yang, L., Xu, J., et al., 2011. Discovery of molecular mechanisms of traditional Chinese medicinal formula Si-Wu-Tang using gene expression microarray and connectivity map. PLoS One 6.

Wetzel, S., Bon, R.S., Kumar, K., Waldmann, H., 2011. Biology-oriented synthesis. Angew. Chemie-Int. Ed. 50, 10800−10826.

Wu, L., Wang, Y., Nie, J., Fan, X., Cheng, Y., 2013. A network pharmacology approach to evaluating the efficacy of Chinese medicine using genome-wide transcriptional expression data. Evid. Based Complement. Alternat. Med. 2013, 915343.

Wu, L., Wang, Y., Li, Z., Zhang, B., Cheng, Y., Fan, X., 2014. Identifying roles of "Jun-Chen-Zuo-Shi" component herbs of QiShenYiQi formula in treating acute myocardial ischemia by network pharmacology. Chin. Med. 9, 24.

Wu, X., Jiang, R., Zhang, M.Q., Li, S., 2008. Network-based global inference of human disease genes. Mol. Syst. Biol. 4, 189.

Xiang, Z., Sun, H., Cai, X., Chen, D., Zheng, X., 2015. The study on the material basis and the mechanism for anti-renal interstitial fibrosis efficacy of rhubarb through integration of metabonomics and network pharmacology. Mol. Biosyst. 11, 1067−1078.

Xu, H., Zhang, Y., Lei, Y., Gao, X., Zhai, H., Lin, N., et al., 2014a. A systems biology-based approach to uncovering the molecular mechanisms underlying the effects of dragon's blood tablet in colitis, involving the integration of chemical analysis, ADME prediction, and network pharmacology. PLoS One 9, e101432.

Xu, H.-Y., Wang, S.-S., Yang, H.-J., Bian, B.-L., Tian, S.-S., Wang, D.-L., et al., 2014b. Study on action mechanism of adjuvant therapeutic effect compound Ejiao slurry in treating cancers based on network pharmacology. Zhongguo Zhong Yao Za Zhi 39, 3148−3151.

Xu, Q., Qu, F., Pelkonen, O., 2011. Network Pharmacology and Traditional Chinese Medicine. In: Hiroshi, Sakagami (Ed.), Alternative medicine. InTech, pp. 277−297.

Yang, H., Xing, L., Zhou, M.-G., et al., 2012. Network pharmacological research of volatile oil from Zhike Chuanbei Pipa Dropping Pills in treatment of airway inflammation. Chinese Traditional and Herbal Drugs 43, 1129−1135.

Yang, M., Chen, J.-L., Xu, L.-W., Ji, G., 2013. Navigating traditional Chinese medicine network pharmacology and computational tools. Evid. Based Complement. Alternat. Med. 2013, 731969.

Yao, X., Hao, H., Li, Y., Li, S., 2011. Modularity-based credible prediction of disease genes and detection of disease subtypes on the phenotype-gene heterogeneous network. BMC Syst. Biol. 5, 79.

Yildirim, M.A., Goh, K., Cusick, M.E., Barabási, A., Vidal, M., 2007. Drug−target network. Nat. Biotechnol. 25, 1119−1126.

Yuan, C.H., Filippova, M., Tungteakkhun, S.S., Duerksen-Hughes, P.J., Krstenansky, J.L., 2012. Small molecule inhibitors of the HPV16-E6 interaction with caspase 8. Bioorg. Med. Chem. Lett. 22, 2125−2129.

Zhang, B., Wang, X., Li, S., 2013. An integrative platform of TCM network pharmacology and its application on a herbal formula, Qing-Luo-Yin. Evid. Based Complement Alternat. Med. 2013.

Zhang, H.-P., Pan, J.-B., Zhang, C., Ji, N., Wang, H., Ji, Z.-L., 2014. Network understanding of herb medicine via rapid identification of ingredient-target interactions. Sci. Rep. 4, 3719.

Zhang, J., Ma, T., Li, Y., Li, S., 2008. dbNEI2.0: building multilayer network for drug-NEI-disease. Bioinformatics 24, 2409−2411.

Zhang, J., Li, Y., Chen, S.-S., Zhang, L., Wang, J., Yang, Y., et al., 2015. Systems pharmacology dissection of the anti-inflammatory mechanism for the medicinal herb folium eriobotryae. Int. J. Mol. Sci. 16, 2913−2941.

Zhang, X., Gu, J., Cao, L., Li, N., Ma, Y., Su, Z., et al., 2014. Network pharmacology study on the mechanism of traditional Chinese medicine for upper respiratory tract infection. Mol. Biosyst. 10.

Zhao, F., Guochun, L., Yang, Y., Shi, L., Xu, L., Yin, L., 2015. A network pharmacology approach to determine active ingredients and rationality of herb combinations of modified-simiaowan for treatment of gout. J. Ethnopharmacol. 168, 1−16.

Zhao, S., Li, S., 2012. A co-module approach for elucidating drug-disease associations and revealing their molecular basis. Bioinformatics 28, 955−961.

Zheng, C., Fu, C., Pan, C., Bao, H., Chen, X., Ye, H., et al., 2015. Deciphering the underlying mechanisms of diesun miaofang in traumatic injury from a systems pharmacology perspective. Mol. Med. Rep.1−8.

Zheng, C.-S., Xu, X.-J., Ye, H.-Z., Wu, G.-W., Li, X.-H., Xu, H.-F., et al., 2013. Network pharmacology-based prediction of the multi-target capabilities of the compounds in Taohong Siwu decoction, and their application in osteoarthritis. Exp. Ther. Med. 6, 125−132.

Zhou, W., Wang, Y., 2014. A network-based analysis of the types of coronary artery disease from traditional Chinese medicine perspective: potential for therapeutics and drug discovery. J. Ethnopharmacol. 151, 66−77.

Zhu, F., Shi, Z., Qin, C., Tao, L., Liu, X., Xu, F., et al., 2012. Therapeutic target database update 2012: a resource for facilitating target-oriented drug discovery. Nucl. Acids Res. 40, 1128−1136.

Zi, T., Yu, D., 2015. A network pharmacology study of Sendeng-4, a Mongolian medicine. Chin. J. Nat. Med. 13, 108−118.

Zimmermann, G.R., Lehár, J., Keith, C.T., 2007. Multi-target therapeutics: when the whole is greater than the sum of the parts. Drug Discov. Today 12, 34−42.

Chapter 6

Genomics-Driven Drug Discovery Process

Rathnam Chaguturu

iDDPartners, Princeton Junction, NJ, United States

HISTORICAL PERSPECTIVE

For millennia, the human race has harbored ailments and has been ravaged by disease(s) of one kind or another. These have been either chronic, infectious, life-style induced or age-related. People turned to nature to seek remedies, and centuries of trial and error, serendipity, and passed-on knowledge gave birth to Ayurveda in India and Traditional Chinese Medicine in China. For the most part, with some exceptions, it has been plant-based remedies, usually an extract of leaves, roots, bark, flowers or fruits from a single plant or a concoction from several plant species with a significantly reasonable outcome. Almost 80% of the world's population relies mainly on these traditional medicines for its primary healthcare. Professor Youyou Tu of the China Academy of Traditional Chinese Medicine was awarded the Nobel Prize in Medicine in 2015 for the discovery of the antimalarial drug artemisinin, inspired by the ancient Chinese texts. This is a long overdue recognition of the traditional approaches to finding cures. Advances in chemistry, a keen insight into pharmacology, and a sharp eye toward a clinical perspective has led to the modernization of age-old explorations in pharmacognosy. Bioactivity-guided fractionations, advances in bioorganic and analytical chemistry principles led to enriched extracts with enhanced and desired pharmacological properties, and at times led to the isolation of the active ingredients that exerted the expected clinical outcome. About 25% of the drugs in use today are based on natural products, with a large percent ($> 70\%$) for anticancer and antibacterial therapeutic areas.

Most of the low-hanging fruit with respect to natural products and therapeutic targets have been relatively well explored and exhausted. With the advent of the industrialization of the drug discovery process along with federal agencies (National Institutes of Health in the United States, Indian Council of Medical Research, etc.) stepping in to support medical research in the public sector, academia across the globe has taken on a major role in the

Innovative Approaches in Drug Discovery. DOI: http://dx.doi.org/10.1016/B978-0-12-801814-9.00006-4
165

discovery of therapeutic targets. With a focus on the patient and the science, the pharmaceutical industry, with significant help from academia, is the driver of the discovery of innovative new drugs, and improvements to the older drugs that are already on the market. Pharma almost always implies that the market size is not relevant, but given the spectrum of drugs discovered and marketed, it is hard to ignore that the market size is not important or relevant—and it may, in fact, be the primary driver.

BASIC RESEARCH DRIVES INNOVATION

Academia has historically been involved in exploring the fundamental aspects of disease targets and in developing tool molecules to better understand the genetic, biological, and biochemical basis of new and novel therapeutic targets (McDonald et al., 2008). The innovative science that forms the foundation of the ensuing innovative products is still the domain of academia, and microbiopharma taking root in the incubator corridors of academia. Although >90% of drugs have historically been discovered by the pharmaceutical industry, harnessing the discoveries made in academic laboratories has become the primary focus for the pharmaceutical industry in the last 15−20 years. Faced with a huge patent cliff, and with the drug pipeline drying up ever so fast and revenues taking a nose dive, pharma has in recent years let go of the NIH ("not invented here") syndrome it has historically practiced, and started enthusiastically embracing academia for new and novel insights into innovative medicines that play a critical role in meeting the unmet medical needs (Chaguturu, 2014). Academic scientists are well equipped to explore and unravel the cellular signal transduction processes and biochemical pathways that enable life at the molecular level as well as in a systems biology context, and the aberrations that result in disease can be defined within this rational context. In the United States, a budget of US$32.0 billion in 2016 funds disease-driven medical research. The funds primarily go to academia, and in recent years, to small biotech companies carrying out cutting edge research by way of Small Business Innovation Research Initiative grants. While this sounds very encouraging, the federal agency is in a way funding only those research areas that it *deems* important. *The academic scientist, primarily defined by independence in pursuing what he/she sees as important and relevant, is now guided, or misguided, by the heavy hand of the federal agency.* The chances of an academic scientist receiving federal funding may or may not be truly based on the merits of the research proposal, but may very well be dependent on the institution where he holds the academic position. The motivation for federal funding is either directed toward addressing a critical unmet need (such as the need to confront a truly rare and neglected disease) or it is a politically motivated one. However, it is clear that without federal funding, academic science falters or could become nonexistent.

The importance of academic research as a driver of innovation is affirmed by the fact that the origins of 90% of the drugs approved by the Food and Drug Administration (FDA) in recent years for new indications can be traced directly to academia (Stevens et al., 2011). Almost 50% of the drugs coming out of academic research collectively treat either cancer or an infectious disease, again affirming the priorities mandated by the federal funding agencies (Stevens et al., 2011).

A committed, collaborative partnership between academia and the pharmaceutical partner appears to be the new norm in discovering new drugs. Pharma, which funds the research, looks for the following key principles:

1. How strong is the science? Are the biochemical principles behind the disease well defined with a reasonable proof-of-principle affirmation?
2. Are the intellectual property rights well defined and protected, with either an outright ownership or a first right of refusal?
3. Does the therapeutic area addresses a critical unmet medical need of a geographic area of interest (such as North America, Africa)?
4. Although not explicitly stated, what is the market size?

DRUG DISCOVERY: SOUP TO NUTS

The discovery and development of a drug is a long arduous road. The pharmaceutical industry is an R&D-intensive business sector, with a higher percentage of net sales, nearly 13%, going to research and development than most other sectors (compare this with 8.4% for computers and electronics and the industry average of 3.5%) (Chaguturu, 2014). Almost a quarter of the research expenditure is spent during the preclinical stage and $\sim 60\%$ during the clinical development phase. Although the total cost from bench to bedside is said to be in excess of US$3 billion, and the length of time it takes is anywhere from 10 to 15 + years, there is no authoritative public disclosure by any company about the true cost of drug development, and of the attrition rates during the different phases of clinical development. The reason for this unsustainable landscape is several-fold, including (1) spiraling R&D costs, (2) demand for greater safety, (3) increased post-marketing surveillance, and most importantly, (4) lower productivity (Chaguturu, 2014). That's the innovation gap. To bridge the innovation gap, pharma needs better strategies for picking new and novel therapeutic targets, tool molecules to probe these drug targets, and smart lead optimization strategies.

The identification of novel, unexplored therapeutic targets and chemical modulators (probes) for the treatment of a disease of interest starts by executing high-throughput small molecules- and shRNA screening in concert with genome-wide association bioinformatics analyses. Extensive scientific evidence is collated to indicate that the disease is an unpredictable, stochastic, evolutionary process characterized by the potential for nearly unlimited genetic and epigenetic diversity. Toward achieving this goal, it is paramount to use, seamlessly, bioinformatics, chemical biology, proteomics, structural biology and medicinal chemistry—based systems biology approaches along with high-throughput cell-free and cell-based assays to identify novel, druggable protein targets, and novel "drug-like" chemical probes. Further validation of the therapeutic potential of the "putative" targets is then achieved via RNAi silencing approaches identified from a comprehensive bioinformatics-based data mining effort and by defining the changes in the expression profile of microRNAs (miRNAs). The screening effort will be augmented by the analysis of genomic profiles of primary disease-relevant cells for proteins with distinct mutation rates or expression levels that are potentially disease related. The engineered cell lines expressing the most promising genes or purified target proteins will then be screened against focused compound sets culled from the institutional chemical libraries that are usually highly diverse and unique. Compounds that modulate target protein activity or are selectively toxic to the disease-relevant cell lines compared to normal cells derived from a comparable tissue, will be considered as starting points for target-specific chemical library expansion and subsequent chemical probe development. Assessment of the therapeutic target as a druggable one comes from the experimental verification that a small molecule can selectively modulate a pathway or the proteins in vivo activity. Innovative structural biology approaches as well as effectiveness in the in vivo disease models need to be undertaken to provide critical insights in to lead optimization strategies, especially for prototypical hard targets that have traditionally been considered undruggable.

A general path in treading the drug discovery process, using the example of ovarian cancer, is presented. The selection of ovarian cancer to describe the drug discovery process has several merits:

- Ovarian cancer is the second most leading gynecological cancer, and one of the deadliest among women. In 2012, ovarian cancer occurred in 239,000 women and resulted in 152,000 deaths worldwide. The overall 5-year survival rate is $\sim 45\%$, and even worse in the developing world. Ovarian cancer is also the most resistant to a chemo- and radiation-therapy regimen.

- Integrated genomic analyses of the ovarian carcinoma have been published (Cancer Genome Atlas Research Network, 2011). This provides a strong starting point to apply systematic, genome-wide, bioinformatics-based, disease-centered, systems biology approaches to identify novel and unexplored therapeutic targets for ovarian cancer.

- This provides the basis to identify and validate a select list of disease-relevant drug targets with distinct mutation, epigenetic, expression, or signature profiles; and the feasibility of cloning, protein expression, stable cell line development and high-throughput screening (HTS) amenable assay for each of these targets.

- It is an ideal target for two drug discovery paradigms, physiology-based and target-based, with forward- and reverse-chemical genomic studies.

- Identification of target-specific chemical probes (drug leads) will help to understand the mechanisms and functional changes underlying the biology of ovarian cancer (proof-of-principle), and provide a novel platform for translating innovative drug target hits to clinical proof of concept unequivocally.

As one reads through the chapter, it should become clear that the path to discovery laid out here is not based only on some generic principles, but on a solid, meticulous path to discovering a therapeutic target from solid genomic and proteomic data that is available and discernible from the literature (for example, Cancer Genome Atlas Research Network, 2011). A detailed process is then presented to identify therapeutically relevant gene candidates and evaluate for (1) the feasibility of cloning, protein expression, stable cell line development and HTS amenable assay for each of these targets, (2) execution of robust biochemical- or cell-based high-throughput screening campaigns against focused libraries, and (3) follow through with mechanistic-based confirmatory (on-target) assays and counter-screens (off-target or selectivity) to select, confirm, and validate the screen hits. Iterative chemoinformatic−, protein structure−guided, and medicinal chemistry−based (targeted synthesis and strategic expansion through acquisition) optimization strategies are then proposed to identify high-quality drug leads (Appendix 1, 2, and 3).

> *Appendix 1* provides a broad outline of for each of the steps involved and decision points for a "go" or "no go" decision to be made to advance the project from target identification all the way to proof of concept studies.
>
> *Appendix 2* outlines the level of effort needed each year over a period of 5 years in accomplishing the three main components of a drug discovery program: (1) target identification and validation, (2) high-throughput screening efforts leading to the identification of confirmed hits and probes, and (3) medicinal chemistry efforts required for screening actives to confirmed hits and quantitative structure-activity-relationship (QSAR) efforts resulting in bona fide leads.
>
> *Appendix 3* shows the critical path flow chart from beginning (target identification) to the end (proof of concept) of a drug discovery (not development) program.

An effort such as the one presented in this chapter gives the reader a comprehensive understanding of the genetic basis for disease (ovarian cancer) phenotypes, and helps the reader to identify truly novel, unexplored, and druggable, 2−3 therapeutically validated disease (ovarian cancer) targets with detailed pharmacology and highly promising, 2−3 drug-like chemical probe/lead series per target with efficacy assessment in small animal models. Identification of target-specific chemical probes (drug leads) will then pave the path to understand the mechanisms and functional changes underlying the biology of the disease (proof-of-principle), and provide a novel platform for translating innovative drug target hits to clinical proof of concept unequivocally.

TARGET IDENTIFICATION

Before embarking on a drug discovery program, a strong argument first and foremost needs to be made based on new cases of the disease and, for the disease in question discussed here, ovarian cancer, instances of occurrence every year and the number of associated deaths. Development of new therapies, especially in the era of targeted treatments and personalized medicine, is typically driven by understanding the underlying biology, molecular biology, and biochemistry of tumor cells and their surrounding microenvironments that target genetic alterations. The evolutionary nature of cancer implies, contrary to conventional wisdom, that the essential features of any therapy for the consistent cure or control of cancer must be independent of the particular pathways of tumor cell evolution, and independent of any particular genetic or epigenetic alterations. Current drug discovery efforts tend to focus on commonly mutated signal transduction pathways, e.g., a series of growth factor receptors and downstream modulators (phosphatases and kinases) that are working in concert to promote growth but are not the central machinery. A nonbiased, disease-centered, systems biology approach will incorporate diverse data sets and varied expertise to identify novel, unexplored, high-quality, therapeutically relevant targets for ovarian cancer, and help discover and develop compounds, with efficacy in small animal models, for ultimate clinical translation.

To identify novel, unique druggable targets and chemical probes to treat ovarian cancer, it is critical to harness the vast institutional drug discovery strengths and invoke a paradigm shift (for academia) by applying the best principles of project management in efficiently managing the research projects to identify novel targets, to validate chemical probes, and to optimize leads using a combination of structure-based screens, in vivo proteomic profiling of drug activity and cell-based assays using primary ovarian tumor cells. It is then essential to employ two drug discovery paradigms—physiology-based and target-based—with forward- and reverse-chemical genomic studies. Results from the extensive mining of ovarian genomic data will then form the basis for the targets and/or target pathways on which one can focus, and the chemically tractable hits coming out of this effort will then be optimized as drug leads with bench-to-bedside translation potential.

Identification of novel, unique, and druggable therapeutic targets through a comprehensive bioinformatics' analysis of the genomic and proteomic profiles, within therapeutically important cellular signaling cascades, of ovarian carcinoma.

As a first approximation, one can use Rough Set (Fang and Grzymala-Busse, 2006a), Random Forest (Breiman, 2001), Support Vector Machine (Vapnik, 1999), Bayesian Neural Network (BNN) (Yu and Chen, 2005) based feature selection (FS) algorithms for mining high-dimensional data, resulting in a list of genes ranked by possibilities/weights. Rough Set−based FS identifies disease-relevant genes using CRS algorithm, an objective approach to mine data with imperfections, and involves computations performed directly on data sets, with no feedback from parameters, such as probability distribution (Fang and Grzymala-Busse, 2006a, b). A shallow feature selection (FS) algorithm assigns each feature a probability of being selected, based on the structure of trained data (Fang and Grzymala-Busse, 2006a). One can then apply BNN-based approaches to identify genes relevant to ovarian cancer from mRNA/miRNA expression profile data. A feature-extraction machine learning approach may then be a good way to analyze "sequencing" datasets (Lee et al., 2011). The following bioinformatics methods are deemed relevant to analyze mRNA signatures from normal and ovarian cancer sequence data: (1) BioMarker Identifier (BMI) methodology, to identify features based on a capacity to discriminate among phenotypes such as diseased vs. normal sequencing datasets. BMI analysis will identify a ranked list of candidates qualified by an informative score measure; (2) Particle Swarm Optimization, a validation tool algorithm to train biomarker models based on BMI-selected features, to define the discriminatory performance of each expressed gene; and (3) Information Gain, a filter-based FS algorithm, to score and validate the resulting models to produce an attribute ranking within the above-described knowledge discovery framework (Netzer et al., 2009).

The genes thus identified should be subjected to comprehensive systems biology analyses (Hanzlik et al., 2009; Salamat-Miller et al., 2006, 2007; Zaidi et al., 2007; Liu et al., 2009; Fang et al., 2009; Thomas, 2010). The BiNGO program (http://www.psb.ugent.be/cbd/papers/BiNGO/Home.html), a plug-in for Cytoscape to assign gene ontology categories for each gene of interest and describe gene products in relation to associated biological processes, cellular components, and molecular functions. The Kolomogorov−Smirnov test and IPA, a commercial software package for pathway analysis, is relevant for discovering gene associations with biological pathways (Han et al., 2009). The Human Protein Reference Database, a protein−protein interaction database (Giuliano et al., 2003) linked to a compendium of signal transduction pathways (netPath), will be analyzed using Cytoscape for visualizing and analyzing biological interaction networks and domain architectures for potential drug candidates.

Validation of the therapeutic potential of targets identified through the systems biology approach using shRNA gene silencing in primary human ovarian tumor cells.

Experimental validation of the potential targets is necessary to determine their relative functional importance and therapeutic potential in relevant clinical samples prior to being nominated for high-throughput drug screening and subsequent drug design. Although it may not be feasible to evaluate all therapeutic candidates, at least 100 should be functionally characterized using shRNA gene silencing approaches. Prioritization will be biology-driven and pathway-based, and will rely on many factors including comparative genomics to gene expression profiling to RNA interference to identify the most promising targets (and equally important, reject undruggable false targets) for drug discovery and development. The goal is to avoid inherent biases and preconceived favorites.

Validation of aberrantly expressed miRNAs that affect gene targets/pathways identified through systems biology and shRNA approaches and establishment of specific miRNA as efficacy biomarkers following drug modulation of target genes.

MicroRNA (miRNA)-mediated posttranscriptional gene regulations play critical roles in normal tissue development and function and in the pathophysiology that leads to cancer. The underlying rationale is that miRNAs are uniquely positioned to have global effects on multiple genes so as to affect cellular and tissue responses in a coordinated manner. Mature miRNAs, unlike typical genes, are thought to more closely correlated with their function, as miRNAs are endpoint regulatory molecules that do not require translation and posttranslational modifications. Thus, comparison of miRNA expression in primary cells before and after target gene silencing should provide valuable insights into the mechanism(s) by which they interact with these genes to change the phenotype of the ovarian cancer cells. miRNA expression analysis of shRNA treated cells should also provide a unique efficacy biomarker panel that is readily and quantitatively measureable following drug modulation of these target genes.

Result: Cancer target identified.

Note: See Appendix 4 (Forward Chemical Genetics) for identifying protein targets of hits discovered from phenotypic screens without a known mechanism of action, for repurposed drugs for which targets might not be known for the new indication, or for natural products with activities of interest.

LEAD IDENTIFICATION

Expression and purification of target proteins and generate HTS-amenable stable cell lines expressing therapeutic candidate genes.

The bioinformatic-shRNA/miRNA—validated gene targets are now ready to be cloned with promoter—reporter constructs or protein expression constructs to engineer cell lines for cell-based, high-throughput screening. Standardized protocols routinely used will need to be refined as necessary to express the proteins in sufficient quantities as needed. Initial characterization of the proteins can be done by circular dichroism, followed by light scattering, and size exclusion chromatography for some general characterization of the oligomeric state and secondary structure. High-throughput protein expression and purification could be achieved using eukaryotic or bacterial expression systems, and the Ligation

Independent Cloning (LIC) system for high-throughput cloning of ORFs to the expression cassettes. LIC technology is highly efficient, with very little background, and no restriction digestion of the ORF is necessary prior to cloning nor enzyme catalyzed ligation into the vector. Cloned ORFs/ reporter constructs are sequenced to confirm the identity, large-scale plasmid preparation is achieved and high-expression yields and efficient purification are demonstrated to generate sufficient quantities of proteins for target verification, ligand screening, and initial structural efforts.

Development of target-specific, pathway-focused, HTS-ready biochemical and cell-based assays, and establish high-throughput screens to identify potent small-molecule modulators of the targets.

Assays: First, assay development considerations will need to be taken on an individual basis for each of the 8 to 12 targets. The wide variety of potential targets is likely lead to a diversity of assay types (Giuliano et al., 2003; Mayr and Bojanic, 2009; Zock, 2009). Where applicable, novel assays should be developed to screen unique targets. In addition to conventional screening methods, extensive use of novel approaches are anticipated for screening targets with unknown function. Where traditional HTS assays are difficult or impossible to develop or no known assay technology/platform exists, extensive use of label-free based technology may be adapted to ease this bottleneck. AlphaScreen technology is quite relevant to study targets involving protein—protein interactions. A high content imaging system may be used to execute phenotypic screens in ovarian cancer cell models.

Chemical libraries: It is essential to have access to a carefully crafted library of compounds optimized for structural diversity, drug-likeness, and compliant with Lipinski Rule of Five (Lipinski et al., 2001). The information-rich compounds synthesized within the institutional Medicinal Chemistry Cores, legacy collection, the NIH Clinical collection, proprietary natural products, and an exhaustive FDA-approved drug library should all be part of this collection. Having a fragment library, an alternative to small-molecule screening, and several pathway-specific focused libraries add diversity to the screening effort. Some of the widely recognized commercial suppliers of high-quality chemical libraries include ChemBridge, ChemDiv, Enamine, Prestwick, TimTec, etc.

As each target is validated, and a screening assay is developed, the assays themselves should be validated by pilot screening. Following assay development, the assay target will be surveyed by executing a pilot screen of using a validation library of 6000 small molecules, which includes an FDA-approved drug library collection, representing structural diversity, and a known biological activity profile. The generalized screening protocol for cell-based assays involves seeding appropriate number of cells into each of the wells of a 384-well microplate, letting them stand overnight, adding compounds (final concentration based upon the target-assay chosen) to quantitate the signal (signal type depends on the assay format), either as kinetic or an end-point readout, after 4-, 24-, 48-, and 72-hour compound exposure. Care is taken to have appropriate controls. This process will validate the screening protocol and would provide a glimpse into how successful a full-scale chemical library screening would be in yielding quality hits. Statistical analysis of the data generated from the pilot library screening will include well-to-well and plate-to-plate variability, using positive and negative controls. This assay validation will confirm that the HTS assay has a signal window that meets or exceeds the requirements for a validated screen with a Z' factor average of 0.70 or greater and an average % CV of 10% or less. Data analysis should be performed in accordance with the established statistical criteria as per the NIH Assay Guidance manual (http://ncgc.nih.gov/guidance). Preliminary hits corresponding to compounds that modulate an assay at greater than/equal to three standard deviations from the plate median should be retested for validation with an eight-point dose response curve to confirm the ability of the HTS assay to identify valid probes before the full HTS campaign. The assay timing will also be tested, to determine the optimal number of plates that can be tested per batch, by day or week, to schedule the full HTS campaign. HTS assay conditions will be optimized to maximize signal and lower assay costs while minimizing liquid handling steps. Established protocols should be implemented in addressing issues concerning false positives and false negatives. Following the HTS assay validation, a full library screening will then be performed for the selected program project targets using their respective HTS assays. Compound library screening will be similar to validation pilot library screening, but on a larger scale. All 384-well plates will include MAX, MID, and MIN positive and negative controls, to provide in-plate controls, and to monitor plate-to-plate and batch-to-batch screening consistency. The HTS screens will rely on the primary assay developed for each specific target or mechanism. Cell-based assays will include reporter–construct expressing stable cell lines, label-free determination of cellular changes, and phenotypic assays monitoring protein expression, regulation, and location through high-content screening. Biochemical assays will include kinetic or end-point assays, and may include protein–protein interaction assays. Before calling a screen hit a *bona fide* one, one should determine the structural integrity and purity of the compounds from the DMSO stocks by LC-Mass-spec, Nuclear Magnetic Resonance (NMR) and high-performance liquid chromatography using institutional analytical core facilities. It is imperative to acquire technical samples of the hits from commercial sources or synthesize in-house and assess structure reconfirmation prior to undertaking lead optimization.

Execution of confirmatory (on-target) assays and counter-screens (off-target) to validate screen hits.

The top 0.5% of screen actives, representing both activity as well as structural diversity need to be cherry-picked and rescreened at eight concentrations to generate IC_{50} values. The specificity of confirmed screen hits is assessed by counter-screening against the primary target (Roy et al., 2009). If the primary assay was not cell-based, a secondary cell-based assay must be used to verify the cellular activity of the probe. Secondary screens are to be established to further validate screen actives, including selectivity screens to eliminate promiscuous compounds that are targeting more than just the target mechanism or protein of interest. An array of cellular assays need to be in place for assessing the selectivity and efficacy of the hits, including growth assays (proliferation-based metabolic read out, biomass, DNA synthesis, live/dead read out), mechanistic assays (cell cycling, apoptosis, immunofluorescence, Western blotting, cellular ELISA, flow cytometry, invasion and migration, and comet), and other special assays (hypoxia, 3D spheroid, phenotypic matrigel, senescence, autophagy, and reactive oxygen species assays), and tumor microenvironment assays. Hit prioritization will rely on the collaborative effort between the medicinal chemistry team and screening groups to perform the iterative task of chemical probe optimization and retesting, to guide structure activity relationship analysis of chemical scaffolds during probe development. Prioritization of screening hits will be performed to guide the selection of compounds for secondary and tertiary screening, and to later guide probe selection and development by the medicinal chemistry team.

LEAD OPTIMIZATION STRATEGIES

Execution of chemoinformatic− and medicinal chemistry−based iterative, optimization studies to develop compounds that potently, efficaciously, and selectively modulate the high-priority therapeutic targets.

Once the target is identified and verified, HTS campaigns executed, and a panel of "hit" compounds collated, traditional lead optimization strategies are employed to transform these hits into tool molecules to probe the mechanistic aspects of target site biology. The following five criteria are recommended to guide probe prioritization:

1. *Novel Structure-Activity Relationships:* Screen select focused compound libraries to identify novel scaffolds;
2. *Novel Probe*: There will likely be current probes for some program project targets. However, it is expected that most of these compounds have poor EC_{50}s in the micromolar range or are nonspecific. For each project, seek a novel probe that uniquely targets the major mechanism of action of the target in its biological pathway;
3. *Potency:* A potent compound would provide the best therapy at low concentrations. An ideal probe would have an EC_{50} in the submicromolar range;
4. *Selectivity:* An ideal probe would be selective for the specific target. It is imperative to develop a highly specific probe that acts through the described mechanism of action; and
5. *Secondary Assays:* Hit compounds are tested in relevant secondary assays to confirm the identified hits are acting through the desired mechanism of action with no or minimal off-target activity.

Prioritization of tractable chemotypes via in silico chemical clustering to form a solid basis for QSAR analysis- as a component of the chemical probe optimization process.

Molecular modeling studies: All hits identified from high-throughput screens should be converted into 3D structures via a software package such as Concord program (The Tripod Associates, 2008), and saved as a Tripos Molecular Spreadsheet within the SYBYL program (8.0 S. The Tripos Associates, 2008). In anticipation of possible downstream lead optimization challenges, all hits are subjected to in silico absorption, distribution, metabolism and excretion (ADME) profiling via the Volsurf program (Cruciani et al., 2003) and toxicological (Sanderson and Earnshaw, 1991) assessment via the DEREK knowledgebase. The hit manifold is now ready to be partitioned based on specific chemotype via in silico chemical clustering. All hits are now loaded into the Selector tool from Tripos (8.0 S. The Tripos Associates, 2008) and subjected to undergo hierarchical, reciprocal nearest neighbor and Jarvis-Patrick clustering (according to default cluster selection Selector parameters programmed into Selector) based on Tanimoto similarity among UNITY fingerprints. Hit chemotype classifications will emerge from a consensus-clustering scheme, whereby chemically analogous compounds coinhabit the same cluster regardless of underlying clustering algorithm. Chemotype clusters with >30 constituent molecules can form a solid basis for QSAR analysis for probe optimization process. Chemotype clusters with fewer representatives but with some of the more potent individual constituent compounds (activity $>4\sigma$ above the mean) will also be considered for subsequent probe optimization. Initial probe optimization will be guided by ligand-based, structure-activity data derived from QSAR analysis. Each well-represented chemotype (>30 hits) from preliminary clustering will be spatially aligned in SYBYL based on conserved chemical functionality using the "Align Database" option. Chemical charges will be constructed according to Gasteiger–Marsili electrostatics (Gasteiger and Marsili, 1980), assuming pH $= 7.4$ protonation states. Since cell permeation tendencies might affect bioactivity measurements, the molecular descriptors of cell membrane permeability (e.g., ClogP, negative solvent accessible surface area) will be determined. QSAR models will be constructed for each well-represented chemotype using the Comparative Molecular Field Analysis (CoMFA) program (Cramer et al., 1988) in SYBYL with the permeation metrics included in the trained model as perturbations. If the resulting model does not achieve adequate self-consistency, recursive refinement will be employed until a model is obtained that meets the minimum internal consistency requirements, or until subsequent iterations fail to improve model performance. If chemotypes other than those used to create the preliminary CoMFA models share those key features, then those additional clusters will be spatially aligned to the CoMFA field, and a new PLS model will be trained based on the merged set. If this superset yields a PLS model satisfying the requisite cross-validation thresholds after recursion, then the merged model will be adopted as a working structure-activity relationship (SAR) framework. The ensuing model will then be applied to rationalize existing activity trends and predict the activity of untested analogs, including species already available as reported in chemical structure databases such as PubChem (The PubChem Compound Database NcfBI, 2005) and the ChemNavigator iResearch (library i, 2009) collection, as well as new synthetically tractable species. All new species identified for follow-up testing will be subjected to the same in silico ADME and toxicology analyses performed for the original hit manifold. If a reasonable structural characterization of the relevant macromolecular receptor is available, the CoMFA model can be replaced with a Comparative Binding Energy (COMBINE) model (Ortiz et al., 1995; Lushington et al., 2007), which generates a receptor-specific model that prioritizes specific ligand-receptor interactions (Goodsell et al., 1996; Jain, 2007) based on their capacity to enhance or interfere with the observed modulative bioactivity, thus enhancing quality of the in silico guidance for practical probe optimization. Once the bound conformers of ligands have been predicted, the COMBINE model can be obtained by computing specific interaction descriptors via COMBSCORE program (Lghwnmg, 2005), followed by validation and refinement steps analogous to those described for CoMFA modeling. If specific chemicals are already known to modulate the target of interest, one may also exploit this prior knowledge toward augmenting the quality of probe optimization guidance achieved from the modeling studies. If previously characterized modulators are chemically similar to specific chemotypes under consideration in our work, bioactivity data from these prior studies can be used to validate the CoMFA or COMBINE models. If the manner in which the bioactivity data from the prior studies closely resembles the screening protocol applied, one may even be able to incorporate the prior data into existing models to provide a stronger basis for predictive rationalization of pharmacophores.

Structure Activity—based iterative medicinal chemistry optimization of tractable screen hits to improve potency, efficacy and specificity.

Target-specific chemical probe optimization: This represents a natural extension of a HTS campaign that typically provides moderately useful hit compounds. Medicinal chemistry optimization is an iterative process that requires good starting points for both biology and chemistry, and requires a clear plan with well-defined end and transition points, technical capabilities in assay design and interpretation, molecular design, and synthetic organic chemistry. Each individual optimization campaign is idiosyncratic in that each combination of biological target and chemical starting point is unique.

The tasks of the Medicinal Chemistry team will be (1) to perform synthesis of known compounds necessary for biochemical studies, (2) to design and synthesize novel drug compounds as probes for ongoing studies, (3) to work with the HTS team in carrying out optimization of screen hits and provide strategically expanded chemical library sets of high value, and (4) to synthesize fluorescent or affinity tagged analogs of existing probes when necessary for cell localization or target identification studies. A set of clear, quantitative goals specific to a project would be defined for potency and selectivity expectations, in vitro pharmacokinetic parameters, aqueous solubility and chemical stability for hit-to-lead optimization programs. A high-quality preliminary data that points at a particular chemical series will provide multiple chemistry starting points. However, hit sets from large-scale, high-profile screening require especially careful validation that entails (1) verification in a low-throughput assay using validated, structure-confirmed compounds, (2) chemical evaluation of the hits to determine their suitability for analoging, and (3) careful examination of the screen for possible nascent SAR. Chemical tractability is then assessed by making a wide range of analogs in early stage exploratory chemistry since the structural requirements are generally better understood in more advanced projects. In early stages, potency milestones will be set for promotion of a given compound set into assays that establish selectivity. If particular chemical properties are required, prospective compounds for synthesis will be examined at the outset using standard chemoinformatics tools for calculated properties such as logP or likely solubility. Each round of SAR will span 2−3 weeks for the synthesis, purification, and compound transfer to HTS team. HTS will generate full dose−response curves, which will be evaluated and planning process undertaken for the next step. The most common outcome of a given round of SAR is that, while some improvement in potency (or other property) may be in hand, the compounds made still do not meet project milestones. In these cases, the new biological results of the SAR set are typically analyzed in the context of those that were already in hand, and a net set of compounds is made. Typically, three full rounds of SAR synthesis/assay/analysis are expected for an "average" probe discovery campaign. Once two to three solid pharmacophores are identified per target, the structural biology team needs to be involved to assess the binding of the probe to a specific target to support structure-based design strategies and achieve target site specificity that is quite paramount in achieving the goal of having probes that specifically target ovarian cancer.

Execution of structure-based drug design strategies to assess protein-ligand interactions and preclinical studies to ascertain proof of concept and efficacy of lead compounds.

NMR structure-based ligand affinity screen: A multistep, structure-based, NMR screen to identify biologically relevant chemical leads among the positive hits from the HTS campaign is quite a powerful strategy. There are four major components to the process: (1) verify good physical properties for the compounds being screened, (2) identify ligands that bind to the protein target, (3) determine binding affinities to prioritize the chemical leads, and (4) determine protein-ligand costructures. The protein-detected NMR screening step filters out nonspecific binders, confirms a stoichiometric interaction, and identifies the ligand-binding site. These NMR spectra are used to rapidly determine a protein-ligand costructure, measure dissociation constant, and verify potential chemical leads, and suggest a common pharmacophore for designing a directed library for further screening.

X-ray crystallography. Once two to three drug leads are identified per target, X-ray crystallography can be used to assess the binding of the lead to the specific target. Purified concentrated target proteins are necessary for crystallization screening using a high-throughput method to setup 96-well screens to maximize the likelihood of obtaining and refining crystals under a variety of crystallization conditions (Cudney et al., 1994). Screens may be set up using Compact Jr. sitting drop vapor diffusion plates and crystallization screens. Crystals are tested for X-ray diffraction using a diffractometer or Bruker X8 Proteum systems and the optimal cryoconditions that yield the highest resolution diffraction are used for subsequent X-ray data collections. High-resolution X-ray diffraction data for structure solution is integrated and scaled with the XDS (Kabsch, 1988) and Scala (Evans, 2006) software packages. Initial structure solution can be attempted by molecular replacement using programs such as Molrep (Vagin and Teplyakov, 1997) or Phaser (McCoy et al., 2007), and homology models are created for molecular replacement searches by comparing the target sequence with known structures from the Protein Databank, and to prepare the search models or by using programs such as ITASSER (Roy et al., 2010; Bazzoli et al., 2011). If molecular replacement proves to be unsuccessful, heavy atom derivatives of the crystals or selenomethionine labeled protein need to be prepared for structure solution using SAD/MAD anomalous scattering phasing methods with Shelx (Sheldrick, 2008) or Phenix (Adams et al., 2010).

For all protein targets, structure refinement should be conducted with either Refmac (Murshudov et al., 1997), Phenix (Adams et al., 2010) or Buster (Blanc et al., 2004) software packages. Once the structure of a particular protein target has been completed, the focus will shift to obtaining structures in complexes with small-molecule modulators, identified from HTS. To obtain an inhibitor-bound complex, either the crystals obtained are soaked in the presence of an inhibitor, or the protein is cocrystallized in the presence of the inhibitors (Chatterjee et al., 2011).

PRECLINICAL STUDIES

The interaction between a druggable target and a small molecule must lead to a modulation in the protein's in vivo activity that results in a positive outcome for treating the disease. Genomic heterogeneity present in human cancers underlies the variable therapeutic responses observed in the clinic. More recently, global gene expression analysis has been successfully used to stratify tumors into subtypes and to predict the clinical efficacy of new therapies

(Cancer Genome Atlas Research Network, 2011; Collisson et al., 2011; Heiser et al., 2009; Neve et al., 2006; Spurdle et al., 2011). Some studies have identified cancer subtypes responsive to specific therapies by using a panel of cultured cell lines (Collisson et al., 2011; Heiser et al., 2009). Preclinical studies are performed to evaluate the efficacy of target-specific shRNAs and optimized, target-specific chemical probes in primary-tumor xenograft models for ovarian cancer. Primary human, serous ovarian tumors are heterotransplanted into NOD−SCID mice to maintain fidelity of the tumors' genomic features. Xenografts of patient biopsies have been shown to retain the morphological and molecular markers of the original tumor even after serial passages through mice (Bankert et al., 2001; Perez-Soler et al., 2000; Rubio-Viqueira et al., 2006).

Primary-Tumor Xenograft Model

To generate viable xenografts, fresh primary serous ovarian tumors are acquired from consenting patients. Portions of the tumor are utilized to: (1) isolate DNA for exome sequencing, (2) isolate RNA for Affymetrix mRNA expression profiling, and (3) to assay the lead compound's target expression by performing immunohistochemistry (IHC). Morphological and histopathological analyses of tumors, in addition to IHC for p53, are performed to verify that tumor xenografts maintain the original tumor characteristics. For each xenotransplantation experiment, nonnecrotic tumor fragments are then surgically implanted, bilaterally, into the flanks of an anesthetized NOD−SCID mouse (Fichtner et al., 2004; Morton and Houghton, 2007). Tumor growth is monitored twice a week for up to 6 months. When palpable tumors are greater than 1 cm^3 or when mice exhibit signs of distress, mice are evaluated by necropsy for localization and extent of tumor burden. Further, tumor tissue will be formalin-fixed and/or snap-frozen for: (1) IHC of p53, the lead compound's target, and critical molecules within the pathways or interaction networks of the target, (2) RT-PCR detection of the β-globin gene to verify the tumor's human origin, and (3) isolation of genomic DNA for sequencing to verify that TP53 mutation status in the xenograft matches the source tumor. Xenografts that grow in vivo are then passaged at least two more times through NOD−SCID mice. For use in subsequent hetero-transplantation experiments, portions of the tumor will be cryopreserved (Elkas et al., 2002). Viable primary-solid-tumor xenografts are established from at least 10 unique tumors to identify a therapeutic agent that has at least a 10% response rate.

Evaluation of Lead Compound Efficacy In Vivo

If the ascites sample used in the shRNA screen has a matched solid tumor sample that was heterotransplanted successfully, then the tumor tissue is ready for xenotransplantation. If not, then the appropriate xeno-graft model has to be selected by comparing the expression of the target molecule and the critical molecules linked to the target by pathway/inter-action network analyses in the successfully xenografted primary tumors and in the ascites-derived cells that were used in the shRNA screen. A pilot study is then performed to evaluate lead compound efficacy by test-ing a single dose based on calculated in vitro IC_{50} values. NOD−SCID mice are xenotransplanted with the appropriate solid tumor and divided into 7 groups (n = 8/arm), where compounds 1a, 1b, and 1c are specific for the first target, and compounds 2a, 2b, and 2c are specific for the sec-ond target. The groups are as follows: (1) vehicle, (2) compound 1a, (3) compound 1b, (4) compound 1c, (5) compound 2a, (6) compound 2b, and (7) compound 2c. Treatment will start when tumors reach 500 mm^3 and will continue for 1−2 months. Three of the eight mice in each group are euthanized at 4, 8, and 24 h postdosing to assay target expression/activ-ity. Caliper measurements of tumors are taken weekly to monitor tumor growth. Mice will also be weighed weekly and observed for signs of distress and therapeutic toxicity. Evaluation at necropsy is performed, in addition to collection of blood samples for analysis of differential blood counts and histological analysis of spleen, lymph node, and thymus. We will select the compound that exhibits the greatest efficacy for each target in the pilot study for a larger preclinical study using 14 mice/arm: (1) vehicle, (2) compound targeting molecule 1, and (3) compound targeting molecule 2. A cohort of four mice is used to analyze target expression/activity at two specific time points determined by our pilot study. The remaining 10 mice will be monitored for tumor growth, and analyses postnecropsy will be performed. Dosing is adjusted based on the results of the pilot study. This larger preclinical study should be repeated using two additional primary-tumor xenograft models to confirm the data.

These preclinical proof of concept studies are critical for developing tractable, "drug like" molecules as drug leads with bench-to-bedside trans-lation potential. The strategies and methodologies described here provide a clear plan to identify and validate novel therapeutic targets and develop novel "drug like" chemical probes for ovarian cancer. Identification of target-specific chemical probes (drug leads) will help to understand the mechanisms and functional changes underlying the biology of ovarian cancer (proof-of-principle), and provide a novel platform for translating innovative drug target hits to clinical proof of concept unequivocally. It must be stressed, however, that the methodologies presented are generic enough to be adapted to identify and validate novel therapeutic targets and develop novel "drug like" chemical probes for any disease one wishes to target.

PRECLINICAL AND CLINICAL DEVELOPMENT OF DRUG CANDIDATES (WWW.FDA.GOV)

Once researchers identify a promising compound for development, experiments are conducted to gather information on:

- How it is absorbed, distributed, metabolized, and excreted
- Its potential benefits and mechanisms of action
- The best dosage
- The best way to give the drug (such as by mouth or injection)
- Side effects (often referred to as toxicity)
- How it affects different groups of people (such as by gender, race, or ethnicity) differently
- How it interacts with other drugs and treatments
- Its effectiveness as compared with similar drugs

In predevelopment, toxicological studies, analytical testing, and pharmacokinetics analysis are first conducted to answer questions about (1) the physico-chemical character of the substance, (2) the metabolic behavior (how the drug is metabolized), (3) bioavailability (how long it unveils its effect), and (4) safety (what potential side effects could occur).

While it is not in the purview of the present chapter to address the preclinical and clinical development of drug candidates in detail, for the sake of completeness, a brief overview of clinical research and the expected outcome are presented here.

CLINICAL DEVELOPMENT

While preclinical research answers basic questions about a drug's safety, it is not a substitute for studies of ways the drug will interact with the human body. "Clinical research" refers to studies, or trials, that are done in people. As the developers design the clinical study, they will consider what they want to accomplish for each of the different Clinical Research Phases and begin the Investigational New Drug Process (IND), a process they must go through before clinical research begins (www.fda.gov). In the IND application, developers must include:

- Animal study data and toxicity (side effects that cause great harm) data
- Manufacturing information
- Clinical protocols (study plans) for studies to be conducted
- Data from any prior human research
- Information about the investigator

The FDA review team has 30 days to review the original IND submission. The process protects volunteers who participate in clinical trials from unreasonable and significant risk in clinical trials. FDA responds to IND applications in one of two ways:

- Approval to begin clinical trials.

- Clinical hold to delay or stop the investigation. FDA can place a clinical hold for specific reasons, including:
  - Participants are exposed to unreasonable or significant risk.
  - Investigators are not qualified.
  - Materials for the volunteer participants are misleading.
  - The IND application does not include enough information about the trial's risks.

A clinical hold is rare; instead, FDA often provides comments intended to improve the quality of a clinical trial. In most cases, if FDA is satisfied that the trial meets federal standards, the applicant is allowed to proceed with the proposed study.

DESIGNING CLINICAL TRIALS (WWW.FDA.GOV)

Researchers design clinical trials to answer specific research questions related to a drug. These trials follow a specific study plan, called a protocol, that is developed by the researcher or manufacturer. Before a clinical trial begins, researchers review prior information about the drug to develop research questions and objectives. Then, they decide:

- Who qualifies to participate (selection criteria)
- How many people will be part of the study
- How long the study will last
- Whether there will be a control group and other ways to limit research bias
- How the drug will be given to patients and at what dosage
- What assessments will be conducted, when, and what data will be collected
- How the data will be reviewed and analyzed

CLINICAL RESEARCH PHASE STUDIES

Clinical trials follow a typical series from early, small-scale, Phase I studies to late-stage, large-scale, Phase III studies.

Phase I (Safety and Dosage): In Phase I clinical trials, doctors usually work with 20−100 healthy volunteers to investigate the absorption, distribution in the human body and excretion of an investigational compound to find its optimal preliminary dosage with the highest short-term tolerability and safety. The percentage of drugs that successfully pass through Phase I is about 70%.

Phase II (Efficacy and Side Effects): Efficacy and safety in the target indication is established with up to several hundred patients suffering from the disease treated for usually several weeks or a few months (Proof of Concept). The final dosage is determined. Only a small percentage ($\sim 33\%$) of the drug candidates entering Phase II pass on to Phase III.

Phase III (Efficacy and Safety): Once the proof of concept of a compound has been confirmed, large clinical trials often with hundreds and thousands (300 to 3000) of patients are conducted. This final stage of the clinical trials confirms and refines the safety and efficacy in large patient populations (several thousands) and long-term treatment appropriate for the indication. The percentage of drugs that move to the next phase is about 25–30%.

FDA Review: Registration and Regulatory Approval

Before filing a marketing application, a developer must have adequate data from two large, controlled clinical trials. If a drug developer has evidence from its early tests and preclinical and clinical research that a drug is safe and effective for its intended use, the company can file an application (New Drug Application, NDA) to market the drug.

A NDA tells the full story of a drug. Its purpose is to demonstrate that a drug is safe and effective for its intended use in the population studied.

A drug developer must include everything about a drug—from preclinical data to Phase III trial data—in an NDA. Developers must include reports on all studies, data, and analyses. Along with clinical results, developers must include:

- Proposed labeling
- Safety updates
- Drug abuse information
- Patent information
- Any data from studies that may have been conducted outside the United States
- Institutional review board compliance information
- Directions for use

The FDA review team of independent experts thoroughly examines all submitted data on the drug and makes a decision on whether or not the drug product should be approved for market entry. In cases where FDA determines that a drug has been shown to be safe and effective for its intended use, it is then necessary to work with the applicant to develop and refine prescribing information. This is referred to as "labeling." Labeling accurately and objectively describes the basis for approval and how best to use the drug.

Phase IV (Life Cycle Management)

The product is further profiled in special patient subgroups and in the context of an even broader concomitant therapeutic environment. These trials may be extremely large (could be as many as 30,000 patients in a trial) and can therefore identify even rare adverse reactions. Approval of the medication for additional indications may be the result.

INDS FOR MARKETED DRUGS

If sponsors want to further develop an approved drug for a new use, dosage strength, new form, or different form (such as an injectable or oral liquid, as opposed to tablet form), or if they want to conduct other clinical research or a postmarket safety study, they would do so under an IND.

CONCLUDING REMARKS

The past few years have witnessed big strides made by the public and private sectors engaged in drug discovery and development. The FDA has approved a record number of new drugs, thus making the rock-bottom approvals experienced over the past decade a distant memory. It is the changed mindset of the pharmaceutical industry and academia that embraced coordinated, collaborative innovation that made it all possible! There are well over 7000 drugs that are in development around the world, with three-fourths being first-in-class drugs. Cancer death rates keep falling, thanks to new treatment options and medicines. Cancer immunotherapy, exemplified by Bristol-Myers Squibb's Opdivo and Merck's Keytruda, is now a reality. The HIV/AIDS death rate has fallen by 80−90% in the last two decades. We now have a near 90% cure rate in treating Hepatitis C. On the down side, the cost to develop a drug is still in excess of US$3 billion, with only 20% of the marketed drugs yielding revenues that either match or exceed the R&D costs incurred. It takes more than 10−15 + years to develop a drug, with fewer than 10−12% of drugs entering clinical trials ever getting FDA approvals. The current failure rate of >80% is unsustainable and we need to find better ways to shepherd clinical candidates toward a successful outcome (Chaguturu, 2016).

The renaissance in pharmacognosy research over the last few years gives us a sense of déjà vu about it. A much desired recognition of the old hat that was the foundation of modern medicine. The mouse model system that we relied so heavily for preclinical proof of concept studies has its own limitations in that it may or may not truly represent or predict the outcome in humans. The newly invented genome editing technology platform by Feng Zhang, CRISPR-Cas system, has taken the field of biomedical research by storm, unlike any since the introduction of PCR. CRISPR, Clustered Regularly Interspaced Short Palindromic Repeats, helps engineer any organism one chooses by modifying its own genome (Chaguturu, 2016). Adaptation of this technology platform in the coming years could pave the way for the discovery and development of new drugs with much better outcome as drug candidates pass through various phases of clinical trials.

ACKNOWLEDGMENTS

The author is indebted Gerry Lushington (LiS Consulting; medchem, chemoinformatics), Jianwen Fang (NIH/University of Kansas; bioinformatics), Scott Lowell (University of Kansas; protein crystallography), Philip Gao (University of Kansas; protein production), Anuradha Roy (University of Kansas; HTS operations), Peter McDonald (University of Kansas), and Andrew Godwin (University of Kansas Medical Center; preclinical animal studies) for their input and personal communications, all of which shaped the author's viewpoints articulated in this chapter.

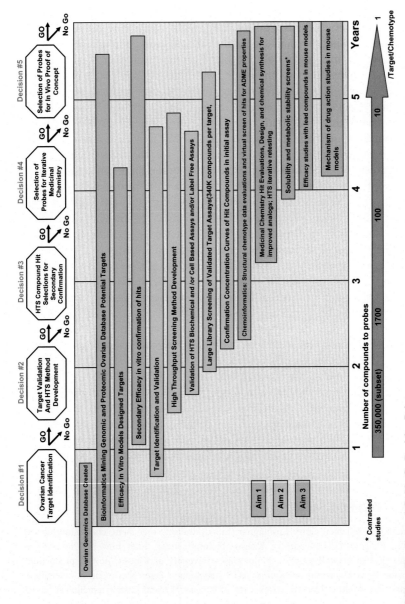

APPENDIX 1 Timeline and Go/No Go Decision Points.

AIM	TASKS	Year 1	Year 2	Year 3	Year 4	Year 5
Aim 1. Target identification and validation	Aim 1A. Bioinformatics	***	**	**	*	*
	Aim 1B. shRNA analysis	***	**	**	*	*
	Aim 1C. miRNA analysis	*	***	**	*	*
Aim 2. HTS: Probe identification from targets	Aim 2A. Protein exp & cell line generation		***	***	**	
	Aim 2B. Primary high through screening		**	***	***	
	Aim 2C. Secondary & counter HTS			***	***	***
Aim 3. Med Chem: Hit-to-probe-to-lead optimization	Aim 3A. Probe prioritization, optimization			**	***	***
	Aim 3B. Iterative QSAR			**	***	***
	Aim 3C. Proof of concept studies			*	**	***

Effort Level:

***	**	*
Very High	High	Medium

APPENDIX 2   Effort scale chart.

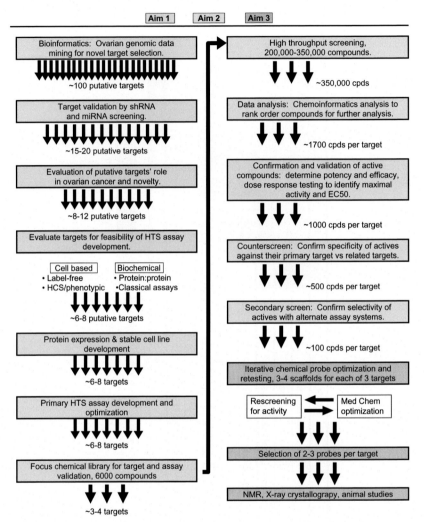

| Aim 1 | Aim 2 | Aim 3 |

Bioinformatics: Ovarian genomic data mining for novel target selection.

~100 putative targets

Target validation by shRNA and miRNA screening.

~15-20 putative targets

Evaluation of putative targets' role in ovarian cancer and novelty.

~8-12 putative targets

Evaluate targets for feasibility of HTS assay development.

Cell based
• Label-free
• HCS/phenotypic

Biochemical
• Protein:protein
• Classical assays

~6-8 putative targets

Protein expression & stable cell line development

~6-8 targets

Primary HTS assay development and optimization

~6-8 targets

Focus chemical library for target and assay validation, 6000 compounds

~3-4 targets

High throughput screening, 200,000-350,000 compounds.

~350,000 cpds

Data analysis: Chemoinformatics analysis to rank order compounds for further analysis.

~1700 cpds per target

Confirmation and validation of active compounds: determine potency and efficacy, dose response testing to identify maximal activity and EC50.

~1000 cpds per target

Counterscreen: Confirm specificity of actives against their primary target vs related targets.

~500 cpds per target

Secondary screen: Confirm selectivity of actives with alternate assay systems.

~100 cpds per target

Iterative chemical probe optimization and retesting, 3-4 scaffolds for each of 3 targets

Rescreening for activity ⇄ Med Chem optimization

Selection of 2-3 probes per target

NMR, X-ray crystallograpy, animal studies

APPENDIX 3   Critical Path Flow Chart: Ovarian Cancer Target Discovery and Chemical Probe Development.

APPENDIX 4

FORWARD CHEMICAL GENETICS

Chemical biology deals with the understanding and unraveling of the myriad effects elicited by bioactive molecules, such as the therapeutically relevant natural products; the identification of the active ingredient(s); and the protein target through which the natural product manifests its effects are a prerequisite to the discovery and development of a drug that eventually leads to FDA approval. Target-based drug discovery involves screening large chemical libraries against a therapeutic target to find the needle in a haystack, but it is likely that such a compound could still have multiple binding partners. Knowing the cellular targets of drugs is crucial for efficient drug discovery. Determining the full spectrum of targets associated with a bioactive small molecule can lead to faster optimization, an understanding of off-target side effects, and the ability to minimize possible toxicities early on in the process. Identifying the protein target of a therapeutically relevant small molecule is still a daunting task. A multifaceted approach to the target identification problem in the context of genome-based drug discovery include (www.broadinstitute.org):

- quantitative proteomics based on mass spectrometry
- genetic complementation of small-molecule effects using RNA interference
- computational inference by connectivity analysis using reference compounds

Identifying the protein target is particularly relevant for hits discovered from phenotypic screens without a known mechanism of action, for repurposed drugs for which targets might not be known for the new indication, or for natural products with activities of interest. Chemical proteomics may also help understand the off-target effects of hits identified from target-based screens as well. It may also be helpful for examining drug polypharmacy, and as a powerful tool for gaining knowledge about off-target effects that lead to toxicity and eventual "valley of death."

Chemical proteomics is a widely used approach involving affinity extraction of proteins that bind the drug of interest, using tandem mass spectrometry to identify interacting proteins, or perturbation of the proteolytic susceptibility of a drug-binding protein upon drug binding. Although affinity chromatography has been one of the most widely used technology platforms (Sato et al., 2010), it poses severe limitation with small molecules that are hard to derivatize. This limitation was adequately addressed with the quantitative capability of SILAC to drastically increase the sensitivity of this approach for target identification (Ong et al., 2009).

A drug affinity responsive target stability (DARTS) method, unlike affinity chromatography, takes advantage of ligand-induced resistance to proteolysis, and helps to identify the direct binding protein targets (and off targets) of small molecules on a proteome scale without requiring chemical modification of the compound. DARTS may be general enough to be used *as a discovery approach* for identifying protein targets binding to small molecules (Lomenick et al., 2009). Additional protein-based target identification platforms include:

- *Proteome-chip based microarrays*, where small molecules are first labeled such that their physical presence and location can be followed upon binding to the proteome chip. However, a current disadvantage shared with affinity chromatography is the need for small-molecule labeling and the requirement that the labeling moiety can be incorporated without abolishing the compound's bioactivity. The power of this approach will be greatly enhanced by the development of label-free binding detection compatible with the proteome array format (Zhu et al., 2001; Lu et al., 2010; Lomenick et al., 2011).

- *Activity-based protein profiling* depends on small molecules with reactive functional groups (mainly electrophiles) that can covalently bind to catalytic residues in an enzyme active site. Such activity-based probes allow the targeted proteins to be labeled for subsequent purification and analysis (Lomenick et al., 2011; Bottcher et al., 2010).

- *Stability of proteins from rates of oxidation* (SPROX) is akin to DARTS in that it detects small molecule-induced changes in the folding and thermodynamic stability of target proteins in complex samples. Instead of using differential proteolysis as a readout, SPROX measures ligand-induced changes in the rate of methionine oxidation for target proteins. The major limiting factor of SPROX is that only the most abundant proteins in each sample can be accurately identified and quantified, has no mechanism to enrich the target proteins from nontarget proteins, and can be applied only to methionine-containing peptides (Lomenick et al., 2011; West et al., 2010).

- Phage Display involves using cloned bacteriophages encoding genes of interest to form fusion proteins with phage coat proteins, and is subsequently allowed to bind to an immobilized compound; putative target proteins interacting with the small molecule of interest are now bound to the bacteriophages. Identity of the bound protein is then achieved by amplification and sequencing of the phage DNA (Takakusagi et al., 2010; Dormán et al., 2016).

Chemical biologists are continually interested in developing experimental tools and techniques for detecting and deconvoluting the interactions between small molecules and proteins. The repertoire of experimental tools outlined here and the ones that are continually being developed are sure to greatly advance the field of pharmacognosy and the phenotypic screens in the coming years (Dormán et al., 2016; Osada, 2009).

REFERENCES

8.0 S. The Tripos Associates, 2008.

Adams, P.D., Afonine, P.V., Bunkoczi, G., Chen, V.B., Davis, I.W., Echols, N., et al., 2010. PHENIX: a comprehensive Python-based system for macromolecular structure solution. Acta Crystallogr. D Biol. Crystallogr. 66 (Pt 2), 213–221.

Bankert, R.B., Egilmez, N.K., Hess, S.D., 2001. Human-SCID mouse chimeric models for the evaluation of anti-cancer therapies. Trends Immunol. 22 (7), 386–393.

Bazzoli, A., Tettamanzi, A.G., Zhang, Y., 2011. Computational protein design and large-scale assessment by I-TASSER structure assembly simulations. J. Mol. Biol. 407 (5), 764–776.

Blanc, E., Roversi, P., Vonrhein, C., Flensburg, C., Lea, S.M., Bricogne, G., 2004. Refinement of severely incomplete structures with maximum likelihood in BUSTER-TNT. Acta Crystallogr. D Biol. Crystallogr. 60 (Pt 12 Pt 1), 2210–2221.

Bottcher, T., Pitscheider, M., Sieber, S.A., 2010. Natural products and their biological targets: proteomic and metabolomic labeling strategies. Angew. Chem. Int. Ed. 49, 2680–2698.

Breiman, L., 2001. Random forests. Mach. Learn. 45 (1), 5–32.

Cancer Genome Atlas Research Network, 2011. Integrated genomic analyses of ovarian carcinoma. Nature 474 (7353), 609–615.

Chaguturu, R., 2014. Collaborative Innovation in Drug Discovery: Strategies for Public and Private Partnerships. Wiley and Sons, New Jersey.

Chaguturu, R., 2016. Editorial: a look back at 2015: hope, hype and hypocrisy. Comb. Chem. High Throughput Screen. 19 (1), 2–3.

Chatterjee, S., Zhong, D., Nordhues, B.A., Battaile, K.P., Lovell, S., De Guzman, R.N., 2011. The crystal structures of the Salmonella type III secretion system tip protein SipD in complex with deoxycholate and chenodeoxycholate. Protein Sci. 20 (1), 75–86.

Collisson, E.A., Sadanandam, A., Olson, P., Gibb, W.J., Truitt, M., Gu, S., et al., 2011. Subtypes of pancreatic ductal adenocarcinoma and their differing responses to therapy. Nat. Med. 17 (4), 500–503.

Cramer, R.D., Patterson, D.E., Bunce, J.D., 1988. Comparative molecular field analysis (CoMFA). 1. Effect of shape on binding of steroids to carrier proteins. J. Am. Chem. Soc. 110 (18), 5959–5967.

Cruciani, G., Meniconi, M., Carosati, E., Zamora, I., Mannhold, R. (Eds.), 2003. VOLSURF: A Tool for Drug ADME-Properties Prediction. Wiley-VCH Verlag GmbH & Co., Weinheim.

Cudney, R., Patel, S., Weisgraber, K., Newhouse, Y., McPherson, A., 1994. Screening and optimization strategies for macromolecular crystal growth. Acta Crystallogr. D Biol. Crystallogr. 50 (Pt 4), 414–423.

Dormán, G., Flachner, B., Hajdú, I., András, C., 2016. Target Identification and Polypharmacology of Nutraceuticals. In: Gupta, R. (Ed.), Neutraceuticals.

Elkas, J.C., Baldwin, R.L., Pegram, M., Tseng, Y., Slamon, D., Karlan, B.Y., 2002. A human ovarian carcinoma murine xenograft model useful for preclinical trials. Gynecol. Oncol. 87 (2), 200–206.

Evans, P., 2006. Scaling and assessment of data quality. Acta Crystallogr. D Biol. Crystallogr. 62 (Pt 1), 72–82.

Fang, J., Koen, Y.M., Hanzlik, R.P., 2009. Bioinformatic analysis of xenobiotic reactive metabolite target proteins and their interacting partners. BMC Chem. Biol. 9, 5.

Fang, J.W., Grzymala-Busse, J.W., 2006a. Leukemia prediction from gene expression data - a rough set approach. Lect. Notes Comput. Sci. 4029, 899–908.

Fang, J.W., Grzymala-Busse, J.W., 2006b. Mining of microRNA expression data - a rough set approach. Lect. Notes Artif. Int. 4062, 758−765.

Fichtner, I., Slisow, W., Gill, J., Becker, M., Elbe, B., Hillebrand, T., et al., 2004. Anticancer drug response and expression of molecular markers in early-passage xenotransplanted colon carcinomas. Eur. J. Cancer 40 (2), 298−307.

Gasteiger, J., Marsili, M., 1980. Partial equalization of orbital electronegativity- a rapid access to atomic changes. Tetrahedron 36, 3219−3228.

Giuliano, K.A., Haskins, J.R., Taylor, D.L., 2003. Advances in high content screening for drug discovery. Assay Drug Dev. Technol. 1 (4), 565−577.

Goodsell, D.S., Morris, G.M., Olson, A.J., 1996. Automated docking of flexible ligands: applications of AutoDock. J. Mol. Recognit. 9 (1), 1−5.

Han, B., Chen, X.W., Wang, X., Michaelis, E.K., 2009. Integrating multiple microarray data for cancer pathway analysis using bootstrapping K-S test. J. Biomed. Biotechnol. 2009, 707580.

Hanzlik, R.R., Fang, J.W., Koen, Y.M., 2009. Filling and mining the reactive metabolite target protein database. Chem. Biol. Interact. 179 (1), 38−44.

Heiser, L.M., Wang, N.J., Talcott, C.L., Laderoute, K.R., Knapp, M., Guan, Y., et al., 2009. Integrated analysis of breast cancer cell lines reveals unique signaling pathways. Genome Biol. 10 (3), R31.

Jain, A.N., 2007. Surflex-Dock 2.1: robust performance from ligand energetic modeling, ring flexibility, and knowledge-based search. J. Comput. Aided Mol. Des. 21 (5), 281−306.

Kabsch, W., 1988. Automatic indexing of rotation diffraction patterns. J. Appl. Crystallogr. 21 (1), 67−72.

Lee, I.-H., Lushington, G., Visvanathan, M., 2011. A filter-based feature selection approach for identifying potential biomarkers for lung cancer. J. Clin. Bioinfor. 1 (1), 11.

Lghwnmg, J.-X., 2005. Reliable prescreening of candidate nerve agent prophylaxes via 3D QSAR. DTIC Monit. Ser. 23, 1−28.

library i, 2009. ChemNavigator Inc., San Diego, CA.

Lipinski, C.A., Lombardo, F., Dominy, B.W., Feeney, P.J., 2001. Experimental and computational approaches to estimate solubility and permeability in drug discovery and development settings. Adv. Drug Deliv. Rev. 46 (1−3), 3−26.

Liu, S., Tang, W., Fang, J., Ren, J., Li, H., Xiao, Z., et al., 2009. Novel regulators of Fgf23 expression and mineralization in Hyp bone. Mol. Endocrinol. 23 (9), 1505−1518.

Lomenick, B., Hao, R., Jonai, N., Chin, R.M., Aghajan, M., Warburton, S., et al., 2009. Target identification using drug affinity responsive target stability (DARTS). Proc. Natl. Acad. Sci. U. S. A. 106, 21984−21989.

Lomenick, B., Olsen, R.W., Huang, J., 2011. Identification of direct protein targets of small molecules. ACS Chem. Biol. 6 (1), 34−46.

Lu, H., Wen, J.A., Wang, X., Yuan, K., Li, W., Lu, H.B., et al., 2010. Detection of the specific binding on protein microarrays by oblique-incidence reflectivity difference method. J. Opt. 12, published online September 6, 2010, http://dx.doi.org/10.1088/2040-8978/12/9/095301.

Lushington, G.H., Guo, J.X., Wang, J.L., 2007. Whither combine? New opportunities for receptor-based QSAR. Curr. Med. Chem. 14 (17), 1863−1877.

Mayr, L.M., Bojanic, D., 2009. Novel trends in high-throughput screening. Curr. Opin. Pharmacol. 9 (5), 580−588.

McCoy, A.J., Grosse-Kunstleve, R.W., Adams, P.D., Winn, M.D., Storoni, L.C., Read, R.J., 2007. *Phaser* crystallographic software. J. Appl. Cryst. 40, 658−674.

McDonald, P., Roy, A., Taylor, B., Price, A., Sittampalam, S., Weir, S., et al., 2008. High throughput screening in academia: drug discovery initiatives at the University of Kansas. Drug Disc. World Fall59−74.

Morton, C.L., Houghton, P.J., 2007. Establishment of human tumor xenografts in immunodeficient mice. Nat. Protocols 2 (2), 247−250.

Murshudov, G.N., Vagin, A.A., Dodson, E.J., 1997. Refinement of macromolecular structures by the maximum-likelihood method. Acta Crystallogr. D Biol. Crystallogr. 53 (Pt 3), 240−255.

Netzer, M., Millonig, G., Osl, M., Pfeifer, B., Praun, S., Villinger, J., et al., 2009. A new ensemble-based algorithm for identifying breath gas marker candidates in liver disease using ion molecule reaction mass spectrometry. Bioinformatics 25 (7), 941−947.

Neve, R.M., Chin, K., Fridlyand, J., Yeh, J., Baehner, F.L., Fevr, T., et al., 2006. A collection of breast cancer cell lines for the study of functionally distinct cancer subtypes. Cancer Cell. 10 (6), 515−527.

Ong, S.E., Schenone, M., Margolin, A.A., Li, X., Do, K., Doud, M.K., et al., 2009. Identifying the proteins to which small-molecule probes and drugs bind in cells. Proc. Natl. Acad. Sci. U. S. A. 106, 4617−4622.

Ortiz, A.R., Pisabarro, M.T., Gago, F., Wade, R.C., 1995. Prediction of drug binding affinities by comparative binding energy analysis. J. Med. Chem. 38 (14), 2681−2691.

Osada, H., 2009. Protein Targeting with Small Molecules: Chemical Biology Techniques and Applications. Wiley, New Jersey.

Perez-Soler, R., Kemp, B., Wu, Q.P., Mao, L., Gomez, J., Zeleniuch-Jacquotte, A., et al., 2000. Response and determinants of sensitivity to paclitaxel in human non-small cell lung cancer tumors heterotransplanted in nude mice. Clin. Cancer Res. 6 (12), 4932−4938.

Roy, A., Taylor, B.J., McDonald, P.R., Price, A.R., Chaguturu, R., 2009. Hit-to-probe-to-lead optimization strategies: a biology perspective to conquer the valley of death. In: Seethala, R., Zhang, L. (Eds.), Drugs and Pharmaceutical Sciences., second ed. Informa Healthcare, New York, NY, pp. 21−55.

Roy, A., Kucukural, A., Zhang, Y., 2010. I-TASSER: a unified platform for automated protein structure and function prediction. Nat. Protocols. 5 (4), 725−738.

Rubio-Viqueira, B., Jimeno, A., Cusatis, G., Zhang, X., Iacobuzio-Donahue, C., Karikari, C., et al., 2006. An in vivo platform for translational drug development in pancreatic cancer. Clin. Cancer Res. 12 (15), 4652−4661.

Salamat-Miller, N., Fang, J.W., Seidel, C.W., Smalter, A.M., Assenov, Y., Albrecht, M., et al., 2006. A network-based analysis of polyanion-binding proteins utilizing yeast protein arrays. Mol. Cell. Proteomics 5 (12), 2263−2278.

Salamat-Miller, N., Fang, J.W., Seidel, C.W., Assenov, Y., Albrecht, M., Middaugh, C.R., 2007. A network-based analysis of polyanion-binding proteins utilizing human protein arrays. J. Biol. Chem. 282 (14), 10153−10163.

Sanderson, D.M., Earnshaw, C.G., 1991. Computer prediction of possible toxic action from chemical structure; the DEREK system. Hum. Exp. Toxicol. 10, 261−273.

Sato, S., Murata, A., Shirakawa, T., Uesugi, M., 2010. Biochemical target isolation for novices: affinity-based strategies. Chem. Biol. 17, 616−623.

Sheldrick, G.M., 2008. A short history of SHELX. Acta Crystallogr. A 64 (Pt 1), 112−122.

Spurdle, A.B., Thompson, D.J., Ahmed, S., Ferguson, K., Healey, C.S., O'Mara, T., et al., 2011. Genome-wide association study identifies a common variant associated with risk of endometrial cancer. Nat. Genet. 43 (5), 451−454.

Stevens, A.J., Jensen, J.J., Wyller, K., Kilgore, P.C., Chatterjee, S., Rohrbaugh, M.L., 2011. The role of public-sector research in the discovery of drugs and vaccines. N. Engl. J. Med. 364 (6), 535–541.

Takakusagi, Y., Takakusagi, K., Sugawara, F., Sakaguchi, K., 2010. Use of phage display technology for the determination of the targets for smallmolecule therapeutics. Expert Opin. Drug Discov. 5, 361–389.

The PubChem Compound Database NcfBI, 2005.

The Tripod Associates, 2008. St. Louis MO [Internet].

Thomas, A.M., 2010. Genome-wide tissue-specific farnesoid X receptor binding in mouse liver and intestine. Hepatology.

Vagin, A.A., Teplyakov, A., 1997. *MOLREP*: an automated program for molecular replacement. J. Appl. Cryst. 30, 1022–1025.

Vapnik, V.N., 1999. An overview of statistical learning theory. IEEE Trans. Neural. Netw. 10 (5), 988–999.

West, G.M., Tucker, C.L., Xu, T., Park, S.K., Han, X., Yates, J.R., et al., 2010. Quantitative proteomics approach for identifying protein-drug interactions in complex mixtures using protein stability measurements. Proc. Natl. Acad. Sci. U. S. A. 107, 9078–9082.

Yu, J.S., Chen, X.W., 2005. Bayesian neural network approaches to ovarian cancer identification from high-resolution mass spectrometry data. Bioinformatics 21, I487–I494.

Zaidi, A., Jiang, L., Fang, J.W., Nichols, D.M., Gogichaeva, N.V., Michaelis, M.L., 2007. Proteomics analysis of age-dependent alterations in synaptic membrane lipid rafts. Free Radic. Biol. Med. 43, S190–S190.

Zhu, H., Bilgin, M., Bangham, R., Hall, D., Casamayor, A., Bertone, P., et al., 2001. Global analysis of protein activities using proteome chips. Science 293, 2101–2105.

Zock, J.M., 2009. Applications of high content screening in life science research. Comb. Chem. High Throughput Screen. 12 (9), 870–876.

Chapter 7

Pharmacogenomics

Yogita A. Ghodke-Puranik[1] and Jatinder K. Lamba[2]

[1]*Mayo Clinic, Rochester, MN, United States,* [2]*University of Florida, Gainesville, FL, United States*

INTRODUCTION

> *If it were not for the great variability among individuals, medicine might as well be a science and not an art.*
>
> Sir William Osler, 1892

Over the years there have been major improvements in the length and quality of life. While infectious diseases are on a decline, noncommunicable and chronic complex diseases are increasing. There have been number of drugs developed for these diseases. However, inter-individual variability in drug response is a major concern in disease management and drug development. Variable drug responses can often be attributed to genetic polymorphism in genes involved in drug pharmacokinetics (PD) and pharmacodynamics (PD). The variability of a drug response can lead to therapeutic failure or adverse effects of drugs in individuals. Unfortunately, prospective identification of those patients who are most likely to benefit from a specific therapy is not routinely possible for many diseases and medications. Drug treatment may be personalized for greater effect if there is a better understanding of the molecular basis of drug action and genetic determinants of drug response. Pharmacogenomics is the study of the role of inheritance in differences in drug responses, and it aims to reveal genetic variants that influence drug responses in order to tailor a patient's treatment based on their genetic makeup. Many pharmacogenetic studies have shown a clear evidence of a causal correlation between genetic polymorphisms and drug responses.

Developments in the field of pharmacogenomics and the concept of personalized medicine are new to the field of modern medical science. However, there is a long-standing tradition regarding this concept of personalized medicine in the Indian medical system of Ayurveda. According to the principles of Ayurvedic medicine, every person has a unique trait, which is defined by specific and permanent composition of doshas at conception called Prakriti. It is one of the important factors for the management of

Innovative Approaches in Drug Discovery. DOI: http://dx.doi.org/10.1016/B978-0-12-801814-9.00007-6

health and diseases. Each Prakriti has certain physical-psychosomatic characteristics, a defined proneness to certain diseases, and specific responses to treatment. These concepts can be integrated with principles of immunogenetics and pharmacogenetics. Overlaying the concept of pharmacogenomics with Ayurveda therapeutics has resulted in origin of this novel field of Ayugenomics. Previous studies have shown that by using the innovative concept of Ayugenomics it is possible to examine Prakriti from a human genome perspective.

In this chapter we will discuss recent advances in the field of pharmacogenomics, its potential use in clinical practice, challenges to future pharmacogenomics, and its translation into individualized medicine. We will further discuss how integrating evidence−based initiatives such as Ayugenomics can potentially facilitate steps toward overcoming some of the challenges to achieve the ultimate goal of individualized medicine.

ABSORPTION, DISTRIBUTION, METABOLISM AND EXCRETION (ADME) OF DRUGS

A therapeutic drug is considered clinically effective based on its efficacy and the level of risk for severe adverse events. The primary goals of drug manufacturers, healthcare providers, and regulators is the evaluation of drug metabolism and optimization of pharmacokinetics (PK) in drug discovery, clinical development, and in routine medical practice to improve the efficacy and safety of drug therapy. The balance between efficacy and safety is influenced by: (1) the drug's absorption, distribution, metabolism, and excretion (ADME), which is also influenced by other factors such as age, sex, health, lifestyle, nutrition, and other environmental factors; (2) drug−drug interactions that are more significant in older patients who are likely to be taking multiple drugs; (3) variability in handling drugs related to an individual's genetic makeup (pharmacogenetics). Although, demographic-, environmental-, and lifestyle-related factors account for some of the inter-individual variability in drug responses, considerable variation remains undefined that can be partially attributed to genetic heterogeneity. Genetic polymorphisms of proteins involved in pharmacodynamics (PD) (i.e., drug targeting) and PK (i.e., drug metabolism and transport) are probably to be the most significant sources of individual variability in drug efficacy (Weinshilboum and Wang, 2004; Roden et al., 2011). For the last decade or so, ADME genes have been studied for the presence of mutations and polymorphisms leading to altered expression levels/activity. These variations have been recurrently and consistently associated with in vitro and in vivo PK properties of a broad range of drugs. While PD genes have been mostly associated with a specific drug target, they are most often only specific to a particular compound's mechanism of action. These genetic variants are very critical especially for drugs with a very narrow therapeutic index where small differences in drug disposition may lead to significant toxicity or loss of efficacy. Ongoing studies further explore how genetic variations are associated with variable clinical outcomes and how we can improve the clinical translation of these genetic markers to improve dose-optimization strategies and reduce adverse drug reactions (ADRs).

ROLE OF ADME GENES IN DRUG RESPONSE AND ADVERSE DRUG REACTIONS

Genetic variation in drug disposition (ADME) can influence pharmacokinetics thereby altering drug levels and clearance of the parent drug or its active metabolites in plasma and target tissue and thereby affect drug action. ADME genes are typically categorized into four types: (1) Phase I (e.g., cytochrome P450s) and II metabolizing enzymes (responsible for the modification of functional groups and conjugation with endogenous moieties, respectively); (2) influx and efflux transporter proteins, responsible for the uptake and excretion of drugs in and out of cells respectively (including, but not restricted to, the ABC family and SLCO1B1); (3) serum binding proteins; and (4) transcription factors (such as RXR retinoid X receptor, orphan nuclear receptors PXR (pregnane X receptor), and CAR (constitutive androstane receptor)) that can are involved in the regulation of expression of ADME genes or other enzymes that affect the biochemistry of ADME enzymes (such as the POR P450 cytochrome oxidoreductase) (Daly, 2010). Phase I enzymes, particularly the cytochrome P450 (CYP) superfamily, has been the most widely studied so far.

Included among the types of genetic variation are single nucleotide polymorphisms (SNPs), structural variants that result from the insertion or deletion of bases (indels), or large copy number variants in addition to complete loss or gain of whole gene. These variations in drug disposition can affect gene expression by altering transcriptional regulations, splicing, or it can affect protein function and levels by causing amino acid changes or truncation of protein coding sequences. Overall, these polymorphisms precipitate into four phenotypic groups with differential metabolic status within a population: poor metabolizers (PM; lack active forms of the enzyme due to presence of deficient alleles on both chromosomes that leads to decreased metabolism) thereby retaining a drug in the body for long time than normal and hence the plasma concentration of the drug is high for a longer period; intermediate metabolizers (IM; carrying combinations of alleles that lead to impaired enzymatic activity toward known probe drugs, a form mostly noted in CYP2D6, but also in other enzymes); extensive metabolizers (EM; carrying two normally functioning alleles) that retain a drug in the body for an optimal period; and ultra-rapid metabolizers (UM; showing an increased capacity for enzymatic metabolism due to increased copies of the functional gene) that retain the drug in the body for less time. Thus, depending on if the drug is a prodrug (a medication after administration is converted within the body into a pharmacologically active drug; prodrugs help to improve bio-availability) or active drug, when an active parent drug undergoes inactivation via a polymorphic drug metabolizing enzyme (DME), reduced function variants can cause drug accumulation and toxicity in PM, while ultra-rapid variants can lead to higher clearance and reduced drug action in UM. On the other hand, when an inactive prodrug needs to be converted to the active drug by a polymorphic DME to exhibit pharmacological activity, reduced function polymorphisms can lead to lack of drug efficacy in PM, whereas ultra-rapid variants can lead to active drug accumulation and toxicity (Evans and Relling, 1999). In addition, there are ethnic differences in the distribution of functional DME variants giving rise to different proportions of PM, IM, EM, and UM subjects within a given population (Ma and Lu, 2011). However, assessing a phenotype based on genotypes of specific DMEs can present major challenges, as these distinctions are not always clear (Gaedigk et al., 2008) making it difficult to directly translate these in clinical practice. Some of the major drugs-metabolizing enzymes with significant contribution to inter-individual variation are discussed below.

PHARMACOGENETICS IN DRUG RESPONSE

An individual's response to a drug is influenced by the complex interaction among environmental and genetic factors. Various studies have been carried out to find out what proportion of drug—response variability is likely to be genetically determined (Wang et al., 2011; Weinshilboum, 2003). Table 7.1 lists the most studied pharmacogenetically important SNPs with their function and with representative examples of clinically significant drugs that is affected by these SNPs covered in this chapter.

PHARMACOGENOMICS OF PHASE I DRUG METABOLIZING ENZYMES

DMEs play central roles in the biotransformation, metabolism and/or detoxification of xenobiotics or foreign compounds, exposed to the human body. For the body to minimize the damage caused by these xenobiotics, various tissues and organs are well equipped with diverse DMEs like various phase I and phase II enzymes that are abundantly present either at the basal level and/or induced after exposure. DMEs catalyze lipophilic drugs to give rise to metabolites with altered activity and increased water solubility or metabolites more suitable to further metabolism by other enzymes. Many of the phase I and phase II DMEs are polymorphic. These polymorphisms cause significant inter-individual differences in drug and metabolite exposure and can determine drug responses as well as the risk for ADRs. Hence, the majority of pharmacogenomic drug labels refers to genes encoding phase I and phase II enzymes (Frueh et al., 2008).

TABLE 7.1 List of Most Studied Pharmacogenetically Important SNPs With Their Function and With Representative Examples of Clinically Significant Drugs That Is Impacted by These SNPs

Gene	refSNP (allele)	Nucleotide Change	Function	Amino Acid Translation	Clinically Significant Impacted Drugs
CYP1A2	rs2069514 (CYP1A2*1C)	G > A	5′-non-coding		Caffeine, antipsychotics, clozapine theophylline
	rs762551 (CYP1A2*1F)	C > A	Intronic		Caffeine, antipsychotics, thioridazine, clozapine
CYP2C19	rs4244285 (CYP2C19*2)	G > A G > C	Synonymous	Pro227Pro	Clopidogrel omeprazole, proton pump inhibitors, mephenytoin, phenytoin, diazepam
	rs4986893 (CYP2C19*3)	G > A	Stop codon	Trp212null	Clopidogrel, mephenytoin, omeprazole, escitalopram
	rs12248560 (CYP2C19*17)	C > T C > A	5′ Flanking		Proton pump inhibitors, mephenytoin, omeprazole, clopidogrel, pantoprazole, escitalopram, imipramine
CYP2C9	rs1799853 (CYP2C9*2)	C > T	Missense	Arg144Cys	Warfarin, phenytoin, sulfonamides, urea derivatives
	rs1057910 (CYP2C9*3)	A > C	Missense	Ile359Leu	Warfarin, phenytoin, antiinflammatory agents, nonsteroids, diclofenac
CYP2D6	rs3892097 (CYP2D6*4)	C > T	Acceptor (splice-3)		Amitriptyline, antidepressants, clomipramine, desipramine, doxepin, imipramine, nortriptyline, or trimipramine, codeine, paroxetine, antidepressants, fluvoxamine, tamoxifen
	rs5030655 (CYP2D6*6)	T > -	Frameshift	Val52Gly	Venlafaxine, metoprolol, antipsychotics
	rs28371725 (CYP2D6*41)	C > T	Missense	Glu242Lys	Tamoxifen
	rs1065852 (part of CYP2D6*4 and CYP2D6*10 haplotype)	G > A	5′ Flanking	Pro34Ser	Citalopram, propranolol, antipsychotics, tamoxifen, escitalopram
CYP3A4	rs2740574 (CYP3A4*1B)	C > T	5′ Flanking		Tacrolimus, docetaxel, cyclophosphamide, indinavir
	rs12721627, rs2242480 (CYP3A4*16B)	G > C	Missense (exonic); intronic	Thr185Ser	Midazolam, paclitaxel
	rs35599367 (CYP3A4*22)	C > T	Intronic		Tacrolimus, cyclosporine A immunosuppressants

(Continued)

TABLE 7.1 (Continued)

Gene	refSNP (allele)	Nucleotide Change	Function	Amino Acid Translation	Clinically Significant Impacted Drugs
CYP3A5	rs776746 (CYP3A5*3)	T > C	Intronic		Cyclophosphamide, tacrolimus, cyclosporine
	rs1026427 (CYP3A5*6)	C > T	Not available	Lys208Lys	Cyclosporine, tacrolimus
TPMT	rs1142345 (TPMT*3C)	T > C	Missense	Tyr240Cys	Cisplatin, purine analogues, cyclophosphamide, mercaptopurine, methotrexate
	rs1800460 (TPMT*3B)	C > T	Missense	Ala154Thr	Cisplatin, mercaptopurine
UGT	rs4148323 (UGT1A1*6)	G > A	Intronic	Gly71Arg	Irinotecan, SN-38
	rs8175347 [UGT1A1*1 (TA)6 repeat (wildtype) UGT1A1*28 (TA)7 repeat]	TA short tandem repeat	Near 5' region		Atazanavir, ritonavir, irinotecan, SN-38
NAT2	rs1801280 (signature SNP for NAT2*5 allelic group)	T > C	Missense	Ile114Thr	Isoniazid, cyclophosphamide, hydrazine
	rs1799931 (signature SNP for NAT2*7 allelic group)	G > A	Missense	Gly286Glu	Isoniazid, rifampin, thalidomide
ABCB1	rs1045642 (ABCB1*6)	A > T A > G	Synonymous	Ile1145Ile	Controversial associations
	rs2032582 (ABCB1*7)	A > T A > C	Missense	Ser893Ala Ser893Thr	Controversial associations
	rs1128503 (ABCB1*8)	A > G	Synonymous	Gly412Gly	Controversial associations
SLCO1B1	rs2306283 (SLCO1B1*1B)	A > G	Missense	Asn130Asp	Pravastatin, pitavastatin, simvastatin, repaglinide, atorvastatin, HMG CoA reductase inhibitors
	rs4149015 (part of SLCO1B1*17-SLCO1B1*21 haplotype)	G > A	5' Flanking		Pravastatin, mycophenolate, mofetil, irinotecan
	rs4149056 (SLCO1B1*5)	T > C	Missense	Val174Ala	Simvastatin, lopinavir, antidiabetic nateglinide

Phase I DMEs primarily consist of the cytochrome (CYP) P450 super-family of microsomal enzymes, which are found in abundance in the liver, gastrointestinal tract, lung, and kidneys. CYP450 superfamily of hemepro-teins are involved in the metabolism of a number of diverse drugs, environ-mental chemicals, and xenobiotics. P450s catalyze the mono oxygenation of hydrophobic drugs to more polar forms. In humans, four CYP gene families (i.e., CYP1, CYP2, CYP3, and CYP4) are believed to play a key role in hepatic as well as extra hepatic metabolism and biotransformation of xeno-biotics and drugs. The details about different human CYP alleles are given in CYP allele nomenclature database (http://www.cypalleles.ki.se). Role of genetic variation in observed inter-individual variation in few of these P450s is discussed below.

CYP1A2

CYP1A2 plays an important role in metabolism of drugs like clozapine, olanzapine, fluvoxamine, haloperidol, theophylline; biotransformation of endogenous compounds like melatonin, bilirubin, estrogens, procarcinogens, aflatoxin B1, and aromatic/heterocyclic amines as well as caffeine (Gunes and Dahl, 2008). Caffeine, a long-known substrate and inducer of CYP1A2, has been used to estimate CYP1A2 activity in human subjects in vivo (Butler et al., 1992). CYP1A2 expression and activity exhibit approximately 40-fold inter-individual variations in human liver (Gunes and Dahl, 2008). Numerous SNPs have been described in the CYP1A2 gene, and most of the nonsynonymous SNPs encode for allozymes (CYP1A2*2 to *21) with reduced enzyme activity than wild-types; however, these SNPs occur at a very low frequency (Gunes and Dahl, 2008; Home page of the Human Cytochrome P450 (CYP) Allele Nomenclature Committee). SNPs in regula-tory regions of CYP1A2 give rise to relatively frequent variant alleles CYP1A2*1C and *1F. CYP1A2*1C has been associated with decreased caf-feine 3-demethylation in Japanese smokers, suggesting decreased inducibility by polycyclic aromatic hydrocarbons in cigarette smoke (Nakajima et al., 1999). CYP1A2*1F allele has been associated with increased caffeine metab-olism in Caucasian smokers (Ghotbi et al., 2007; Sachse et al., 1999). These results are further supported by independent, genome wide−association stud-ies (GWAS) and a meta-analysis study confirming an association between CYP1A2 variation and the habitual consumption of caffeine (Cornelis et al., 2011; Sulem et al., 2011; Amin et al., 2012; Cornelis et al., 2014). Studies have shown that CYP1A locus was also associated with blood pressure (Newton-Cheh et al., 2009; Ehret et al., 2011; Palatini et al., 2009). A recent study also found a relationship of the CYP1A2*1F allele with increased caffeine intake and reduced risk of hypertension among non-smokers (Guessous et al., 2012). The authors postulate that the increased caf-feine intake, which is caused by CYP1A2 polymorphism, accounts for the genetic impact of CYP1A2 on blood pressure, and that CYP1A2 induction by smoking reduces these genetic effects. In conclusion, these studies support a role of CYP1A2 in the regulation of blood pressure, while further studies are needed to investigate the mechanistic aspects.

CYP2C19

CYP2C19 catalyzes the metabolism of more than 12 clinically important drugs, such as omeprazole (antiulcerative), (S)-mephenytoin (anticonvulsant), and diazepam (anxiolytic), etc. (Lee, 2012). It plays an important role in the proton pump—inhibitor therapy for peptic ulcer and gastroesophageal reflux diseases. Among the 34 variants of CYP2C19, two principle alleles CYP2C19*2 and CYP2C19*3 have been reported with PM phenotypes in most cases. The prevalence of PMs varies from 15% to 25% in Chinese, Japanese, Korean, and Indian subjects, and 3% to 5% in European white subjects (Ghodke et al., 2007). It has been shown that a higher concentration of omeprazole in PMs results in great gastric acid suppression as compared with EMs (Chang et al., 1995). Cure rates for *Helicobacter pylori* in patients receiving omeprazole and amoxicillin were found to be 28% in homozygous EMs (CYP2C19*1/*1), 60% in heterozygous EMs (CYP2C19*1/*2 and *1/*3), and 100% in PMs (CYP2C19*2/*2 and *2/*3), indicating the importance of dose adjustment in the cases of EMs (Furuta et al., 1998). Individuals homozygous for the defective CYP2C19*2 allele has longer plasma half-lives of diazepam (84 hour) than subjects homozygous for the wild-type allele (20 hour), or individuals heterozygous for one CYP2C19 defective allele (64 hour) (Wan et al., 1996; Qin et al., 1999). The half-life of the metabolite desmethyldiazepam was also longer in homozygous CYP2C19 PMs. Proguanil is an inactive antimalarial prodrug that requires a biotransformation to its therapeutically active metabolite cycloguanil, which is predominantly catalyzed by CYP2C19 and to minor extent by CYP3A4 (Birkett et al., 1994; Funck-Brentano et al., 1997). A reduced activation of proguanil to cycloguanil in CYP2C19 PMs may result in failure of malaria chemoprophylaxis (Xie et al., 1999). The antiplatelet agent clopidogrel is a prodrug requiring activation through CYP2C19 to exert its therapeutic effect to prevent ischemic events particularly in patients with coronary syndromes, percutaneous coronary intervention, and myocardial infarction. Role of CYP2C19 genetic variation in variability in clinical response to clopidogrel has been extensively studies by different groups. In a GWAS study in healthy subjects, CYP2C19 SNPs were the only genetic variation that reached genome-wide significance with respect to drug levels, and CYP2C19*2 allele was associated with increased risk of cardiovascular events in patients (Shuldiner et al., 2009). In recent years, the clinical significance of CYP2C19 genotype on clopidogrel treatment has been extensively studied, and various meta-analyses have addressed the influence of the defective CYP2C19 alleles (mainly CYP2C19*2 alleles) on clopidogrel treatment response (Holmes et al., 2011; Bauer et al., 2011; Zabalza et al., 2012; Hulot et al., 2010; Sofi et al., 2011). Few studies have observed that rapid CYP2C19 metabolism caused by the CYP2C19*17 allele is associated with reduced risk of cardiovascular events as well as increased risk of bleedings (Zabalza et al., 2012; Harmsze et al., 2012; Li et al., 2012); however, contradictory results have also been reported (Bauer et al., 2011). The studies so far on CYP2C19-clopidogrel pair had resulted in development of guidelines by the Clinical Pharmacogenetics Implementation Consortium (CPIC) recommending an alternative antiplatelet therapy (e.g., prasugrel, ticagrelor) for CYP2C19 poor or IM if there is no contraindication (Scott et al., 2013).

CYP2C9

CYP2C9 constitutes approximately 20% of the total human liver microsome P-450 content and metabolizes many of therapeutically important drugs, such as tolbutamide (hypoglycemic agent), glipizide (hypoglycemic agent), phenytoin (anticonvulsant), and flurbiprofen (antiinflammatory agent), and (S)-warfarin (anticoagulant), which has a narrow therapeutic index. More than 55 variants of CYP2C9 have been identified (http://www.cypalleles.ki.se) of which CYP2C9*2 and CYP2C9*3 are the two most common variant alleles that show largely reduced enzymatic activities that lead to poor metabolism. A difference in allelic frequencies has been well documented in populations with diverse ethnic origins. The allele frequencies of CYP2C9*2 and CYP2C9*3 generally tend to be higher in white populations than Asian populations (Xie et al., 2002). Thus, CYP2C9 exhibits marked inter-individual and inter-ethnic variability in its expression and catalytic activity and can result in either drug toxicity (e.g., warfarin-induced bleeding complications) or therapeutic failure in some patients who take standard doses of CYP2C9 substrate drugs (Aithal et al., 1999; Schwarz, 2003; Sim et al., 2013). Clinical problems with toxicity and dosage adjustment of both warfarin and phenytoin have been found in CYP2C9 PMs (Steward et al., 1997; Ninomiya et al., 2000). In patients with at least one wild-type CYP2C9*1 (S)-warfarin is cleared from the body normally, whereas in CYP2C9 PMs with CYP2C9*2 and/or CYP2C9*3 alleles there is an impaired metabolism of (S)-warfarin. These patients have a two- to fourfold higher risk of having an adverse event than those with the wild-type allele on warfarin therapy, thus requiring dosage adjustments.

Information gained so far on the impact of CYP2C9 and warfarin has been used to develop CPIC guidelines to guide warfarin therapy in patients (Johnson et al., 2011). The United States Food and Drug Administration (USFDA) has also updated the warfarin drug package insert to include information on CYP2C9 genetic polymorphisms and recommendations on reducing warfarin doses (http://www.fda.gov/Drugs/ScienceResearch/ResearchAreas/Pharmacogenetics/ucm083378.htm).

CYP2D6

Though CYP2D6 constitutes only small proportion of the total hepatic CYP content, it is responsible for the metabolism of approximately 20% to 25% of all marketed drugs (Weinshilboum, 2003). Typical drug substrates of CYP2D6 include antipsychotics, antiarrhythmics, ß-adrenergic receptor blockers, antidepressants, and antiestrogens such as tamoxifen (Weinshilboum, 2003). In contrast to other CYPs, CYP2D6 expression is not induced by drugs and chemicals (Weinshilboum, 2003). CYP2D6 is one of the most extensively studied and highly polymorphic among P450s, with more than 100 allelic variants described to date (Frueh et al., 2008; Gunes and Dahl, 2008). Variant alleles of CYP2D6 are classified on the basis of enzymatic activities (Ingelman-Sundberg, 2005). CYP2D6 PM phenotype occurs in five to 10% of Caucasians and one to two% in Asians due to major variant alleles like CYP2D6*3,*4, *5, and *6 causing enzyme inactivation. Drug doses need to be reduced in PM, as they exhibit high plasma drug levels and risk of drug-related side effects. CYP2D6*9,*10, and *41 variants are responsible for the IM phenotype that causes low residual enzyme activity and subsequent lower-dose requirements for some patients. While CYP2D6 EM phenotype requires standard dosing for most of the patients. CYP2D6 also exhibits gene duplication (2 to 13 copies), which is responsible for the UM phenotype. The frequency of UM phenotype is 1% to 2% in Caucasians, 30% in Ethiopians, whereas this phenotype is absent in Asians. A UM phenotype leads to a very high enzyme activity, very low therapeutic plasma level that results in loss of drug efficacy and consequently a higher drug dose requirement. Methods for rapid, effective clinical testing of the variants are available, and knowing the CYP2D6 phenotype of an individual patient would allow physicians to prescribe a safe and effective dose of the drug to the patient.

Evidence gathered so far on PK data for CYP2D6 substrates has resulted in recommendations for dose adjustments for several antidepressants (Kirchheiner et al., 2004). Several tricyclic antidepressants require dose adjustments in CYP2D6 PMs, IMs, and UMs. Studies have shown that poor response to antidepressants is associated with CYP2D6 UM phenotype (Rau et al., 2004; Kawanishi et al., 2004; Lobello et al., 2010; Tsai et al., 2010; Penas-Lledo et al., 2013) while CYP2D6 PMs were over-represented in patients who experienced adverse events (Rau et al., 2004). This shows CYP2D6 clearly influences PK component of these drugs. Similarly, for a number of psychotic agents, dose adjustments of varying degree have been recommended; this is especially important in subjects with CYP2D6 PM and UM phenotype (Kirchheiner et al., 2004).

CYP2D6 is also involved in the activation of codeine into the active analgesic substance morphine. UMs of CYP2D6 thus are at risk of excessive morphine levels, which can cause sedation and respiratory depression both in adults and in infants of CYP2D6 UM breastfeeding mothers. On the other hand no benefit has been observed in CYP2D6 PMs due to reduced activation of codeine to morphine (Sulem et al., 2011; Amin et al., 2012). A study using a novel combination of maternal genetic markers to predict codeine toxicity in infants and their mothers revealed that the maternal CYP2D6 genotype increased the risk of infant CNS depression (OR = 17, P = 0.043) (Cornelis et al., 2014). Based on these effects of CYP2D6 variants on codeine metabolism, the FDA has included codeine drug label information on increased bioactivation in CYP2D6 UMs and recommended lower doses for the shortest period of time in breast-feeding mothers as well as in the general population, to avoid overdose symptoms such as sleepiness, confusion, or shallow breathing (Newton-Cheh et al., 2009).

Antiestrogenic tamoxifen treatment has long been a standard for estrogen receptor (ER)-positive breast cancer. Conversion of prodrug tamoxifen into the high-affinity ER antagonist endoxifen and 4-hydroxytamoxifen is catalyzed to a large extent by CYP2D6. Both metabolites have significantly higher affinity for the drug target and greater ability to inhibit cell proliferation in endocrine therapy than the parent drug (Jin et al., 2005). Many studies support the observation that the formation of endoxifen is highly linked to CYP2D6 polymorphism (Irvin et al., 2011; Kiyotani et al., 2012; Madlensky et al., 2011), whereas the effect of CYP2D6 genotype on the pharmacodynamic response to tamoxifen has not been well defined (Madlensky et al., 2011). Due to multiple copies of functional alleles of CYP2D6, patients with UM allele had higher mean plasma concentrations of endoxifen than those without UM allele (Borges et al., 2006). CYP2D6*4 is the most common null allele contributing to the CYP2D6 PM phenotype in white persons. In a retrospective study of a prospective adjuvant tamoxifen trial in postmenopausal women with surgically resected ER-positive breast cancer, patients with the CYP2D6*4/*4 genotype (PM) had shorter relapse free time and worse disease-free survival compared with patients with either one or no *4 alleles (Goetz et al., 2005). On the other hand, higher incidence of moderate or severe hot flashes were found in patients with one or no *4 alleles (20%) compared with homozygotes of the *4 allele (0%). Recent reports on a large cohort of patients have reported a significant effect of CYP2D6 polymorphism on tamoxifen treatment response and thus breast cancer recurrence with an overall odds ratio of between two and three for PM (Schroth et al., 2009, 2010; Thompson et al., 2011). More details about important pharmacogenetic variants are given on PharmGKB website (https://www.pharmgkb.org/gene/PA128#tabview=tab3&subtab=31).

In conclusion, differences in CYP2D6 mediated formation of active metabolites between PM and EM patients were the probable cause for the differential therapeutic efficacy and side effects observed in these patients.

CYP3A4 and CYP3A5

CYP3As are the most abundant CYPs in human liver and are accountable for the metabolism of more than 50% of clinical drugs. Important substrates include immunosuppressants (cyclosporine A, tacrolimus), calcium channel blockers, macrolide antibiotics, HMG-CoA reductase inhibitors, and anti-HIV inhibitors. CYP3A4 thought to dominate in whites and CYP3A5 in African Americans. More than 20 CYP3A4 variants have been known and many of the variants have altered enzyme activities, ranging from a modest to significant loss in catalytic efficiency (Ma and Lu, 2011; Miyazaki et al., 2008). However, there is no clear distinction between groups of slow or rapid metabolizers. Many of the coding region variants in CYP3A4 exists in low frequencies and are unlikely to account for the 10-fold differences in CYP3A4 activities observed in vivo (Lamba et al., 2002). CYP3A5 may contribute to the complexity of these unexplained observations as almost all CYP3A4 substrates, with a few exceptions, are also metabolized by CYP3A5. Supporting this, a study in cancer patients carrying CYP3A4*1B showed a higher rate of docetaxel clearance, and so a lower exposure to docetaxel (Tran et al., 2006). though this is possibly due to linkage disequilibrium with CYP3A5*1. Thus involvement of this dual pathway potentially complicates the clinical effects of CYP3A4 variants in human studies. Overall, CYP3A4 genotype variation contributes only to minor extent or only in rare cases to the inter-individual differences in the CYP3A4 phenotype (Werk and Cascorbi, 2014). So far, there is some evidence indicating reduced activity due to CYP3A4*16. In a study on Japanese cancer patients receiving paclitaxel, heterozygous *16B carriers showed a 20% reduced median area under curve of the metabolite 3'-p-hydroxypacitaxel compared with wild-type carriers (Nakajima et al., 2006). Recently, CYP3A4*22 seems to be the most important genetic variant, as it results in up to a 50% reduction in mRNA expression and subsequent reduction in enzyme activity (Werk and Cascorbi, 2014). Clinical studies in Caucasian subjects have demonstrated association of CYP3A4*22 with reduced clearance of tacrolimus, cyclosporine A, and immunosuppressants such as everolimus in renal transplant patients (Werk and Cascorbi, 2014).

The active enzyme for CYP3A5 is encoded by wild-type allele CYP3A5*1 while CYP3A5*3, *6, *7 variants result in nonfunctional proteins (Zanger and Schwab, 2013). Subjects with at least one allele CYP3A5*1 (functional CYP3A5) are classified as CYP3A5 expressers, while the variants result in allele CYP3A5 nonexpresser phenotypes. Few clinical studies examined the effect of CYP3A5 variants in combination with SNPs in CYP3A4 on PK of the immunosuppressant tacrolimus in kidney-transplant patients. CYP3A5 polymorphisms plays an important role in tacrolimus dose requirements to reach target trough blood concentrations (C_0) and CYP3A5 expressers require a higher dose of tacrolimus to achieve the targeted whole-blood concentrations (Hesselink et al., 2003). In a randomized, controlled trial that compared the efficacy of tacrolimus dosing on the basis of individual CYP3A5 genotypes with a standard tacrolimus dosing regimen that was based on body weight, the pharmacogenetic adaptation of the daily dose of tacrolimus is found to be associated with improved achievement of the target C_0 (Thervet et al., 2010).

PHARMACOGENOMICS OF PHASE II DRUG METABOLIZING ENZYMES

The Phase II DMEs consist of a superfamily of enzymes such as sulfotransferases (SULTs), UDP-glucuronosyltransferases (UGTs), and DT-diaphorase or NAD(P)H: quinone oxidoreductase (NQO) or NAD(P)H: menadione reductase (NMO), epoxide hydrolases (EPH), glutathione S-transferases (GST) and N-acetyltransferases (NAT). Phase II enzymes conjugate phase I metabolites, other intermediates, or the parent compound for renal or biliary excretion. Phase II DMEs has potential influence on the metabolism, PK/PD, toxicokinetics/dynamics, and drug–drug interactions of many therapeutic agents as well as their potential to protect the human body against exposure to environmental xenobiotics.

TPMT

Thiopurine methyltransferase or thiopurine S-methyltransferase (TPMT) catalyzes S-methylation of thiopurine prodrugs such as mercaptopurine, azathioprine, and thioguanine to inactive metabolites, which are used in the treatment of acute lymphoblastic anemia, autoimmune disorders, and inflammatory bowel disease. Polymorphisms in the TPMT gene has been reported, and defective TPMT alleles, such as *3A, *3B, *3C, and *2, result in significant decreases in levels of TPMT protein; therefore, enzyme activity due to enhanced degradation of TPMT allozymes is encoded by these alleles (Zhou et al., 2008; Tai et al., 1997). This leads to an accumulation of higher levels of cytotoxic thiopurine nucleotides in patients carrying defective TPMT alleles and subsequent severe hematological toxicity with standard doses of the parent drugs. CPIC guidelines and the FDA recommend genotyping and phenotyping for TPMT to identify patients at risk for toxicity and subsequent dose reduction or alternative treatment in these patients (https://www.pharmgkb.org/gene/PA356#tabview=tab0&subtab=31).

UGTs

UGTs catalyze the glucuronidation of numerous lipophilic xenobiotics to more hydrophilic forms and thereby enhance their elimination. Polymorphisms have been described for UGT1A1 and UGT2B7 that leads to variation in drug metabolism due to altered UGT activity. Polymorphisms in coding region and promoter region of UGT1A1 in particular UGT1A1*28 is a thymine-adenine (TA) repeat polymorphism with six or seven repeats with six TA repeats being wild-type and seven TA repeats as polymorphism resulting in lower mRNA expression and hence enzyme activity (Zhang et al., 2007). In humans, UGT1A1*28 cause various forms of inherited, unconjugated hyperbilirubinemia such as Crigler-Najjar syndrome and Gilbert's syndrome, respectively (Kadakol et al., 2000). The severity of the hyperbilirubinemia correlates with the enzymatic activities of the polymorphic UGT1A1 resulting in either complete absence of bilirubin glucuronidation, as in case of Crigler-Najjar type I syndrome, or reduced activity of bilirubin conjugation ($\sim$ 10 to 30% of the normal level), as observed in Crigler Najjar type II syndrome resulting in altered serum levels of unconjugated bilirubin. While in patients with the Gibert's syndrome, a genetic polymorphism in the UGT1A1promoter region UGT1A1*28 gives rise to reduced expression of UGT1A1 and, consequently, the syndrome. Similarly, the HIV-protease inhibitor atazanavir reduces hepatic UGT activity and can precipitate hyperbilirubinemia in patients with UGT1A1*28 variant (Rodriguez-Novoa et al., 2006).

Additionally, UGT1A1*28 and *6 alleles have shown associations with the development of irinotecan toxicities (Hu et al., 2010; Hoskins et al., 2007; Onoue et al., 2009). The anticancer prodrug irinotecan is converted to its active metabolite SN-38 in the liver and further conjugated primarily by UGT1A1 for elimination in bile and urine (Bandres et al., 2007). The dose-limiting toxicities of irinotecan are attributed to increased levels of the active metabolite SN-38 due to reduced expression UGT1A1 caused by polymorphisms of the gene (Palomaki et al., 2009). This results in lower SN-38 glucuronidation and increased incidence of toxicity. About 7% of patients that undergo irinotecan treatment and present with severe neutropenia and fever will die due to these complications (Obradovic et al., 2008). UGT1A1*28 genotype is associated with an increased risk irinotecan-related toxicity. The FDA suggests a reduction by at least one level in the starting dose of irinotecan for patients homozygous for the UGT1A1*28 allele.

Similarly, idiosyncratic hepatotoxicity that progresses to jaundice caused by diclofenac has been attributed to presence of UGT2B7 polymorphisms (Daly et al., 2007).

NATs

N-Acetyltransferases catalyze the acetylation of aromatic amines and hydrazines. The drug acetylation polymorphisms in humans was first revealed during the initial clinical trials of isoniazid (INH) for the treatment for tuberculosis (Evans et al., 1960). Although the drug was very effective in tuberculosis treatment, a high percentage of patients receiving isoniazid developed severe neurotoxicity that correlated with elevated serum levels of the drug. Two distinct phenotypes of acetylation were identified as "rapid acetylators" and "slow acetylators" that were later recognized to be differences in the enzymatic activities of NAT1 and NAT2. For both NAT genes more than 25 polymorphic forms exist but null alleles of NAT2 are more frequent. NAT2*5A, NAT2*6A, and NAT2*7A are associated with the slow acetylator phenotype in humans (Zhou et al., 2008) and show inter-ethnic differences in the occurrence of the slow acetylation form. Many studies have reported that due to reduced metabolism, NAT2 slow acetylators have increased exposure to INH and hydrazine and hence have been associated with an increased risk of hepatotoxicity/liver injury/hepatitis induced by anti-TB drug treatment as compared to rapid acetylators (and sometimes intermediates) (https://www.pharmgkb.org). Since NAT2 isozyme catalyzes both activation and deactivation of arylamine, hydrazine drugs, and carcinogens, NAT2 polymorphisms are also associated with higher incidences of cancer and drug toxicity (Agundez, 2008). There are still inconsistencies for NAT2 and NAT1 genotype-phenotype associations and further studies are essential to examine clinical utility of NAT2 genotyping for determining a patient's dosage for treatment efficacy and to avoid drug toxicity.

GSTs

GSTs play an important role in chemical detoxification by a combination of glutathione with electrophilic chemicals and metabolites that are further metabolized by hepatic and renal enzymes to final a excreted form of drug conjugates. Seven cytosolic GST families have been identified in humans based on sequence and immunochemical relatedness and substrate specificity, and a number of polymorphic alleles have been described for some GSTs (Iyer and Ratain, 1998). In colorectal cancer patients genetic polymorphisms in GSTs genes have been linked to increased chemotherapeutic treatment benefit (Yiannakopoulou, 2013).

PHARMACOGENOMICS OF DRUG TRANSPORTERS

Membrane transport proteins are involved in the translocation of various physiological substances, chemicals, and drugs into and out of cells using active and passive mechanisms. These transporters can be classified in two broad categories as influx or efflux transporters. Influx transporters include organic anion transporters (OATs and OATPs), organic cation transporters (OCTs), and oligopeptide transporters. Efflux transporters include ATP-binding cassette transporter family (ABC) and multidrug toxin extrusion proteins (MATES) (Giacomini et al., 2010). Transporters modulate the absorption, distribution, and elimination of drugs by controlling the influx and efflux of drugs in cells and can affect drug efficacy and toxicity. There is increased evidence indicating that genetic polymorphisms of transporters have a significant impact on drug disposition, drug efficacy, and drug safety (Giacomini et al., 2010). Few drug transporters are described below.

ABCB1

The ABCB1 gene encodes the P-glycoprotein (Pgp, ABCB1, multidrug resistance 1) that transports many important drugs such as chemotherapeutic agents, tyrosine kinase inhibitors, HIV protease inhibitors, HMG-CoA inhibitors, and toxic xenobiotics out of cells. P-gp has an important role in limiting entry of various drugs into the central nervous system. ABCB1 is highly polymorphic: more than 50 SNPs affecting ABCB1 gene function have been reported, and some of these variants exhibit ethnicity-dependent distribution. A number of studies showed inconsistent results in establishing the role of ABCB1 genotypes in different phenotypes such as P-gp function, expression, drug response, and disease susceptibility. The three most common SNPs in the ABCB1 protein coding region, rs1128503 (1236T > C), rs2032582 (2677T > G/A), and rs1045642 (3435T > C) (Wang et al., 2005), are the most studied SNPs for many pharmacokinetic and disease associations; however, results are controversial (Leschziner et al., 2007). ABCB1 SNPs have also been implicated in drug-related adverse events in case of clopidogrel and taxane treatment (Ghodke et al., 2007). Further studies are needed to validate these associations.

The discrepancy on the effect of ABCB1 polymorphisms on drug disposition and drug efficacy could be due to a high genetic variation of ABCB1 in different populations, a variable effect of a given SNP on ABCB1 expression/function in different organs, and a variety of substrates that ABCB1 transport. In addition, physiology and disease influence drug transport (Ghodke et al., 2007).

ABCG2

ABCG2 breast cancer—resistance protein (BCRP) is an ABC transporter that plays an important role in the intestinal absorption and biliary excretion of drugs, drug metabolites, and some toxic xenobiotics (Gradhand and Kim, 2008). Inter-individual differences in ABCG2 function may contribute to variable bioavailability, exposure (AUC and C_{max}), and pharmacological response of drugs that are ABCG2 substrates (Giacomini et al., 2010). The most substantial clinical effects are likely to be for drugs that have a narrow therapeutic index and have a low bioavailability. ABCG2 overexpression leads to enhanced drug efflux and subsequent resistance to a variety of anticancer agents, including anthracyclines, mitoxantrone, and the camptothecins (Ni et al., 2010). In addition, recent studies have demonstrated that subjects with reduced BCRP expression levels, correlating with the Q141K variant, are at increased risk for gefitinib-induced diarrhea and altered PK of irinotecan, sulphasalazine, 9-aminocamptothecin, diflomotecan, rosuvastatin, and topotecan (Giacomini et al., 2010).

OATs, OATPs, and OCTs

OATs and OATPs are the superfamily of solute carrier transporters that transport organic anions, including drugs and metabolites, across the cell membrane. OATs transport the smaller and more hydrophilic organic anions, while OATPs transport the large and hydrophobic anions (Roth et al., 2012). OATPs are encoded by genes in the SLCO/Slco superfamily. The SLCO/OATP family drug transporters are mainly influx transporters of drugs into cells like hepatocytes and renal tubular cells (Yiannakopoulou, 2013). Many studies have shown associations between altered OATP expression levels and disease conditions as well as documented effects of various alleles and SNPs in OATPs on drug disposition. The most significant SNP studies in SLCO1B1 includes a nonsynonymous SNP resulting in change of amino acid at position 174 from Valine to alalnine-V174A (rs4149056, 625T > C). This change has been associated with a decreased cholesterol lowering effect of multiple statins as well an increased systemic exposure of the HIV protease inhibitor lopinavir and antidiabetic nateglinide (Kalliokoski and Niemi, 2009). The FDA recommends an 80 mg daily dosage of simvastatin. In patients with the C allele at SLCO1B1 rs4149056, there are modest increases in myopathy risk even at lower simvastatin doses (40 mg daily); if optimal efficacy is not achieved with a lower dose, alternate agents should be considered (https://www.pharmgkb.org/gene/PA134865839#tabview = tab0&subtab = 31). Another SLCO1B1 coding SNP resulting in change of amino acid at position 130 from N (Asparagine) to D (Aspartic acid) has been associated with altered PK of pravastatin and pitavastatin. This polymorphism decreases the capacity of OATPB1 to transport active statins from the portal circulation resulting in markedly increased plasma concentration of statin and thus enhancing risk of statin induced myopathy and reducing therapeutic index of statins (Roth et al., 2012; Kalliokoski and Niemi, 2009).

In addition, certain OATPB1 variants are associated with an enhanced clearance of methotrexate and increase risk of gastrointestinal toxicity by methotrexate in the treatment of children with acute lymphoblastic leukemia (Yiannakopoulou, 2013). There is limited data on the clinical significance of other OATPs polymorphisms, with some evidence of OATP1A2 polymorphisms associated with imatinib clearance (Yamakawa et al., 2011) and OATP2B1 polymorphisms with fexofenadine PK (Akamine et al., 2010). SNPs have been described for OATs; however, the clinical impact of these SNPs is unclear and needs to be further explored.

The OCT family consists of three facilitated transporter subtypes: OCT1 (encoded by SLC22A1 gene), OCT2 (SLC22A2), and OCT3 (SLC22A3) (Roth et al., 2012). For the majority of times, OCTs are associated with risk of adverse drug—drug interactions. It has been observed that OCT1 polymorphisms are associated with altered PK of the antidiabetic drug metformin and the tyrosine kinase inhibitor imatinib, whereas a wide range of drugs have been implicated in potential drug—drug interactions (Fahrmayr et al., 2010).

PHARMACOGENOMICS OF DRUG TARGETS

Drug targets can be classified into three main categories: the direct protein target of the drug, signal transduction cascades or downstream proteins, and proteins involved in disease pathogenesis. Genetic variation in drug targets can have a considerate effect on drug response; few such examples are discussed below.

Methylenetetrahydrofolate reductase (MTHFR) pathway is the target of several antifolate drugs such as methotrexate (MTX). MTHFR reduces 5,10-CH2- to 5-CH3-tetrahydrofolate and thus interacts with folate-dependent one-carbon synthesis reactions, as well as pyrimidine/purine synthesis and homocysteine/methionine metabolism. The two most significant nonsynonymous MTHFR polymorphisms—677C > T (Ala222Val) and 1298A > C (Glu429Ala)—are responsible for the vast majority of MTHFR deficiencies and exhibit ethnic differences (Goyette et al., 1994; Ghodke et al., 2011a). These polymorphisms may not alter drug PK, but it does appear to modulate PD by predisposing ADRs to the antifolate drug MTX. Clinical studies have linked the presence of the variant c.677C > T to methotrexate-related drug response (toxicity and efficacy) in various cancerous and noncancerous pathologies (Owen et al., 2013; Muhl and Pfeilschifter, 2011; Toffoli and De Mattia, 2008; Ghodke et al., 2008; Ghodke-Puranik et al., 2015). The molecular basis for MTX-related enhanced toxicity and altered drug efficacy is not clearly understood, but it could be attributed to increased plasma homocysteine levels and higher serum MTX concentrations; however, additional studies are needed to completely understand the molecular mechanisms underlying the associations observed for these SNPs (Toffoli and De Mattia, 2008).

Angiotensin-converting enzyme (ACE) inhibitors and β-adrenoceptor antagonists (β-blockers) are drugs that play a central role in the treatment of hypertension and heart failure. The β-2 adrenoreceptor is a target for β agonists and is encoded by the ADRB2 gene. Genetic variants of the ADRB2 are responsible for altered process of signal transduction by these receptors (Liggett, 2000; Dishy et al., 2001). SNPs in ADRB2 have been linked to altered expression and down regulation in response to β 2-adrenoreceptor agonists (Liggett, 2000). Relatively common SNPs (such as amino acids changes as Arg16Gly and Gln27Glu) have been shown to have significant functional impact on drug treatment. It has been reported that individual homozygous for Arg16/Arg16 exhibits a larger and more rapid bronchodilation response to β agonist albuterol than carriers of the Gly16 allele (Arg16/Gly16 and Gly16/Gly16) (Lima et al., 1999). Another study of agonist-mediated vasodilatation and desensitization demonstrated that the Arg16 polymorphism of the ADRB2 is linked with enhanced agonist−mediated desensitization in the vasculature, while Glu27 polymorphism is linked with increased agonist-mediated responsiveness (Dishy et al., 2001). The ACE gene encodes an angiotensin I-converting enzyme that catalyzes the transformation of decapeptide angiotensin I to a potent vasoconstrictor octapeptide angiotensin II and the degradation of a potent vasodilator bradykinin. ACE is a principal target in the treatment of hypertension, congestive heart failure, and diabetic nephropathy. Insertion polymorphisms in the ACE gene are linked with increased ACE serum levels, while deletion polymorphism is associated with decreased ACE levels, indicating that insertion/deletion polymorphism can account for the total phenotypic variance of serum ACE (Rigat et al., 1990). In a separate study, a pharmacogenetic score combining three SNPs in the angiotensin-II type I receptor gene and bradykinin type 1 receptor gene predicted patients that are most possibly benefited from ACE-inhibitor therapy (Brugts et al., 2010).

Warfarin is the most frequently prescribed oral anticoagulant worldwide. It is used for the treatment and prevention of thrombotic disorders. Warfarin exerts its effect by inhibiting the vitamin K-dependent clotting pathway. The primary genes contributing to warfarin dose requirements are vitamin K epoxide reductase complex 1 (VKORC1) and CYP2C9. The VKORC1 is the target protein for warfarin. Warfarin inhibits VKORC1 by preventing reduction of vitamin K to vitamin KH2, a necessary cofactor for carboxylation and activation of clotting factors. Though efficacious, warfarin has a narrow therapeutic index and exhibit inter-individual variability in its response. Excess use of the drug will result in hemorrhage, while a drug dose that is too low will result in undesired coagulation. Several polymorphisms in the coding region of VKORC1 that affect the warfarin response have been identified of which 1173C/T and promoter polymorphism 1639G/A have been the most extensively studied (Limdi and Veenstra, 2008). A promoter 1639G > A SNP in the VKORC1 that alters its transcription factor binding site can predict dose requirements across various ethnic groups (Limdi et al., 2010). The 1639A minor allele is linked to lower gene expression and considerably low warfarin dose requirements as compared to wild-type G allele (Rieder et al., 2005). There are ethnic differences in the frequency of the A allele: Asians with the high frequency followed by Europeans (intermediate) and African Americans (lowest). These allele frequency differences accounts for the lower dose requirements generally observed in Asian populations and higher requirements in Africans compared to Europeans. Recent clinical studies demonstrated that individuals with the A allele require a 28% decrease in the therapeutic warfarin dose per allele, and this SNP is the most important predictor of an initiation dose for warfarin (Gage et al., 2008). It is predicted that VKORC1 genotype accounts for 15% to 30% of the variability in warfarin response, thereby making it the single biggest predictor for warfarin dosing (Geisen et al., 2005) (https://www.pharmgkb.org/gene/PA133787052?tabType = tabVip#tabview = tab3&subtab =).

Information gained so far on the impact of CYP2C9, VKORC1, and warfarin has been used to develop dosing guidelines for warfarin therapy (http://www.warfarindosing.org; IWPC Pharmacogenetic Dosing Algorithm). In addition, based on warfarin pharmacogenomics data, the FDA modified the warfarin label, stating that CYP2C9 and VKORC1 genotypes may be useful in determining the optimal initial dose of warfarin in 2007 (Gage and Lesko, 2008). The label was further updated in 2010 to include a table describing recommendations for dosing ranges for patients with different combinations of CYP2C9 and VKORC1 genotype.

GENETIC VARIABILITY AFFECTING ADVERSE DRUG REACTIONS

Serious ADRs are among the major decisive factors responsible for the preclusion of potential drugs for entering the market and for postmarketing withdrawal of approved drugs (Charlab and Zhang, 2013). All genetic factors that influence drug response (discussed in previous sections) and genes that indirectly affect drug action can modify drug toxicity and related ADRs. Pharmacogenomic strategies can be applied to uncover potential gene(s) linked to the adverse events and develop biomarkers for screening patients at risk (Ma and Lu, 2011). In this section we will discuss few such examples in which a genetic marker was associated to ADR.

Drug-Induced Liver Injury

DILI is the most common cause of clinical trial termination and drug withdrawal from the market. Idiosyncratic DILI is responsible for approximately 13% of acute liver failure in the United States and 75% patients either die or need a liver transplant (Ma and Lu, 2011), thus underlying the importance of recognizing patients at risk. The pathogenesis of most DILI remains unclear; however, for few drugs a genetic association of individual susceptibility is well known. Most of the conclusive genetic association studies in DILI are related to the human leukocyte antigen (HLA) gene variants or gene variants relevant to drug metabolism and transport (Wang et al., 2011; Andrade et al., 2009). Flucloxacillin is an antibiotic widely used for the treatment of staphylococcal infection but is linked to a typical cholestatic hepatitis. In a multicenter GWAS, a missense SNP in the major histocompatibility complex, rs2395029 which is in complete linkage disequilibrium with HLA-B*5701, showed a very strong association (odd's ratio 81) with flucloxacillin-induced hepatic injury (Daly et al., 2009). A retrospective study found a genetic association between ximelagatran (thrombin inhibitor)-related elevated alanine transaminases and HLA-DRB1*07 and HLA-DQA1*02 (Kindmark et al.,

2008) and thus failed to establish a favorable safety profile. Lumiracoxib, a selective COX-2 inhibitor effective in the symptomatic treatment of osteoarthritis and acute pain, was either not approved or withdrawn from the market worldwide due to hepatotoxicity concerns. A common HLA haplotype (HLA-DRB1*1501-HLA-DQB1*0602-HLA-DRB5*0101-HLA-DQA1*0102) was found to be strongly associated with lumiracoxib-related liver injury (Singer et al., 2010). Difficulties in obtaining well-characterized, large sample size of patients with these ADR for GWA scale studies, involvement of multiple genes, and complex gene−environment interactions, makes it challenging to replicate these associations in an attempt to potentially "revive the drugs" (Pirmohamed, 2010).

Drug Hypersensitivity (Ma and Lu, 2011)

Drug hypersensitivity reactions (DHRs) are the adverse effects of the drug that are immune-mediated and clinically look similar to allergies. DHRs can be life-threatening, require or prolong hospitalization, or need changes in the drug prescription. Although DHRs are unpredictable and pathogenic events for several DHRs are unclear, genetic polymorphisms of certain genes can increase the susceptibility of patients to drug allergy. A potent anti-HIV-1 drug, abacavir, can lead to a serious, possibly fatal hypersensitivity syndrome characterized by multisystem involvement in approximately five to nine of the patients (Ma and Lu, 2011). The hypersensitivity was strongly associated with HLA-B*5701 polymorphism and its combination with a haplotype polymorphism of Hsp-70-Hom (Mallal et al., 2008). Among the most convincing applications of pharmacogenomics, a double-blind, prospective, randomized multicenter study indicated that prospective HLA-B*5701 pre-screening reduced the risk of hypersensitivity reaction to abacavir (Mallal et al., 2008). The FDA-approved label for abacavir states that genetic screening for the HLA-B*5701 allele is required prior to initiating or reinitiating treatment with abacavir in patients of unknown HLA-B*5701 status. Abacavir is contraindicated in patients with the HLA-B*5701 allele due to risk for abacavir hypersensitivity reactions. Additionally, CPIC guidelines also emphasize that abacavir is not recommended in HLA-B*5701-positive individuals and should be considered only under exceptional circumstances (Martin et al., 2014). This screening is now applied in many countries and has reduced the incidence of skin reactions to this drug. Similarly, carbamazepine (CBZ), a commonly prescribed first line anticonvulsant for treatment of seizures, can cause serious DHRs including maculopapular eruption, hypersensitivity syndrome, Stevens−Johnson syndrome (SJS), and toxic epidermal necrosis (TEN). CBZ induced SJS/TEN was strongly associated with a HLA polymorphism HLA-B*1502 in Han Chinese (Hung et al., 2006), supporting HLA-B*1502 genotyping in this population. HLA-B*1502 is most frequently found in Asian populations but only 1% to 2% in white populations, which explains the lower incidence of CBZ-SJS in white populations compared with Asian populations. According to the FDA's carbamazepine labeling and CPIC guidelines, "patients with ancestry in populations in which HLA-B*1502 may be present" should be screened for the allele before therapy (Leckband et al., 2013). Patients testing HLA-B*1502-positive should not be given carbamazepine "unless the benefit clearly outweighs the risk." However, caution should be exercised in deciding which patients to screen due to the high inter- and intra-ethnic variability in the HLA-B*1502 occurrence. Recently, GWAS studies have also identified an association of HLA-A*3101 with CBZ-induced ADRs in persons of Northern European ancestry (McCormack et al., 2011) and in the Japanese (Ozeki et al., 2011), underscoring the variability of the genetic markers among ethnic groups.

Irinotecan-Induced Myelosuppression

Irinotecan is a chemotherapeutic agent used for the treatment of lung and colorectal cancers. Irinotecan gets converted to the active metabolite SN-38 in liver, which is further metabolized primarily through glucuronidation by the polymorphic UGT1A1 enzyme. High levels of SN-38 due to impaired glucuronidation can lead to severe ADRs such as severe myelosuppression in 15% to 20% and severe delayed-type diarrhea in 20% to 25% of patients on irinotecan therapy (Ma and Lu, 2011). Several prospective and retrospective studies have shown that subjects carrying UGT1A1-diminished function alleles such as UGT1A1*28 are at higher risk of developing severe bone marrow and gastrointestinal ADRs due to SN-38 if treated with a normal dose of irinotecan for cancer therapy (Ma and Lu, 2011; Zhang et al., 2007). Hence, the FDA now recommends a reduced initial dose for patients known to be homozygous for UGT1A1*28. Similarly, ABCC2 polymorphisms also appear to impact the incidence of irinotecan-related diarrhea (de Jong et al., 2007).

CLINICAL IMPLEMENTATION OF PHARMACOGENOMICS

Pharmacogenomics has the potential to influence clinically relevant outcomes in drug dosing, efficacy, and toxicity that can result in subsequent recommendations for testing. For many routinely used drugs, pharmacogenomics has provided inconclusive evidence for such testing. A probable reason could be the involvement of both genetic and nongenetic factors and their extent of contribution that determines the clinical relevance of some drugs. Therefore, identification of genetic markers associated with drug responses does not always link to clinically useful predictors of adverse outcomes, and most of the time require independent replication of genotype—phenotype association before pursuing clinical implementation.

Lack of readily available resources, feasibility, utility, level of evidence, provider knowledge, cost effectiveness, and ethical, legal, and social issues further adds to the limitations and challenges to implementing pharmacogenomic testing in clinical practice. In order for a genetic marker to be implicated in clinical practice, an association of a genetic marker to a particular trait requires screening of tissues from several individuals, and corresponding functional studies are needed to establish probable association with the trait/phenotype. However, to overcome these challenges there are some pharmacogenomic tests for drugs currently used in clinical practice that have applied value in predicting ADRs and/or drug efficacy. Table 7.2 lists some of these clinically valuable pharmacogenomics tests. These tests are based on distinct genetic variants that have well-validated reproducible and significant impact on the drug therapy. These tests have a strong causal association between genetic polymorphisms and drug responses: a strong indication for clinical utility and high prognostic value. The tests are available both commercially and in academic settings, with many of these tests having clinical guidelines for dose adjustment and alternative medications (Wei et al., 2012). In addition, various international pharmacogenomic consortia have been developed recently to supervise drug response studies.

A list of current pharmacogenomic guidelines from these consortiums along with a well-annotated pharmacogenomic database has been consolidated into one curated database known as Pharmacogenomics Knowledge Base (PharmGKB) (Thorn et al., 2010). PharmGKB is available via an online portal where users can search on the website by gene, drug, metabolic pathway, and disease. To boost the clinical application of pharmacogenetics and address the barriers to implementation of pharmacogenetic tests into clinical practice CPIC was formed as a shared project between PharmGKB and the Pharmacogenomics Research Network (https://cpicpgx.org). CPIC provides freely available, peer-reviewed, updatable, and detailed gene/drug clinical practice guidelines that enable the translation of genetic laboratory test results into actionable prescribing decisions for specific drugs. The guidelines can focus on genes (e.g., thiopurine methyltransferase and its implications for thiopurines) or around drugs (e.g., warfarin and CYP2C9 and VKORC1). Efforts like PharmGKB and CPIC can help to overcome the confusion created about various pharmacogenetic tests and can help clinical decision making. In addition, the FDA has created a table of Pharmacogenomic Biomarkers in Drug Labeling that lists FDA-approved drugs with pharmacogenomic information in their labeling (http://www.fda.gov/Drugs/ScienceResearch/ResearchAreas/Pharmacogenetics/ucm083378.htm). This biomarker table provides up to date information on genomic markers that have been referred in FDA package inserts for different drugs. Various biomarkers are included in this table, e.g., germ-line or somatic gene variants, functional deficiencies, expression changes, and chromosomal

TABLE 7.2 Examples of Clinically Valuable Application of Pharmacogenomics Tests in Predicting Drug Response (Efficacy and Toxicity)

Affected Pathways/ Conditions	Genetic Markers	Drugs	Clinical Action	Type of Effect (PK, PD, Efficacy, Toxicity)	Clinical Use Recommendation/Notes
Phase I DMEs	CYP2C9	Celecoxib	Nonsteroidal antiinflammatory drug	Toxicity	To prevent adverse cardiovascular and gastrointestinal events in PM (*3/*3) consider starting treatment at half the lowest recommended dose
	CYP2C9 + VKORC1	Warfarin	Anticoagulant	PK and PD and subsequent efficacy and toxicity	To acquire efficacy and prevent bleeding complications dose adjustment should be done based on CYP2C9 and VKORC1 genotypes. FDA guidelines are available
	CYP2C19	Clopidogrel	Antithrombotic	PK	Alternative therapy is advised for PM (*2/*2) to avoid bleeding complications. FDA guidelines are available
	CYP2D6	Codeine	Analgesic	PK	UM (*1/*1 and *1/*2) should avoid use due to probable drug toxicity and preference to choose lower doses for shortest time period in breast-feeding mothers. FDA guidelines are available
Phase II DMEs	TPMT	Azathioprine, mercaptopurine	Immunosuppressant; antineoplastic	PK, toxicity	TPMT genotype based dose adjustment to achieve efficacy and prevent bone-marrow suppression for carriers with nonfunctional TPMT alleles *2, *3A, and *3C. FDA recommends TPMT genotyping or phenotyping (RBC TPMT activity)
	UGT1A1	Irinotecan	Antineoplastic	PK, toxicity	To achieve efficacy and avoid neutropenia, a dose adjustment requirement, based on UGT1A1 genotype (UGT1A1*28). FDA guidelines are available
Drug transporters	SLCO1B1	Simvastatin	Lipid-lowering drug	PK, toxicity	To avoid myopathy, dose adjustment recommendations, based on SLCO1B1 genotype (C allele of rs4149056 SLCO1B1). FDA guidelines are available

Drug targets	Gefitinib	EGFR	Antineoplastic	Efficacy	First EGFR-targeted category approved for nonsmall cell lung cancer depending on pharmacogenomics findings during drug development
	Trastuzumab	ERBB2 (HER2)	Antineoplastic	Efficacy	Cardiac toxicity to be considered in benefit: risk analysis in HER2 positive tumors
	Ivacaftor	CFTR (G551D mutation)	To treat cystic fibrosis	Efficacy	Pharmacogenomics-guided drug development
Drug induced liver injury	HLA-B*1502	Carbamazepine, phenytoin	Antiepileptic/ anticonvulsant	PK, PD	To prevent SJS/TEN occurrence, avoid drug use in HLA-B*1502 carriers. FDA guidelines are available for carbamazepine
Drug induced skin injury	HLA-B*5701	Abacavir, flucloxacillin	Antiretroviral; antibiotic	PD, toxicity	Carriers of HLA-B*5701 should avoid drug use to prevent hepatotoxicity FDA/clinical pharmacogenetics implementation consortium guidelines are available for abacavir
	HLA-B*5801	Allopurinol	Antihyperurecemia and antigout	PD, toxicity	Carriers of HLA-B*5801 should avoid drug use to inhibit severe cutaneous adverse reactions. Clinical pharmacogenetics implementation consortium guidelines are available
Inborn errors of metabolism	G6PD deficiency	Chloroquine; dapsone; rasburicase	Antimalarial; antibiotic	Toxicity	Contraindicated in G6PD-deficient patients to prevent hemolysis
	DPD deficiency	Capecitabine; fluorouracil	Antineoplastic	Toxicity	Contraindicated in DPD-deficient patients to prevent severe drug-related adverse events FDA guidelines are available for fluorouracil

abnormalities as well as selected protein biomarkers that need to be tested before starting treatment in a selected subset of patients. Moreover, with continued integration of pharmacogenomics in clinical trials and drug development, novel important genes and variants that can predict drug efficacy and toxicity will be identified and can be implemented in clinical practice.

PHARMACOGENOMICS IN DRUG DEVELOPMENT

The pharmaceutical companies have a keen interest in utilizing pharmacogenomic information to improve time-consuming and a very costly drug-development process. Pharmacogenomics knowledge can be applied at various levels of drug discovery and development right from target/candidate selection, different phases of clinical development, and drug approval until postmarketing surveillance. In early clinical development, efficacy/safety pharmacogenomics, if applied in phase I and IIa, can help to stratify patients who need a different dosage to achieve efficacy or fewer ADRs. Phase IIa efficacy trials generally involve a relatively small number of patients and might have an insufficient statistical significance for genetic influence. However, generated results can be used for a predictive hypothesis development that can be tested in subsequent trials (Roses, 2008). This will help in the preselection of a patient for trials based on their genotype, efficacy, and safety profile. If such prospective PGx data is accessible beforehand or between the phase IIa and phase IIb trials, this will considerably shorten phase III, thereby increasing a success rate that can lead to better therapeutic outcomes.

Drug regulatory authorities like the FDA are dynamically exploring the utilization of PGx data for understanding drug responses (especially toxicity) in drug development (dose selection) and are making this information widely available to investigators and physicians. As a step toward this, the FDA has released graft-guidance document about clinical pharmacogenomics that discusses premarketing assessments in early-phase clinical studies (Draft Guidance for Industry on Clinical Pharmacogenomics). These guidelines will assist the pharmaceutical industry and investigators to collect better-quality data during new drug development. Additionally, it will help to establish stronger genotype–phenotype (clinical pharmacology, drug response) associations. Finally, even though pharmacogenomics has the potential to improve the drug discovery pipeline, there is a need to fill the knowledge gap between industry, health care professional/providers, and academic researchers. A new collaborative platform needs to be created where these three sectors can interact with each other to improve drug development strategies and gene discoveries using newer technologies.

CONCEPT OF PERSONALIZED MEDICINE IN TRADITIONAL INDIAN MEDICAL SYSTEM: AYURVEDA

A good physician knows individual variations and specific treatment accordingly

Charaka Samhita. (Sutra 1/ 62)

Ayurveda (Ayu: life; Veda: knowledge) means science or knowledge of life that has a strong philosophical, experiential, logical foundation and has history of more than 5000 years of practice. It is one of the most ancient living traditions that addresses health holistically. Ayurveda is practiced widely in India, Sri Lanka, and other countries (Chopra and Doiphode, 2002). Indian healthcare consists of medical pluralism, and Ayurveda still remains dominant compared to modern medicine, particularly for treatment of a variety of chronic disease conditions (Waxler-Morrison, 1988). The core concept of health and disease in Ayurveda is built on a strong belief in the uniqueness of the individual. Ayurveda applies a Tridosha (three types of doshas, or humors) theory consisting of Vata (V, associated to motion); Pitta (P, associated to metabolism); and Kapha (K, associated to lubrication and structure) as discrete phenotype groups for determining a person's mind—body classification (Patwardhan and Bodeker, 2008). Depending on the relative proportions of each dosha, Ayurveda categorizes all individuals into different "Prakriti" types. Prakriti is specific for each individual. It is mostly determined at the time of conception, has influence of environmental factors including maternal diet, lifestyle, and remains unaltered during the lifetime. It is therefore supposed to have strong genetic mechanisms. In Ayurveda, the Prakriti classification of an individual's constitution is based on differences in physical, physiological, and psychological characteristics, and is independent of racial, ethnic, or geographical considerations (Swoboda, 1996). Prakriti specific treatment including prescription of medications, diet, and lifestyle is a distinctive feature of Ayurveda (Patwardhan and Bodeker, 2008). A quantitative measure of Tridosha level (V, P, K) is obtained by applying an algorithmic heuristic approach to the exhaustive list of qualitative features/factors that are used by Ayurvedic physicians. Tridosha could thus be quantitatively estimated from qualitative characterization using core diagnostic criteria of Ayurveda (Joshi, 2004). Decision support software like AyuSoft has been developed for optimal applications of Ayurveda knowledge (Patwardhan, 2005). This will help in the correct assessment of Prakriti of subjects and help to control possible variations. Thus Tridoshas being substances that are quantifiable in nature, they could be considered as qualitative and quantitative traits.

Ayurvedic therapeutics is based on philosophy of maintaining equilibrium or homeostasis. Ayurvedic pharmacological classification of drugs describes drug actions based on the certain attributes present in the drug such as Rasa (taste), Guna (property), Virya (potency), Vipaka (postdigestive taste), and Prabhava (effect), whereas in modern pharmacology the drug action is ascribed to the chemical structure of a molecule (Rastogi, 2010). These Ayurvedic pharmacological principles takes into consideration the Prakriti of the person as well as the PD and PK properties of a drug when treating patients unlike modern medicine treatments that can lead to variable inter-individual response for the same drug for the same disease. In order to understand and practice personalized medicine, a systematic classification of the human population is essential. Conversely, modern medicine classifies human populations based on ethnicity and geographic patterns, which demonstrate frequent, inter-individual variations in drug responses (Wilson et al., 2001). The science of Ayurveda and the concept of Prakriti-based Ayurvedic classification can be explored to effectively fill this void. The Ayurvedic concept of Prakriti plays a principal role in understanding health and disease, which is very comparable to the concept of pharmacogenetics. The fundamental principles of the Ayurvedic system of medicine can be used to create designer medicines (Patwardhan, 2000). Determining the genetic basis for Prakriti constitutes a step toward this. Establishing relationships between Prakriti and genome is thus essential. This can be functionally achieved by generating three organized databases capable of logically collaborating with each other to give a customized prescription, human constitution (genotype), disease constitution (phenotype), and drug constitution (traditional medicine PG). The "Golden Triangle" of Ayurveda, modern medicine, and modern science will converge to form a real discovery engine that can result in newer, safer, cheaper, and effective therapies (Patwardhan and Mashelkar, 2009). Various traditional systems of medicine including Ayurveda, traditional Chinese medicine, and Korean medicine have distinct systems of constitutional types for prescribing medications that have well-defined similarities to modern pharmacogenomics (Joshi et al., 2010). Hence, applying genomic approaches to investigate constitutional differences in various traditional systems of medicine is therefore worth exploring for effective personalized treatment.

TRADITIONAL MEDICINE TO MODERN PHARMACOGENOMICS: AYUGENOMICS

The human genome project has revealed the complexity in the relationship between genotypes and phenotypes. A better understanding of the human genome has helped in understanding the scientific basis of individual variations. It is possible to examine the Ayurvedic concept of Prakriti from a human genome perspective. Permutations and combinations of V, P, and K attributes' characters along with other host factors, such as tissue status (Dhatusarata), twenty Guna, psychological nature (Manas Prakriti), habitat (Desha), season (Kaala), and digestive capacity (Agni), lead to an infinite number indicating every individual has unique constitution. This is how Ayurveda describes the basis of individual variation (Patwardhan et al., 2004; Hankey, 2001). The integration of the Prakriti concept of Ayurveda with genomics nomenclature as Ayugenomics (also spelled as Ayurgenomics) is worth exploring to unravel many challenges in genomics, therapeutics, and personalized medicine.

Ayugenomics a Tool for Classifying Human Population

Every individual is unique. It is essential to identify factors that govern the "individuality" of a person: the genotypes linked to phenotypes and classification of the human population. Classification (genotypic or phenotypic) of human populations is crucial for better understanding of disease pathogenesis (Pearson et al., 2003), in drug responses (Meyer, 2000; Kirchheiner et al., 2001), and the like. Existing classifications of human populations is roughly based on geographical location; ethnicity, or self-reported ancestry, are inaccurate ways to represent genetic clusters (Wilson et al., 2001) and have had limited success in phenotype correlations. Thus, classifying human populations is a major challenge to biomedical sciences (Palatini et al., 2009).

Ayurveda has been explored for this purpose. As a proof of concept, in a pilot study 76 subjects were evaluated both for their Prakriti and HLA DRB1 types (Bhushan et al., 2005; Patwardhan and Ghodke, 2006). The study observed a reasonable correlation between HLA-type and Prakriti-type and concluded that Ayurveda-based phenomes may also provide a model for the study of multigenic traits. It could even propose a novel approach for correlating genotypes with phenotypes for human classification. However, more scientific investigations are necessary to validate these findings in large populations of different ethnic groups and in terms of Prakriti-specific differential gene expression analysis in major Prakriti types to identify the genes that are up- or down regulated.

Ayurveda Prakriti Type Associated With the Metabolic Variability (Ghodke et al., 2011b)

The three major constitution types described in Ayurveda have unique putative metabolic activities, K being slow, P fast, while V is considered to have a variable metabolism. We hypothesized that this might relate to drug metabolism and genetic polymorphism of DMEs and can be translated in terms of modern science, e.g., to different phenotypic subpopulations of drug metabolizers. Metabolic variability in different Prakriti types was studied using the DMEs CYP2C19 gene polymorphism model. The distribution of CYP2C19 genotypes was investigated in 132 healthy individuals of different Prakriti classes. The results obtained suggest a possible association of CYP2C19 gene polymorphism with Prakriti phenotypes. EM genotypes were predominant in P Prakriti while PM genotypes were highest in K. It is interesting to note that a *1/*3 genotype specific to the EM group was present only in P, while the *2/*3 genotype typical of the PM group was observed in K as expected. Similarly, in the case of gene polymorphism, we observed that the occurrence of EM genotypes was significantly higher in P Prakriti. Our study thus demonstrated a probable genomic basis for metabolic differences attributable to Prakriti, possibly providing a new approach to pharmacogenomics. Its results should be validated with a larger sample size.

Other Studies on Traditional Medicine

Recently, various studies have explored Ayurveda for possible genetic associations in healthy as well as disease conditions (Patwardhan and Bodeker, 2008; Dey and Pahwa, 2014; Rizzo-Sierra, 2011). Genome-wide expression and biochemical differences between Ayurveda-based Prakriti types have been studied, revealing differentially expressed genes related to biological processes across different Prakriti types (Prasher et al., 2008). Overexpression of genes related to immune responses was seen in Pitta, whereas the Vata group showed differences in expression of genes related to cellular processes. Kapha males showed an up regulation of genes involved in cellular biosynthesis. A study has been carried out to integrate the knowledge of traditional Ayurvedic concepts with contemporary science. This study demonstrated analysis of Prakriti classification and its association with BMI and the place of birth with the implications to one of the ways for human classification (Rotti et al., 2014b).

In another study, immunophenotyping of normal individuals classified on the basis of human dosha Prakriti identified significant differences in the expression of CD14, CD25, and CD56 markers between three different Prakriti (Rotti et al., 2014a). This study reported an increased level of CD25 and CD56 in Kapha Prakriti, suggesting an ability to stimulate a better immune response, which is in accordance with textual references in Ayurveda. An investigation of normal healthy individuals to examine if the platelet aggregatory response and its inhibition by aspirin varied in the different Prakriti subtypes reported that ADP-induced maximal platelet aggregation (MPA) was highest among the Vata–Pitta prakriti individuals as compared to the other Prakriti types and these individuals responded better to a lower dose of aspirin compared to other Prakriti types, indicating Prakriti classifications may help in individualizing therapy or predicting proneness to a disease (Bhalerao et al., 2012). To evaluate the potential of an Ayugenomics approach in complex traits research, an exploratory study on rheumatoid arthritis observed discrete causal pathways for RA etiology in Prakriti-based subgroups thereby validating the concepts of Prakriti and personalized medicine in Ayurveda (Juyal et al., 2012).

Apart from the above-mentioned studies, an attempt has also been made to integrate Ayurveda with functional genomics to identify pathways associated with activity of crude and active components of an herb, Ashwagandha, which is used for cancer treatment (Deocaris et al., 2008). Similarly, a study on pharmacogenomics of medicinal plants has also been undertaken (Chavan et al., 2006). There are several similarities between Ayurveda and other traditional systems of medicine in Asia such as traditional Chinese, Korean (Sasang constitution medicine), Japanese (Kampo) medicine, including holistic and individual classification systems. These traditional medicine systems have also been explored for their basis of personalized medicine, and some positive leads have been found. Thus, data generated to support genetic basis for traditional medicine indicates this traditional knowledge can be utilized to create a system of predictive, preventive, and personalized medicine so that instead of a generalized symptomatic approach, the practice of medicine takes an individual approach based on one's genetic makeup (Joshi et al., 2010).

PERSPECTIVES AND CONCLUSIONS

Recent advances in understanding of the factors that affect gene expression, both regulation by transcription factors and by microRNA and epigenetic factors, have added to an understanding of variation in expression of ADME and drug-target genes. Studies using both conventional and novel approaches including GWAS and next-generation-sequencing technologies have provided new insights into the field of pharmacogenetics. This has led to a significant number of successful modifications to the clinical practice, increased advances in pharmacogenomic tests, pharmacogenomics-guided drug regulation and drug development that subsequently encouraged the FDA to include pertinent pharmacogenomic information and recommendations in the revised drug labels for certain drugs.

Despite all the above facts, inconsistent results across genotype−phenotype association studies, due to inaccurate genotype/phenotype classification of humans or phenotypic heterogeneity, is a major challenge in the field of complex chronic disease pharmacogenomics. A long-standing tradition regarding the concept of "personalized medicine" in Ayurveda and other traditional health practices can be explored further for this purpose. Moving forward, studies have already started reporting that integrating evidence-based and innovative initiatives such as Ayugenomics can potentially facilitate steps toward overcoming some of the challenges to achieve the ultimate goal of individualized medicine.

REFERENCES

Agundez, J.A., 2008. Polymorphisms of human N-acetyltransferases and cancer risk. Curr. Drug Metab. 9, 520–531.

Aithal, G.P., Day, C.P., Kesteven, P.J., Daly, A.K., 1999. Association of polymorphisms in the cytochrome P450 CYP2C9 with warfarin dose requirement and risk of bleeding complications. Lancet 353, 717–719.

Akamine, Y., Miura, M., Sunagawa, S., Kagaya, H., Yasui-Furukori, N., Uno, T., 2010. Influence of drug-transporter polymorphisms on the pharmacokinetics of fexofenadine enantiomers. Xenobiotica 40, 782–789.

Amin, N., Byrne, E., Johnson, J., Chenevix-Trench, G., Walter, S., Nolte, I.M., et al., 2012. Genome-wide association analysis of coffee drinking suggests association with CYP1A1/CYP1A2 and NRCAM. Mol. Psychiatry 17, 1116–1129.

Andrade, R.J., Robles, M., Ulzurrun, E., Lucena, M.I., 2009. Drug-induced liver injury: insights from genetic studies. Pharmacogenomics 10, 1467–1487.

Bandres, E., Zarate, R., Ramirez, N., Abajo, A., Bitarte, N., Gariia-Foncillas, J., 2007. Pharmacogenomics in colorectal cancer: the first step for individualized-therapy. World J. Gastroenterol. 13, 5888–5901.

Bauer, T., Bouman, H.J., van Werkum, J.W., Ford, N.F., ten Berg, J.M., Taubert, D., 2011. Impact of CYP2C19 variant genotypes on clinical efficacy of antiplatelet treatment with clopidogrel: systematic review and meta-analysis. BMJ 343, d4588.

Bhalerao, S., Deshpande, T., Thatte, U., 2012. Prakriti (Ayurvedic concept of constitution) and variations in platelet aggregation. BMC Complement. Altern. Med. 12, 248.

Bhushan, P., Kalpana, J., Arvind, C., 2005. Classification of human population based on HLA gene polymorphism and the concept of Prakriti in Ayurveda. J. Altern. Complement. Med. 11, 349–353.

Birkett, D.J., Rees, D., Andersson, T., Gonzalez, F.J., Miners, J.O., Veronese, M.E., 1994. In vitro proguanil activation to cycloguanil by human liver microsomes is mediated by CYP3A isoforms as well as by S-mephenytoin hydroxylase. Br. J. Clin. Pharmacol. 37, 413–420.

Borges, S., Desta, Z., Li, L., Skaar, T.C., Ward, B.A., Nguyen, A., et al., 2006. Quantitative effect of CYP2D6 genotype and inhibitors on tamoxifen metabolism: implication for optimization of breast cancer treatment. Clin. Pharmacol. Ther. 80, 61–74.

Brugts, J.J., Isaacs, A., Boersma, E., van Duijn, C.M., Uitterlinden, A.G., Remme, W., et al., 2010. Genetic determinants of treatment benefit of the angiotensin-converting enzyme-inhibitor perindopril in patients with stable coronary artery disease. Eur. Heart J. 31, 1854–1864.

Butler, M.A., Lang, N.P., Young, J.F., Caporaso, N.E., Vineis, P., Hayes, R.B., et al., 1992. Determination of CYP1A2 and NAT2 phenotypes in human populations by analysis of caffeine urinary metabolites. Pharmacogenetics 2, 116–127.

Chang, M., Dahl, M.L., Tybring, G., Gotharson, E., Bertilsson, L., 1995. Use of omeprazole as a probe drug for CYP2C19 phenotype in Swedish Caucasians: comparison with S-mephenytoin hydroxylation phenotype and CYP2C19 genotype. Pharmacogenetics 5, 358–363.

Charlab, R., Zhang, L., 2013. Pharmacogenomics: historical perspective and current status. Methods Mol. Biol. 1015, 3–22.

Chavan, P., Joshi, K., Patwardhan, B., 2006. DNA microarrays in herbal drug research. Evid. Based Complement. Altern. Med. 3, 447–457.

Chopra, A., Doiphode, V.V., 2002. Ayurvedic medicine. Core concept, therapeutic principles, and current relevance. Med. Clin. North Am. 86, 75–89, vii.

Cornelis, M.C., Byrne, E.M., Esko, T., Nalls, M.A., Ganna, A., Paynter, N., et al., 2014. Genome-wide meta-analysis identifies six novel loci associated with habitual coffee consumption. Mol. Psychiatry.

Cornelis, M.C., Monda, K.L., Yu, K., Paynter, N., Azzato, E.M., Bennett, S.N., et al., 2011. Genome-wide meta-analysis identifies regions on 7p21 (AHR) and 15q24 (CYP1A2) as determinants of habitual caffeine consumption. PLoS Genetics 7, e1002033.

Daly, A.K., 2010. Pharmacogenetics and human genetic polymorphisms. Biochem. J. 429, 435–449.

Daly, A.K., Aithal, G.P., Leathart, J.B., Swainsbury, R.A., Dang, T.S., Day, C.P., 2007. Genetic susceptibility to diclofenac-induced hepatotoxicity: contribution of UGT2B7, CYP2C8, and ABCC2 genotypes. Gastroenterology 132, 272–281.

Daly, A.K., Donaldson, P.T., Bhatnagar, P., Shen, Y., Pe'er, I., Floratos, A., et al., 2009. HLA-B*5701 genotype is a major determinant of drug-induced liver injury due to flucloxacillin. Nat. Genetics 41, 816–819.

de Jong, F.A., Scott-Horton, T.J., Kroetz, D.L., McLeod, H.L., Friberg, L.E., Mathijssen, R.H., et al., 2007. Irinotecan-induced diarrhea: functional significance of the polymorphic ABCC2 transporter protein. Clin. Pharmacol. Ther. 81, 42–49.

Deocaris, C.C., Widodo, N., Wadhwa, R., Kaul, S.C., 2008. Merger of ayurveda and tissue culture-based functional genomics: inspirations from systems biology. J. Transl. Med. 6, 14.

Dey, S., Pahwa, P., 2014. Prakriti and its associations with metabolism, chronic diseases, and genotypes: possibilities of new born screening and a lifetime of personalized prevention. J. Ayurveda Integr. Med. 5, 15–24.

Dishy, V., Sofowora, G.G., Xie, H.G., Kim, R.B., Byrne, D.W., Stein, C.M., et al., 2001. The effect of common polymorphisms of the beta2-adrenergic receptor on agonist-mediated vascular desensitization. New Engl. J. Med. 345, 1030–1035.

Draft Guidance for Industry on Clinical Pharmacogenomics: Premarketing Evaluation in Early Phase Clinical Studies. Availability.

Ehret, G.B., Munroe, P.B., Rice, K.M., Bochud, M., Johnson, A.D., Chasman, D.I., et al., 2011. Genetic variants in novel pathways influence blood pressure and cardiovascular disease risk. Nature 478, 103–109.

Evans, D.A., Manley, K.A., Mc, K.V., 1960. Genetic control of isoniazid metabolism in man. Br. Med. J. 2, 485–491.

Evans, W.E., Relling, M.V., 1999. Pharmacogenomics: translating functional genomics into rational therapeutics. Science 286, 487–491.

Fahrmayr, C., Fromm, M.F., Konig, J., 2010. Hepatic OATP and OCT uptake transporters: their role for drug-drug interactions and pharmacogenetic aspects. Drug Metab. Rev. 42, 380–401.

Frueh, F.W., Amur, S., Mummaneni, P., Epstein, R.S., Aubert, R.E., DeLuca, T.M., et al., 2008. Pharmacogenomic biomarker information in drug labels approved by the United States food and drug administration: prevalence of related drug use. Pharmacotherapy 28, 992–998.

Funck-Brentano, C., Becquemont, L., Lenevu, A., Roux, A., Jaillon, P., Beaune, P., 1997. Inhibition by omeprazole of proguanil metabolism: mechanism of the interaction in vitro and prediction of in vivo results from the in vitro experiments. J. Pharmacol. Exp. Therap. 280, 730–738.

Furuta, T., Ohashi, K., Kamata, T., Takashima, M., Kosuge, K., Kawasaki, T., et al., 1998. Effect of genetic differences in omeprazole metabolism on cure rates for Helicobacter pylori infection and peptic ulcer. Ann. Int. Med. 129, 1027–1030.

Gaedigk, A., Simon, S.D., Pearce, R.E., Bradford, L.D., Kennedy, M.J., Leeder, J.S., 2008. The CYP2D6 activity score: translating genotype information into a qualitative measure of phenotype. Clin. Pharmacol. Ther. 83, 234–242.

Gage, B.F., Lesko, L.J., 2008. Pharmacogenetics of warfarin: regulatory, scientific, and clinical issues. J. Thromb. Thrombolysis 25, 45−51.

Gage, B.F., Eby, C., Johnson, J.A., Deych, E., Rieder, M.J., Ridker, P.M., et al., 2008. Use of pharmacogenetic and clinical factors to predict the therapeutic dose of warfarin. Clin. Pharmacol. Ther. 84, 326−331.

Geisen, C., Watzka, M., Sittinger, K., Steffens, M., Daugela, L., Seifried, E., et al., 2005. VKORC1 haplotypes and their impact on the inter-individual and inter-ethnical variability of oral anticoagulation. Thromb. Haemost. 94, 773−779.

Ghodke, Y., Joshi, K., Arya, Y., Radkar, A., Chiplunkar, A., Shintre, P., et al., 2007. Genetic polymorphism of CYP2C19 in Maharashtrian population. Eur. J. Epidemiol. 22, 907−915.

Ghodke, Y., Chopra, A., Joshi, K., Patwardhan, B., 2008. Are Thymidylate synthase and Methylene tetrahydrofolate reductase genes linked with methotrexate response (efficacy, toxicity) in Indian (Asian) rheumatoid arthritis patients? Clin. Rheumatol. 27, 787−789.

Ghodke, Y., Chopra, A., Shintre, P., Puranik, A., Joshi, K., Patwardhan, B., 2011a. Profiling single nucleotide polymorphisms (SNPs) across intracellular folate metabolic pathway in healthy Indians. Indian J. Med. Res. 133, 274−279.

Ghodke, Y., Joshi, K., Patwardhan, B., 2011b. Traditional Medicine to Modern Pharmacogenomics: Ayurveda Prakriti Type and CYP2C19 Gene Polymorphism Associated with the Metabolic Variability. Evid. Based Complement. Altern. Med. 2011, 249528.

Ghodke-Puranik, Y., Puranik, A.S., Shintre, P., Joshi, K., Patwardhan, B., Lamba, J., et al., 2015. Folate metabolic pathway single nucleotide polymorphisms: a predictive pharmacogenetic marker of methotrexate response in Indian (Asian) patients with rheumatoid arthritis. Pharmacogenomics 16, 2019−2034.

Ghotbi, R., Christensen, M., Roh, H.K., Ingelman-Sundberg, M., Aklillu, E., Bertilsson, L., 2007. Comparisons of CYP1A2 genetic polymorphisms, enzyme activity and the genotype-phenotype relationship in Swedes and Koreans. Eur. J. Clin. Pharmacol. 63, 537−546.

Giacomini, K.M., Huang, S.M., Tweedie, D.J., Benet, L.Z., Brouwer, K.L., Chu, X., et al., 2010. Membrane transporters in drug development. Nat. Rev. Drug Discov. 9, 215−236.

Goetz, M.P., et al., 2005. Pharmacogenetics of tamoxifen biotransformation is associated with clinical outcomes of efficacy and hot flashes. J Clin Oncol 23, 9312−9318.

Goyette, P., Sumner, J.S., Milos, R., Duncan, A.M., Rosenblatt, D.S., Matthews, R.G., et al., 1994. Human methylenetetrahydrofolate reductase: isolation of cDNA, mapping and mutation identification. Nat. Genetics 7, 195−200.

Gradhand, U., Kim, R.B., 2008. Pharmacogenomics of MRP transporters (ABCC1-5) and BCRP (ABCG2). Drug Metab. Rev. 40, 317−354.

Guessous, I., Dobrinas, M., Kutalik, Z., Pruijm, M., Ehret, G., Maillard, M., et al., 2012. Caffeine intake and CYP1A2 variants associated with high caffeine intake protect non-smokers from hypertension. Hum. Mol. Genetics 21, 3283−3292.

Gunes, A., Dahl, M.L., 2008. Variation in CYP1A2 activity and its clinical implications: influence of environmental factors and genetic polymorphisms. Pharmacogenomics 9, 625−637.

Hankey, A., 2001. Ayurvedic physiology and etiology: Ayurvedo Amritanaam. The doshas and their functioning in terms of contemporary biology and physical chemistry. J. Altern Complement. Med. 7, 567−574.

Harmsze, A.M., van Werkum, J.W., Hackeng, C.M., Ruven, H.J., Kelder, J.C., Bouman, H.J., et al., 2012. The influence of CYP2C19*2 and *17 on on-treatment platelet reactivity and bleeding events in patients undergoing elective coronary stenting. Pharmacogenet. Genomics 22, 169−175.

Hesselink, D.A., van Schaik, R.H., van der Heiden, I.P., van der Werf, M., Gregoor, P.J., Lindemans, J., et al., 2003. Genetic polymorphisms of the CYP3A4, CYP3A5, and MDR-1 genes and pharmacokinetics of the calcineurin inhibitors cyclosporine and tacrolimus. Clin. Pharmacol. Ther. 74, 245–254.

Holmes, M.V., Perel, P., Shah, T., Hingorani, A.D., Casas, J.P., 2011. CYP2C19 genotype, clopidogrel metabolism, platelet function, and cardiovascular events: a systematic review and meta-analysis. JAMA 306, 2704–2714.

Home page of the Human Cytochrome P450 (CYP) Allele Nomenclature Committe.

Hoskins, J.M., Goldberg, R.M., Qu, P., Ibrahim, J.G., McLeod, H.L., 2007. UGT1A1*28 genotype and irinotecan-induced neutropenia: dose matters. J. Natl. Cancer Inst. 99, 1290–1295.

Hu, Z.Y., Yu, Q., Pei, Q., Guo, C., 2010. Dose-dependent association between UGT1A1*28 genotype and irinotecan-induced neutropenia: low doses also increase risk. Clin. Cancer Res. Off. J. Am. Assoc. Cancer Res. 16, 3832–3842.

Hulot, J.S., Collet, J.P., Silvain, J., Pena, A., Bellemain-Appaix, A., Barthelemy, O., et al., 2010. Cardiovascular risk in clopidogrel-treated patients according to cytochrome P450 2C19*2 loss-of-function allele or proton pump inhibitor coadministration: a systematic meta-analysis. J. Am. Coll. Cardiol. 56, 134–143.

Hung, S.I., Chung, W.H., Jee, S.H., Chen, W.C., Chang, Y.T., Lee, W.R., et al., 2006. Genetic susceptibility to carbamazepine-induced cutaneous adverse drug reactions. Pharmacogenet. Genomics 16, 297–306.

Ingelman-Sundberg, M., 2005. Genetic polymorphisms of cytochrome P450 2D6 (CYP2D6): clinical consequences, evolutionary aspects and functional diversity. Pharmacogenomics J. 5, 6–13.

Irvin Jr., W.J., Walko, C.M., Weck, K.E., Ibrahim, J.G., Chiu, W.K., Dees, E.C., et al., 2011. Genotype-guided tamoxifen dosing increases active metabolite exposure in women with reduced CYP2D6 metabolism: a multicenter study. J. Clin. Oncol. Off. J. Am. Soc. Clin. Oncol. 29, 3232–3239.

Iyer, L., Ratain, M.J., 1998. Pharmacogenetics and cancer chemotherapy. Eur. J. Cancer 34, 1493–1499.

Jin, Y., Desta, Z., Stearns, V., Ward, B., Ho, H., Lee, K.H., et al., 2005. CYP2D6 genotype, antidepressant use, and tamoxifen metabolism during adjuvant breast cancer treatment. J. Natl. Cancer Inst. 97, 30–39.

Johnson, J.A., Gong, L., Whirl-Carrillo, M., Gage, B.F., Scott, S.A., Stein, C.M., et al., 2011. Clinical pharmacogenetics implementation consortium guidelines for CYP2C9 and VKORC1 genotypes and warfarin dosing. Clin. Pharmacol. Ther. 90, 625–629.

Joshi, K., Ghodke, Y., Shintre, P., 2010. Traditional medicine and genomics. J. Ayurveda Integr. Med. 1, 26–32.

Joshi, R.R., 2004. A biostatistical approach to ayurveda: quantifying the tridosha. J. Altern. Complement. Med. 10, 879–889.

Juyal, R.C., Negi, S., Wakhode, P., Bhat, S., Bhat, B., Thelma, B.K., 2012. Potential of ayurgenomics approach in complex trait research: leads from a pilot study on rheumatoid arthritis. PloS One 7, e45752.

Kadakol, A., Ghosh, S.S., Sappal, B.S., Sharma, G., Chowdhury, J.R., Chowdhury, N.R., 2000. Genetic lesions of bilirubin uridine-diphosphoglucuronate glucuronosyltransferase (UGT1A1) causing Crigler-Najjar and Gilbert syndromes: correlation of genotype to phenotype. Hum. Mutat. 16, 297–306.

Kalliokoski, A., Niemi, M., 2009. Impact of OATP transporters on pharmacokinetics. Br. J. Pharmacol. 158, 693–705.

Kawanishi, C., Lundgren, S., Agren, H., Bertilsson, L., 2004. Increased incidence of CYP2D6 gene duplication in patients with persistent mood disorders: ultrarapid metabolism of antidepressants as a cause of nonresponse. A pilot study. Eur. J. Clin. Pharmacol. 59, 803–807.

Kindmark, A., Jawaid, A., Harbron, C.G., Barratt, B.J., Bengtsson, O.F., Andersson, T.B., et al., 2008. Genome-wide pharmacogenetic investigation of a hepatic adverse event without clinical signs of immunopathology suggests an underlying immune pathogenesis. Pharmacogenomics J. 8, 186–195.

Kirchheiner, J., Brosen, K., Dahl, M.L., Gram, L.F., Kasper, S., Roots, I., et al., 2001. CYP2D6 and CYP2C19 genotype-based dose recommendations for antidepressants: a first step towards subpopulation-specific dosages. Acta Psychiatry Scand 104, 173–192.

Kirchheiner, J., Nickchen, K., Bauer, M., Wong, M.L., Licinio, J., Roots, I., et al., 2004. Pharmacogenetics of antidepressants and antipsychotics: the contribution of allelic variations to the phenotype of drug response. Mol. Psychiatry 9, 442–473.

Kiyotani, K., Mushiroda, T., Nakamura, Y., Zembutsu, H., 2012. Pharmacogenomics of tamoxifen: roles of drug metabolizing enzymes and transporters. Drug Metab. Pharmacokinet. 27, 122–131.

Lamba, J.K., Lin, Y.S., Thummel, K., Daly, A., Watkins, P.B., Strom, S., et al., 2002. Common allelic variants of cytochrome P4503A4 and their prevalence in different populations. Pharmacogenetics 12, 121–132.

Leckband, S.G., Kelsoe, J.R., Dunnenberger, H.M., George Jr., A.L., Tran, E., Berger, R., et al., 2013. Clinical pharmacogenetics implementation consortium guidelines for HLA-B genotype and carbamazepine dosing. Clin. Pharmacol. Ther. 94, 324–328.

Lee, S.J., 2012. Clinical application of CYP2C19 pharmacogenetics toward more personalized medicine. Front. Genetics 3, 318.

Leschziner, G.D., Andrew, T., Pirmohamed, M., Johnson, M.R., 2007. ABCB1 genotype and PGP expression, function and therapeutic drug response: a critical review and recommendations for future research. Pharmacogenomics J. 7, 154–179.

Li, Y., Tang, H.L., Hu, Y.F., Xie, H.G., 2012. The gain-of-function variant allele CYP2C19*17: a double-edged sword between thrombosis and bleeding in clopidogrel-treated patients. J. Thromb. Haemost. 10, 199–206.

Liggett, S.B., 2000. beta(2)-adrenergic receptor pharmacogenetics. Am. J. Respir. Crit. Care Med. 161, S197–201.

Lima, J.J., Thomason, D.B., Mohamed, M.H., Eberle, L.V., Self, T.H., Johnson, J.A., 1999. Impact of genetic polymorphisms of the beta2-adrenergic receptor on albuterol bronchodilator pharmacodynamics. Clin. Pharmacol. Ther. 65, 519–525.

Limdi, N.A., Veenstra, D.L., 2008. Warfarin pharmacogenetics. Pharmacotherapy 28, 1084–1097.

Limdi, N.A., Wadelius, M., Cavallari, L., Eriksson, N., Crawford, D.C., Lee, M.T., et al., 2010. Warfarin pharmacogenetics: a single VKORC1 polymorphism is predictive of dose across 3 racial groups. Blood 115, 3827–3834.

Lobello, K.W., Preskorn, S.H., Guico-Pabia, C.J., Jiang, Q., Paul, J., Nichols, A.I., et al., 2010. Cytochrome P450 2D6 phenotype predicts antidepressant efficacy of venlafaxine: a secondary analysis of 4 studies in major depressive disorder. J. Clin. Psychiatry 71, 1482–1487.

Ma, Q., Lu, A.Y., 2011. Pharmacogenetics, pharmacogenomics, and individualized medicine. Pharmacol. Rev. 63, 437–459.

Madlensky, L., Natarajan, L., Tchu, S., Pu, M., Mortimer, J., Flatt, S.W., et al., 2011. Tamoxifen metabolite concentrations, CYP2D6 genotype, and breast cancer outcomes. Clin. Pharmacol. Ther. 89, 718–725.

Mallal, S., Phillips, E., Carosi, G., Molina, J.M., Workman, C., Tomazic, J., et al., 2008. HLA-B*5701 screening for hypersensitivity to abacavir. New Engl. J. Med. 358, 568–579.

Martin, M.A., Hoffman, J.M., Freimuth, R.R., Klein, T.E., Dong, B.J., Pirmohamed, M., et al., 2014. Clinical pharmacogenetics implementation consortium guidelines for HLA-B genotype and abacavir dosing: 2014 update. Clin. Pharmacol. Ther. 95, 499−500.

McCormack, M., Alfirevic, A., Bourgeois, S., Farrell, J.J., Kasperaviciute, D., Carrington, M., et al., 2011. HLA-A*3101 and carbamazepine-induced hypersensitivity reactions in Europeans. New Engl. J. Med. 364, 1134−1143.

Meyer, U.A., 2000. Pharmacogenetics and adverse drug reactions. Lancet 356, 1667−1671.

Miyazaki, M., Nakamura, K., Fujita, Y., Guengerich, F.P., Horiuchi, R., Yamamoto, K., 2008. Defective activity of recombinant cytochromes P450 3A4.2 and 3A4.16 in oxidation of midazolam, nifedipine, and testosterone. Drug Metab. Dispos. Biol. Fate Chem. 36, 2287−2291.

Muhl, H., Pfeilschifter, J., 2011. Pharmacogenetics and pharmacogenomics of methotrexate. Current status and novel aspects. Z. Rheumatol. 70, 101−107.

Nakajima, M., Yokoi, T., Mizutani, M., Kinoshita, M., Funayama, M., Kamataki, T., 1999. Genetic polymorphism in the 5'-flanking region of human CYP1A2 gene: effect on the CYP1A2 inducibility in humans. J. Biochem. 125, 803−808.

Nakajima, Y., Yoshitani, T., Fukushima-Uesaka, H., Saito, Y., Kaniwa, N., Kurose, K., et al., 2006. Impact of the haplotype CYP3A4*16B harboring the Thr185Ser substitution on paclitaxel metabolism in Japanese patients with cancer. Clin. Pharmacol. Ther. 80, 179−191.

Newton-Cheh, C., Johnson, T., Gateva, V., Tobin, M.D., Bochud, M., Coin, L., et al., 2009. Genome-wide association study identifies eight loci associated with blood pressure. Nat. Genetics 41, 666−676.

Ni, Z., Bikadi, Z., Rosenberg, M.F., Mao, Q., 2010. Structure and function of the human breast cancer resistance protein (BCRP/ABCG2). Curr. Drug Metab. 11, 603−617.

Ninomiya, H., Mamiya, K., Matsuo, S., Ieiri, I., Higuchi, S., Tashiro, N., 2000. Genetic polymorphism of the CYP2C subfamily and excessive serum phenytoin concentration with central nervous system intoxication. Ther. Drug Monit. 22, 230−232.

Obradovic, M., Mrhar, A., Kos, M., 2008. Cost-effectiveness of UGT1A1 genotyping in secondline, high-dose, once every 3 weeks irinotecan monotherapy treatment of colorectal cancer. Pharmacogenomics 9, 539−549.

Onoue, M., Terada, T., Kobayashi, M., Katsura, T., Matsumoto, S., Yanagihara, K., et al., 2009. UGT1A1*6 polymorphism is most predictive of severe neutropenia induced by irinotecan in Japanese cancer patients. Int. J. Clin. Oncol. 14, 136−142.

Owen, S.A., Lunt, M., Bowes, J., Hider, S.L., Bruce, I.N., Thomson, W., et al., 2013. MTHFR gene polymorphisms and outcome of methotrexate treatment in patients with rheumatoid arthritis: analysis of key polymorphisms and meta-analysis of C677T and A1298C polymorphisms. Pharmacogenomics J. 13, 137−147.

Ozeki, T., Mushiroda, T., Yowang, A., Takahashi, A., Kubo, M., Shirakata, Y., et al., 2011. Genome-wide association study identifies HLA-A*3101 allele as a genetic risk factor for carbamazepine-induced cutaneous adverse drug reactions in Japanese population. Hum. Mol. Genetics 20, 1034−1041.

Palatini, P., Ceolotto, G., Ragazzo, F., Dorigatti, F., Saladini, F., Papparella, I., et al., 2009. CYP1A2 genotype modifies the association between coffee intake and the risk of hypertension. J. Hypertens. 27, 1594−1601.

Palomaki, G.E., Bradley, L.A., Douglas, M.P., Kolor, K., Dotson, W.D., 2009. Can UGT1A1 genotyping reduce morbidity and mortality in patients with metastatic colorectal cancer treated with irinotecan? An evidence-based review. Genetics Med. Off. J. Am. Coll. Med. Genetics 11, 21−34.

Patwardhan, B., 2000. Ayurveda: the designer medicine. Indian Drugs 37, 213−227.

Patwardhan, B., Bodeker, G., 2008. Ayurvedic genomics: establishing a genetic basis for mind-body typologies. J. Altern. Complement. Med. 14, 571–576.

Patwardhan, B., Mashelkar, R.A., 2009. Traditional medicine-inspired approaches to drug discovery: can Ayurveda show the way forward?. Drug Discov. Today 14, 804–811.

Patwardhan, B., Joshi, K., Ghodke, Y., 2006. Genetic basis to concept of Prakriti. Curr. Sci. 90, 896.

Patwardhan, B., Vaidya, A.D.B., Chorghade, M., 2004. Ayurveda and natural product drug discovery. Curr. Sci. 86, 789–790.

Patwardhan, B.D.M., 2005. Ayusoft-A decision support system. In: CDAC and Univerisity of Pune: Ministry of Information Technology, Government of India.

Pearson, E.R., Starkey, B.J., Powell, R.J., Gribble, F.M., Clark, P.M., Hattersley, A.T., 2003. Genetic cause of hyperglycaemia and response to treatment in diabetes. Lancet 362, 1275–1281.

Penas-Lledo, E.M., Trejo, H.D., Dorado, P., Ortega, A., Jung, H., Alonso, E., et al., 2013. CYP2D6 ultrarapid metabolism and early dropout from fluoxetine or amitriptyline monotherapy treatment in major depressive patients. Mol. Psychiatry 18, 8–9.

Pirmohamed, M., 2010. Pharmacogenetics of idiosyncratic adverse drug reactions. Handb.Exp. Pharmacol.477–491.

Prasher, B., Negi, S., Aggarwal, S., Mandal, A.K., Sethi, T.P., Deshmukh, S.R., et al., 2008. Whole genome expression and biochemical correlates of extreme constitutional types defined in Ayurveda. J. Transl. Med. 6, 48.

Qin, X.P., Xie, H.G., Wang, W., He, N., Huang, S.L., Xu, Z.H., et al., 1999. Effect of the gene dosage of CgammaP2C19 on diazepam metabolism in Chinese subjects. Clin. Pharmacol. Ther. 66, 642–646.

Rastogi, S., 2010. Building bridges between Ayurveda and modern science. Int. J. Ayurveda Res. 1, 41–46.

Rau, T., Wohlleben, G., Wuttke, H., Thuerauf, N., Lunkenheimer, J., Lanczik, M., et al., 2004. CYP2D6 genotype: impact on adverse effects and nonresponse during treatment with antidepressants-a pilot study. Clin. Pharmacol. Ther. 75, 386–393.

Rieder, M.J., Reiner, A.P., Gage, B.F., Nickerson, D.A., Eby, C.S., McLeod, H.L., et al., 2005. Effect of VKORC1 haplotypes on transcriptional regulation and warfarin dose. N Engl. J. Med. 352, 2285–2293.

Rigat, B., Hubert, C., Alhenc-Gelas, F., Cambien, F., Corvol, P., Soubrier, F., 1990. An insertion/deletion polymorphism in the angiotensin I-converting enzyme gene accounting for half the variance of serum enzyme levels. J. Clin. Invest. 86, 1343–1346.

Rizzo-Sierra, C.V., 2011. Ayurvedic genomics, constitutional psychology, and endocrinology: the missing connection. J. Altern. Complement. Med. 17, 465–468.

Roden, D.M., Wilke, R.A., Kroemer, H.K., Stein, C.M., 2011. Pharmacogenomics: the genetics of variable drug responses. Circulation 123, 1661–1670.

Rodriguez-Novoa, S., Barreiro, P., Jimenez-Nacher, I., Soriano, V., 2006. Overview of the pharmacogenetics of HIV therapy. Pharmacogenomics J. 6, 234–245.

Roses, A.D., 2008. Pharmacogenetics in drug discovery and development: a translational perspective. Nat. Rev. Drug Discov. 7, 807–817.

Roth, M., Obaidat, A., Hagenbuch, B., 2012. OATPs, OATs and OCTs: the organic anion and cation transporters of the SLCO and SLC22A gene superfamilies. Br. J. Pharmacol. 165, 1260–1287.

Rotti, H., Guruprasad, K.P., Nayak, J., Kabekkodu, S.P., Kukreja, H., Mallya, S., et al., 2014a. Immunophenotyping of normal individuals classified on the basis of human dosha prakriti. J. Ayurveda Integr. Med. 5, 43–49.

Rotti, H., Raval, R., Anchan, S., Bellampalli, R., Bhale, S., Bharadwaj, R., et al., 2014b. Determinants of prakriti, the human constitution types of Indian traditional medicine and its correlation with contemporary science. J. Ayurveda Integr. Med. 5, 167–175.

Sachse, C., Brockmoller, J., Bauer, S., Roots, I., 1999. Functional significance of a C-- > A polymorphism in intron 1 of the cytochrome P450 CYP1A2 gene tested with caffeine. Br. J. Clin. Pharmacol. 47, 445–449.

Schroth, W., Goetz, M.P., Hamann, U., Fasching, P.A., Schmidt, M., Winter, S., et al., 2009. Association between CYP2D6 polymorphisms and outcomes among women with early stage breast cancer treated with tamoxifen. JAMA 302, 1429–1436.

Schroth, W., Hamann, U., Fasching, P.A., Dauser, S., Winter, S., Eichelbaum, M., et al., 2010. CYP2D6 polymorphisms as predictors of outcome in breast cancer patients treated with tamoxifen: expanded polymorphism coverage improves risk stratification. Clin. Cancer Res. Off. J. Am. Assoc. Cancer Res. 16, 4468–4477.

Schwarz, U.I., 2003. Clinical relevance of genetic polymorphisms in the human CYP2C9 gene. Eur. J. Clin. Invest. 33 (Suppl. 2), 23–30.

Scott, S.A., Sangkuhl, K., Stein, C.M., Hulot, J.S., Mega, J.L., Roden, D.M., et al., 2013. Clinical pharmacogenetics implementation consortium guidelines for CYP2C19 genotype and clopidogrel therapy: 2013 update. Clin. Pharmacol. Ther. 94, 317–323.

Shuldiner, A.R., O'Connell, J.R., Bliden, K.P., Gandhi, A., Ryan, K., Horenstein, R.B., et al., 2009. Association of cytochrome P450 2C19 genotype with the antiplatelet effect and clinical efficacy of clopidogrel therapy. JAMA 302, 849–857.

Sim, S.C., Kacevska, M., Ingelman-Sundberg, M., 2013. Pharmacogenomics of drug-metabolizing enzymes: a recent update on clinical implications and endogenous effects. Pharmacogenomics J. 13, 1–11.

Singer, J.B., Lewitzky, S., Leroy, E., Yang, F., Zhao, X., Klickstein, L., et al., 2010. A genome-wide study identifies HLA alleles associated with lumiracoxib-related liver injury. Nat. Genetics 42, 711–714.

Sofi, F., Giusti, B., Marcucci, R., Gori, A.M., Abbate, R., Gensini, G.F., 2011. Cytochrome P450 2C19*2 polymorphism and cardiovascular recurrences in patients taking clopidogrel: a meta-analysis. Pharmacogenomics J. 11, 199–206.

Steward, D.J., Haining, R.L., Henne, K.R., Davis, G., Rushmore, T.H., Trager, W.F., et al., 1997. Genetic association between sensitivity to warfarin and expression of CYP2C9*3. Pharmacogenetics 7, 361–367.

Sulem, P., Gudbjartsson, D.F., Geller, F., Prokopenko, I., Feenstra, B., Aben, K.K., et al., 2011. Sequence variants at CYP1A1-CYP1A2 and AHR associate with coffee consumption. Hum. Mol. Genetics 20, 2071–2077.

Swoboda, R.E., 1996. Prakriti: Your Ayurvedic Constitution. Motilal Banarasidass Publishers, India.

Tai, H.L., Krynetski, E.Y., Schuetz, E.G., Yanishevski, Y., Evans, W.E., 1997. Enhanced proteolysis of thiopurine S-methyltransferase (TPMT) encoded by mutant alleles in humans (TPMT*3A, TPMT*2): mechanisms for the genetic polymorphism of TPMT activity. Proc. Natl. Acad. Sci. U. S. A. 94, 6444–6449.

Thervet, E., Loriot, M.A., Barbier, S., Buchler, M., Ficheux, M., Choukroun, G., et al., 2010. Optimization of initial tacrolimus dose using pharmacogenetic testing. Clin. Pharmacol. Ther. 87, 721–726.

Thompson, A.M., Johnson, A., Quinlan, P., Hillman, G., Fontecha, M., Bray, S.E., et al., 2011. Comprehensive CYP2D6 genotype and adherence affect outcome in breast cancer patients treated with tamoxifen monotherapy. Breast Cancer Res. Treat. 125, 279–287.

Thorn, C.F., Klein, T.E., Altman, R.B., 2010. Pharmacogenomics and bioinformatics: PharmGKB. Pharmacogenomics 11, 501–505.

Toffoli, G., De Mattia, E., 2008. Pharmacogenetic relevance of MTHFR polymorphisms. Pharmacogenomics 9, 1195–1206.

Tran, A., Jullien, V., Alexandre, J., Rey, E., Rabillon, F., Girre, V., et al., 2006. Pharmacokinetics and toxicity of docetaxel: role of CYP3A, MDR1, and GST polymorphisms. Clin. Pharmacol. Ther. 79, 570−580.

Tsai, M.H., Lin, K.M., Hsiao, M.C., Shen, W.W., Lu, M.L., Tang, H.S., et al., 2010. Genetic polymorphisms of cytochrome P450 enzymes influence metabolism of the antidepressant escitalopram and treatment response. Pharmacogenomics 11, 537−546.

Wan, J., Xia, H., He, N., Lu, Y.Q., Zhou, H.H., 1996. The elimination of diazepam in Chinese subjects is dependent on the mephenytoin oxidation phenotype. Br. J. Clin. Pharmacol. 42, 471−474.

Wang, D., Johnson, A.D., Papp, A.C., Kroetz, D.L., Sadee, W., 2005. Multidrug resistance polypeptide 1 (MDR1, ABCB1) variant 3435C > T affects mRNA stability. Pharmacogenet. Genomics 15, 693−704.

Wang, L., McLeod, H.L., Weinshilboum, R.M., 2011. Genomics and drug response. New Engl. J. Med. 364, 1144−1153.

Waxler-Morrison, N.E., 1988. Plural medicine in Sri Lanka: do Ayurvedic and Western medical practices differ? Soc. Sci. Med. 27, 531−544.

Wei, C.Y., Lee, M.T., Chen, Y.T., 2012. Pharmacogenomics of adverse drug reactions: implementing personalized medicine. Hum. Mol. Genetics 21, R58−65.

Weinshilboum, R., 2003. Inheritance and drug response. N Engl. J Med. 348, 529−537.

Weinshilboum, R., Wang, L., 2004. Pharmacogenomics: bench to bedside. Nat. Rev. Drug Discov. 3, 739−748.

Werk, A.N., Cascorbi, I., 2014. Functional gene variants of CYP3A4. Clin. Pharmacol. Ther. 96, 340−348.

Wilson, J.F., Weale, M.E., Smith, A.C., Gratrix, F., Fletcher, B., Thomas, M.G., et al., 2001. Population genetic structure of variable drug response. Nat. Genetics 29, 265−269.

Xie, H.G., Kim, R.B., Stein, C.M., Wilkinson, G.R., Wood, A.J., 1999. Genetic polymorphism of (S)-mephenytoin 4'-hydroxylation in populations of African descent. Br. J. Clin. Pharmacol. 48, 402−408.

Xie, H.G., Prasad, H.C., Kim, R.B., Stein, C.M., 2002. CYP2C9 allelic variants: ethnic distribution and functional significance. Adv. Drug Deliv. Rev. 54, 1257−1270.

Yamakawa, Y., Hamada, A., Shuto, T., Yuki, M., Uchida, T., Kai, H., et al., 2011. Pharmacokinetic impact of SLCO1A2 polymorphisms on imatinib disposition in patients with chronic myeloid leukemia. Clin. Pharmacol. Ther. 90, 157−163.

Yiannakopoulou, E., 2013. Pharmacogenomics of phase II metabolizing enzymes and drug transporters: clinical implications. Pharmacogenomics J. 13, 105−109.

Zabalza, M., Subirana, I., Sala, J., Lluis-Ganella, C., Lucas, G., Tomas, M., et al., 2012. Meta-analyses of the association between cytochrome CYP2C19 loss- and gain-of-function polymorphisms and cardiovascular outcomes in patients with coronary artery disease treated with clopidogrel. Heart 98, 100−108.

Zanger, U.M., Schwab, M., 2013. Cytochrome P450 enzymes in drug metabolism: regulation of gene expression, enzyme activities, and impact of genetic variation. Pharmacol. Therap. 138, 103−141.

Zhang, D., Cui, D., Gambardella, J., Ma, L., Barros, A., Wang, L., et al., 2007. Characterization of the UDP glucuronosyltransferase activity of human liver microsomes genotyped for the UGT1A1*28 polymorphism. Drug Metab. Dispos. Biol. Fate Chem. 35, 2270−2280.

Zhou, S.F., Di, Y.M., Chan, E., Du, Y.M., Chow, V.D., Xue, C.C., et al., 2008. Clinical pharmacogenetics and potential application in personalized medicine. Curr. Drug Metab. 9, 738−784.

Chapter 8

Transcriptomics and Epigenomics

Preeti Chavan-Gautam[1], Tejas Shah[2] and Kalpana Joshi[2]
[1]Bharati Vidyapeeth Deemed University, Pune, Maharashtra, India, [2]Sinhgad College of Engineering, Pune, Maharashtra, India

INTRODUCTION

Drug discovery, for several years, has mainly focused on the single-target paradigm, also known as the "lock and key model." Advances in molecular biology and the reductionist view of systems biology have aided in identifying and developing selective ligands for single-target drugs while avoiding unwanted side effects. The pursuit of suitable ligands for single targets led to the development of in vitro high-throughput screening (HTS) approaches and advances in the design and synthesis of extensive combinatorial libraries (Houghten et al., 1999) that enabled the screening of a vast repertoire of biogenically designed compounds in a relatively short timeframe (Medina-Franco et al., 2008). Despite the successful applications of in vitro HTS (Roy et al., 2010), the lack of clinical efficacy of the hits identified remains a major drawback of this approach, since most diseases are the consequence of disturbed intercellular and intracellular networks linking different tissues and organ systems. Systems biology and polypharmacology (drugs acting on multiple targets or disease pathways) are emerging as important paradigms in drug discovery. There is a need to design drugs that act on individual targets as well as pathway networks, thereby modulating the disturbed network structure back its original state (Galizzi et al., 2013; Hood and Perlmutter, 2004). The emerging biological approaches in drug discovery, such as genomics (Ricke et al., 2006), transcriptomics, epigenomics (Joshi et al., 2012; Chen and Xie, 2012), chemogenomics (Cases and Mestres, 2009), and phenotypic (Main et al., 2014; Ko and Gelb, 2014) approaches, offer a platform to explore systematically not only the molecular complexity of a particular disease, leading to the identification of disease mechanisms and pathways, but also for identifying disease targets and therapeutic ligands. Integrated, multidisciplinary approaches are essential for the management and interpretation of the huge data sets arising from these studies (Hopkins, 2008; Ashburn and Thor, 2004).

Innovative Approaches in Drug Discovery. DOI: http://dx.doi.org/10.1016/B978-0-12-801814-9.00008-8
235

A direct application of polypharmacology is drug repurposing (also called drug repositioning), which is an increasingly growing approach to speed up the drug discovery process by identifying a new clinical use for an existing approved drug (Ashburn and Thor, 2004; Aubé, 2012). In addition, there is growing interest into searching systematically for potential targets of natural products (Rollinger, 2009; Lauro et al., 2011). Herbal remedies or compounds used in traditional Chinese medicine (TCM), Ayurveda, and other traditional medicine systems are known to be effective for the treatment of many diseases. The advent of large compound collections, such as the TCM database (Chen, 2011), has opened up the possibility to search the targets of the active components using computational approaches (Tsai et al., 2011). Recent analysis of the molecular complexity, structural diversity, and molecular properties of the TCM database reveals that this collection is a rich source of molecules to expand the traditional medicinally relevant chemical space (López-Vallejo et al., 2012).

This chapter focuses on transcriptomics and epigenomics in drug discovery. Recent advances in these technologies along with their applications in traditional herbal medicine research and development are discussed. The challenges and pitfalls in these approaches are highlighted.

TRANSCRIPTOMICS

The transcriptome is the complete set of transcripts in a cell, and their quantity, for a specific developmental stage or physiological condition. Transcriptomics is the study of the transcriptome—the complete set of RNA transcripts that are produced by the genome under specific circumstances or in a specific cell. Transcriptomic discovery approaches include microarray-based technologies as well as sequencing-based technologies. Transcriptomic experiments provide dynamic information about gene expression at the tissue level. Comparison of transcriptomes allows the identification of genes that are differentially expressed in distinct cell populations, or in response to different treatments.

The popularity of genomic, high-throughput technologies has caused a transformation in biomedical research, especially in drug discovery and development. Omic's approach has offered a model to understand the substantial human genetic heterogeneity revealed by genomics sequencing in the context of the network of functional regulatory mechanisms and protein drug interactions (Dopazo, 2014). Pharmaceutical and biotechnology organizations have started to reorient their drug discovery strategies to consider human genetic heterogeneity. High-throughput and deep sequencing technologies have and are still providing a valuable support by yielding enormous amounts of omics data and have contributed to understanding the molecular mechanisms responsible for drug action (Kadioglu and Efferth, 2014).

As stated earlier, drug discovery and development is a lengthy and highly taxing process with various stringent requirements. This has been challenging for the pharmaceutical companies, despite the fact that time and expenditure on drug research and development (R&D) have increased annually, with a steady decline in R&D efficiency, as evidenced by the stagnation of the number of newly approved drugs for the past 15−20 years, mainly because of their failure in clinical phase 2 trials (Mullard, 2012).

Pharmaceutical and biotechnology organizations use a range of technologies for assessing the biological effects of compounds. These technologies are often used to gather information about compound-target interactions, and animal-based readouts in later stages, or the detection of adverse effects (Verbist et al., 2015).

The Interrogation of the Transcriptome

The data acquired from genomic analysis of genetic mutation and polymorphisms have static information. To capture physiological fluctuations, expression profiles that are dynamic in nature are required at tissue level. This resultant expression analysis is a signature of cellular states and can be used to distinguish subtle differences. Thus, cell lineage makes a greater footprint than biochemical assays, and in turn much greater than individual gene effect, if any. Both microarrays and sequence-based assays are used to study the transcriptome. These technologies have the ability to distinguish disease classes that standard clinical assays and assessments cannot. Understanding the transcriptome is essential for interpreting the functional elements of the genome and revealing the molecular constituents of cells and tissues, and also for understanding the progression of a disease.

The key aim of transcriptomics is to catalog all species of transcript, including mRNAs, noncoding RNAs, and small RNAs, to determine the transcriptional structure of genes in terms of their start sites, $5'$ and $3'$ ends, splicing patterns, and other posttranscriptional modifications and to quantify the changing expression levels of each transcript during development and under different conditions.

Small Interfering RNAs (siRNA), as Therapeutic Agents

Small interfering RNA (siRNA), also known as short interfering RNA or silencing RNA, is a class of double-stranded RNA molecules (20−25 bp length) and interferes with the expression of specific genes with complementary nucleotide sequences. RNAi has been a promising therapeutic approach for diseases with aberrant protein production. RNAi can also be applied to inhibit the expression or replication of pathogenic viruses, such as HIV and hepatitis C virus.

Double-stranded RNA-mediated interference (RNAi) is a simple and rapid method of silencing gene expression. The principle behind gene silencing is to degrade the RNA into short RNAs so as to activate ribonucleases and target homologous mRNA. The resulting genotypes are either similar to those of genetic null mutants or resemble an allelic series of mutants. RNAi-induced gene silencing is a two-step method. The first step involves degradation of dsRNA into RNAs (siRNAs), by an RNase III-like activity. In the second step, the siRNAs links to an RNase complex, (RISC) RNA-induced silencing complex, which acts on the cognate mRNA and degrades it. Various important components for their roles in RNAi process *viz.* Dicer, RNA-dependent RNA polymerase, helicases, and dsRNA endonucleases have been identified in different organisms. Few of these components have also been known to regulate the developmental process of many organisms by processing many noncoding RNAs, called micro-RNAs. The biogenesis and function of micro-RNAs resemble RNAi activities to a large extent.

Recent studies indicate that RNAi may play an important role in epigenetic modifications like DNA methylation, heterochromatin formation, and programmed DNA elimination. As a result of these changes, the silencing effect of gene functions is exercised as tightly as possible. Due to properties like specificity and efficiency, RNAi is considered as a fundamental approach not only in field of functional genomics, but also for gene-specific therapeutic activities that target the mRNAs of disease-related genes (Agrawal et al., 2003).

Challenges

As described earlier, due to potential specificity and efficiency RNAi has been extremely promising in therapeutics by silencing genes as demonstrated in selected in vitro and in vivo studies. However, for more beneficiary application, several intracellular and extracellular barriers still need to be overcome to explore the broader potential of this technology.

1. Stability and Targeting

     Extracellularly, siRNA are extremely susceptible to degradation by enzymes found in serum and tissues. The half-life of siRNAs is from few minutes to an hour in serum (Behlke, 2006), therefore the required therapeutic accretion on target site remains a major challenge. For successful intervention of siRNAs they must not only pull through the serum but also need to be reached at target cells that express the abnormal gene/genes of interest. The larger size and negative charge of siRNAi hinders their diffusion across the plasma membrane and decreases intracellular accumulation. The effect of *RNAse* on degradation of siRNA needs to integrated with RISC for better efficacy.

2. Off-Target Silencing

     Beside the problem of target delivery, the RNAi epitome of specific gene silencing unfortunately crumples at times in reality (Krol et al., 2010). There are instances where microarray analysis have shown that siRNA treatment may result in off-target gene silencing, i.e., inhibiting genes other than the desired gene targets. Off-target silencing is undesirable, as it can lead to dangerous mutations of gene expression and unexpected cell transformation. While designing siRNA, off-target silencing cannot be ignored, and the potency of therapeutic siRNA-candidate sequences must be thoroughly analyzed for perturbation of normal protein expression profiles.

3. Particle size

Particle size plays a crucial role while designing intravenous administration of siRNA polyplex to prevent clogging of the capillary. Also, extravasation of siRNA complexes through fenestrations of tumor capillaries requires certain size requirements (Buyens et al., 2008). Small particles less than 6 nm are readily eliminated by the kidney, whereas large cells are taken up by liver and spleen for phagocytic mechanism. Hence, the ability to precisely determine the size of siRNA polyplexes is key to their rational design, formulation, and safe application in vivo.

4. Internalization

Internalization pathways determine the intracellular fate of complexes. Reineke et al. scrutinized the mechanisms involved in the cellular internalization and trafficking. Carbohydrate-based poly(glycoamidoamine) polymers can bind and compact nucleic acids into polyplexes that facilitate effective intracellular pDNA delivery with lesser toxicity (Ingle et al., 2011). Xiang et al. briefed the uptake mechanisms of nonviral gene delivery systems and classified uptake mechanisms of nonviral gene delivery, factors for pathway selection and the inhibitors or tools for the study of these pathways. The uptake pathways of nonviral gene complexes are usually determined by not only the gene/carrier interaction, but also by the interaction between complexes and target cells (Xiang et al., 2012). In spite of the progress mentioned above, a detailed understanding of uptake mechanisms is lacking because only simple molecules have been developed and studied.

5. Endosomal escape

Bartlett and Davis reported the kinetics of gene silencing in both unmodified and nuclease stabilized siRNAs both in vitro and in vivo experiments (Bartlett and Davis, 2006, 2007). Upon endosomal escape many formulations such as PEGylated liposomes allow direct release of siRNA into the cytoplasm. Since all endosomes will not rupture at the same time, the release of siRNA into the cytoplasm could be sustained for longer than required for efficient gene silencing at a relatively low concentration. The release from endosomes may therefore result in prolonged effects of siRNA (Gao and Huang, 2013).

6. Mathematical models

Mathematical models can help to create effective siRNA treatment regimens by designing models that can withstand important properties of siRNA therapeutics. Raab et al. (Raab and Stephanopoulos, 2004) demonstrated some of the principal characteristics of RNAi as a tool for gene silencing such as the RNA dose level, RNA complex exposure time, and the time of transfection relative to gene induction, in the context of silencing a green fluorescent protein reporter gene in mouse hepatoma cells. The authors established a model that may help determining key parameters in virtual complex silencing experiments and explore alternative gene silencing protocols (Raab and Stephanopoulos, 2004). More detailed mathematical models are required which should include RNAi-specific parameters such as intracellular siRNA stability, activation of RISC, the kinetics of siRNA−RISC−mRNA complexes, and formulation kinetics of siRNA release (Gao and Huang, 2013).

The Role of RNAi in Identification and Validation of Drug Targets

RNAi has the potential to affect multiple stages of drug discovery (Fig. 8.1). Target validation is a broad and it includes several phenomenon and roles to understand, the roles of disease-related signature genes, and genes involved in the initiation of disease phenotypes. Primarily, target validation is mostly performed in cell culture systems and then further carried forward to preclinical stages. The advantage of target validation is that it associates a functional relationship rather than a correlative link. Target validation in cell culture systems has several essential requirements. Importantly, the cell-based system should mimic facets of the disease under the study. Mostly two types of RNAi are used in cell culture−based systems. Most prominently used is commercially synthesized short double-stranded RNA molecules called as siRNA or siRNAs. The second one used is shRNA, expressed as short hairpin RNAs (shRNAs). They are produced inside the cells after transfection process with plasmid or viral expression vectors (Miller, 2005).

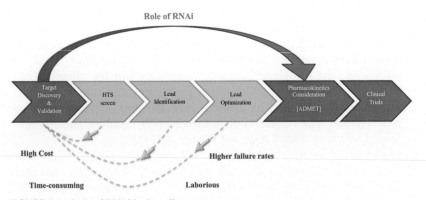

FIGURE 8.1 Role of RNAi in drug discovery process.

Van Den Haute et al. developed human immunodeficiency virus type 1-derived LVs encoding an shRNA specific for enhanced green fluorescent protein (EGFP) mRNA that were capable of inhibiting EGFP expression in mammalian cells. EGFP knockdown persisted after multiple passages of the cells. Especially, RNAi LVs were equally effective in the inhibition and prevention of EGFP expression after stereotactic injection in an adult mouse brain, thereby indicating a promising aid to probe gene function in vivo and for gene therapy for diseases related to central nervous system (Van den Haute et al., 2003).

Mackeigan et al. systematically screened for the kinase- and phosphatase-encrypting factors of the human genome and identified new regulators of apoptosis and chemo-resistance using a customized set of libraries of siRNAs that were designed to include two siRNA duplexes for each gene target. In total, identified kinase library was directed against 650 target genes, and their phosphatase library was directed against 222 genes. The development of inhibitors that target these kinases or phosphatases may help in discovering new anticancer strategies (MacKeigan et al., 2005).

Bernsetal reported the construction of a set of retroviral vectors that encode 23,742 distinct shRNAs and target 7914 different human genes. The authors used their human cells library to identify one known and five previously unknown modulators of arrest of the p53-dependent proliferation. Suppression of these genes conferred resistance to the arrest of both the p53-dependent and the p19ARF-dependent proliferation of cells, and abolished the DNA damage-induced arrest of the cell cycle at G1 (Berns et al., 2004).

Applications of RNAi in Various Diseases

1. Central Nervous System Disorders

The development, design, and delivery of epigenetic therapeutic products have several hurdles into stem cell generative areas and site of ischemic injuries in the CNS. Yet technologies like nanotechnology have potential to overcome the problems of permeability of the blood−brain barrier and to allow selective and subcellular utilization of combinations of oligonucleotides, small molecules, and proteins in the CNS (Kubinová and Syková, 2010; Modi et al., 2009; Orive et al., 2009; Provenzale and Silva, 2009).

For instance, magnetic and optical properties of iron oxide and quantum dot nanoparticles has enabled to track pathophysiological processes involved in the study and treatment of stroke. Further, imaging techniques can be used to study and monitor the activation and migration of neural stem and progenitor cells to the sites of ischemic brain injury and will also help to explore and understand process. The combination of RNAi therapy and imaging techniques will be beneficial in the understanding and treatment of CNS diseases in the future (Gao and Huang, 2013).

2. Pulmonary Disorders

Respiratory diseases in the developing world are a major burden in terms of morbidity and mortality; RNAi strategies therefore have attracted particular attention. Due to easy accessibility through nasal route and/or inhalation, it allows the design of effective treatments. However, the delivery of siRNA to the lungs remains a hurdle due to number of barriers, including the mucus layer secreted by goblet cells, apical membrane glycol conjugates, etc. (Gao and Huang, 2013). Despite these barriers, polyethyleneimine (PEI) has shown promising delivery of pDNA when it was administered to the lungs by inhalation (Bragonzi et al., 2000; Rudolph and Mu, 2002; Densmore, 2000).

3. Cardiac disorders

It is hoped that RNAi will play an important role in the treatment of heart diseases illustrating from functions of various cardiac genes and to attenuate cold ischemia injuries to prolong the preservation time of donor hearts for transplantation procedures (Zheng et al., 2009). A substitute approach for the treatment of coronary artery disease such as atherosclerosis is the delivery of potential angiogenic factors to trigger new vessel growth using gene transfer (Ylä-Herttuala and Alitalo, 2003). With a better understanding of the mechanism of endogenous RNAi and their delivery systems, in the near future new therapeutic applications are expected.

a. The impact of RNAi on drug discovery

RNAi has shown a promising approach to improve the efficacy of target validation. It should be noted that there are many other criteria that influence whether a target will advance beyond the initial stages of drug discovery other than RNAi. Factors that may serve as influences include target class and druggability, therapeutic rationale, market size and strategic fit, risk analysis and IP positions all come into play, and in fact will override even the most solid target-validation data. Most research utilizes RNAi as a tool for making good decisions regarding target validation. A thorough understanding and more exploratory research on RNAi is ongoing to explore if RNAi can be used for assay selection of molecule optimization (Miller, 2005).

Haibin Xia et al. established a principle by markedly reducing expression of exogenous and endogenous genes in vitro and in vivo in the brain and liver, and further applied this strategy to a model system of a major class of neurodegenerative disorders, the polyglutamine diseases, to show reduced polyglutamine aggregation in cells. This viral-mediated strategy can prove useful in reducing expression of target genes to model biological processes or to provide therapy for dominant human diseases (Xia et al., 2002).

Ramsingh et al. using NGS identified genetic variants of miRNA genes, screened for alterations in miRNA binding sites in a patient with acute myeloid leukemia. RNA sequencing of leukemic myeloblasts or

CD34$^+$ cells pooled from healthy donors indicated that 472 miRNAs were expressed, including seven novel miRNAs, some of which displayed differential expression. Sequencing of all known miRNA disclosed several unidentified germline polymorphisms. Further analysis of the 3′-untranslated regions (UTRs) of all coding genes discovered a single somatic mutation in the 3′-UTR of *TNFAIP2*, a known target of the *PML-RAR*α oncogene. This mutation resulted in translational suppression of a reporter gene in a Dicer-dependent fashion. This study represents the first complete characterization of the "miRNAome" in a primary human cancer and indicates that the generation of miRNA binding sites in the UTR regions of genes is another potential mechanism by which somatic mutations may affect gene expression (Ramsingh et al., 2010).

Silvia Calo et al. depicted that the human fungal pathogen *Mucor circinelloides* develops spontaneous resistance to the antifungal drug FK506 (tacrolimus) via two distinct mechanisms. One involving Mendelian mutations that confer stable drug resistance and the second occurs via an RNAi-mediated pathway leading to unstable drug resistance. The peptidyl-prolyl-isomerase FKBP12 interacts with FK506 forming a complex that inhibits the protein phosphatase calcineurin. Calcineurin inhibition by FK506 blocks *M. circinelloides* transition to hyphae and enforces yeast growth. Mutations in the fkbA gene encoding FKBP12 or the calcineurin cnbR or cnaA genes confer FK506 resistance and restore hyphal growth. In parallel, RNAi is spontaneously triggered a silence of the fkbA gene, giving rise to drug-resistant epimutants. FK506-resistant epimutants readily reverted to the drug-sensitive wild-type phenotype when grown without exposure to the drug. The establishment of these epimutants is accompanied by generation of abundant fkbA small RNAs and requires the RNAi pathway as well as other factors that constrain or reverse the epimutant state. Silencing involves the generation of a double-stranded RNA trigger intermediate using the fkbA mature mRNA as a template to produce antisense fkbA RNA. This study uncovers a novel epigenetic RNAi-based epimutation mechanism controlling phenotypic plasticity, with possible implications for antimicrobial drug resistance and RNAi-regulatory mechanisms in fungi and other eukaryotes (Calo et al., 2014).

A majority of the studies of host–pathogen interactions have focused on pathogen-specific virulence causal factors. Agaisse et al. reported a genome-wide RNA interference screen to identify host factors involved in intracellular bacterial pathogenesis. Using Drosophila cells and the cytosolic pathogen *Listeria monocytogenes*, authors identified 305 double-stranded RNAs targeting a wide range of cellular functions that altered *L. monocytogenes* infection. Comparison to a similar screen with *Mycobacterium fortuitum*, a vacuolar pathogen, identified host factors that may play a general role in intracellular pathogenesis and factors that specifically affect access to the cytosol by *L. monocytogenes* (Agaisse et al., 2005). Using RNAi libraries, Futami et al. were able to identify some unexpected and novel pathways in thapsigargin-induced apoptosis, and the results provided evidence for the efficacy and utility of the comprehensive analysis of signaling networks and pathways with a library of siRNA-expression vectors (Futami et al., 2005).

Advantages of RNAi

RNA interference—RNAi has shown potentially significant advantages over traditional- and complementary-based approaches for treating diseases.

Broad Applicability—RNA interference-based drugs can be used for identifying causative genes involved in diseases or as an important contributing factor.

Therapeutic Precision—As RNAi therapeutics will be designed for inhibiting diseases causative genes and targeted genes it will reduce the side effects associated with other medicines.

Target RNA Destruction—RNAi drugs are designed to destroy the target RNA compared to most other drugs that only temporarily prevent targeted protein function, and therefore stop the association of undesirable protein production involved in disease progression.

Limitations of RNAi technology

Although there is great potential for the application of RNAi technology in drug target identification and validation, certain drawbacks of the technology have come into light. After more than a decade of experimentation and trials, RNAi screening is still surrounded by doubt due to lack of reproducibility of data sets from different research groups, off-target effects, and lack of positive therapeutic outcome. As an example, Lipardi and Paterson had to retract their RNAi screening article due to misinterpretation of their screening data analysis (Bhinder and Djaballah, 2013).

Considering all these concerns, the scientific world has started losing faith in the merits of novel gene candidates due to this hit-or-miss approach of RNAi screening process, and this has raised the necessity for validations of results.

Transcriptome Technologies

1. SAGE

Serial analysis of gene expression, or SAGE, is an experimental technique designed to acquire direct quantification of gene expression. The principle is to isolate a unique sequence tags (9−10 bp in length) from individual mRNAs and linkage of tags serially into long DNA molecules for lump-sum sequencing. The SAGE method can be applied to the studies exploring virtually any kind of biological phenomena in which the changes in cellular transcription are responsible. SAGE is a highly efficient technology that not only generates a global expression profile but also identifies a set of specific genes responsible for cellular conditions by comparing profiles within healthy and diseased groups (Yamamoto et al., 2001).

The main setback of SAGE is the requirement of relatively high amount of mRNA and the difficulty in constructing tag libraries.

2. Microarray Technologies

Microarray experiments include two components: probe and target. These thousands of probes are fixed to a surface, and RNA samples (the targets) are labeled with fluorescent dyes for hybridization to the microarray. Probes are constructed using cDNA or presynthesized oligonucleotides and are fixed upon silicon wafers using photolithography or printed onto a glass slide. There are many microarray platforms that differ in array fabrication and usage of dye. After hybridization, laser lights are used to excite the fluorescent dye. The hybridization intensity is represented by the amount of fluorescent emission, which gives an estimate of the relative amounts of the different transcripts that are represented.

In cDNA microarrays, mRNA from biological samples is reversed transcribed and simultaneously labeled with Cy3 and Cy5. After hybridization, Cy3 and Cy5 fluorescence is measured separately, and captured in two images, which is further merged to produce a composite image.

High-density oligonucleotides microarrays involve shorter probe sequences (approx. 25 bp) and use only a single fluorescence color, as the mRNA sample is converted to biotinylated cRNA and only one target is hybridized to each array (Freedman and Loscalzo, 2009).

Microarray technology represents a wonderful opportunity for biomedical research, significant issues must be considered. Although microarray-related studies can monitor global changes in gene expression, these studies are limited by access and cost. There is also a lack of rigorous standards for data collection, analysis, and validation (Russo et al., 2003). An additional limitation of this technology is that each microarray can only provide information about the genes that are included on the array.

3. Sequencing Technologies

The world has now embarked into a new era of omics since the continued advancements in the next generation of high-throughput sequencing (NGS) technologies, which includes sequencing assays like synthesis-fluorescent in situ sequencing (FISSEQ), pyrosequencing sequencing, Sequencing by Oligonucleotide Ligation and Detection (SOLiD), sequencing by hybridization along with sequencing by ligation, and nanopore technology (Yadav et al., 2014). NGS is believed to make advances and make the drug discovery process more rapid.

NGS technologies have several applications ranging from genetic applications like comparative genomics, metagenomics, high-throughput polymorphism detection, mutation detection, analysis of small RNAs, transcriptome profiling, methylation profiling, and chromatin remodeling. The major measurements for the success of the NGS technology are large sequences (read length), sequence quality, high throughput, and comparatively lower cost.

The various assays involved in NGS technologies are described below:

a. *Sequencing by Synthesis (SBS)*

Flurophore-labeled, reversible nucleotide is one of the most common platforms of sequencing by synthesis (SBS). It is also referred as FISSEQ. Ronaghi et al. at Stanford University, developed pyrosequencing technology and is now another SBS technology in use (Ronaghi et al., 1996). The principle is based on the detection of pyrophosphate (PPi) released during DNA synthesis when inorganic PPi is released after a nucleotide incorporation by DNA polymerase. The released PPi is then converted to ATP by ATP sulfurylase. A luciferase reporter enzyme uses the ATP to generate light, which is then detected by a charged couple device camera. Pyrosequencing has been upgraded into an NGS technology, with the composite of several technologies involving template carrying microbeads attached to picoliter-sized reaction wells connected to the optical fibers (Shendure et al., 2004). 454 Life Sciences/Roche Diagnostic has a Genome Sequencer 20 System and Genome Sequencer FLX System, two high-throughput commercial sequencing platforms, and DNA helices are fractionated into 300−500 bp fragments and linkers are added to their 3' and 5' ends. Single-stranded DNA is isolated and captured on beads. The beads with DNAs are then emulsified in a "water-in-oil" mixture with amplification reagents to create micro reactors for emulsion PCR (emPCR). Finally, beads with amplified DNAs are loaded onto a picotitre plate for sequencing (Yadav et al., 2014).

b. *Polony Sequencing*

This high-throughput method was developed at Harvard University, at George Church's Laboratory based on polony amplification and FISSEQ (Shendure and Ji, 2008). In polony amplification DNA is amplified in situ on a thin polyacrylamide film (Mitra and Church, 1999). The DNA movement is limited in the polyacrylamide gel, so the amplified DNAs are localized in the gel and form the so-called polonies, that is, polymerase colonies. Up to five million polonies (i.e., five million PCRs) can be formed on a single glass microscope slide.

Kim et al. developed a technology named Polony Multiplex Analysis of Gene Expression, which blends polony amplification and a sequence-by-ligation method, to sequence 14-base tags (Kim and Porreca, 2007). Up to 5 million polonies can be sequenced in parallel.

c. *Single Molecule DNA Sequencing*

Most current sequencing technologies are based on sequencing many identical copies of DNA molecules (often amplified). However, the main drawback associated with sequencing amplified multiple copies of identical DNAs is achieving the synchronous priming of each copy of the multiple DNA by the sequencing primers (Lin et al., 2008). This problem can be overcome by performing SBS methods discussed earlier in the chapter. Here DNA is attached to solid support to form single molecule arrays, and the single DNA molecule is then sequenced directly. Applera Corp. invented fluorescent intercalators that are occupied as a donor in fluorescence resonance energy transfer for use in single-molecule-sequencing reactions (Sun, 2007).

d. *Nanopore Sequencing*

This sequencing technology is one of the most promising technologies because of rapidity, real-time assay, and true single-molecule DNA sequencing. It involves the usage of nanopores, which are nanometer-scale pores (Rhee and Burns, 2006). The principle behind this technology is noticing the change in the ionic current in nanopores when molecules cross through a nanopore and is used for the detection, counting, and characterization of single molecules (Meller and Branton, 2002; Meller et al., 2000). Recent progress has made a big step toward ultrafast sequencing using nanopore technologies. Lagerqvist et al. proposed and theoretically demonstrated a novel idea to measure the electric current perpendicular to the DNA backbone (Lagerqvist et al., 2006). Further, Zhao et al. showed that a single nucleotide polymorphism (SNP) can be detected by a change in the threshold voltage of a nanopore (Zhao et al., 2007).

e. *Sequencing by Ligation*

Lynx Therapeutics Inc. released the first NGS by ligation, the technology involved massively parallel signature sequencing (Brenner et al., 2000). The method was upgraded to ultra-fast and NGS at Church's laboratory at Harvard Medical School (Kim and Porreca, 2007; Myllykangas et al., 2012). They converted an epifluorescence for rapid DNA sequencing. DNA molecules were amplified in parallel onto microbeads by an emulsion polymerase chain reaction. Millions of beads were immobilized in a polyacrylamide gel and sequenced using sequencing a ligation method. Applied Biosystem Inc. acquired Agencourt Personal Genomics, which developed the SOLiD for high-throughput DNA sequencing (Yadav et al., 2014).

4. RNA-seq Technology

RNA-seq technology is based on a deep sequencing technology and, compared to microarray, is a newer method to interrogate single cell transcriptome. The substantial advantage is that it allows direct access to sequences of mRNA; also, variations due to hybridization and labeling efficiencies are reduced. In addition, RNA-seq also allows the detection of RNA editing events, like alternative splicing, the most important source of phenotypic diversity in eukaryotes (Malone and Oliver, 2011). In an RNA-seq experiment, total RNA is first extracted from cell samples.

As the bulk of cellular RNA is contained of rRNA, it becomes necessary to reduce the quantity of rRNA to maximize diversity of the sequences retrieved from sequencing. The rRNA quantity in the sample is reduced by the enrichment of polyadenylated RNA or by the deletion of the rRNA quantity (Wilhelm et al., 2010). The sample is treated with DNase to remove any remaining DNA followed by cDNA synthesis. Before loading onto the platform, this cDNA is labeled using a variety of creation procedures depending upon the sequencing technology, platform, and analysis technique (Wilhelm et al., 2010; Tang et al., 2009). At present various sequencing platforms used for single cell transcriptome are from Pacific Biosciences, Illumina, and Complete Genomics. Mainly RNA-seq technology is used for three main applications:

1. Sequence mapping
2. Transcriptome Reconstruction
3. Expression Profiles

APPLICATIONS OF TRANSCRIPTOMICS IN DRUG DISCOVERY

After the completion of the Human Genome Project, there has been a great interest among scientists and researchers toward exploring the role played by multiple genes in managing complex cellular functions and addressing molecular mechanism pathways. NGS technologies is being used for various applications such as whole genome sequencing, re-sequencing, SNP detection, structural variation discovery, mRNA and noncoding RNA profiling, and protein-nucleic acid interaction assays. NGS technologies are becoming a potential tool for gene expression analysis (Fig. 8.2).

DNA microarrays have been specially used to study genetic variations in a sample or to determine the expression levels in genes. The expression profiles of a gene is linked to its biological role; microarray studies provide important information on the biochemical pathways involved, sites of gene expression, and, most importantly, the function of the gene in a particular organ as well as whole organism. Additionally, the microarray technique is used for assays involved in the description of the genes involved in the

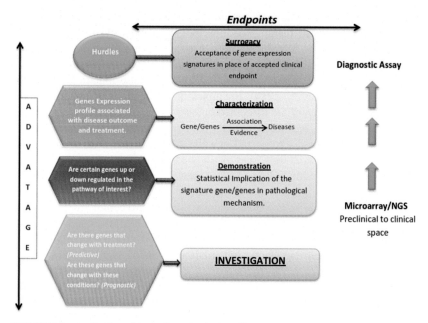

FIGURE 8.2 Application of transcriptomics in drug discovery.

physiological and pathological processes, and identification of disease specific genes. Signature genes related to diseases may act as a target for therapeutic interventions and monitoring (Azad et al., 2008).

Transcriptomics in Herbal Drug Discovery

There are estimated 250,000—500,000 plant species. The World Health Organization (WHO) has suggested there are about 21,000 plant species with potential medicinal values. Only a small percentage of these species have been investigated phytochemically and even fewer for their pharmacological properties (Kumar, 2012). Various transcriptome technologies discussed above have potential applications in discovery of new therapeutic targets, target screening, understanding mechanisms of action at the transcriptome level, lead optimization, and toxicity studies. The field of transcriptomics also offers the scope of developing molecules to target defects in the transcriptional machinery. An example of this is Ataluren, developed by PTC Therapeutics. Ataluren (PTC124) is a novel, orally administered small molecule compound used for treatment of patients with genetic disorders due to a nonsense mutation. Ataluren interacts with ribosome, enabling it to neglect premature nonsense stop signals on mRNA and thereby allowing the cell to produce a full-length, functional protein. As a result, Ataluren has the potential to be an important therapy for muscular dystrophy, cystic fibrosis, and other genetic disorders for which a nonsense mutation is the cause of the disease. Ataluren is in clinical development for the treatment of Duchenne muscular dystrophy and cystic fibrosis caused by a nonsense mutation (McElroy et al., 2013; Kerem et al., 2014). Examples of applications of trancriptomics on herbal drug discovery are discussed below:

For instance, the leaf extract (EGb 761) from the *Ginkgo biloba* leaf is widely used for neurodisorders and is a top selling herbal drug in the world (Mahadevan and Park, 2008). Su et al. showed that gene expression profiling of mice brain fed with EGb761, an extract of *G. biloba*, showed that it affects neuroactive ligand-receptor interaction pathway and upregulates the subgroup of dopamine receptors, especially dopamine receptor 1a. This probably explains why EGb761 can be used to treat neurodisorders and its potential use (Su et al., 2009). Further to the established efficacy of EGb761 in neurodisorders, novel therapeutic potentials of EGb761 can be predicted by microarray analysis.

Further research by Bidon et al. shows that EGb 761 reactivates a juvenile profile in the skeletal muscle of sarcopenic rats by transcriptional reprogramming. It plays an important role in the gain of muscular mass, improves muscular performances, and it can be used for sarcopenia. On DNA microarray analysis it showed that these modifications are contributed by genes related to myogenesis via transforming growth factor-β signaling pathway and to the energy production via fatty acids and glucose oxidation (Bidon et al., 2009).

In 1980, Govindarajan proved that curcumin is a major chemical component of Curcuma longa rhizome, which has been used as a spice to give a specific flavor and yellow color to curry (Govindarajan, 1980). Huang et al. (1988) discovered that curcumin exhibits anticarcinogenic properties in mice. Further, in 2004 a microarray analysis indicated that curcumin exhibits a novel antimetastatic effect via regulating the expression of certain genes involved in metastasis (Chen et al., 2004).

Extracts prepared from medicinal plants/herbs contain various molecules with potent biological activities. However, it is difficult to analyze the biological activities of these extracts because of their complex constituents. To overcome this issue, Cheng et al. linked the formulae-altered genes with drug- or compound-regulated genes by Connectivity Map (Cheng et al., 2010). Connectivity map compares lists of differential expressed genes to a library of experiments evaluating the effects of small molecules and genetic events on gene expression. Connectivity Map looks for connections among molecules sharing similar mechanisms of action. By connecting the gene expression signatures of formulae with those of drugs, we can predict the novel therapeutic potential of medicinal plants/ herbs and further identify the phytochemical candidate for drug development (Lo et al., 2012).

Transcriptomics for Lead Optimization

There is a requirement of a multidimensional assay that measures a diversity of biological effects during lead optimization that will be highly desirable for making the right decisions in the early phase of drug development process and would save considerable amounts of time and money. Gene expression profiling is one of the assays that has gained considerable attention in the past decade. Gene expression profiling simultaneously measures many of the biological effects of a compound on the transcriptional level, giving a comprehensive snapshot of the biological state of a living system (Verbist et al., 2015).

Veen et al. showed that keratinocyte based prediction assays may provide an essential information on the skin-sensitizing potential of chemicals (Van Der Veen et al., 2013). Further, Natsch et al. and Vandebriel et al. confirmed the importance of the previously identified Nrf2-Keap1 and MAP Kinase signaling pathways in the skin sensitizing after gene expression profiling of keratinocytes exposed to sensitizers (Natsch, 2010; Vandebriel and Van Loveren, 2010). Ng et al. (2010) demonstrated the first successful application of exome sequencing to discover the gene for a rare Mendelian disorder of unknown cause, Miller syndrome. Sanger sequencing confirmed the presence of DHODH mutations in three additional families with Miller syndrome. Exome sequencing of a small number of unrelated affected individuals is a powerful, efficient strategy for identifying the genes underlying rare Mendelian disorders and will likely transform the genetic analysis of monogenic traits (Zhou et al., 2009).

Zheng et al. constructed a siRNA library comprising of 8000 human genes. The authors inserted gene-specific siRNA sequences between two different opposing polymerase III promoters: the mouse U6 and human H1 promoters. The library was arrayed on a plate and an HTS was performed by cotransfection of the siRNA cassettes with a pNF-kB-Luc reporter plasmid into HEK293T cells for identification of potential NF-kB regulators. Luciferase reporter activity was measured as an indicator of NF-kB activity and TNFa was used to stimulate transfected cells. Various known and unknown regulators of NFkB activity were explored and identified from the library screening. NF-kB is known to be involved in multiple cell signaling pathways and plays a key role in diseases such as cancer and inflammation, the discovered novel regulators of NF-kB can have potential therapeutic value (Zheng et al., 2004).

The identification of the cellular targets of small molecules with anticancer activity is crucial for further development as drug molecules. Brummelkamp et al. presented the application of a large-scale RNA interference-based shRNA barcode screen to gain insight in the mechanism of action of nutlin-3. Nutlin-3 is a cytotoxic and activates the p53 pathway. Nutlin-3 showed a potential antitumor effect in mice, with few unexpected side effects on normal tissues. The authors also identified 53BP1 as a critical mediator of nutlin-3-induced cytotoxicity. 53BP1 is part of a signaling network induced by DNA damage that is frequently activated in cancer but not in healthy tissues. This study proposed that nutlin-3's tumor specificity may result from its ability to turn a cancer cell—specific property into a weakness that can be exploited therapeutically (Brummelkamp et al., 2006).

Yang et al. constructed an siRNA library in the pHUMU vector using partially randomized sequences targeting the consensus region in the ZnF_C4 signature motif of the nuclear hormone receptors and further against the entire receptor superfamily. The authors adapted a reporter assay for screening of this library for receptors that might be involved in reducing amyloid β peptide accumulation. The screen identified siRNA vectors that specifically increase the Aβ40/42 cleavage and pointed to a potential receptor target, ROR-γ. siRNAs targeting other regions of ROR-γ not only confirmed the observed reporter activity but also reduced the level of the toxic Aβ peptides. The results demonstrated a general principle for the creation and application of RNAi library approach for functional gene discovery within a predefined protein family. The discovered negative effect of ROR-γ on the degradation of the toxic Aβ peptides may provide a potential drug target or targetable pathway for intervention of Alzheimer's disease (Yang et al., 2006).

Transcriptomics for Avoiding Toxicity Pathways

Ritonavir, an HIV protease inhibitor (PI) on detailed liver transcriptome analysis, exhibited several key roles in cellular pathways (Bai et al., 2013). These results were then compared to a gene expression profile of 52 unrelated compounds and other PIs such as atazanavir and two experimental HIV PIs. The results depicted showed that ritonavir played a role in signature genes involved in cholesterol and fatty acid biosynthesis. In 2011, Bhat et al. reported that ritonavir upregulated the ubiquitin proteasome system (UPS) as well, which contains multiple proteasomal subunit transcripts and genes involved in ubiquitination (Bhat and Greer, 2011). Thus, the association between proteasomal induction and lipid elevations was established for the first time and was further taken into consideration while screening for the novel PIs that do not induce the UPS.

Transcriptomics in Toxicogenomics

Toxicogenomics can be used to analyze the gene expression profile of several thousand genes to identify changes associated with drug-induced toxicities. It is believed that toxicogenomics analysis can be a substitute or complementary approach to study the safety of a molecule at preclinical stage or to predict molecule-induced toxicities.

Use of Toxicogenomics in Risk Assessment (The National Academy of Sciences, 2007):

Exposure Assessment: Toxicogenomics is used to identify genetic patterns linked to genetic exposure due to any chemicals or other mixtures. Standardized methods for identifying these signatures will be needed.

Hazard Screening: Toxicogenomics is used for rapid screening of the potential toxicity of molecule/entity during drug discovery purposes.

Variability in Susceptibility: Susceptibility to toxic effects of chemical exposures varies from person to person depending upon genotype. Toxicogenomic technologies offer the potential to use genetic information to identify susceptible subpopulations and assess differences in susceptibility in larger populations. Further, toxicogenomics would be able to address regulatory processes to susceptibility within a population.

Mechanistic Information: Toxicogenomics offers an insight to explore the molecular mechanisms to identify mode of action, especially in the case of traditional medicines.

Cross-Species Extrapolation: Traditionally animals were used to study toxicity , but animal-to-human toxicity extrapolations introduce uncertainty into risk assessment. Toxicogenomics extends the potential to significantly enhance the confidence of such extrapolations by using human cells.

Dose-Response Relationships: Toxicogenomics studies can help in improving the understanding of dose–response relationships of toxicants, particularly at low levels of exposure.

Developmental Exposures: Toxicogenomic technologies are expected to reveal the potential health effects of exposure to toxic substances in early development.

Ying Jiang et al. showed that a diagnosis of kidney proximal tubule toxicity, measured by pathology, can successfully be achieved even with study design of fewer samples, using algorithm applied for the classification of toxicogenomics diagnosis was SVM (Support Vector Machine). Instead of applying cross-validation methods, the authors used an independent testing set by dividing the studies or samples into independent training and testing sets to evaluate the diagnostic performance. Result of the study showed achievement of 88% of sensitivity and 91% of specificity. The diagnosis performance emphasizes the potential application of toxicogenomics in a preclinical lead optimization process of drugs entering into development (Ng et al., 2010).

Limitations and Further Scope

Even though the instrumentation prices of microarray/sequencer are lower, the financial investment and maintenance remains high. Costs per base are generally higher than for standard instruments, and a very similar overall infrastructure is still required. Often the choice of an appropriate sequencing platform is project-specific and sometimes combinations can be advantageous.

In the future, a database needs to be constructed to contain large-scale expression profiles of quality herbs or species recommended by WHO to analyze the biological events induced by herbs, to predict the therapeutic potential of herbs, to evaluate the safety of herbs, and to identify the drug candidate of herbs. In addition, such a database can be served as a translational platform between traditional Chinese herbal medicine and Western medicine.

Requisite to continuing successful transition will be a further sequencing-cost reduction, improved read accuracy, more streamlined sample preparation, and perhaps more importantly, computer-based analytics for data acquisition, management, validation, analyses, and biological interpretation.

EPIGENOMICS

The postgenomics era has seen the rapid emergence of the field of epigenetics. It is now clear that the genome alone cannot completely explain many physiological and pathophysiological observations such as variability in phenotypes, drug responses, discordance between monozygotic twins for the same trait or disorder, and disease susceptibility of an individual. Epigenetic modifications of genome could underlie many of these phenomena (Shastry, 2012). There is increasing evidence that epigenetic changes play a critical role in the development of human diseases. Epigenetics can be defined as heritable, potentially reversible modifications of DNA and DNA-binding proteins that do not involve changes in the DNA sequence. Epigenetics refers to both heritable changes in gene activity and expression (in the progeny of cells or of individuals) and also stable, long-term alterations in the transcriptional potential of a cell that may not be heritable. While epigenetics refers to the study of single genes or groups of genes, epigenomics refers to the analyses of epigenetic changes across the entire genome. They can be modulated by a variety of environmental and lifestyle factors. The major epigenetic alterations that have been identified are DNA methylation, histone modifications, and gene silencing through microRNA (miRNA) or siRNA.

Epigenetic modifications are involved in normal mammalian development. Epigenomic pathways are essential for normal cellular functions with abnormalities in their programming leading to complex disorders. Despite being heritable, epigenetic modifications are potentially reversible, thereby opening up the scope for development of epigenetic therapies for diseases. Epigenetic alterations can thus serve as molecular markers to predict diseases and also the responsiveness of diseases to therapy. Epigenomic changes and identification of factors that mediate these alterations may lead to new drug targets and therapies. Thus, epigenomic approaches to drug discovery are gaining importance. The NIH Roadmap-Epigenomics Mapping Consortium was launched with the goal of producing a public resource of human epigenomic data to catalyze basic biology and disease-oriented research.

An understanding of the different epigenetic modifications is necessary in order to understand their role in disease pathogenesis and as therapeutic targets. Here, we briefly describe the different epigenetic mechanisms and discuss their role in disease mechanisms and therapeutics.

DNA methylation

DNA methylation involves the addition of a methyl group or hydroxymethyl group at the C-5 position in the cytosine residues, mainly, but not exclusively within CpG dinucleotides and is an important epigenetic mark associated with gene repression. In vertebrates three DNA methyltransferases (DNMTs) are involved in the establishment and maintenance of DNA methylation. Dnmt3a and Dnmt3b are responsible for de novo methylation while Dnmt1 acts on newly synthesized DNA and is involved in maintenance of DNA methylation marks (Pradhan et al., 1999). Another member of this family, Dnmt2, is primarily a tRNA methyltransferase with only a weak DNMT activity (Schaefer and Lyko, 2010).

Recently, the existence of a "6th base," 5-hydroxymethylcytosine (5-hmC) has been discovered in mammalian genomes (Munzel et al., 2011; Tahiliani et al., 2009) that further complicates the epigenetic code. Like 5-methylcytosine, 5-hmC is not truly a new nucleotide, but a nucleotide that arises from the hydroxylation of 5-mC to 5-hmC by members of the ten−eleven translocation (TET) protein family. The Tet protein family consists of three members: Tet1, Tet2, and Tet3 that converts 5-mC to 5-hmC. Global changes in 5-hmC levels may contribute to disease; however, more research is required to biologic significance.

HISTONE MODIFICATIONS

The core of the nucleosome is made up of eight proteins, consisting of two of each of the following histone proteins: H2A, H2B, H3, and H4. Histones are proteins with an inherent positive charge that bind to the negatively charged DNA and form the nucleosome. The amino terminal tails of these histone proteins undergo posttranslational histone modifications such as phosphorylation, acetylation, or methylation that affect the electrostatic charge of the histones, thereby altering the association between the histone proteins and the DNA. Depending on the electrostatic change, the posttranslational modification may promote a condensed chromatin state or a relaxed chromatin state. Histone modifications are highly dynamic and play a role in regulating gene expression during a cell cycle, changes in intracellular conditions, or in response to different stimuli. They are added or removed by chromatin-modifying enzymes, which, in turn, are subject to transcriptional and posttranslational regulation. The histone acetylases (HATs) catalyze the transfer of an acetyl group to a lysine amino acid in a histone protein. Histone acetylation is a widely studied, reversible, posttranslation modification that regulates transcription (Struhl, 1998). Histone methyltransferases (HMTs) catalyze the transfer of methyl groups to amino acids in the histone tails. Histone deacetylases HDAC promotes the removal of the acetyl group from acetyl–lysine (Ac–Lys). Histone acetylation is traditionally a sign of open chromatin structure and transcriptional activation. Histone deacetylation, and HDAC activity, is characteristic of transcriptional repression and structurally repressive chromatin. Lysine-specific demethylase 1 (LSD1, also known as BHC110 and KDM1A) catalyzes the removal of methyl groups from histone 3 lysine 4 (H3K4) mono and dimethyllysines in a complex where it is associated with the CoREST protein. Although histone methylation and acetylation are most widely studied, histone proteins also undergo a number of other posttranslational modifications including: ADP-ribosylation, citrullination, clipping, phosphorylation, sumoylation, ubiquitination, and others (Ray-Gallet and Almouzni, 2010; Lister et al., 2009; Hassan et al., 2002; Sanchez and Zhou, 2009).

Posttranslational modifications may create binding sites for proteins like chromatin regulators or remodeling complexes that may further affect chromatin structure and/or gene expression. For example, bromodomain proteins can bind to acetylated histones, and these bromodomain proteins may form part of a protein complex that further regulates chromatin structure and gene transcription (Hassan et al., 2002; Sanchez and Zhou, 2009).

EPIGENOMICS METHODOLOGIES

Over the years several methodologies have been developed for analyzing the 5-methylcytosine content of DNA. Following purification of DNA from cells, the overall DNA 5-methylcytosine content can be determined using high-performance capillary electrophoresis (HPCE) or high-performance liquid chromatography (HPLC), or the DNA methylation of specific candidate genes can be detected with methylation-sensitive methods. An alternative approach for profiling DNA methylation patterns is based on the extraction of mRNA, followed by microarray expression analysis. Analysis of the same sample in the presence or absence of a demethylating agent helps to identify genes showing increased expression due to the removal of DNA methylation marks. Other widely used methodologies include restriction landmark genomic scanning (RLGS), which uses restriction digestion methylation-specific enzymes followed by size-fractionation; amplification of intermethylated sites (AIMS), which uses arbitrary primed PCR and does not rely on prior knowledge of sequence information; and differential methylation hybridization (DMH) in which genomic DNA from the tissue of interest is digested with methylation-sensitive enzymes and the digestion products are used as templates for linker PCR. The resulting oligonucleotides are used as probes to screen for hyper-methylated sequences within the CpG-island library; methylated DNA immunoprecipitation (methyl-DIP) in which DNA is immunoprecipitated with an antibody against 5-methylcytosine can be used as a probe for hybridization of genomic microarray platforms. Methodologies in which sodium bisulphite—treated DNA is sequenced using NGS; MALDI-TOF mass spectrometry are also widely used (Callinan and Feinberg, 2006).

Histone modifications in candidate genes can be detected using mass spectrometry or single-gene chromatin immunoprecipitation (ChIP) using antibodies against specific histone modifications. For global profiling, ChIP is combined with DNA arrays (ChIP-on-chip) to detect patterns across the genome. Chromatin immunoprecipitation (ChIP) can be used to study a protein of interest from the transcription machinery, accessory factors, modified histones, or DNA sequence-specific transcription factors along with its associated genomic DNA fragments when combined with deep sequencing using next-generation sequencing (NGS) platforms (Welboren et al., 2009). Serial analysis of chromatin occupancy (SACO) is an alternative approach to mapping transcription factor—binding proteins based on the SAGE technique of identifying mRNA transcripts (Impey et al., 2004). The hypersensitivity of regulatory sequences to endonuclease DNase I has been employed to predict, via the analysis of chromatin structure, the location of regulatory sequences in complex genomes (Dorschner et al., 2004). Stunnenberg et al. have used a synergistic model of quantitative mass spectrometry-based interactomics and high-throughput genomic profiling for epigenetic research (Stunnenberg and Vermeulen, 2011).

Epigenetic Modifications in Infectious Diseases

In order to infect mammalian hosts, bacterial pathogens evolved an array of mechanisms that serve to create an environment conducive for survival, replication, and spread. It is now well recognized that bacterial and viral pathogens can reprogram host gene expression through epigenetic modifications (Sinclair et al., 2014; Li et al., 2014) and has contributed to the emergence of the field called patho-epigenetics (Cossart and Lebreton, 2014). Some of the strategies employed by pathogens to modulate the host genome include the prevention of chromatin remodeling, thereby maintaining a silenced chromatin state, formation of heterochromatin, displacement of chromatin associated proteins, expression of proteins that directly bind DNA to induce or prevent transcription, modulation of histone posttranslational modifications through manipulation of host enzymes, or directly through secreted effector enzymes (Silmon de Monerri and Kim, 2014). The epigenetic machinery involved in the development and reproduction of schistosomes, the parasites responsible for schistosomiasis, and the potential for the development of novel drug treatments targeting these epigenetic mechanisms have been reviewed recently (Cabezas-Cruz et al., 2014). Studies also point toward the role of epigenetic mechanisms in determining the variation in the host's immune response to infections (Pacis et al., 2014).

Epigenetic Modifications in Lifestyle Diseases

In recent years there has been a rise in the incidence of lifestyle diseases like hypertension, diabetes mellitus, dyslipidemia, and overweight/obesity associated with cardiovascular diseases. The epigenetic basis of these noncommunicable diseases is increasingly recognized. According to the concept of developmental programming of adult diseases, any insult during the intrauterine period can lead to changes in tissue structure, physiological function, and metabolism thereby increasing the susceptibility to diseases in later life (Barker, 1995). The epigenetic basis for DOHaD originates from studies that show how alterations in the maternal diet during pregnancy can result in changes in the methylation patterns of the offspring, thereby contributing to disease (Heijmans et al., 2008; Estampador and Franks, 2014). Our studies have shown alterations in maternal global DNA methylation patterns (Gadgil et al., 2014) and placental global (Chavan-Gautam et al., 2011; Kulkarni et al., 2011) and gene-specific DNA methylation (Sundrani et al., 2013, 2014) patterns in adverse pregnancy outcomes like preeclampsia and preterm birth. These alterations may have long-term implications for health of the mother and baby in later life. The contribution of DNA methylation and histone modifications in cardiac development and disease has been reviewed (Nührenberg et al., 2014). The role of miRNAs in cardiovascular disease is receiving a lot of attention (Mishra et al., 2013). There is ample evidence from human and animal studies for the role of epigenomic mechanisms in the transgenerational transmission of programmed obesity and metabolic syndrome (Ge et al., 2014; Desai et al., 2015). Several studies point toward underlying epigenetic mechanisms for the link between maternal hyperglycemia and adverse long-term outcome in the offspring (Ma et al., 2015) and also for the link between obesity and reproductive disorders (Crujeiras and Casanueva, 2015). A recent study has shown that altered DNA methylation in human pancreatic islets contributes to disturbed hormone secretion and the pathogenesis of type 2 diabetes (Dayeh et al., 2014).

Epigenetic Modifications in Degenerative Diseases

Epigenetic processes are also considered important mechanisms through which environmental and stochastic stressors promote numerous pathologies in humans. Epigenetic factors are also important mediators of development and aging; therefore, their role in complex, late-onset, degenerative disorders are highly researched. Epigenetic mechanisms underlie the high plasticity of the brain in response to experience and the ability to integrate and store new information to shape future neuronal and behavioral response. Disruptions in these processes can lead to neurodegeneration affecting cognition, learning, and memory (Landgrave-Gómez et al., 2015). Major epigenetic mechanisms such as DNA methylation; histone modifications (acetylation, methylation, phosphorylation, sumoylation, ubiquitylation, glycosylation, ADP-ribosylation, biotinylation); and chromatin remodeling and noncoding RNA regulation have been reported to contribute to the pathology of neurodegenerative disorders like Alzheimer's disease (Bennett et al., 2015; Cacabelos et al., 2014), dementia (Woldemichael et al., 2014), Parkinson's disease (Ammal et al., 2013; Feng et al., 2015), and schizophrenia (Diwadkar et al., 2014; Mahgoub and Monteggia, 2013; Guidotti et al., 2014). Elevated levels of 5-hmC have been found in neurons of the brain in Alzheimer's disease (Coppieters et al., 2013).

The major pathogenesis of degenerative disorders like osteoporosis and osteoarthritis is the deregulation of bone remodeling. Epigenetic mechanisms are involved in bone remodeling and bone homeostasis, and hence these conditions are considered to have a strong epigenetic component (Vrtačnik et al., 2014; Im and Choi, 2013).

Epigenetic Modifications in Cancer

Epigenetic change is part of the carcinogenic process with a huge potential for biomarker discovery. Clinically relevant methylation changes are known in common human cancers such as cervix, prostate, breast, colon, bladder, stomach, and lung cancers (Lorincz, 2014). In cancer, overall DNA hypomethylation, concomitant with hypermethylation of tumor suppressor genes at CpG islands in the promoter regions, has been observed (Feinberg, 2007). The role DNA methylation and histone modification in cancer is well reviewed in literature (Hattori and Ushijima, 2014). The role of TETs and 5-hmC in cancer has been reviewed recently (Kinney and Pradhan, 2013). Loss of 5-hmC has been shown to correlate with poorer prognosis in some types of cancer (Yang et al., 2013; Jawert et al., 2013; Orr et al., 2012), and loss of 5-hmC and TET expression has been observed in melanoma (Lian et al., 2012; Gambichler et al., 2013). Low levels of 5-hmC associated with anaplasia are reported in brain tumors (Kraus et al., 2012), while another study shows increased 5-hmC and reduced 5-mC in pediatric brain tumors (Ahsan et al., 2014). Impaired 5-hmC levels and TET function are also reported in myeloid leukemias (Ko et al., 2010; Rampal et al., 2014).

Epigenetic Machinery as Therapeutic Target

Epigenetic modifications, despite being heritable and stably maintained, are also potentially reversible, and there is scope for the development of epigenetic therapies for diseases. DNA methylation and demethylation pathways and chromatin remodeling processes may be useful targets for developing new drugs aimed at preventing or limiting the impact of various diseases. Dnmt inhibitors are the most widely used therapeutic strategies for targeting DNA methylation. Several of them, such as 5-fluoro-2′-deoxycytidine (FdCyD) with tetrahydrouridine (THU), (−)-epigallocatechin-3-gallate (EGCG), ASTX727, cc-486, CP-4200, decitabine (Dacogen), hydralazine, MG98, procainamide and procaine (ester analog of procainamide), Psammaplin A, RG108 (*N*-Phthaloyl-L-tryptophan)/RG108 analogs, RRx-001, SGI-1027, SGI-110, Vidaza (5-azacytidine), zebularine, are in preclinical and clinical trials. Of these decitabine and 5-azacytidine are approved by FDA and EMEA (Hamm and Costa, 2015). The enzyme, activation-induced cytidinede aminase (AID), initiates a process that ultimately leads to DNA demethylation through the replacement of a 5-mC with an unmethylated cytosine. AID may promote aberrant gene expression by decreasing the promoter DNA methylation of specific genes (Munoz et al., 2013; Isobe et al., 2013). Some of the Dnmt inhibitors such as zebularine, ASTX727, and THU also act as inhibitors of AID.

In the field of epigenetic modifiers, histone deacetylase inhibitors have also shown much promise. There are four different classes of HDACs (I, II, III, and IV), which are established based on function and similarity to yeast proteins. HDACs are involved in the deacetylation not only of chromatin proteins, which can lead to altered gene transcription regulation, but also of nonhistone proteins, which regulate important functions that, in turn, regulate cellular homeostasis (cell cycle progression, differentiation, and apoptosis). Many of these pathways are abnormal in tumor cells and consequently can be targeted by HDAC inhibitor therapy (Ahmad et al., 2012). HDAC inhibitors have been shown, in a preclinical setting, to be effective anticancer agents via multiple mechanisms, by upregulating expression of tumor suppressor genes, inhibiting oncogenes, inhibiting tumor angiogenesis and upregulating the immune system. HDAC inhibitors for glioblastoma therapy have been reviewed recently (Lee et al., 2015). Suberanilo-hydroxamic acid (SAHA) (vorinostat) is one of the most well-known and best-studied HDAC inhibitors, which has also been approved for the treatment of cutaneous T-cell lymphoma by the FDA in 2006. Valproate is a Class I and IIa HDAC inhibitor that have been approved by the FDA. Belinostat, an HDAC class I and class II inhibitor has been approved by the FDA for the treatment of relapsed or refractory peripheral T-cell lymphoma. Boks et al. have reviewed the effect of several antipsychotics, antidepressants, and mood stabilizers on epigenetic processes such as DNA methylation and histone modifications (Boks et al., 2012).

The FDA approval of some of the drugs targeting epigenetic machinery highlights the validity of the epigenome as a therapeutic target, and this is slowly emerging as a major therapeutic strategy.

EPIGENOMICS AND ETHNOPHARMACOLOGY

Many recent studies on traditional medicines are now focusing their effect on the epigenetic machinery, such as histone modification, DNA methylation, and siRNA- or miRNA-based silencing. The effect of dietary phytochemicals such as curcumin on epigenetic modifications and their role in cancer therapy and prevention have been reviewed. Epigenetic patterns have recently been used to differentiate between natural and the ex situ medicinal plant, Rhodiola sachalinensis (Zhao et al., 2014). Treatment of middle- and late-stage tumor patients receiving chemotherapy with a Chinese medicine, Dujieqing Oral Liquid (DJQ), has been shown to reduce the promoter methylation of the O6-methylguanine-DNA methyltransferase (MGMT) gene (Rong et al., 2012). Treatment with arsenic-containing Chinese herbal formulas resulted in significant genome-wide demethylation in myelodysplastic syndrome patients (Shuzhen et al., 2012). The herbal compound cryptotanshinone from the Chinese herb *Salvia miltiorrhiza* has been shown to down regulate androgen receptor signaling by modulating LSD1 function in prostate cancer patients (Wu et al., 2012). Tanshinone IIA was found to improve cell resistance to hypoxic insult by upregulating miR-133 expression in neonatal cardiomyocytes (Zhang et al., 2012). It was also shown to repress miR-1 in a rat model of myocardial infarction (Shan et al., 2009). The TCM medicine berberine has been suggested to suppress multiple myeloma cell growth by down regulating miR-21 levels (Luo et al., 2014). Another study suggests that berberine treatment results in p53-dependent up regulation of miR-23, which is responsible for its antihepatocellular carcinoma effect (Wang et al., 2014b). The TCM TianMai Xiaoke tablet, which is used to treat type 2 diabetes, has been shown to improve blood glucose in diabetic rats, which involved increasing the expression of miR-375 and miR-30d to activate an insulin synthesis in islet (Zhang et al., 2014). The TCM Jian Jing has been reported to regulate differential miRNA expression in serum of patients with Myasthenia gravis, thereby affecting clinical symptoms of patients (Jiang et al., 2014). The traditional Asian medicine sho-saiko-to, used for chronic liver diseases, was found to affect the expression of genes from the cell cycle pathway, metabolism-related and immune-related pathways through regulation of micro-RNAs in primary mouse hepatocytes (Song et al., 2014).

Modulation of miRNA expression has been suggested to be an important mechanism of inhibiting breast cancer cell growth by Aidi injection, which is a Chinese herbal preparation with an anticancer activity (Zhang et al., 2011). miR-21 has been suggested to be one of the therapeutic targets for the TCM tongxinluo used to treat diabetic nephropathy (Wang et al., 2014a).

In our work on asthma, we have observed that an Ayurvedic regimen treatment brings epigenetic changes manifesting modulation of circulating cytokines and reduction in plasma IgE (Joshi et al., 2016). Bioinformatics is one of the in silico tools to predict epigenetic targets of medicinal herbs. A materia-medica—wide, bioinformatic analysis of TCM medicines was carried out to identify constituent chemicals that interact with human histone-modifying enzymes. This study showed that 1170 or 36% of the 3294 TCM medicines interact with human histone-modifying enzymes (Hsieh et al., 2013).

LIMITATIONS AND SCOPE

Epigenetic mechanisms are largely studied in isolation, despite the fact that neither histone modifications nor DNA methylation act independently. Simultaneous studies on these different levels of epigenetic modification would provide a better insight into relevant epigenetic interactions, their role in disease etiopathology, and also aid in designing therapeutic strategies. Further, epigenetic mechanisms such as ubiquitination, sumoylation, RNA- and polycomb-based mechanisms are not yet fully understood, and so more research is required in this direction. Issues such as delivery of miRNAs to localized areas remain unaddressed (Byrne et al., 2014).

There has been much focus on epigenetic therapies in cancer, and a similar emphasis on epigenetic alterations that underlie the pathology of a number of diseases ranging from infectious to noninfectious and chronic is much needed.

Although several epigenome-based drug targets and therapies have been researched, their progression from bench to bedside has been limited. This is mainly because many of the epigenetic therapies have nonspecific actions and may have unwanted side effects. Designing a specific drug for a given target is a major challenge faced by researchers (Joshi et al., 2012).

Several ongoing clinical trials are examining novel epigenetic therapies that may provide greater specificity and fewer side effects than the current FDA-approved epigenetic therapies. There is also increased interest in investigating the role of dietary components (Szarc vel et al., 2010) and traditional medicines in regulating epigenetic events.

REFERENCES

Agaisse, H., Burrack, L., Philips, J., Rubin, E., Perrimon, N., Higgins, D., 2005. Genome-wide RNAi screen for host factors required for intracellular bacterial infection. Science 309 (5738), 1248−1251.

Agrawal, N., Dasaradhi, P.V.N., Mohmmed, A., Malhotra, P., Bhatnagar, R.K., Mukherjee, S.K., 2003. RNA interference: biology, mechanism, and applications. Microbiol. Mol. Biol. Rev. 67 (4), 657−685. Available from: <http://mmbr.asm.org/cgi/doi/10.1128/MMBR.67.4.657-685.2003>.

Ahmad, M., Hamid, A., Hussain, A., Majeed, R., Qurishi, Y., Bhat, J., et al., 2012. Understanding histone deacetylases in the cancer development and treatment: an epigenetic perspective of cancer chemotherapy. DNA Cell. Biol. 31 (Suppl. 1), S62−S71.

Ahsan, S., Raabe, E., Haffner, M., Vaghasia, A., Warren, K., Quezado, M., et al., 2014. Increased 5-hydroxymethylcytosine and decreased 5-methylcytosine are indicators of global epigenetic dysregulation in diffuse intrinsic pontine glioma. Acta Neuropathol. Commun. 2, 59.

Ammal, K.N., Tarannum, S., Thomas, B., 2013. Epigenetic landscape of Parkinson's disease: emerging role in disease mechanisms and therapeutic modalities. Neurotherapeutics 10 (4), 698−708.

Ashburn, T., Thor, K., 2004. Drug repositioning: identifying and developing new uses for existing drugs. Nat. Rev. Drug Discov. 3, 673−683.

Aubé, J., 2012. Drug repurposing and the medicinal chemist. ACS Med. Chem. Lett. 3, 442−444.

Azad, N., Krishnan, A., Iyer, V., Rojanasakul, Y., 2008. DNA microarrays in drug discovery and development. In: Wu-Pong, S., Rojanasakul, Y. (Eds.), Biopharmaceutical Drug Design and Development. Humana Press, New Jersey, pp. 47−66.

Bai, J.P.F., Alekseyenko, A.V., Statnikov, A., Wang, I.M., Wong, P.H., 2013. Strategic applications of gene expression: from drug discovery/development to bedside. AAPS J. 15 (2), 427−437.

Barker, D., 1995. Fetal origins of coronary heart disease. BMJ 311, 171−174.

Bartlett, D.W., Davis, M.E., 2006. Insights into the kinetics of siRNA-mediated gene silencing from live-cell and live-animal bioluminescent imaging. Nucleic. Acids Res. 34 (1), 322−333.

Bartlett, D.W., Davis, M.E., 2007. Effect of siRNA nuclease stability on the in vitro and in vivo kinetics of siRNA-mediated gene silencing. Biotechnol. Bioeng. 97 (4), 909−921.

Behlke, M., 2006. Progress towards in vivo use of siRNAs. Mol. Ther. 13 (4), 644−670.

Bennett, D., Yu, L., Yang, J., Srivastava, G., Aubin, C., De Jager, P., 2015. Epigenomics of Alzheimer's disease. Transl. Res. 165 (1), 200−220.

Berns, K., Hijmans, E., Mullenders, J., Brummelkamp, T., Velds, A., Heimerikx, M., et al., 2004. A large-scale RNAi screen in human cells identifies new components of the p53 pathway. Nature 428, 431−437.

Bhat, K.P., Greer, S.F., 2011. Proteolytic and non-proteolytic roles of ubiquitin and the ubiquitin proteasome system in transcriptional regulation. Biochim. Biophys. Acta 1809 (2), 150−155.

Bhinder, B.D., Djaballah, H., 2013. A decade of RNAi screening: too much hay & very few needles. Drug Disc. World 14, 31−41.

Bidon, C., Lachuer, J., Molgó, J., Wierinckx, A., Porte de la, S., Pignol, B., et al., 2009. The extract of Ginkgo biloba EGb 761 reactivates a juvenile profile in the skeletal muscle of sarcopenic rats by transcriptional reprogramming. PLoS ONE 4 (11), e7998.

Boks, M., de Jong, N., Kas, M., Vinkers, C., Fernandes, C., Kahn, R., et al., 2012. Current status and future prospects for epigenetic psychopharmacology. Epigenetics 7 (1), 20−28.

Bragonzi, A., Dina, G., Villa, A., Calori, G., Biffi, A., Bordignon, C., et al., 2000. Biodistribution and transgene expression with nonviral cationic vector/DNA complexes in the lungs. Gene. Ther. 7 (20), 1753−1760.

Brenner, S., Williams, S., Vermaas, E., Storck, T., Moon, K., McCollum, C., et al., 2000. In vitro cloning of complex mixtures of DNA on microbeads: physical separation of differentially expressed cDNAs. Proc. Natl. Acad. Sci. USA. 97 (4), 1665−1670.

Brummelkamp, T.R., Fabius, A.W.M., Mullenders, J., Madiredjo, M., Velds, A., Kerkhoven, R.M., et al., 2006. An shRNA barcode screen provides insight into cancer cell vulnerability to MDM2 inhibitors. Nat. Chem. Biol. 2 (4), 202−206.

Buyens, K., Lucas, B., Raemdonck, K., Braeckmans, K., Vercammen, J., Hendrix, J., et al., 2008. A fast and sensitive method for measuring the integrity of siRNA-carrier complexes in full human serum. J. Control. Release 126 (1), 67−76.

Byrne, M., Murphy, R., Ryan, A., 2014. Epigenetic modulation in the treatment of atherosclerotic disease. Front Genet. 5, 364.

Cabezas-Cruz, A., Lancelot, J., Caby, S., Oliveira, G., Pierce, R., 2014. Epigenetic control of gene function in schistosomes: a source of therapeutic targets? Front Genet. 10 (5), 317.

Cacabelos, R., Torrellas, C., López-Muñoz, F., 2014. Epigenomics of Alzheimer's disease. J. Exp. Clin. Med. 6 (3), 75−82.

Callinan, P., Feinberg, A., 2006. The emerging science of epigenomics. Hum. Mol. Genet. 15 (1), R95−101.

Calo, S., Shertz-Wall, C., Lee, S.C., Bastidas, R.J., Nicolás, F.E., Granek, J.A., et al., 2014. Antifungal drug resistance evoked via RNAi-dependent epimutations. Nature 513 (7519), 555−558.

Cases, M., Mestres, J., 2009. A chemogenomic approach to drug discovery: focus on cardiovascular diseases. Drug. Discov. Today 14 (9-10), 479−485.

Chavan-Gautam, P., Sundrani, D., Pisal, H., Nimbargi, V., Mehendale, S., Joshi, S., 2011. Gestation-dependent changes in human placental global DNA methylation levels. Mol. Reprod. Dev. 78 (3), 150.

Chen, C.-C., 2011. TCM database@Taiwan: the world's largest traditional Chinese medicine database for drug screening in silico. PLoS ONE 6, e15939.

Chen, H., Yu, S., Chen, J.J.W., Li, H., Lin, Y., Yao, P., et al., 2004. Anti-invasive gene expression profile of curcumin in lung adenocarcinoma based on a high throughput microarray analysis. Mol. Pharmacol. 65 (1), 99−110.

Chen, J., Xie, J., 2012. Progress on RNAi-based molecular medicines. Int. J. Nanomed. 7, 3971−3980.

Cheng, H.M., Li, C.C., Chen, C.Y., Lo, H.Y., Cheng, W.Y., Lee, C.H., et al., 2010. Application of bioactivity database of Chinese herbal medicine on the therapeutic prediction, drug development, and safety evaluation. J. Ethnopharmacol. 132 (2), 429−437.

Coppieters, N., Dieriks, B.V., Lill, C., Faull, R.L., Curtis, M.A., Dragunow, M., 2013. Global changes in DNA methylation and hydroxymethylation in Alzheimer's disease human brain. Neurobiol. Aging 6, 1334−1344.

Cossart, P., Lebreton, A., 2014. A trip in the "New Microbiology" with the bacterial pathogen *Listeria monocytogenes*. FEBS Lett. 588 (15), 2437−2445.

Crujeiras, A., Casanueva, F., 2015. Obesity and the reproductive system disorders: epigenetics as a potential bridge. Hum. Rehprod. Update 21 (2), 249−261.

Dayeh, T., Volkov, P., Salö, S., Hall, E., Nilsson, E., Olsson, A., et al., 2014. Genome-wide DNA methylation analysis of human pancreatic islets from type 2 diabetic and non-diabetic donors identifies candidate genes that influence insulin secretion. PLoS Genet. 10 (3), e1004160.

Densmore, C., 2000. Aerosol delivery of robust polyethyleneimine−DNA complexes for gene therapy and genetic immunization. Mol. Ther. 1 (2), 180−188. Available from: <http://www.nature.com/doifinder/10.1006/mthe.1999.0021>.

Desai, M., Jellyman, J., Ross, M., 2015. Epigenomics, gestational programming and risk of metabolic syndrome. Int. J. Obes. 39 (4), 633−641.

Diwadkar V, Bustamante, A., Rai, H., Uddin, M., 2014. Epigenetics, stress, and their potential impact on brain network function: a focus on the schizophrenia diatheses. Front Psychiatry 5, 71.

Dopazo, J., 2014. Genomics and transcriptomics in drug discovery. Drug. Discov. Today 19 (2), 126–132.

Dorschner, M., Hawrylycz, M., Humbert, R., Wallace, J., Shafer, A., Kawamoto, J., et al., 2004. High-throughput localization of functional elements by quantitative chromatin profiling. Nat. Methods 1 (3), 219–225.

Estampador, A., Franks, P., 2014. Genetic and epigenetic catalysts in early-life programming of adult cardiometabolic disorders. Diabetes Metab. Syndr. Obes. 1 (7), 575–586.

Feinberg, A., 2007. Phenotypic plasticity and the epigenetics of human disease. Nature 447, 433–440.

Feng, Y., Jankovic, J., Wu, Y., 2015. Epigenetic mechanisms in Parkinson's disease. J. Neurol. Sci. 349 (1-2), 3–9.

Freedman, J.D., Loscalzo, J., 2009. In: Freedman, J.E., Loscalzo, J. (Eds.), In new therapeutic agents in thrombosis and thrombolysis, third ed. Informa Healthcare, CRC Press, New York.

Futami, T., Miyagishi, M., Taira, K., 2005. Identification of a network involved in thapsigargin-induced apoptosis using a library of small interfering RNA expression vectors. J. Biol. Chem. 280 (1), 826–831.

Gadgil, M.S., Joshi, K.S., Naik, S.S., Pandit, A.N., Otiv, S.R., Patwardhan, B.K., 2014. Association of homocysteine with global DNA methylation in vegetarian Indian pregnant women and neonatal birth anthropometrics. J. Matern. Neonatal. Med. 27 (17), 1749–1753. Available from: <http://www.tandfonline.com/doi/full/10.3109/14767058.2013.879702>.

Galizzi, J., Lockhart, B., Bril, A., 2013. Applying systems biology in drug discovery and development. Drug Metab. Drug Interact. 28 (2), 67–78.

Gambichler, T., Sand, M., Skrygan, M., 2013. Loss of 5-hydroxymethylcytosine and teneleven translocation 2 protein expression in malignant melanoma. Melanoma. Res. 23, 218–220.

Gao, K., Huang, L., 2013. Achieving efficient RNAi therapy: progress and challenges. Acta Pharm. Sin. B 3 (4), 213–225.

Ge, Z., Zhang, C., Schatten, H., Sun, Q., 2014. Maternal diabetes mellitus and the origin of non-communicable diseases in offspring: the role of epigenetics. Biol. Reprod. 90 (6), 139.

Govindarajan, V.S., 1980. Turmeric—Chemistry, Technology and Quality. Crit. Rev. Food. Sci. Nutr. 12 (3), 199–301.

Guidotti, A., Auta, J., Davis, J., Dong, E., Gavin, D., Grayson, D., et al., 2014. Toward the identification of peripheral epigenetic biomarkers of schizophrenia. J. Neurogenet. 28 (1–2), 41–52.

Hamm, C.A., Costa, F.F., 2015. Epigenomes as therapeutic targets. Pharmacol Ther 151, 72–86.

Hassan, A.H., Prochasson, P., Neely, K.E., Galasinski, S.C., Chandy, M., Carrozza, M.J., et al., 2002. Function and selectivity of bromodomains in anchoring chromatin-modifying complexes to promoter nucleosomes. Cell 111, 369–379.

Hattori, N., Ushijima, T., 2014. Compendium of aberrant DNA methylation and histone modifications in cancer. Biochem. Biophys. Res. Commun. 455 (1–2), 3–9.

Heijmans, B., Tobi, E., Stein, A., Putter, H., Blauw, G., Susser, E., et al., 2008. Persistent epigenetic differences associated with prenatal exposure to famine in humans. Proc. Natl. Acad. Sci. U. S. A. 105, 17046–17049.

Hood, L.L., Perlmutter, R., 2004. The impact of systems approaches on biological problems in drug discovery. Nat. Biotechnol. 22, 1215–1217.

Hopkins, A.L., 2008. Network pharmacology: the next paradigm in drug discovery. Nat. Chem. Biol. 4, 682–690.

Houghten, R., Pinilla, C., Appel, J., Blondelle, S., Dooley, C., Eichler, J., et al., 1999. Mixture-based synthetic combinatorial libraries. J. Med. Chem. 42, 3743−3778.

Hsieh, H., Chiu, P., Wang, S., 2013. Histone modifications and traditional Chinese medicinals. BMC Compl. Altern. Med. 13, 115.

Huang, M., Smart, R.C., Wong, C., Conney, A.H., 1988. Inhibitory effect of curcumin, chlorogenic acid, caffeic acid, and ferulic acid on tumor promotion in mouse skin by 12-O-Tetradecanoylphorbol-13-acetate. Cancer Res. 48 (21), 5941−5946.

Im, G., Choi, Y., 2013. Epigenetics in osteoarthritis and its implication for future therapeutics. Expert. Opin. Biol. Ther. 13 (5), 713−721.

Impey, S., McCorkle, S.R., Cha-Molstad, H., Dwyer, J.M., Yochum, G.S., Boss, J.M., et al., 2004. Defining the CREB regulon: a genome-wide analysis of transcription factor regulatory regions. Cell 119, 1041−1054.

Ingle, N.P., Malone, B., Reineke, T.M., 2011. Poly(glycoamidoamine)s: a broad class of carbohydrate-containing polycations for nucleic acid delivery. Trends Biotechnol. 29 (9), 443−453.

Isobe, T., Song, S.N., Tiwari, P., Ito, H., Yamaguchi, Y., Yoshizaki, K., 2013. Activation induced cytidine deaminase auto-activates and triggers aberrant gene expression. FEBS Lett. 587, 2487−2492.

Jawert, F., Hasseus, B., Kjeller, G., Magnusson, B., Sand, L., Larsson, L., 2013. Loss of 5-hydroxymethylcytosine and TET2 in oral squamous cell carcinoma. Anticancer Res. 33, 4325−4328.

Jiang, C., Liu, P., Zhang, J., Bao, W., Qiu, S., Liang, Y., et al., 2014. Clinical study of effects of Jian Ji Ning, a Chinese herbal medicine compound preparation, in treating patients with Myasthenia gravis via the regulation of differential MicroRNAs expression in serum. Evid. Based Compl. Altern. Med. 2014, 518942.

Joshi, K., Bhat, S., Deshpande, P., Sule, M., Satyamoorthy, K., 2012. Epigenetic mechanisms and degenerative diseases. Open J. Genet. 2, 173−183.

Joshi K., Nesari T., Dedge A., Dhumal V., Shengule S., Gadgil M., et al., Dosha Phenotype specific Ayurveda intervention ameliorates asthma symptoms through cytokine modulations: Results of whole system clinical trial. J. Ethnopharmacol. Available from: <http://dx.doi.org/10.1016/j.jep.2016.07.071>.

Kadioglu, O., Efferth, T., 2014. Contributions from emerging transcriptomics technologies and computational strategies for drug discovery. Invest. New Drugs 32 (6), 1316−1319.

Kerem, E., Konstan, M.W., De Boeck, K., Accurso, F.J., Sermet-Gaudelus, I., Wilschanski, M., et al., 2014. Ataluren for the treatment of nonsense-mutation cystic fibrosis: a randomised, double-blind, placebo-controlled phase 3 trial. Lancet Respir. Med. 2 (7), 539−547. Available from: <http://dx.doi.org/10.1016/S2213-2600(14)70100-6>.

Kim, J.B., Porreca, G.J., 2007. Polony multiplex analysis of gene expression (PMAGE) in mouse hypertrophic cardiomyopathy. Science 316 (5830), 1481−1484.

Kinney, S., Pradhan, S., 2013. Ten eleven translocation enzymes and 5-hydroxymethylation in mammalian development and cancer. Adv. Exp. Med. Biol. 754, 57−79.

Ko, H., Gelb, B., 2014. Concise review: drug discovery in the age of the induced pluripotent stem cell. Stem Cells Transl. Med. 3 (4), 500−509.

Ko, M., Huang, Y., Jankowska, A., Pape, U., Tahiliani, M., Bandukwala, H., et al., 2010. Impaired hydroxylation of 5-methylcytosine in myeloid cancers with mutant TET2. Nature 468 (7325), 839−843.

Kraus, T.F., Globisch, D., Wagner, M., Eigenbrod, S., Widmann, D., Munzel, M., et al., 2012. Low values of 5-hydroxymethylcytosine (5hmC), the sixth base, are associated with anaplasia in human brain tumors. Int. J. Cancer 31 (7), 1577–1590.

Krol, J., Loedige, I., Filipowicz, W., 2010. The widespread regulation of microRNA biogenesis, function and decay. Nat. Rev. Genet. 11 (9), 597–610.

Kubinová, Š., Syková, E., 2010. Nanotechnology for treatment of stroke and spinal cord injury. Nanomedicine 5 (1), 99–108.

Kulkarni, A., Chavan-Gautam, P., Mehendale, S., Yadav, H., Joshi, S., 2011. Global DNA methylation patterns in placenta and its association with maternal hypertension in pre-eclampsia. DNA Cell. Biol. 30 (2), 79–84.

Kumar, A., Asthana, M., Sharma, S., Roy, P., Amdekar, S., Singh, V., et al., 2012. Importance of using DNA microarray in studying medicinal plant. Webmed Central Molecular Biology 3 (12). Available from: < http://dx.doi.org/10.9754/journal.wmc.2012.003876; https://www.webmedcentral.com/article_view/3876>.

Lagerqvist, J., Zwolak, M., Di Ventra, M., 2006. Fast DNA sequencing via transverse electronic transport. Nano. Lett. 6 (4), 779–782.

Landgrave-Gómez, J., Mercado-Gómez, O., Guevara-Guzmán, R., 2015. Epigenetic mechanisms in neurological and neurodegenerative diseases. Front Cell Neurosci. 27 (9), 58.

Lauro, G., Romano, A., Riccio, R., Bifulco, G., 2011. Inverse virtual screening of antitumor targets: pilot study on a small database of natural bioactive compounds. J. Nat. Prod. 74, 1401–1407.

Lee, P., Murphy, B., Miller, R., Menon, V., Banik, N., Giglio, P., et al., 2015. Mechanisms and clinical significance of histone deacetylase inhibitors:epigenetic glioblastoma therapy. Anticancer Res. 35 (2), 615–625.

Li, S., Kong, L., Yu, X., Zheng, Y., 2014. Host-virus interactions: from the perspectives of epigenetics. Rev. Med. Virol. 24 (4), 223–241.

Lian, C.G., Xu, Y., Ceol, C., Wu, F., Larson, A., Dresser, K., et al., 2012. Loss of 5-hydroxymethylcytosine is an epigenetic hallmark of melanoma. Cell 150, 1135–1146.

Lin, B., Wang, J., Cheng, Y., 2008. Recent patents and advances in the next-generation sequencing technologies. Recent Pat. Biomed. Eng. 2008 (1), 60–67. Available from: <http://www.ncbi.nlm.nih.gov/pubmed/3122325; http://www.ncbi.nlm.nih.gov/pmc/articles/PMC3122325; http://www.pubmedcentral.nih.gov/articlerender.fcgi?artid=3122325&tool=pmcentrez&rendertype=abstract>.

Lister, R., Pelizzola, M., Dowen, R.H., Hawkins, R.D., Hon, G., Tonti-Filippini, J., et al., 2009. Human DNA methylomes at base resolution show widespread epigenomic differences. Nature 462, 315–322.

Lo, H.Y., Li, C.C., Huang, H.C., Lin, L.J., Hsiang, C.Y., Ho, T.Y., 2012. Application of transcriptomics in Chinese herbal medicine studies. J. Tradit. Compl. Med. 2 (2), 105–114.

López-Vallejo, F., Giulianotti, M., Houghten, R., Medina-Franco, J., 2012. Expanding the medicinally relevant chemical space with compound libraries. Drug Discov. Today 17, 718–726.

Lorincz, A., 2014. Cancer diagnostic classifiers based on quantitative DNA methylation. Expert. Rev. Mol. Diagn. 14 (3), 293–305.

Luo, X., Gu, J., Zhu, R., Feng, M., Zhu, X., Li, Y., et al., 2014. Integrative analysis of differential miRNA and functional study of miR-21 by seed-targeting inhibition in multiple myeloma cells in response to berberine. BMC Syst. Biol. 8, 82.

Ma, R., Tutino, G., Lillycrop, K., Hanson, M., Tam, W., 2015. Maternal diabetes, gestational diabetes and the role of epigenetics in their long term effects on offspring. Prog. Biophys. Mol. Biol. S0079–6107 (15), 00035–00038.

MacKeigan, J.P., Murphy, L.O., Blenis, J., 2005. Sensitized RNAi screen of human kinases and phosphatases identifies new regulators of apoptosis and chemoresistance. Nat. Cell. Biol. 7 (6), 591−600.

Mahadevan, S., Park, Y., 2008. Multifaceted therapeutic benefits of *Ginkgo biloba* L: chemistry, efficacy, safety, and uses. J. Food Sci. 73 (1), R14−R19. Available from: <http://www.ncbi.nlm.nih.gov/pubmed/18211362>.

Mahgoub, M., Monteggia, L., 2013. Epigenetics and psychiatry. Neurotherapeutics 10 (4), 734−741.

Main, H., Munsie, M., O'Connor, M., 2014. Managing the potential and pitfalls during clinical translation of emerging stem cell therapies. Clin. Transl. Med. 3, 10.

Malone, J.H., Oliver, B., 2011. Microarrays, deep sequencing and the true measure of the transcriptome. BMC Biol. 9, 34.

McElroy, S.P., Nomura, T., Torrie, L.S., Warbrick, E., Gartner, U., Wood, G., et al., 2013. A lack of premature termination codon read-through efficacy of PTC124 (Ataluren) in a diverse array of reporter assays. PLoS Biol. 11 (6).

Medina-Franco, J.L., Martinez-Mayorga, K., Giulianotti, M.A., Houghten, R.A., Pinilla, C., 2008. Visualization of the chemical space in drug discovery. Curr. Comput. Aided Drug Des. 4, 322−333.

Meller, A., Branton, D., 2002. Single molecule measurements of DNA transport through a nanopore. Electrophoresis 23 (16), 2583−2591.

Meller, A., Nivon, L., Brandin, E., Golovchenko, J., Branton, D., 2000. Rapid nanopore discrimination between single polynucleotide molecules. Proc. Natl. Acad. Sci. U. S. A. 97 (3), 1079−1084. Available from: <http://www.pnas.org/cgi/doi/10.1073/pnas.97.3.1079>.

Miller C., The impact of RNAi on drug discovery, Target Validation, Drug Discovery World Spring 2005, 41−46.

Mishra, P., Givvimani, S., Chavali, V., Tyagi, S., 2013. Cardiac matrix: a clue for future therapy. Biochim. Biophys. Acta 1832 (12), 2271−2276.

Mitra, R.D., Church, G.M., 1999. In situ localized amplification and contact replication of many individual DNA molecules. Nucleic. Acids Res. 27, 24.

Modi, G., Pillay, V., Choonara, Y.E., Ndesendo, V.M.K., Toit, L.C., du, Naidoo, D., 2009. Nanotechnological applications for the treatment of neurodegenerative disorders. Prog. Neurobiol. 88 (4), 272−285.

Mullard, A., 2012. 2011 FDA drug approvals. Nat. Rev. Drug Discov.(11), 91−94.

Munoz, D.P., Lee, E.L., Takayama, S., Coppe, J.P., Heo, S.J., Boffelli, D., et al., 2013. Activation-induced cytidine deaminase (AID) is necessary for the epithelial−mesenchymal transition inmammary epithelial cells. Proc. Natl. Acad. Sci. U. S. A. 110, E2977−E2986.

Munzel, M., Globisch, D., Carell, T., 2011. 5-hydroxymethylcytosine, the sixth base of the genome. Angew. Chem. Int. Ed. Engl. 50, 6460−6468.

Myllykangas, S., Buenrostro, J., Ji, H.P., 2012. Overview of sequencing technology platforms. Bioinformatics for High Throughput Sequencing. Springer, New York, NY, pp. 11−25.

National Research Council (US) Committee on Applications of Toxicogenomic Technologies to Predictive Toxicology, 2007. Applications of Toxicogenomic Technologies to Predictive Toxicology and Risk Assessment. National Academies Press (US), Washington (DC). Available from: < http://www.ncbi.nlm.nih.gov/books/NBK10219/; http://dx.doi:10.17226/12037>.

Natsch, A., 2010. The Nrf2-Keap1-ARE toxicity pathway as a cellular sensor for skin sensitizers--functional relevance and a hypothesis on innate reactions to skin sensitizers. Toxicol. Sci. 113 (2), 284−292.

Ng, S.B., Buckingham, K.J., Lee, C., Bigham, A.W., Tabor, H.K., Dent, K.M., et al., 2010. Exome sequencing identifies the cause of a mendelian disorder. Nat. Genet. 42 (1), 30−35.

Nührenberg, T., Gilsbach, R., Preissl, S., Schnick, T., Hein, L., 2014. Epigenetics in cardiac development, function, and disease. Cell Tissue Res. 356 (3), 585−600.

Orive, G., Anitua, E., Pedraz, J.L., Emerich, D.F., 2009. Biomaterials for promoting brain protection, repair and regeneration. Nat. Rev. Neurosci. 10 (9), 682−692.

Orr, B.A., Haffner, M.C., Nelson, W.G., Yegnasubramanian, S., Eberhart, C., 2012. Decreased 5-hydroxymethylcytosine is associated with neural progenitor phenotype in normal brain and shorter survival in malignant glioma. PLoS ONE 7, e41036.

Pacis, A., Nédélec, Y., Barreiro, L., 2014. When genetics meets epigenetics: deciphering the mechanisms controlling inter-individual variation in immune responses to infection. Curr. Opin. Immunol. 29, 119−126.

Pradhan, S., Bacolla, A., Wells, R.D., Roberts, R., 1999. Recombinant human DNA (cytosine-5) methyltransferase I. Expression, purification, and comparison of de novo and maintenance methylation. J. Biol. Chem. 274, 33002−33010.

Provenzale, J.M., Silva, G.A., 2009. Uses of nanoparticles for central nervous system imaging and therapy. AJNR Am. J. Neuroradiol. 30 (7), 1293−1301. Available from: <http://www.ncbi.nlm.nih.gov/pubmed/19617446>.

Raab, R.M., Stephanopoulos, G., 2004. Dynamics of gene silencing by RNA interference. Biotechnol. Bioeng. 88 (1), 121−132.

Rampal, R., Alkalin, A., Madzo, J., Vasanthakumar, A., Pronier, E., Patel, J., et al., 2014. DNA hydroxymethylation profiling reveals that WT1 mutations result in loss of TET2 function in acute myeloid leukemia. Cell Rep. 9 (5), 1841−1855.

Ramsingh, G., Koboldt, D., Trissal, M., Chiappinelli, K., Wylie, T., Koul, S., et al., 2010. Complete characterization of the microRNAome in a patient with acute myeloid leukemia. Blood 116 (24), 5316−5326.

Ray-Gallet, D., Almouzni, G., 2010. Nucleosome dynamics and histone variants. Essays Biochem. 48, 75−87.

Rhee, M., Burns, M.A., 2006. Nanopore sequencing technology: research trends and applications. Trends Biotechnol. 24 (12), 580−586.

Ricke, D., Wang, S., Cai, R., Cohen, D., 2006. Genomic approaches to drug discovery. Curr. Opin. Chem. Biol. 10 (4), 303−308.

Rollinger, J., 2009. Accessing target information by virtual parallel screening−the impact on natural product research. Phytochem. Lett. 2, 53−58.

Ronaghi, M., Karamohamed, S., Pettersson, B., Uhlén, M., Nyrén, P., 1996. Real-time DNA sequencing using detection of pyrophosphate release. Anal. Biochem. 242 (1), 84−89.

Rong, Z., Xu, Y., Mo, C., 2012. Effects of dujieqing oral liquid on the promoter methylation of the MGMT gene in middle-and-late stage tumor patients receiving chemotherapy. Chin. J. Integr. Tradit. West Med. 32 (12), 1611−1615.

Roy, A., McDonald, P., Sittampalam, S., Chaguturu, R., 2010. Open access high throughput drug discovery in the public domain: a Mount Everest in the making. Curr. Pharm. Biotechnol. 11, 764−778.

Rudolph, C., Müller, R.H., Rosenecker, J., 2002. Jet nebulization of PEI/DNA polyplexes: physical stability and in vitro gene delivery efficiency. J. Gene. Med. 4 (1), 66−74.

Russo, G., Zegar, C., Giordano, A., 2003. Advantages and limitations of microarray technology in human cancer. Oncogene 22 (42), 6497−6507.

Sanchez, R., Zhou, M., 2009. The role of human bromodomains in chromatin biology and gene transcription. Curr. Opin. Drug. Discov. Devel. 12, 659−665.

Schaefer, M., Lyko, F., 2010. Solving the Dnmt2 enigma. Chromosoma 119 (1), 35−40.

Shan, H., Li, X., Pan, Z., Zhang, L., Cai, B., Zhang, Y., et al., 2009. Tanshinone IIA protects against sudden cardiac death induced by lethalarrhythmias via repression of microRNA-1. Br. J. Pharmacol. 158 (5), 1227−1235.

Shastry, B.S., 2012. Role of Epigenomics in Drug Discovery and Therapies. Drug. Develop. Res 73 (8), 513−517.

Shendure, J., Ji, H., 2008. Next-generation DNA sequencing. Nat. Biotechnol. 26 (10), 1135−1145.

Shendure, J., Mitra, R.D., Varma, C., Church, G.M., 2004. Advanced sequencing technologies: methods and goals. Nat. Rev. Genet. 5 (5), 335−344.

Shuzhen, S., Rou, M., Xiaomei, H., Xiao-Hong, Y., Yong-Gang, X., Hongzhi, W., et al., 2012. Karyotype and DNA-methylation responses in myelodysplastic syndromes following treatment with traditional Chinese formula containing arsenic. Evid. Based Compl. Altern. Med. 2012, 969476.

Silmon de Monerri, N., Kim, K., 2014. Pathogens hijack the epigenome: a new twist on host-pathogen interactions. Am. J. Pathol. 184 (4), 897−911.

Sinclair, S., Rennoll-Bankert, K., Dumler, J., 2014. Effector bottleneck: microbial reprogramming of parasitized host cell transcription by epigenetic remodeling of chromatin structure. Front Genet. 5, 274.

Song, K., Kim, Y., Kim, B., 2014. Sho-saiko-to, a traditional herbal medicine, regulates gene expression and biological function by way of microRNAs in primary mouse hepatocytes. BMC Compl. Altern. Med. 14, 14.

Struhl, K., 1998. Histone acetylation and transcriptional regulatory mechanisms. Genes Dev. 12, 599−606.

Stunnenberg, H., Vermeulen, M., 2011. Towards cracking the epigenetic code using a combination of high-throughput epigenomics and quantitative mass spectrometry-based proteomics. Bioessays 33, 547−551.

Su, S.-Y., Hsieh, C.-L., Wu, S.-L., Cheng, W.-Y., Li, C.-C., Lo, H.-Y., et al., 2009. Transcriptomic analysis of EGb 761-regulated neuroactive receptor pathway in vivo. J. Ethnopharmacol. 123, 68−73.

Sun, H., 2007. US20070202521A1.

Sundrani, D.P., Reddy, U.S., Joshi, A.A., Mehendale, S.S., Chavan-Gautam, P.M., Hardikar, A.A., et al., 2013. Differential placental methylation and expression of VEGF, FLT-1 and KDR genes in human term and preterm preeclampsia. Clin. Epigenetics 5 (1), 6. Available from: <http://www.pubmedcentral.nih.gov/articlerender.fcgi?artid = 3640948&tool = pmcentrez rendertype = abstract>.

Sundrani, D.P., Reddy, U.S., Chavan-Gautam, P.M., Mehendale, S.S., Chandak, G.R., Joshi, S. R., 2014. Altered methylation and expression patterns of genes regulating placental angiogenesis in preterm pregnancy. Reprod. Sci. 21 (12), 1508−1517. Available from: <http://rsx.sagepub.com/cgi/doi/10.1177/1933719114532838>.

Szarc vel, S.K., Ndlovu, M., Haegeman, G., Vanden, B.W., 2010. Nature or nurture: let food be your epigenetic medicine in chronic inflammatory disorders. Biochem. Pharmacol. 80, 1816−1832.

Tahiliani, M., Koh, K.P., Shen, Y., Pastor, W.A., Bandukwala, H., Brudno, Y., et al., 2009. Conversion of 5-methylcytosine to 5-hydroxymethylcytosine in mammalian DNA by MLL partner TET1. Science 324, 930−935.

Tang, F., Barbacioru, C., Wang, Y., Nordman, E., Lee, C., Xu, N., et al., 2009. mRNA-Seq whole-transcriptome analysis of a single cell. Nat. Methods 6 (5), 377−382.

Tsai, T., Chang, K., Chen, C., 2011. iScreen: world's first cloud-computing web server for virtual screening and de novo drug design based on TCM database@Taiwan. J. Comput. Aided Mol. Des. 25, 525–531.

Van den Haute, C., Eggermont, K., Nuttin, B., Debyser, Z., Baekelandt, V., 2003. Lentiviral vector-mediated delivery of short hairpin RNA results in persistent knockdown of gene expression in mouse brain. Hum. Gene. Ther. 14 (18), 1799–1807.

Van Der Veen, J.W., Pronk, T.E., Van Loveren, H., Ezendam, J., 2013. Applicability of a keratinocyte gene signature to predict skin sensitizing potential. Toxicol. Vitro 27 (1), 314–322.

Vandebriel, R.J., van Loveren, H., 2010. Non-animal sensitization testing: state-of-the-art. Crit. Rev. Toxicol. 40 (5), 389–404.

Verbist, B., Klambauer, G., Vervoort, L., Talloen, W., Shkedy, Z., Thas, O., et al., 2015. Using transcriptomics to guide lead optimization in drug discovery projects: Lessons learned from the QSTAR project. Drug Discov. Today00(00). Available from: <http://www.ncbi.nlm.nih.gov/pubmed/25582842>.

Vrtačnik, P., Marc, J., Ostanek, B., 2014. Epigenetic mechanisms in bone. Clin. Chem. Lab. Med. 52 (5), 589–608.

Wang, J., Gao, Y., Zhang, N., Zou, D., Xu, L., Zhu, Z., et al., 2014a. Tongxinluo ameliorates renal structure and function by regulating miR-21-induced epithelial-to-mesenchymal transition in diabetic nephropathy. Am. J. Physiol. Ren. Physiol. 306 (5), F486–F495.

Wang, N., Zhu, M., Wang, X., Tan, H., Tsao, S., Feng, Y., 2014b. Berberine-induced tumor suppressor p53 up-regulation gets involved in the regulatory network of MIR-23a in hepatocellular carcinoma. Biochim. Biophys. Acta 1839 (9), 849–857.

Welboren, W., van Driel, M., Janssen-Megens, E., van Heeringen, S., et al., 2009. ChIP-Seq of ERalpha and RNA polymerase II defines genes differentially responding to ligands. EMBO J. 28, 1418–1428.

Wilhelm, B.T., Marguerat, S., Goodhead, I., Bähler, J., 2010. Defining transcribed regions using RNA-seq. Nat. Protoc. 5 (2), 255–266.

Woldemichael, B., Bohacek, J., Gapp, K., Mansuy, I., 2014. Epigenetics of memory and plasticity. Prog. Mol. Biol. Transl. Sci. 122, 305–340.

Wu, C., Hsieh, C., Huang, K., Chang, C., Kang, H., 2012. Cryptotanshinone down-regulates androgen receptor signaling by modulating lysine-specific demethylase 1 function. Int. J. Cancer 131 (6), 1423–1434.

Xia, H., Mao, Q., Paulson, H.L., Davidson, B.L., 2002. siRNA-mediated gene silencing in vitro and in vivo. Nat. Biotechnol. 20 (10), 1006–1010.

Xiang, S., Tong, H., Shi, Q., Fernandes, J.C., Jin, T., Dai, K., et al., 2012. Uptake mechanisms of non-viral gene delivery. J. Control Release 158 (3), 371–378.

Yadav, N.K., Shukla, P., Omer, A., Pareek, S., Singh, R.K., 2014. Next generation sequencing: potential and application in drug discovery. Sci. World J. 2014, 802437.

Yamamoto, M., Wakatsuki, T., Hada, A., Ryo, A., 2001. Use of serial analysis of gene expression (SAGE) technology. J. Immunol. Methods 250 (1–2), 45–66.

Yang, H., Liu, Y., Bai, F., Zhang, J.Y., Ma, S.H., Liu, J., et al., 2013. Tumor development is associated with decrease of TET gene expression and 5-methylcytosine hydroxylation. Oncogene 32, 663–669.

Yang, J.P., Fan, W., Rogers, C., Chatterton, J.E., Bliesath, J., Liu, G., et al., 2006. A novel RNAi library based on partially randomized consensus sequences of nuclear receptors: identifying the receptors involved in amyloid beta degradation. Genomics 88 (3), 282–292.

Ylä-Herttuala, S., Alitalo, K., 2003. Gene transfer as a tool to induce therapeutic vascular growth. Nat. Med. 9 (6), 694–701.

Zhang, H., Zhou, Q., Lu, Y., Du, J., Su, S., 2011. Aidi injection alters the expression profiles of microRNAs in human breast cancer cells. J. Tradit. Chin. Med. 31 (1), 10−16.

Zhang, L., Wu, Y., Li, Y., Xu, C., Li, X., Zhu, D., et al., 2012. Tanshinone IIA improves miR-133 expression through MAPK ERK1/2 pathway in hypoxic cardiac myocytes. Cell. Physiol. Biochem. 30 (4), 843−852.

Zhang, Q., Xiao, X., Li, M., Li, W., Yu, M., Zhang, H., et al., 2014. miR-375 and miR-30d in the effect of chromium-containing Chinese medicine moderating glucose metabolism. J. Diabetes Res. 2014, 862473.

Zhao, Q., Sigalov, G., Dimitrov, V., Dorvel, B., Mirsaidov, U., Sligar, S., et al., 2007. Detecting SNPs using a synthetic nanopore. Nano Lett. 7 (6), 1680−1685. Available from: <http://www.pubmed-central.nih.gov/articlerender.fcgi?artid = 2565804&tool = pmcentrez&rendertype = abstract>.

Zhao, W., Shi, X., Li, J., Guo, W., Liu, C., Chen, X., 2014. Genetic, epigenetic, and HPLC fingerprint differentiation between natural and ex situ populations of Rhodiola sachalinensis from Changbai Mountain, China. PLoS ONE 9 (11), e112869.

Zheng, L., Liu, J., Batalov, S., Zhou, D., Orth, A., Ding, S., et al., 2004. An approach to genomewide screens of expressed small interfering RNAs in mammalian cells. Proc. Natl. Acad. Sci. U. S. A. 101 (1), 135−140.

Zheng, X., Lian, D., Wong, A., Bygrave, M., Ichim, T.E., Khoshniat, M., et al., 2009. Novel small interfering RNAp-containing solution protecting donor organs in heart transplantation. Circulation 120 (12), 1099−1107. Available from: <http://circ.ahajournals.org/cgi/doi/10.1161/CIRCULATIONAHA.108.787390>.

Zhou, Q., Zhang, H., Lu, Y., Wang, X., Su, S., 2009. Curcumin reduced the side effects of mitomycin C by inhibiting GRP58-mediated DNA cross-linking in MCF-7 breast cancer xenografts. Cancer Sci. 100 (11), 2040−2045.

Chapter 9

Proteomics

Kalpana Joshi[1] and Dada Patil[2]

[1]*Savitribai Phule Pune University, Pune, Maharashtra, India,* [2]*Serum Institute of India Pvt Ltd., Pune, Maharashtra, India*

INTRODUCTION

The pharmaceutical industry has witnessed a steadily declining R&D efficiency resulting in fewer drugs reaching the market despite increased investment. A major cause for this low efficiency is the failure of drug candidates in late-stage development owing to safety issues or previously undiscovered side effects. Omics technologies provide some insights in predicting the risk of drug failure. Gene expression profiles offer clues in understanding the observed biological effects of drugs across disease areas, therapeutic targets and chemical scaffolds, and, in turn, de-risk drug development in early phases. Gene expression profiling can detect adverse effects of compounds, and is a valuable tool in early-stage drug discovery decision making (Verbist et al., 2015). Gene expression data has successfully been used to support go/no-go decisions for selected drug discovery projects within a global pharmaceutical company.

Recent advances in omics sciences, such as genomics, transcriptomics, proteomics, and metabolomics, have been used to provide alternate perspectives on quality, safety, and in understanding the mode of action (MOA) of drugs at systems level (Joshi et al., 2010; Mohd Fauzi et al., 2013). This central dogma of molecular biology forms the basis of omics trilogy (genomics, transcriptomics, and proteomics) with the addition of metabolomics and epigenomics (Joshi et al., 2012). Proteomics includes identification and quantification of proteins and also their localization, modifications, interactions, activities, and, ultimately, defining their function. Unlike DNA, proteins undergo complex biochemical modifications at the cotranslational or posttranslational level. A single gene can encode multiple proteins by means of alternative splicing of the messenger RNA or by multiples genes that encode for a single protein. Such possibilities result in a proteome that is more complex than the genome.

Innovative Approaches in Drug Discovery. DOI: http://dx.doi.org/10.1016/B978-0-12-801814-9.00009-X

273

RECENT ADVANCES IN PROTEOMICS TECHNOLOGIES

Proteomics, through techniques including isotope-coded affinity tags, stable isotopic labeling by amino acids in cell cultures, isobaric tags for relative and absolute quantification, multidirectional protein-identification technology, activity-based probes, protein/peptide arrays, phage displays, and two-hybrid systems are used in multiple areas throughout the drug development pipeline including target and lead identification, compound optimization, and clinical trials.

Currently, two approaches based on mass spectrometry are the most frequently used for global quantitative protein profiling: (1) two-dimensional electrophoresis (2-DE) followed by staining, selection, and identification by mass spectrometry and (2) isotope tags to label proteins, separation by multidimensional liquid chromatography, and mass spectrometry analysis (Cho, 2007).

Two-Dimensional Gel Electrophoresis

Two-dimensional gel electrophoresis (2-DE) is a key tool for comparative proteomics research. In 2-DE, mixtures of proteins are separated by charge (isoelectric point, pI) in the first dimension and further separated by mass in the second dimension on 2-D gels. Coupling 2-DE with immobilized pH gradients, IPG-Dalt, has provided higher resolution, improved reproducibility, and higher loading capacity for preparative purposes (O'Farrell, 1975). The 2-DE can achieve the separation of several thousand different proteins in one gel. Stains such as Coomassie Brilliant Blue, silver, SYPRO Ruby, and Deep Purple can be employed to visualize the proteins (Nilsson et al., 2000). Unfortunately, 2-DE technique is a time-consuming and labor-intensive process. Conventional 2-DE is restricted to the detection of denatured proteins in the size range of $10 \sim 200$ kDa at pH $3.5 \sim 11.5$. Traditionally, vertical and horizontal streaking of proteins can obscure analysis, and membrane proteins are usually under-represented due to extraction and insolubility problems. Furthermore, 2-DE is ineffective at distinguishing low-abundant proteins and small molecular weight proteins (<10 kDa). In recent years, some modified 2-DE platforms have been developed to detect nondenatured proteins in extreme size and pI. Moreover, significant improvements have been made in 2-DE technology with the development of two-dimensional fluorescence difference gel electrophoresis, which can be used to reduce gel-to-gel variations. Proteins are first labeled with one of three spectrally resolvable fluorescent cyanine dyes before being separated over the first and second dimensions according to their charge and size, respectively. It builds on 2-DE by adding a highly accurate quantitative dimension, which enables multiple protein extracts to be separated on the same 2-D gel. When used in conjunction with automated analysis packages, this multiplexing approach can accurately and reproducibly quantify protein expression for control and experimental groups. Differentially expressed proteins can be subsequently identified by mass spectrometric methods (Marouga et al., 2005).

ELECTROSPRAY IONIZATION

Electrospray ionization (ESI) involves the release of ions achieved by spraying the sample using an electrical field so that charged droplets are formed. As the solvent gradually evaporates from these droplets, freely hovering stark-naked protein molecules remain. Because the molecules take on strong positive charges, the mass/charge ratio becomes small enough to allow the substances to be analyzed in ordinary mass spectrometers. Another advantage is that the same molecule causes a series of peaks since each can take up a varying number of charges, which gives information that makes identification easier. In recent years, a novel linear ion trap (LIT) mass spectrometer with ESI and matrix-assisted laser desorption/ionization (MALDI) has been built in the MALDI-LIT-ESI configuration. The design features two independent ion source/ion optical channels connected to opposite ends of a single mass analyzer (Smith et al., 2007).

MATRIX-ASSISTED LASER DESORPTION/IONIZATION

Ionization by MALDI involves a laser pulse striking the sample which, unlike in the spray method, is in a solid or viscous phase. When the sample takes up the energy from the 914 W.C.-S. CHO laser pulse, it is blasted into small bits. The molecules let go of one another, released as intact hovering ions with a low charge, which are then accelerated by an electrical field and detected as described above by recording their time-of-flight (TOF). The technology is able to analyze proteins down to attomole quantities. It can tolerate small amounts of contaminants. The information obtained from MALDI analysis can be automatically submitted to a database search for further examination. Currently, efforts are underway for the direct analysis and MALDI imaging of formalin-fixed, paraffin-embedded tissue sections using the strategy based on in situ enzymatic digestion of the tissue section after paraffin removal. This approach provides access to massive amounts of archived samples in the clinical pathology setting (Lemaire et al., 2007).

SURFACE-ENHANCED LASER DESORPTION/IONIZATION

The surface-enhanced laser desorption/ionization (SELDI)-TOF MS is a technological breakthrough combining chromatographic active surfaces with an interface chip for MALDI. Using as little as one microliter per sample, a high-resolution mass spectrum following a complete chromatographic separation can be performed. The development of SELDI technology holds much promise for future protein analysis. It can be used for protein purification, expression profiling, or protein interaction profiling. There are many types of substances bound to the protein arrays, including antibodies, receptors, ligands, nucleic acids, carbohydrates, or chromatographic surfaces (e.g., cationic, anionic, hydrophobic, or hydrophilic). Some surfaces have a broad specificity that binds the whole classes of proteins, while others are highly specific in which only a few proteins from a complex sample are bound. After the capture step, the array is washed to reduce nonspecific binding. When subjected to short bursts of a laser beam, the retained proteins are uncoupled from the array surface and analyzed by laser desorption/ionization TOF MS.

Some protein arrays contain antibodies covalently immobilized onto the array surface that capture corresponding antigens from a complex mixture. Many analyses can be followed, e.g., analysis of proteolytic digests of the proteins bound to the array can disclose the antigenic determinant, other proteins of interest can be immobilized on the array, bound receptors can reveal ligands, and binding domains for protein−protein interactions can be detected. The proteins must often remain folded in the correct conformation during the preparation and incubation with the array for protein−protein interactions to occur (Cho, 2006).

PROTEIN MICROARRAY TECHNOLOGY

The microarray format provides a robust and convenient platform for the simultaneous analysis of thousands of individual protein samples, facilitating the design of sophisticated and reproducible biochemical experiments under highly specific conditions (Gouriet et al., 2008). Protein chips similar to DNA chips are likely be the next major evolution in proteomics and offer another solution for high-throughput proteomic analyses and detection of low-abundant proteins (Zhu et al., 2006). Protein chips can only provide data on a set of proteins selected by the investigator (Jones et al., 2006). These protein chips are used to study the biochemical activities of an entire proteome in a single experiment. They are used to study numerous protein interactions, such as protein−protein, protein−DNA, protein−RNA, protein−phospholipid, and protein−small molecule interactions (Zhu et al., 2001).

Antibody arrays are proteins captured on an antibody microarray substrates such as nylon membranes, plastic microwells, planar glass slides, gel-based arrays, and beads are detected by a cocktail of detection antibodies. High-throughput multiplex antibody arrays are immunoassays that quantitatively measure hundreds of known proteins in complex biological matrices for diagnostic discovery and biomarker-assisted drug development.

APPLICATIONS OF PROTEOMICS IN DRUG DISCOVERY

Proteomic technologies have advanced various areas of drug discovery and development through the comparative assessment of normal and diseased-state tissues, transcription and/or expression profiling, side effect profiling, pharma-cogenomics, and the identification of biomarkers. The majority of small molecule drugs and biologics act on protein targets. These proteins do not act in isolation but are embedded in cellular pathways and networks and are thus tightly interconnected with many other proteins and subcellular components. Given this complexity, it seems natural to apply proteomics in the drug discovery process. Target-based approaches start with the selection of a protein target based on its presumed or validated role in the relevant disease. Biochemical or biophysical assays, typically using purified protein, are developed to monitor modulation of target activity and to identify hits in high-throughput screens using large libraries of small molecules. After a hit validation, lead compounds are selected and further optimized with regard to potency, selectivity, pharmacodynamics, and pharmacokinetic properties, and are then tested for in vivo efficacy in the respective-disease model (Schirle et al., 2012). Proteomics technologies have successfully been used in biomarker discovery, target identification and validation, lead optimization, and MOA to toxicity prediction (Fig. 9.1).

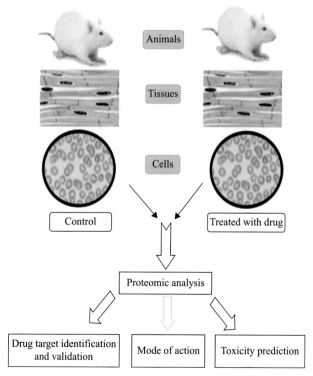

FIGURE 9.1 Protemics workflow in drug discovery.

BIOMARKER DISCOVERY AND IDENTIFICATION OF POTENTIAL THERAPEUTIC TARGETS

According to the US Food and Drug Administration (USFDA), a biomarker is a characteristic that is objectively measured and evaluated as an indicator of normal biologic or pathogenic processes or pharmacological responses to a therapeutic intervention. It may also be defined as an in vivo derived molecule present at levels deviating significantly from the average in association with specific conditions of health (Atkinson et al., 2001; Zhang et al., 2007).

Some Key Examples

Increased levels of liver transaminases in blood indicates destruction of liver cells, the prostate specific antigen (PSA) for prostate cancer (Wang et al., 1981), or the troponin I and T for acute myocardial infarction (Mair et al., 1992; Antman et al., 1996). However, such markers exist in limited numbers and in quite low concentrations, and it can be hoped that a wide search for tissue-leakage markers should provide some new and interesting candidates (Amacher, 1998; Hsich et al., 1996; Ahmed et al., 2004). Proteomics has facilitated the cataloging of protein profiles in different tissues and biological fluids (Honda et al., 2013); however, identification of clinical biomarkers remains one of the most challenging applications (Altelaar et al., 2013). Current biomarkers or biomarker candidates struggle with limited reliability and proper validation as well as with limited sensitivity and specificity (Barbosa et al., 2012). This limitation is mainly due to the dynamic nature of proteome where proteins are continually undergoing changes, e.g., binding to the cell membrane, partnering with other proteins to form complexes, or undergoing synthesis and degradation.

In cancer, proteomics enabled the identification of several promising candidates from tissue, blood, cerebrospinal fluid, cell lines, or even animal models using 2-DE and MS, SELDI-TOF, protein microarrays, LC-MS/MS, ELISA, and so forth (Hudler et al., 2014). Signature proteins like PSA and CA-125, are the current best markers for prostate and ovarian cancer, respectively (Velonas et al., 2013; Mai et al., 2011).

Proteome analysis of normal human vitreous humor using high-resolution Fourier transform mass spectrometry should facilitate biomedical research into pathological conditions of the eye including diabetic retinopathy, retinal detachment, and cataract (Murthy et al., 2014). A quantitative proteomic profiling of synovial fluid obtained from rheumatoid arthritis (RA) and osteoarthritis (OA), using iTRAQ labeling followed by high-resolution mass spectrometry analysis, a total of 575 proteins were identified out of which 135 proteins were found to be differentially expressed by $\geq$ 3-fold in RA and OA synovial fluid.

Proteins not previously reported to be associated with RA including, coronin-1A (CORO1A), fibrinogen like-2 (FGL2), and macrophage-capping protein (CAPG) were found to be upregulated in RA. Proteins such as CD5 molecule-like protein (CD5L), soluble scavenger receptor cysteine-rich domain-containing protein (SSC5D), and TTK protein kinase (TTK) were found to be upregulated in the synovial fluid of osteoarthritis patients. Pathway analysis of differentially expressed proteins revealed a significant enrichment of genes involved in glycolytic pathway in RA which, in turn, might aid in early diagnosis and prognosis as well as in the evaluation of the disease progression of RA and OA. These novel proteins need to be explored further for their role in the disease pathogenesis of RA and osteoarthritis (Balakrishnan et al., 2014).

Despite the substantial advances in our understanding of the molecular basis of disease, there is a paucity of approved biomarkers. Protein biomarkers in biological fluids in particular have the potential to inform regarding risk of disease or to allow early detection for more effective treatment. There is an equally appalling lack of other types of biomarkers, whether for disease classification for individualized therapy or for other applications. The challenge for the next decade is to implement road maps that fast track the development of biomarkers, whether protein, nucleic acid, or metabolite-based, to reach the clinic in an efficient manner (Hanash, 2011).

Drug targets are proteins or signal-transduction pathways in which proteins are involved. Therapeutic relevancy of the chosen target must be proven first prior to initiating other processes in drug discovery. Tyrosine kinase receptor (PDGFR, VEGFR2, FGFR1), Aurora kinases and TANK-binding kinase-1 are identified as targets for tumor vascularization. Aldehyde dehydrogenase-1 and quinine reductase-2 in malaria, RICK (Rip-like interacting kinase), CLARP (caspase-like apoptosis-regulatory protein kinase), GAK (cyclin-G associated kinase), and CK1α are some of the targets used for drug discovery (Kopec et al., 2005; Katayama and Oda, 2007). A new drug molecule is being searched against the chosen target that usually involves high-throughput screening, wherein large libraries of chemicals are tested to determine their ability to modify the target.

UNDERSTANDING DISEASE MECHANISMS—MOA (MODE OF ACTION)

Comparative proteomics or protein–protein interaction studies can be used to elucidate mechanisms of action by which a drug can modulate target activity. Differential protein expressions observed with and without a compound treatment, either on cells or tissues or animals, allow the identification of compound-sensitive proteins and their interactions (Fig. 9.2). Proteomic analysis of SAHA treated and untreated cancer cells was used for target identification. Using tagged subunits of the SIN3A HDAC complex, Smith

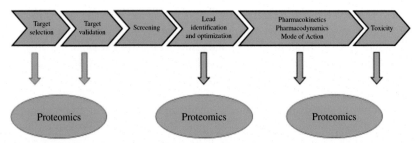

FIGURE 9.2 Proteomics in drug discovery pipeline.

and colleagues found that SAHA, the first FDA-approved HDAC inhibitor for the treatment of cancer, causes dissociation of the ING2 subunit from this complex. Absence of ING2 leads to loss of binding of the SIN3A complex to the p21 promoter and, thus, directly contributes to the growth inhibitory effect of SAHA (Smith et al., 2010).

Another example is the identification of the interaction of tagged cAMP-dependent protein kinase (PKA) subunit Cb1 and CAP1, which was shown to be sensitive to an ATP-competitive PKA inhibitor (Erlbruch et al., 2010). Developing large-scale protein interaction maps of complete disease-related signaling pathways could also be challenging but useful in the identification of druggable targets. Protein—protein interaction mapping of around 32 members of the pro-inflammatory TNF-a-induced NKkB pathway was done, resulting in 80 novel protein interactions; 10 of these proteins were confirmed to have a modulatory role in TNF-a signaling (Bouwmeester et al., 2004). Selective binding of the HSP90 inhibitor PU-H71 to cancer-specific oncoprotein-HSP90 complexes was identified using an immobilized PU-H71 matrix (Moulick et al., 2011). Differential phosphoproteomic analyses using selective small molecule inhibitors of particular kinases such as MAPK inhibitors U0126 and SB202190, the clinical BCR-ABL inhibitor Dasatinib, and inhibitors of Aurora and Polo-like kinases have been used to identify substrates in human cell lines and to characterize the effect of inhibition on signaling events (Pan et al., 2009; Kettenbach et al., 2011).

Quantitative proteomics has been used successfully in many cases to study the effect of small molecule inhibitors by monitoring protein acetylation and methylation. Quantitative effects of the HDAC inhibitor trichostatin A was studied in a similar manner on the histone modification state in a murine model of systemic lupus erythematosus (Garcia et al., 2005). Lee and colleagues used label-free mass spectrometry to quantify the effect of HDAC inhibitors of varying degrees of selectivity on histone acetylation (Lee et al., 2008). Proteomic approaches have been used to study the effect of inhibition of the histone demethylase JMJD2A by pyridine-2,4-dicarboxylic acid derivatives (MacKeen et al., 2010) as well as the histone methyltransferases G9A and GLP by the small molecule inhibitor UNC0638 (Vedadi et al., 2011). The potential value of proteomics in drug development, especially in elucidating MOA, has been demonstrated in many successful examples. Proteomic approaches have been recognized as promising techniques that can facilitate the systematic characterization of a drug action and side effect prediction, thereby helping to reduce the typically high attrition rates in discovery projects.

PROTEOMICS IN LEAD OPTIMIZATION

Pharmacokinetics (PK) and pharmacodynamics (PD) are an integral part of drug development. Drug efficacy, drug toxicity, and the therapeutic index of a drug are important criteria for lead optimization. A panel of in vitro and in vivo assays are applied to shortlist compounds post discovery. Proteomics technologies have potential to monitor global protein expressions as a surrogate for the effect of the applied treatment (Kraus et al., 2007). It is also possible to map the pharmacological loss of function of one protein that causes the cell to express increased levels of another protein with a redundant function (Kraus et al., 2007). Global expression proteomics mainly captures the alterations in effect or pairs it with a specific cellular treatment.

Phosphoproteomics is used for selective applications such as assessing the selectivity of compounds in discovery of kinase inhibitors. For protein kinases the conserved ATP-binding site has been used to generate a nonselective protein kinase panel that provide selectivity assessments for up to 150 kinase targets in a single experiment (Schirle et al., 2012). Such selectivity matrices have been successfully used to profile clinical BCR-ABL inhibitors in the chronic myeloid leukemia cell line K562 (Bantscheff et al., 2007), EGFR inhibitors in HeLa cells (Sharma et al., 2009), and a range of investigational and clinical multikinase inhibitors in patient-derived primary chronic lymphocytic leukemia cells (Kruse et al., 2011). Immobilized kinase inhibitors have also been successfully used to identify targets in head and neck cancers by analyzing the kinase complement across 34 squamous cell carcinoma lines established from patients (Wu et al., 2011).

The lead optimization process aims at improving the hit/lead molecules properties for ADME. Lead optimization process is the balancing between multiple properties such as PK/PD without compromising efficacy, although complicated proteomics has been shown to have a potential for ex vivo lead optimization.

PROTEOMICS FOR EVALUATING DRUG TOXICITY

Drug safety is an utmost important consideration during the process of drug discovery and development. A large proportion of failures in drug discovery and development projects are not due to limited efficacy but result from toxicity: many approved drugs are later withdrawn from the market because of issues of toxicity (Scannell et al., 2012). Prediction of toxicity at an early stage of drug development is crucial for the loss due to drugs failure at later stages. Attempts have been made to compare genomics and proteomics of safe drugs with that of drugs under investigation to predict activity and toxicity (Searfoss et al., 2005). Few findings have been published on how gene expression facilitates go/no-go decisions during lead optimization (van der Veen et al., 2013; Magkoufopoulou et al., 2012; Jiang et al., 2007). Drug induced renal toxicity, prediction of genotoxicity, and prediction of skin sensitizing potential are some of the examples of use of transcriptomic technology in lead optimization. Baum et al. investigated off-target effects and were able to prioritize compounds based on transcriptional profiles (Baum et al., 2010). Although transcriptomics data have been shown to support decision making in a number of projects, they also have their limitations. Conceptually, transcriptional profiling is limited in its nature because it cannot detect changes at the metabolite or protein level.

Cancer therapeutic agents such as anthracycline and doxorubicin are reported to have cardiotoxicity in 14% to 49% of patients treated for lymphoma. Novel targeted anticancer agents such as trastuzumab, imatinib, and sunitinib, often induce adverse effects on the heart in a small population of patients. The successful use of anthracyclines like doxorubicin in chemotherapy is limited by their severe cardiotoxicity. Despite decades of clinical application, a satisfying description of the molecular mechanisms involved and a preventive treatment have not yet been achieved. Doxorubicin-induced changes in cell signaling as a novel potential mediator of doxorubicin toxicity was addressed by applying a non-biased screen of the cardiac phosphoproteome. Two-dimensional gel electrophoresis, phosphorspecific staining, quantitative image analysis, and MALDI-TOF/TOF mass spectrometry were combined to identify (de)phosphorylation events occurring in the isolated rat heart upon Langendorff-perfusion with clinically relevant (5 μM) and supraclinical concentrations (25 μM) of doxorubicin. This approach identified 22 proteins with a significantly changed phosphorylation status and these results were validated by immunoblotting for selected phosphosites. Overrepresentation of mitochondrial proteins (> 40%) identified this compartment as a prime target of doxorubicin. Identified proteins were mainly involved in energy metabolism (e.g., pyruvate dehydrogenase and acyl-CoA dehydrogenase), sarcomere structure and function (e.g., desmin), or chaperone-like activities (e.g., α-crystallin B chain and prohibitin). Changes in phosphorylation of pyruvate dehydrogenase, regulating pyruvate entry into the Krebs cycle, and desmin, maintaining myofibrillar array, are relevant for the main symptoms of cardiac dysfunction related to doxorubicin treatment, namely energy imbalance and myofibrillar disorganization (Gratia et al., 2012).

Complex proteomic signature of chronic anthracycline cardiotoxicity was revealed through translational proteomics approach. In addition to mitochondrial proteins, a marked drop in myosin light-chain isoforms, activation of proteolytic machinery (including the proteasome system), increased abundance of chaperones and proteins involved in chaperone-mediated autophagy, membrane repair as well as apoptosis were found. Dramatic changes in proteins of basement membrane and extracellular matrix were documented. In conclusion, and for the first time, this enhances our understanding of the basis for this phenomenon and it may enhance efforts in targeting its reduction (Štěrba et al., 2011).

Serum Proteomic Pattern Diagnostics is a new type of proteomic platform in which patterns of proteomic signatures from high-dimensional mass spectrometry data are used as a diagnostic classifier at the critical initial stages of toxicity (Petricoin et al., 2004).

A drug targets the desired protein, but the induced loss or gain of function exhibits undesirable biological effects limiting the usefulness of the treatment. Well-known examples for this category include drugs targeting the p38 MAP kinase in inflammatory diseases (Hammaker and Firestein, 2009). Toxicoproteomic studies on drug selectivity and MOA can, therefore, often highlight potential toxicity issues early on and, thus, provide a valuable source for identifying lead molecules (Kennedy, 2002). Liver toxicity is a particularly problematic issue and is indeed frequently observed.

Global proteome profiling of human hepatocytes or rodent livers exposed to a drug can be employed to obtain an appreciation of the effects the treatment may impose. Troglitazone, a once-marketed first-generation thiazolidinedione used for the treatment of type-II diabetes mellitus, was withdrawn from the market owing to unacceptable idiosyncratic hepatotoxicity risks even though troglitazone did not cause hepatotoxicity in normal healthy rodents and monkeys in preclinical drug safety assessments and long-term studies.

To understand idiosyncratic hepatotoxicity mechanistically, Lee et al. used MS-based proteomics to characterize mitochondrial protein changes to track the involvement of specific mitochondrial proteins in troglitazone-induced hepatotoxicity in a mouse model (Lee et al., 2013). By combining high-throughput, MS-based, mitoproteome-wide profiling, biochemical endpoints, and network biology, the authors demonstrated that the hepatic mitochondrial proteome followed a two-phase response to a repeated troglitazone administration that culminated in liver injuries by the fourth week.

Meierhofer et al. demonstrated the power of protein set analysis to gain insights into the regulation of cell and tissue homeostasis during a high-fat diet feeding and medication with two antidiabetic compounds (Meierhofer et al., 2013). GSEA allowed for more sensitive detection of low-level but coordinated protein-expression changes, and the functional modules showed a higher correlation than individual genes/proteins when comparing proteomics and transcriptomics data. Suter et al. characterized the effect of 16 test compounds using conventional toxicological parameters in the integrated EU Framework 6 Project: Predictive toxicology (PredTox) (Suter et al., 2011).

Toxicoproteomics using proteomic pattern technology can have important direct applications within the drug development pipeline as well as potentially powerful bedside applications. We can envision a future in which the specific serum/urine/plasma mass spectral proteomic portraits of a variety of major organ toxicities such as hepatotoxicity, nephro-toxicity, cardiotoxicity, and reprotoxicity, are used to rapidly screen against experimental compounds, either for toxic liability or for protective-intervention efficacy.

MS-based proteomics is maturing into a robust technology for the measurement of proteome-wide exposure effects. The benefits of including proteomic data to understand exposure effects have already been demonstrated in several case studies. Although some challenges still exist to make full use of the richness of proteomic datasets (van Vliet, 2011; Merrick and Witzmann, 2009; Martin et al., 2013), there is overall a great opportunity for proteomics to contribute to an improved understanding of toxicant action, the linkages to accompanying dysfunction and pathology, and the development of predictive biomarkers and signatures of toxicity (Titz et al., 2014).

PROTEOMICS IN ETHNOPHARMACOLOGY RESEARCH

Investigating MOA Botanical Drugs

Traditional botanical medicine preparations have been used for centuries for their health and therapeutic benefits. However, the molecular mechanisms of underlying their efficacies remain largely unclear. Resveratrol (RVT), a polyphenolic compound, has been used extensively for decades as a potential therapy or as a preventive agent for various chronic conditions such as cancer, cardiovascular atherosclerosis, hypertension, and diabetes. The underlying biological processes and molecular pathways by which RVT induces these beneficial effects remains largely undefined. Recently, few studies using proteomics approaches (2-DE combined with MS/MS) have been undertaken to explore the molecular mechanisms of RVT in the amelioration of cancer and endothelial dysfunction in human ovarian cancer cell lines and human umbilical vein endothelial cells, respectively. The cancer cell proteomic analysis found a down regulation of the protein cyclin D1 and the phosphorylation levels of protein kinase B (Akt) and glycogen synthase kinase-3b (GSK-3b) targeting signaling pathways involved in cell proliferation and drug resistance (Vergara et al., 2012). Another study on human umbilical vein endothelial proteomics found the down regulation of elongation factor 2 (EEF2), carboxymethyl-cofilin-1 (cofilin-1), acetyl-eukaryotic translation initiation factor 5A-1 (acetyl-EIF5A) and barrier-to-autointegration factor, and upregulation of heat shock protein beta-1 (HSP27), phospho-HSP27, phospho-stathmin, Nicotinate-nucleotidepyrophosphorylase, and 1, 2-dihydroxy-3-keto-5-methylthiopentene dioxygenase after RVT exposure (Shao et al., 2012). The study also demonstrated that several protein species with posttranscriptional modification (carboxymethyl, acetyl, and phospho) were found to be altered following exposure to RVT. These findings of cancer and endothelial proteome analysis could help in our understanding of the molecular mechanisms underlying the pleiotropic effects of RVT. Quercetin, a flavonoid abundantly present in plants, is widely used as a phytotherapy in prostatitis and prostate cancer. Quercetin has been reported to have a number of therapeutic effects; the cellular target(s) responsible for its anticancer action has not yet been clearly elucidated, but it is understood that anticancer effects of quercetin are mediated, in part, by impairing functions of hnRNPA1, insights that were obtained using a chemical proteomics strategy (Ko et al., 2014).

Withania somnifera, a popular Ayurvedic rasayana botanical (a medicinal plant having immunomodulatory activity) has been used as an immunomodulator and in the management of cancer. Several cellular studies on bioactive compound; withaferin A (WA) from *W. somnifera* has demonstrated that the anticancer potential is due to the modulation of processes such as apoptosis, inflammation, angiogenesis, and cell proliferation either by upregulation or downregulation of numerous proteins (Patil et al., 2013). The underline mechanistic study using proteomics with 2-DE followed by MALDITOF/TOF technologies demonstrated that WA could regulate total of 65 proteins including downregulation of many glycolysis-related proteins such as M2-type pyruvate kinase, phosphoglycerate kinase, and fructose-bisphosphate aldolase A isoform 2 in mammary tumor tissue samples (Hahm et al., 2013). The proteomic analysis suggested that the possible MOA WA-mediated mammary cancer prevention could be due to the suppression of glycolysis process in the cancer cells.

Guggulsterone (GS) is a natural hypolipidemic drug extracted from the gum resin of tree *Commiphora mukul*. The gum resin guggul has been used since ancient times for the treatment of various ailments including obesity, arthritis, inflammation and lipid disorders as an Ayurvedic medicine. Extensive molecular mechanism studies on GS showed apoptosis inducing and antiinflammatory activities have a role in obesity, arterial thrombosis, inflammatory bowel diseases, and different types of cancers. Recent proteomics analysis studies on 3T3-L1 preadipocytes treated with GS using 2-DE with MALDITOF/TOF technologies showed the upregulation of Annexin 5, marker protein of apoptosis (Pal et al., 2013).

Siwu decoction is an ancient traditional Chinese herbal medicine (*Rehmannia glutinosa, Angelica sinensis, Paeonia lacitflora, Ligusticum chuanxiong*) used to replenish blood, stimulate the hemopoiesis of the bone marrow for a blood-deficient subject as well as increase the peripheral blood count. With proteomics technologies including 2-DE, image analysis, in-gel digestion, MALDI-TOF MS, and bioinformatics, has shown that Siwu decoction could regulate the protein expression of the bone marrow of blood-deficient mice, including lymphocyte specific protein 1, proteasome 26S ATPase subunit 4, hematopoietic cell protein-tyrosine phosphatase, glyceraldehyde-3-phosphate dehydrogenase, growth factor receptor binding protein 14, and lgals12. The proteome analysis provided a possible explanation of the mechanism underlying Siwu decoction in the hemopoiesis process (Guo et al., 2004).

Diabetes mellitus is a chronic progressive disease with metabolic disorder of the endocrine system. *Panax ginseng* has been used to treat diabetes mellitus since ancient time. Studies on ginsenoside Re, an active compound of *Panax ginseng* has demonstrated significant antidiabetic actions mainly as an antiinflammatory and through the reduction in insulin-resistance activities. Recent proteomics studies employing high-throughput SELDI-TOF MS and bioinformatics technologies used to explore the possible proteins involved in the antidiabetic actions of ginsenoside Re (Cho et al., 2006; Gao et al., 2013). The proteomic analysis of Cho et al. showed the presence of 293 potential biomarkers differentiating between diabetes and control normal rats. C-reactive protein, a marker protein, was found to be altered in ginsenoside Re-treated diabetic rats and was validated by ELISA. Studies by Gao et al., using a genomics and proteomics approach, demonstrated a reduction in insulin-resistance activity of ginsenoside Re through activation of PPAR-γ pathway and inhibition of TNF-α production. These findings indicate that ginsenoside Re might be beneficial to patients suffering from diabetes mellitus and its complications by alleviating inflammation and insulin resistance.

These examples have shed light on connecting the exploration of traditional medicines with powerful proteomics tools and serve as an ideal integration for discovering new treasures within herbal medicine and thereby bringing traditional medicine research to a new horizon.

QUALITY CONTROL AND STANDARDIZATION

Quality control and standardization of herbal drugs remains one of the bottlenecks in herbal drug development (Warude and Patwardhan, 2005). There are several approaches based on morphology, microscopy, preliminary qualitative phytochemistry. Phytochemical investigations based on total chromatographic fingerprint analysis or quantitative estimations that target secondary metabolites in crude, processed extracts and final formulations as well as the use of gene expressions studies using microarrays have been used for monitoring the quality of herbal drugs (Chitlange et al., 2009; Joshi et al., 2004; Patil et al., 2009). Monitoring the quality of herbal drugs based on the spectrum analysis of only secondary metabolites is not enough to reflect the quality of an entire product. Therefore, there is a need to monitor the quality of the product based on primary metabolites as well secondary metabolites. There are reports on monitoring the quality based on primary metabolites such as polysaccharides, proteins and glycoproteins, all of which have been documented. *Panax ginseng* and *Panax quinquefolius* are two widely used valuable TCMs. However, conventional separation methods cannot distinguish different parts (main root, lateral roots, rhizome head, and skin) of the two species. The 2-DE maps have been applied to identify different ginseng samples containing distinct and common protein spots to permit easy discrimination. The use of these potential biomarkers might help to speed up the identification process of herbal drug development (Lum et al., 2002).

TOXICOKINETICS AND HERB–DRUG INTERACTIONS

There are increasing incidences of herb–drug interactions affecting the safety and efficacy of treatment mainly though pharmacokinetic and/or pharmacodynamic modulation. The concomitant administration of herbs with conventional therapeutics has shown a modulatory effect (inhibitory or inducing) on metabolizing enzymes, such as cytochrome P450s (CYPs), or transporter proteins like P glycoprotein (p-gp), organic anionic transporter peptides, or organic cationic transporter polypeptides that leads to pharmacokinetic interactions. Assessment of these interactions in the early stage of herbal drug development is an important step recommended by various international regulatory agencies such as the USFDA and the European Medicines Agency (EMA) (USFDA, 2004; EMA, 2010). There are reports available on traditional Chinese herbal medicines and Japanese herbal medicines on the early prediction of clinically relevant herb–drug interactions based on CYP modulation and transport proteins using proteomics with the aid of genomics and metabolomics approaches (Mrozikiewicz et al., 2010; Shord et al., 2009). *Ginkgo biloba* extract is one of the most popular herbal ingredients used for improvement of cognitive function and peripheral arterial disease. Bilobalide has been identified as major constituent responsible for induction of CYPs suggesting potential for HDIs. Western blot analysis and a real-time PCR study demonstrated a dose-dependent induction of CYP2B protein (Taki et al., 2009). Another study using CYP activity mediated through probe drug substrate metabolite formation showed induction of multiple CYPs such as CYP1A1 CYP2C and demonstrates significant reduction of plasma warfarin (substrate of CYP 2C9) concentration affecting its anticoagulant efficacy through pharmacokinetic interaction (Taki et al., 2012).

So far CYP enzymes have been studied using a variety of different bioanalytical methods including immunoblotting, PCR, and enzyme-activity assays. The studies performed have not provided definitive data on the protein levels of individual CYP isoforms. Although the application of RT-PCR to quantify, e.g., CYP2E1 mRNA, was successful, the result does not necessarily translate to the protein level (Haufroid et al., 2001). Western blot analysis can be performed at the protein level, but is dependent on the availability of specific antibodies, and may not assure 100% selectivity (Guengerich and Turvy, 1991). Additionally, only one CYP-isoform can be quantified per analysis. CYP protein levels have also been investigated indirectly by studying their enzymatic activity, e.g., CYP2E1 via metabolism of chlorzoxazon (Tanaka et al., 2003). However, there remains the problem that more than one CYP-isoform can catalyze a given reaction. In recent years LC-MS/MS has gained popularity in the qualitative and quantitative determination of proteins. For CYP analysis, LC-MS/MS has been mainly used in a discovery mode, where the goal is one of protein identification. However, quantitative analysis is also possible (Wang et al., 2008).

A recent proteomic study using 2-DE coupled with MS/MS identified and quantified a total of 18 major CYP isoenzymes responsible for metabolism of more than 90% of pharmaceuticals in human liver samples (Seibert and Davidson, 2008). These findings suggest that the recent advancement in quantitative proteomics and mass spectrometry could provide useful information on absolute estimation of proteins and more accurate prediction of HDIs. Since proteomics aids in understanding the complex mechanisms of traditional herbal medicines at the cellular and molecular levels, it has great meanings to the modernization and internationalization of traditional herbal medicines.

LIMITATIONS AND FUTURE PROSPECTIVE

Despite of the rapid advancements acquired by proteomics in past years, there are also some disadvantages: low reproducibility and a difficult separation of proteins of a big or small isoelectric point. Moreover, some hydrophobic proteins, insoluble membrane proteins, and large molecular weight, low-abundance proteins may be ignored in the process of examination. It is noteworthy that the proteomics community has identified four major areas for strengthening the proteomics. These include (1) the need to provide high-quality standardized, sensitive, specific, quantitative, and readily accessible protein, peptide, or other biomarkers of health, disease, response to therapy into the approval processes of regulatory agencies (e.g., FDA), and obtain approval from the relevant agencies for their use in a clinical or other test settings; (2) implement standard processes for collecting, processing, and storing human clinical samples in biorepositories and enforcement of measures to ensure subject integrity including informed consent for the downstream use of samples and in registrations of subject identities within study databases; (3) test and validate mass spectrometry technology platforms that hold much promise for creating opportunities for obtaining new and important knowledge at levels of detection previously not achievable; and (4) organize clinical discovery operations and activities in an intuitive manner to meet the challenges of increased interests in the science and diminishing levels of centrally financed resources and infrastructure support (Fehniger et al., 2014).

Successful use of key proteomic technologies will provide in-depth understanding of the molecular and cellular mechanisms of drugs. How these proteins interact with each other at cellular level and express the phenotype remains complex. Mapping of such "interactome networks" and the transition of omic data, including proteomics to interactomics, will require ongoing continued development to understand health, disease, and drug action (Vidal et al., 2011).

REFERENCES

Ahmed, N., Barker, G., Oliva, K.T., Hoffmann, P., Riley, C., Reeve, S., et al., 2004. Proteomic-based identification of haptoglobin-1 precursor as a novel circulating biomarker of ovarian cancer. Br. J. Cancer 91 (1), 129–140.

Altelaar, A.F.M., Munoz, J., Heck, A.J.R., 2013. Next-generation proteomics: towards an integrative view of proteome dynamics. Nat. Rev. Genet. 14 (1), 35–48.

Amacher, D.E., 1998. Serum transaminase elevations as indicators of hepatic injury following the administration of drugs. Regul. Toxicol. Pharmacol. 27 (2), 119–130.

Antman, E.M., Tanasijevic, M.J., Thompson, B., Schactman, M., McCabe, C.H., Cannon, C.P., et al., 1996. Cardiac-specific troponin I levels to predict the risk of mortality in patients with acute coronary syndromes. N. Engl. J. Med. 335 (18), 1342–1349.

Atkinson, A.J., Colburn, W.A., DeGruttola, V.G., DeMets, D.L., Downing, G.J., Hoth, D.F., et al., 2001. Biomarkers and surrogate endpoints: preferred definitions and conceptual framework. Clin. Pharmacol. Ther. 69 (3), 89–95.

Balakrishnan, L., Bhattacharjee, M., Ahmad, S., Nirujogi, R.S., Renuse, S., Subbannayya, Y., et al., 2014. Differential proteomic analysis of synovial fluid from rheumatoid arthritis and osteoarthritis patients. Clin. Proteomics 11 (1), 1.

Bantscheff, M., Eberhard, D., Abraham, Y., Bastuck, S., Boesche, M., Hobson, S., et al., 2007. Quantitative chemical proteomics reveals mechanisms of action of clinical ABL kinase inhibitors. Nat. Biotechnol. 25 (9), 1035–1044.

Barbosa, E.B., Vidotto, A., Polachini, G.M., Henrique, T., de Marqui, A.B.T., Helena Tajara, E., 2012. Proteomics: methodologies and applications to the study of human diseases. Rev da Assoc. Médica Bras. 58 (3), 366–375.

Baum, P., Schmid, R., Ittrich, C., Rust, W., Fundel-Clemens, K., Siewert, S., et al., 2010. Phenocopy--a strategy to qualify chemical compounds during hit-to-lead and/or lead optimization. PLoS One 5 (12), e14272.

Bouwmeester, T., Bauch, A., Ruffner, H., Angrand, P.-O., Bergamini, G., Croughton, K., et al., 2004. A physical and functional map of the human TNF-alpha/NF-kappa B signal transduction pathway. Nat. Cell Biol. 6 (2), 97–105.

Chitlange, S.S., Kulkarni, P.S., Patil, D., Patwardhan, B., Nanda, R.K., 2009. High-performance liquid chromatographic fingerprint for quality control of Terminalia arjuna containing Ayurvedic churna formulation. J. AOAC Int. 92 (4), 1016–1020.

Cho, W.C.S., 2006. Research progress in SELDI-TOF MS and its clinical applications. China J. Biotechnol. 22 (6), 871–877.

Cho, W.C.S., 2007. Application of proteomics in Chinese medicine research. Am. J. Chin. Med. 35 (6), 911–922.

Cho, W.C.S., Yip, T.T., Chung, W.S., Lee, S.K.W., Leung, A.W.N., Cheng, C.H.K., et al., 2006. Altered expression of serum protein in ginsenoside Re-treated diabetic rats detected by SELDI-TOF MS. J. Ethnopharmacol. 108 (2), 272–279.

EMA, 2010. Guideline on the Investigation of drug interactions.

Erlbruch, A., Hung, C.-W., Seidler, J., Borrmann, K., Gesellchen, F., König, N., et al., 2010. Uncoupling of bait-protein expression from the prey protein environment adds versatility for cell and tissue interaction proteomics and reveals a complex of CARP-1 and the PKA Cbeta1 subunit. Proteomics 10 (16), 2890–2900.

Fehniger, T.E., Boja, E.S., Rodriguez, H., Baker, M.S., Marko-Varga, G., 2014. Four areas of engagement requiring strengthening in modern proteomics today. J. Proteome Res. 13 (12), 5310–5318.

Fields, S., 2001. PROTEOMICS: proteomics in Genomeland. Science 291 (5507), 1221–1224.

Gao, Y., Yang, M.F., Su, Y.P., Jiang, H.M., You, X.J., Yang, Y.J., et al., 2013. Ginsenoside Re reduces insulin resistance through activation of PPAR- pathway and inhibition of TNF-production. J. Ethnopharmacol. 147 (2), 509–516.

Garcia, B.A., Busby, S.A., Shabanowitz, J., Hunt, D.F., Mishra, N., 2005. Resetting the epigenetic histone code in the MRL-lpr/lpr mouse model of lupus by histone deacetylase inhibition. J. Proteome Res. 4 (6), 2032–2042.

Gouriet, F., Samson, L., Delaage, M., Mainardi, J.L., Meconi, S., Drancourt, M., et al., 2008. Multiplexed whole bacterial antigen microarray, a new format for the automation of serodiagnosis: the culture-negative endocarditis paradigm. Clin. Microbiol. Infect. 14 (12), 1112–1118.

Gratia, S., Kay, L., Michelland, S., Sève, M., Schlattner, U., Tokarska-Schlattner, M., 2012. Cardiac phosphoproteome reveals cell signaling events involved in doxorubicin cardiotoxicity. J. Proteomics 75 (15), 4705–4716.

Guengerich, F., Turvy, C., 1991. Comparison of levels of several human microsomal cytochrome P-450 enzymes and epoxide hydrolase in normal and disease states using immunochemical analysis of surgical liver samples. J. Pharmacol. Exp. Ther. 256, 1189–1194.

Guo, P., Ma, Z.C., Li, Y.F., Liang, Q.D., Wang, J.F., Wang, S.Q., 2004. Effects of siwu tang on protein expression of bone marrow of blood deficiency mice induced by irradiation. China J. Chinese Mater. Medica. 29 (9), 893–896.

Hahm, E.-R., Lee, J., Kim, S.-H., Sehrawat, A., Arlotti, J. a, Shiva, S.S., et al., 2013. Metabolic alterations in mammary cancer prevention by withaferin A in a clinically relevant mouse model. J. Natl. Cancer Inst. 105 (15), 1111–1122.

Hammaker, D., Firestein, G.S., 2009. "Go upstream, young man": lessons learned from the p38 saga. Ann. Rheum. Dis. 69 (Suppl. 1), i77–i82.

Hanash, S.M., 2011. Why have protein biomarkers not reached the clinic? Genome Med. 3 (10), 66.

Haufroid, V., Toubeau, F., Clippe, A., Buysschaert, M., Gala, J.-L., Lison, D., 2001. Real-time quantification of cytochrome P4502E1 mRNA in human peripheral blood lymphocytes by reverse transcription-PCR: method and practical application. Clin. Chem. 47 (6), 1126–1129.

Honda, K., Ono, M., Shitashige, M., Masuda, M., Kamita, M., Miura, N., et al., 2013. Proteomic approaches to the discovery of cancer biomarkers for early detection and personalized medicine. J. Clin. Oncol. 43 (2), 103–109.

Hsich, G., Kenney, K., Gibbs, C., Lee, K., Harrington, M., 1996. The 14-3-3 brain protein in cerebrospinal fluid as a marker for transmissible spongiform encephalopathies. N. Engl. J. Med. 335 (13), 924–930.

Hudler, P., Kocevar, N., Komel, R., 2014. Proteomic approaches in biomarker discovery: new perspectives in cancer diagnostics. Sci. World J. 2014, 260348.

Jiang, Y., Gerhold, D.L., Holder, D.J., Figueroa, D.J., Bailey, W.J., Guan, P., et al., 2007. Diagnosis of drug-induced renal tubular toxicity using global gene expression profiles. J. Transl. Med. 5, 47.

Jones, R.B., Gordus, A., Krall, J.A., MacBeath, G., 2006. A quantitative protein interaction network for the ErbB receptors using protein microarrays. Nature 439 (7073), 168–174.

Joshi, K., Bhat, S., Deshpande, P., Sule, M., Satyamoorthy, K., 2012. Epigenetics mechanisms and degenerative diseases. Open J. Genet. 2 (4), 173–183.

Joshi, K., Chavan, P., Warude, D., Patwardhan, B., 2004. Molecular markers in herbal drug technology. Curr. Sci. 87 (2), 159–165.

Joshi, K., Ghodke, Y., Shintre, P., 2010. Traditional medicine and genomics. J. Ayurveda Integr. Med. 1 (1), 26–32.

Katayama, H., Oda, Y., 2007. Chemical proteomics for drug discovery based on compound-immobilized affinity chromatography. J. Chromatogr. B Anal. Technol. Biomed. Life Sci. 855 (1), 21–27.

Kennedy, S., 2002. The role of proteomics in toxicology: identification of biomarkers of toxicity by protein expression analysis. Biomarkers 7 (4), 269–290.

Kettenbach, A.N., Schweppe, D.K., Faherty, B.K., Pechenick, D., Pletnev, A.A., Gerber, S.A., 2011. Quantitative phosphoproteomics identifies substrates and functional modules of Aurora and Polo-like kinase activities in mitotic cells. Sci. Signal 4 (179), rs5.

Ko, C.C., Chen, Y.J., Chen, C.T., Liu, Y.C., Cheng, F.C., Hsu, K.C., et al., 2014. Chemical proteomics identifies heterogeneous nuclear ribonucleoprotein (hnRNP) A1 as the molecular target of quercetin in its anti-cancer effects in PC-3 cells. J. Biol. Chem. 289 (32), 22078–22089.

Kopec, K.K., Bozyczko-Coyne, D., Williams, M., 2005. Target identification and validation in drug discovery: the role of proteomics. Biochem. Pharmacol. 69 (8), 1133–1139.

Kraus, M., Rückrich, T., Reich, M., Gogel, J., Beck, A., Kammer, W., et al., 2007. Activity patterns of proteasome subunits reflect bortezomib sensitivity of hematologic malignancies and are variable in primary human leukemia cells. Leukemia 21 (1), 84–92.

Kruse, U., Pallasch, C.P., Bantscheff, M., Eberhard, D., Frenzel, L., Ghidelli, S., et al., 2011. Chemoproteomics-based kinome profiling and target deconvolution of clinical multi-kinase inhibitors in primary chronic lymphocytic leukemia cells. Leukemia 25 (1), 89–100.

Lee, A.Y.H., Paweletz, C.P., Pollock, R.M., Settlage, R.E., Cruz, J.C., Secrist, J.P., et al., 2008. Quantitative analysis of histone deacetylase-1 selective histone modifications by differential mass spectrometry. J. Proteome Res. 7 (12), 5177–5186.

Lee, Y.H., Goh, W.W., Bin, Ng, C.K., Raida, M., Wong, L., Lin, Q., et al., 2013. Integrative toxicoproteomics implicates impaired mitochondrial glutathione import as an off-target effect of troglitazone. J. Proteome Res. 12 (6), 2933–2945.

Lemaire, R., Desmons, A., Tabet, J.C., Day, R., Salzet, M., Fournier, I., 2007. Direct analysis and MALDI imaging of formalin-fixed, paraffin-embedded tissue sections. J. Proteome Res. 6, 1295–1305.

Lum, J.H.-K., Fung, K.-L., Cheung, P.-Y., Wong, M.-S., Lee, C.-H., Kwok, F.S.-L., et al., 2002. Proteome of Oriental ginseng Panax ginseng C. A. Meyer and the potential to use it as an identification tool. Proteomics 2 (9), 1123–1130.

MacKeen, M.M., Kramer, H.B., Chang, K.H., Coleman, M.L., Hopkinson, R.J., Schofield, C.J., et al., 2010. Small-molecule-based inhibition of histone demethylation in cells assessed by quantitative mass spectrometry. J. Proteome Res. 9 (8), 4082–4092.

Magkoufopoulou, C., Claessen, S.M.H., Tsamou, M., Jennen, D.G.J., Kleinjans, J.C.S., Van delft, J.H.M., 2012. A transcriptomics-based in vitro assay for predicting chemical genotoxicity in vivo. Carcinogenesis 33 (7), 1421–1429.

Mai, P.L., Wentzensen, N., Greene, M.H., 2011. Challenges related to developing serum-based biomarkers for early ovarian cancer detection. Cancer Prev. Res. 4 (3), 303–306.

Mair, J., Dienstl, F., Puschendorf, B., 1992. Cardiac troponin T in the diagnosis of myocardial injury. Crit. Rev. Clin. Lab. Sci. 29 (1), 31−57.

Marouga, R., David, S., Hawkins, E., 2005. The development of the DIGE system: 2D fluorescence difference gel analysis technology. Anal. Bioanal. Chem. 382 (3), 669−678.

Martin, S.F., Falkenberg, H., Dyrlund, T.F., Khoudoli, G.A., Mageean, C.J., Linding, R., 2013. PROTEINCHALLENGE: crowd sourcing in proteomics analysis and software development. J. Proteomics 88, 41−46.

Meierhofer, D., Weidner, C., Hartmann, L., Mayr, J.A., Han, C.-T., Schroeder, F.C., et al., 2013. Protein sets define disease states and predict in vivo effects of drug treatment. Mol. Cell Proteomics 12 (7), 1965−1979.

Merrick, B.A., Witzmann, F.A., 2009. The role of toxicoproteomics in assessing organ specific toxicity. EXS 99, 367−400.

Mohd Fauzi, F., Koutsoukas, A., Lowe, R., Joshi, K., Fan, T.P., Glen, R.C., et al., 2013. Chemogenomics approaches to rationalizing the mode-of-action of traditional chinese and ayurvedic medicines. J. Chem. Inf. Model. 53 (3), 661−673.

Moulick, K., Ahn, J.H., Zong, H., Rodina, A., Cerchietti, L., Gomes DaGama, E.M., et al., 2011. Affinity-based proteomics reveal cancer-specific networks coordinated by Hsp90. Nat. Chem. Biol. 7 (11), 818−826.

Mrozikiewicz, P.M., Bogacz, A., Karasiewicz, M., Mikolajczak, P.L., Ozarowski, M., Seremak-Mrozikiewicz, A., et al., 2010. The effect of standardized Echinacea purpurea extract on rat cytochrome P450 expression level. Phytomedicine 17 (10), 830−833.

Murthy, K.R., Goel, R., Subbannayya, Y., Jacob, H.K., Murthy, P.R., Manda, S., et al., 2014. Proteomic analysis of human vitreous humor. Clin. Proteomics 11 (1), 29.

Nilsson, C.L., Larsson, T., Gustafsson, E., Karlsson, Ka, Davidsson, P., 2000. Identification of protein vaccine candidates from Helicobacter pylori using a preparative two-dimensional electrophoretic procedure and mass spectrometry. Anal. Chem. 72 (9), 2148−2153.

O'Farrell, P.H., 1975. High resolution two-dimensional electrophoresis of proteins. J. Biol. Chem. 250, 4007−4021.

Pal, P., Kanaujiya, J.K., Lochab, S., Tripathi, S.B., Sanyal, S., Behre, G., et al., 2013. Proteomic analysis of rosiglitazone and guggulsterone treated 3T3-L1 preadipocytes. Mol. Cell Biochem. 376 (1-2), 81−93.

Pan, C., Olsen, J.V., Daub, H., Mann, M., 2009. Global effects of kinase inhibitors on signaling networks revealed by quantitative phosphoproteomics. Mol. Cell Proteomics 8 (12), 2796−2808.

Patil, D., Gautam, M., Mishra, S., Kulkarni, P., Suresh, K., Gairola, S., et al., 2009. Quantitative determination of protoberberine alkaloids in Tinospora cordifolia by RP-LC-DAD. Chromatographia 71 (3-4), 341−345.

Patil, D., Gautam, M., Mishra, S., Karupothula, S., Gairola, S., Jadhav, S., et al., 2013. Determination of withaferin A and withanolide A in mice plasma using high-performance liquid chromatography-tandem mass spectrometry: application to pharmacokinetics after oral administration of Withania somnifera aqueous extract. J. Pharm. Biomed. Anal. 80, 203−212.

Petricoin, E., Rajapaske, V., Herman, E., Arekani, A., Ross, S., Johann, D., et al., 2004. Toxicoproteomics: serum proteomic pattern diagnostics for early detection of drug induced cardiac toxicities and cardioprotection. Toxicol. Pathol. 32 (Suppl. 1), 122−130.

Scannell, J.W., Blanckley, A., Boldon, H., Warrington, B., 2012. Diagnosing the decline in pharmaceutical R&D efficiency. Nat. Rev. Drug Discov. 11 (3), 191−200.

Schirle, M., Bantscheff, M., Kuster, B., 2012. Mass spectrometry-based proteomics in preclinical drug discovery. Chem. Biol. 19 (1), 72−84.

Schirle, M., Petrella, E.C., Brittain, S.M., Schwalb, D., Harrington, E., Cornella-Taracido, I., et al., 2012. Kinase inhibitor profiling using chemoproteomics. Methods Mol. Biol. 795, 161−177.

Searfoss, G., Ryan, T., Jolly, R., 2005. The role of transcriptome analysis in pre-clinical toxicology. Curr. Mol. Med. 5 (1), 53−64.

Seibert, C., Davidson, B., 2008. Multiple-approaches to the identification and quantification of cytochromes P450 in human liver tissue by mass spectrometry. J. Proteome Res. 8 (4), 1672−1681.

Shao, B., Tang, M., Li, Z., Zhou, R., Deng, Y., Nie, C., et al., 2012. Proteomics analysis of human umbilical vein endothelial cells treated with resveratrol. Amino Acids 43 (4), 1671−1678.

Sharma, K., Weber, C., Bairlein, M., Greff, Z., Kéri, G., Cox, J., et al., 2009. Proteomics strategy for quantitative protein interaction profiling in cell extracts. Nat. Methods 6 (10), 741−744.

Shord, S.S., Shah, K., Lukose, A., 2009. Drug-botanical interactions: a review of the laboratory, animal, and human data for 8 common botanicals. Integr. Cancer Ther. 8 (3), 208−227.

Smith, K.T., Martin-Brown, S.A., Florens, L., Washburn, M.P., Workman, J.L., 2010. Deacetylase inhibitors dissociate the histone-targeting ING2 subunit from the Sin3 complex. Chem. Biol. 17 (1), 65−74.

Smith, S.A., Blake, T.A., Ifa, D.R., Cooks, R.G., Ouyang, Z., 2007. Dual-source mass spectrometer with MALDI-LIT-ESI configuration. J. Proteome Res. 6 (2), 837−845.

Štěrba, M., Popelová, O., Lenčo, J., Fučíková, A., Brčáková, E., Mazurová, Y., et al., 2011. Proteomic insights into chronic anthracycline cardiotoxicity. J. Mol. Cell Cardiol. 50 (5), 849−862.

Suter, L., Schroeder, S., Meyer, K., Gautier, J.-C., Amberg, A., Wendt, M., et al., 2011. EU framework 6 project: predictive toxicology (PredTox)--overview and outcome. Toxicol. Appl. Pharmacol. 252 (2), 73−84.

Taki, Y., Yamazaki, Y., Shimura, F., Yamada, S., Umegaki, K., 2009. Time-dependent induction of hepatic cytochrome P450 enzyme activity and mRNA expression by bilobalide in rats. J. Pharmacol. Sci. 109 (3), 459−462.

Taki, Y., Yokotani, K., Yamada, S., Shinozuka, K., Kubota, Y., Watanabe, Y., et al., 2012. Ginkgo biloba extract attenuates warfarin-mediated anticoagulation through induction of hepatic cytochrome P450 enzymes by bilobalide in mice. Phytomedicine 19 (2), 177−182.

Tanaka, E., Kurata, N., Yasuhara, H., 2003. How useful is the "cocktail approach" for evaluating human hepatic drug metabolizing capacity using cytochrome P450 phenotyping probes in vivo? J. Clin. Pharm. Ther. 28 (3), 157−165.

Titz, B., Elamin, A., Martin, F., Schneider, T., Dijon, S., Ivanov, N.V., et al., 2014. Proteomics for systems toxicology. Comput. Struct. Biotechnol. J. 11 (18), 73−90.

USFDA, 2004. Guidance for Industry Botanical Drug Products. U.S. Department of Health and Human Services Food and Drug Administration Center for Drug Evaluation and Research (CDER).

van der Veen, J.W., Pronk, T.E., van Loveren, H., Ezendam, J., 2013. Applicability of a keratinocyte gene signature to predict skin sensitizing potential. Toxicol. Vitro 27 (1), 314−322.

van Vliet, E., 2011. Current standing and future prospects for the technologies proposed to transform toxicity testing in the 21st century. ALTEX Altern zu Tierexperimenten 28 (1), 17−44.

Vedadi, M., Barsyte-Lovejoy, D., Liu, F., Rival-Gervier, S., Allali-Hassani, A., Labrie, V., et al., 2011. A chemical probe selectively inhibits G9a and GLP methyltransferase activity in cells. Nat. Chem. Biol. 7 (8), 566−574.

Velonas, V.M., Woo, H.H., dos Remedios, C.G., Assinder, S.J., 2013. Current status of biomarkers for prostate cancer. Int. J. Mol. Sci. 14 (6), 11034−11060.

Verbist, B., Klambauer, G., Vervoort, L., Talloen, W., Shkedy, Z., Thas, O., et al., 2015. Using transcriptomics to guide lead optimization in drug discovery projects: lessons learned from the QSTAR project. Drug Discov. Today 20 (5), 505−513.

Vergara, D., Simeone, P., Toraldo, D., Del Boccio, P., Vergaro, V., Leporatti, S., et al., 2012. Resveratrol downregulates Akt/GSK and ERK signalling pathways in OVCAR-3 ovarian cancer cells. Mol. Biosyst. R. Soc. Chem. 8 (4), 1078−1087.

Vidal, M., Cusick, M.E., Barabasi, A.L., 2011. Interactome networks and human disease. Cell 144, 986−998.

Wang, M.C., Papsidero, L.D., Kuriyama, M., Valenzuela, L.A., Murphy, G.P., Chu, T.M., 1981. Prostate antigen: a new potential marker for prostatic cancer. Prostate 2 (1), 89−96.

Wang, Y., Muneton, S., Sjövall, J., Jovanovic, J.N., Griffiths, W.J., 2008. The effect of 24S-hydroxycholesterol on cholesterol Homeostasis in neurons: quantitative changes to the cortical neuron proteome. J. Proteome Res. 7 (4), 1606−1614.

Warude, D., Patwardhan, B., 2005. Botanicals: quality and regulatory issues. J. Sci. Ind. Res. (India) 64 (2), 83−92.

Wasinger, V.C., Cordwell, S.J., Cerpa-Poljak, A., Yan, J.X., Gooley, A.A., Wilkins, M.R., et al., 1995. Progress with gene-product mapping of the Mollicutes: mycoplasma genitalium. Electrophoresis 16 (7), 1090−1094.

Wu, Z., Doondeea, J.B., Gholami, A.M., Janning, M.C., Lemeer, S., Kramer, K., et al., 2011. Quantitative chemical proteomics reveals new potential drug targets in head and neck cancer. Mol. Cell Proteomics 10 (12), M111.011635.

Zhang, H., Liu, A.Y., Loriaux, P., Wollscheid, B., Zhou, Y., Watts, J.D., et al., 2007. Mass spectrometric detection of tissue proteins in plasma. Mol. Cell Proteomics 6 (1), 64−71.

Zhu, H., Bilgin, M., Bangham, R., Hall, D., Casamayor, A., Bertone, P., et al., 2001. Global analysis of protein activities using proteome chips. Science 293 (5537), 2101−2105.

Zhu, H., Hu, S., Jona, G., Zhu, X., Kreiswirth, N., Willey, B.M., et al., 2006. Severe acute respiratory syndrome diagnostics using a coronavirus protein microarray. Proc. Natl. Acad Sci. U. S. A. 103 (11), 4011−4016.

Chapter 10

Chemical Informatics

Gerald H. Lushington[1] and Rathnam Chaguturu[2]

[1]LiS Consulting, Lawrence, KS, United States, [2]iDDPartners, Princeton Junction, NJ, United States

The process of drug discovery is like a stream. A hypothesis springs from a headwater source based somewhere in an area of fundamental biological knowledge, and winds its gradual way downhill over a terrain of logic and testing, toward the ideal destination—a fresh channel sustaining the reservoir of public health. As is rendered fancifully in Fig. 10.1, the gradual course of the stream is augmented by various tributaries, including data to validate the hypothesis, as well as specific therapeutic chemistries that can translate the hypothesis into a practical biochemical modulation. A great many streams in the drug discovery landscape wash into stagnant mires of poor efficacy, or dry up in deserts of toxicological and delivery complications. Fortunately, some steer viable courses through the landscape, sustained by the provenance of favorable data and suitable chemical modulators, and ultimately avail themselves to the betterment of humanity.

Informatics, a diverse and important collection of computational tools aimed at generating and resolving data inferences, provides a means for systematically mapping the landscape and incumbent pharmacological strata to plot paths of opportunity of least resistance in pursuit of the ultimate goal of safe, effective, and disease-specific drug formulations. Navigation to a suitable formulation entails the identification of a suitable route (e.g., biochemical pathway) for which the topographical incline (i.e., biochemical kinetics) is suitable, and for which flow-sustaining tributaries (corroborative physiological evidence and amenable therapeutic candidates) are manifest. Even for such a favorable route, the chance of success remains marginal unless your informatics analysis ascertains that the underlying bed of pharmacodynamics and toxicology is favorable, and verifies the flow of corroborative data and optimizable chemotypes is adequate.

Just as a hydrogeological engineer designing a complex canal system would need to consult with a variety of authorities in different fields of geology and engineering, the drug discovery process may at many stages require a diverse array of algorithms to characterize and assess the practical obstacles

Innovative Approaches in Drug Discovery. DOI: http://dx.doi.org/10.1016/B978-0-12-801814-9.00010-6
295

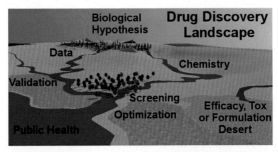

FIGURE 10.1 Successful drug discovery is a flowing process from biological hypothesis to successful impact on public health.

and perceive plausible solutions. Examples of relevant computational analyses include clustering and feature selection methods to identify the genetic underpinnings of an etiology, numerical integration to quantitatively appreciate genetic interdependencies relative to proposed targets, statistical validation techniques to perceive real small-molecule modulators of proposed targets, machine learning to rationalize structure-activity relationships (SARs) among analogous modulators, and ultimately Newtonian physics and statistical mechanics to recognize how biochemical structures imbue these SARs.

Since bioinformatics methods are discussed in other chapters, our immediate focus here will be on chemical informatics—a field that can be thought of as the formulation of quantifiable representations of chemical compounds, their properties, and their relationships with the world around them. Within the general context of drug discovery, chemical informatics comes to embrace the application of a diverse collection of computational algorithms for probing the way structural and physical properties of compounds influence medically relevant aspects of human physiology. This paradigm thus enables computational prediction, assessment and validation of therapeutic prospects, and limitations of drug candidates. Since the focus of this book is to explore innovative approaches in drug discovery, the object of this subsection will be to relate how new and emerging informatics techniques are refining the strategies by which novel therapeutics are currently being sought. For a much more general discussion of chemical informatics in drug discovery (including a mix of common traditional and emerging methods) the reader is referred to an excellent book edited by Oprea (Oprea, 2005).

Chemical informatics methods offer promise toward drug design projects outside of the conventional chemotype-specific lead optimization path. The field of pharmacognosy, which in some practical ways mirrors more basic pharmacology, poses distinct challenges for informatics-based knowledge gathering and optimization. However, many of the basic concepts are harmonious, thus a discussion will be presented to map out possible tactics for enhancing the computational redress of drug development efforts involving natural product extracts.

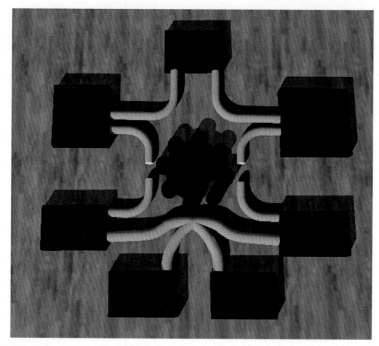

FIGURE 10.2 Key decision points in drug discovery are interconnected, and for each nexus, a reliable transit it facilitated by informatics analysis.

KEY INFORMATICS CHALLENGES IN DRUG DISCOVERY

Perhaps the best angle to approach innovations in chemical informatics techniques is to examine challenging decision points within the drug discovery process and to question whether or not computational techniques are emerging that might ease a project past these junctures. As summarized briefly in Fig. 10.2, some key decision points include the following:

When specifying a chemical screening deck for a preliminary screen, are there practical ways to home in on chemotypes that are more likely to produce hits?

If your screen is phenotypic, is it possible to identify the specific biochemicals that are being modulated in order to produce the observed bioactivity?

From your screening results, is it possible to group the modulators according to subsets whose components exhibit shared mechanism of action?

What are some reliable ways to infer SAR from screening data?

How can you confidently achieve a structure-based activity rationalization?

Which resources and techniques are available for selecting hits with enhanced prospects for target specificity?

Can toxicology be accurately predicted for pharmacologically promising hits?

These decision points are all interrelated as portions of the gradual flow from hypothetical biology to practical medicine and, as will be elaborated in subsequent sections, each step can be addressed with confidence if the corresponding analysis is backed by rigorous, well-validated informatics analysis. The prospects for successful consummation of each step are further enhanced as the rigor and informational underpinnings of such analyses continue to grow.

EFFICIENT SCREEN FOCUSING

High-throughput screens that subject specific assays to hundreds of thousands of compounds, although in vogue a decade ago, have fallen into recent disfavor due to a cost-benefit ratio that has failed to live up to expectations. This failure arises from multiple factors, but perhaps the two most prominent include high rates of false positives and false negatives, and a de facto shortage of legitimately interesting chemical compounds within the screening deck (Lushington and Chaguturu, 2014). The former problem is a technical issue that arises at least in part from cutting analytical corners in order to expedite high-throughput processing of a large number of chemical compounds. This tends to bolster an argument that higher cost-benefit ratios might emerge from more exacting treatment of a smaller number of compounds. The second issue, that of screening large numbers of compounds doomed in advance to be of minimal biochemical interest, suggests a criterion to help guide us in identifying smaller compound sets to screen—the best cost-benefit ratio is likely to be achieved if the screening set is dominated by compounds that have good prospects for demonstrating biologically interesting properties. This latter strategy is further augmented if one has some way of identifying compounds in advance that have some predisposition toward being active in the specific screen of interest.

Identification of intelligent, biologically relevant screening sets is not difficult to do in a general sense. Such strategic compound selections may be readily implemented through molecular information mining techniques, including chemical database filters designed to virtually screen for compounds with inherent similarity to peptides, natural products, metabolites, and an ever-evolving set of privileged scaffolds that reflects not only organic molecules that have historically proven to have interesting biological activity, but also novel scaffolds that have more recently demonstrated promise (Lushington and Chaguturu, 2014; Zhang et al., 2011).

Finer-grained tailoring of screening sets to predispose toward activity is a greater inherent challenge, although there are varying degrees of rigor to which one might choose to pursue such refinements. For example, finding subsets of compounds that will at least distribute to the correct general tissue type is not difficult. There are some very basic filters that may be implemented, based on quantities such as cLogP (Mannhold et al., 2008), volume of distribution, and other pharmacodynamic predictions (Martini et al., 2011), that enable chemotype prioritization according to preferred physiological environments.

Depending on the precise target of interest, more precise gene-specific chemotype selection can range between easy differentiation (e.g., preselected screening sets are sold by numerous vendors for well-documented target classes such as kinases, proteases, ion channels, and G-Protein Coupled Receptor (GPCRs)) to much less accessible ones. The availability of prior screening data is, of course, the key determining factor for being able to identify in advance a subset of compounds with some elevated prospects for producing interesting biochemical outcomes in relation to a specific target.

Given the results of previous screens, a diverse arsenal of informatics techniques may be available to translate sparse inhomogeous data into useful, testable inferences regarding the relationships between different substructural and physicochemical attributes and the propensities for corresponding chemotypes to modulate targets. Data normalization techniques can be productively applied to massage together the information content of multiple distinct experimental protocols. Interpolation methods can help to approximately overcome some minor holes in the structure-activity landscape. Significance evaluation metrics are available for sifting through inconsistencies across different data sets, producing ranks of features that sustain high-confidence decision-making criteria, and de-emphasizing properties that are more likely to be discrepant. Finally, there are numerous machine learning techniques available for training and validating models that relate substructural and physical attributes to bioactivity trends in a consistent and meaningful manner.

Many artificial intelligence techniques bear little resemblance to the old-fashioned linear regression models that have been standbys within traditional quantitative structure-activity relationship (QSAR) methodology (Mitchell, 2014). The introduction of these new, nonlinear model-generation paradigms has proven especially useful in enhancing our ability to realistically and meaningfully assess a diverse array of compounds according to their prospects for modulating given target classes.

In order to appreciate why nonlinear modeling can be so important, we might consider the example of molecular volume—a fundamental property with some (often profound, but frequently complicated) degree of influence on ligand bioactivity. In a given receptor cavity, a certain class of organic heterocycles might exhibit a pseudolinear relationship between molecular volume and binding affinity, such that within a series of highly similar ligands an increasing sidechain volume might correspond to progressively compatible fit with a given hydrophobic pocket. At a certain point (e.g., perhaps for a fairly large substituent such as adamantyl) the pocket volume may pass a saturation point and a sharply inverse relationship between activity and volume could begin to manifest. Somewhat similar chemotypes with comparable binding modes may exhibit analogous behavior. However, a completely different scaffold (e.g., linear peptides) may demonstrate completely different trends, or even no detectible trend at all. Such a scenario, dominated by nonlinearities and complex contingencies, is often of no value whatsoever to the linear regression perspective incumbent in simple QSAR, but may well be resolved and exploited productively by more flexible, adaptive machine learning techniques.

The fuel for such modeling efforts, whether they be linear QSAR or higher-order machine learning strategies, is bioactivity data spanning a variety of different chemotypes and pharmaceutical end points. A potent informational basis for such informatics manipulations is gradually accruing in the form of open-access databases that report both the structure and observed biochemical effects of different bioactive chemicals. This review must emphasize that the world of open-access data is constantly evolving. However, a snapshot of some of the most useful resources available as of spring 2015 would include the following:

PubChem (http://pubchem.ncbi.nlm.nih.gov/): the largest current compendium of chemical biology data of our time, with over 90 million compound entries (a reasonable effort is made to slant toward unique compounds, although many entries vary only by ionization state or other physiologically indistinguishable variations), and more than 1.2 million assay entries (these are by no means unique—large numbers of assay entries are functionally identical and only vary by specific compounds screened in a given entry). PubChem has various drawbacks, including a curation quality that has varied substantially over time, relatively slow search and retrieval rates for bioactivity information, and decidedly cumbersome routes to achieving some forms of information. Nonetheless, it is a data resource of unparalleled magnitude and value.

ChemBank (http://chembank.broadinstitute.org/): a collection of screening data and associated chemical structures that, although much smaller in scope than PubChem, is more carefully curated and focuses heavily on cell-based screens. It is thus of direct relevance to biomedical phenotypes and general understanding of chemical effects on key physiological pathways.

DrugBank (http://www.drugbank.ca): a compendium of structures and biomedically relevant data for known drug molecules (including FDA-approved therapeutics, experimental drugs, withdrawn drugs, illicit drugs, and nutraceuticals). Documented associations are provided between these chemical entities and (where available) their identified protein targets (more than 4100 unique biochemicals).

ChemMine (http://chemminedb.ucr.edu): in terms of information content, this is of similar scope relative to PubChem, but it is substantially smaller but nonetheless worth mentioning because the data collection is better curated, and on-site data analysis tools appear to be faster and more sophisticated.

BindingDB (http://www.bindingdb.org/bind/index.jsp): another resource that combines chemical structure and screening data, this database merits consideration because it includes a substantial amount of chemical biology data derived not just from HTS measurements uploaded en masse to data management utilities, but also based on carefully curated information culled from lower-throughput studies reported in the literature.

The above five resources provide the informational basis for intelligently focusing a screening set to produce meaningful and interesting screening results but, in and of themselves, they are not ideally suited for directly answering the question of what screening subset one should subject a given assay to. The techniques and protocols for this are still evolving, but at the present time it is worth mentioning two online utilities that take rather different approaches to addressing this challenge, plus a third that has not quite matured yet but may well soon prove to be valuable. These include:

STITCH (http://stitch.embl.de/): is a resource that provides plausible chemical-protein interaction pairs, based on a combination of definitive and inferential evidence. Given a specific compound of interest, STITCH will report back a list of potential protein targets that the chemical might be expected to modulate. Given a protein target, the utility provides a list of proposed chemical modulators that could be taken as a basis for constructing a screening set. The algorithm for assessing relationships entails associative machine learning methods that evaluate a combination of large screening data sets, interactions reported explicitly in the literature, inferential associations obtained from text mining, chemical similarity to know modulators of a given target, and target orthology to proteins known to associate specific chemotypes (Kuhn et al., 2014).

DockBlaster (http://blaster.docking.org/): augments STITCH via a structure-based design paradigm in which a chemical screening set is proposed according to the results of molecular docking calculations for a diverse collection of representative chemotypes into any prospective target of interest, as long as that target can be reasonably represented by a three-dimensional atomic structure. The docking studies are automated in all respects (Irwin et al., 2009), including an intelligent selection of prospective small-molecule binding sites via the PocketPicker algorithm (Coleman and Sharp, 2010).

Drugable (http://drugable.com/): is a database composed of proteins and proposed small-molecule binders that has been assembled based on a comprehensive interaction matrix produced by a massive docking campaign (approximately 600,000 chemicals screened against ∼7000 unique receptors, as computed using hundreds of millions of CPU hours, sponsored by Google). As of time of writing, the research underlying

Drugable has not yet been published, and it has been subject to some thought-provoking criticism (Jogalekar, 2013). Consequently, the authors herein will not yet endorse the resource, but will nonetheless point it out as a utility that may emerge in importance in the future.

TARGET IDENTIFICATION

Although cell-based assays tend to be more technically demanding than conventional target-specific biochemical assays, they have gained substantial favor for quantitative assessment of ligand efficacy and potency (Wang, 2014). The drawback with cell-based assays from a strategic perspective is that the target-specific information that they frequently obscure is often of substantial analytical value in pharmacophore perception and lead optimization. Fortunately, informatics methods that utilize powerful target-specific resources (such as those described in the previous section) may greatly facilitate the process of target rationalization. This may be accomplished by objectively comparing (i.e., through statistical assessment) the activity profile of hits from the cell-based assay with predicted or observed profiles for targets or target classes (Schenone et al., 2013). Some cell-based assays will likely produce comparable hits that act over different underlying targets. In general, informatics methods should be capable of accommodating such ambiguities, although to some extent the successful prosecution of such analyses can require significant skill in the choice and appropriate application of clustering and classification algorithms.

One of the most widely used resources for facilitating target identification is the PASS tool (http://www.pharmaexpert.ru/passonline/index.php) (Filimonov et al., 2014). Based on training-to-modulation data on more than 300,000 organic compounds, as gauged against more than four thousand distinct measures of bioactivity, PASS purports to achieve qualitatively accurate predictions (i.e., active vs inactive) more than 95% of the time. An article by Drakakis et al., however, questions the validity of this statistic in terms of statistically driven issues such as justifiable selection of thresholds for distinguishing between active and inactive assignments of different ligand-target pairs (Drakakis et al., 2015). Additional technical questions raised by Drakakis et al. include the pitfalls in attempting to establish global standard thresholds for assigning actives, as well as the practical issue of how effective a given chemical training set is for producing a predictive activity model for compounds whose functional compositions stray from the chemotypes used in the original model training (Drakakis et al., 2015).

Ultimately, the question of how best to assemble models for predicting which biochemical targets a given compound may interact with is intricately tied in with the specific scientific question to be addressed. If the goal is to identify strong prospects for modulation of a given target, one may wish to set a conservative threshold for bioactive prediction, thus potentially leaving out some marginal-activity compounds but minimizing the likelihood of selecting inactives. Specification of a targeted yet speculative screening set might dictate a more liberal threshold, which reduces the chances of omitting potentially interesting chemotypes from a more definitive analytical evaluation. Finally, prescreens intended to flag prospective off-target (and potentially toxic) interactions might set the bar even more liberally, under the assumption that questionable flags for undesired collateral effects may be checked more definitively via toxicology assays or counterscreens.

MECHANISM OF ACTION PERCEPTION

Meaningful SAR analysis is often used as a means for rationalizing the informatically provided capacity to reliably perceive a common biochemical target from within a phenotypic screen. This, in turn, can be a key first step toward classifying hits according to a shared mechanism of action. Once a common target has been identified, analyses similar to those for target resolution (Schenone et al., 2013) may be applied in order to identify compounds subsets that appear to share common SAR trends (and thus, by inference, probable shared mechanism of action). Other techniques that specifically seek to sift through complex multimodal data for mechanistically consistent subsets are emerging, including the biclustering protocol described by Smalter–Hall and Lushington (Aaron Smalter-Hall and Lushington, 2012).

RELIABLE STRUCTURE-ACTIVITY RELATIONSHIP (SAR) ELABORATION

Given a set of screened compounds for which consistent bioactivity data has been quantified, and for which one has reasonable confidence of a conserved mechanism of action, one may proceed toward intelligently optimizing the activity. One popular framework for this optimization is QSAR analysis, but as has been emphasized earlier in this chapter, researchers should always be prepared to explore new options that emerge. An example of this are powerful machine learning methods (as discussed earlier and reviewed elsewhere (Mitchell, 2014)) available for resolving meaningful multivariate relationships with greater flexibility and adaptivity than traditional linear regression methods.

A QSAR model based on well-validated linear regression fitting can provide valuable insight into the underlying structural trends that dictate observed bioactivity but, more often than not, lead optimization studies attempt to employ such QSAR models outside of the models' rather limited zones of applicability. Specifically, the assumed linear-dependence between observed activity and a given molecular property is usually approximately valid only for a certain range of values for that property. Any structural modification taken that places a compound of interest outside of that applicability range effectively invalidates the model for the purposes of activity prediction. This happens very easily when following even relatively basic medicinal chemistry lead optimization strategies. The unsuspecting chemist may thus conceive of several potentially interesting variants to an earlier hit, use the trained, validated (and potentially peer-reviewed and published) QSAR model to evaluate the expected activities of these analogs, and prioritize them for synthesis—only to later obtain disappointing or seemingly illogical results.

Given that many machine learning techniques can embrace nonlinear variable dependence and have a much greater capacity for achieving broader zones of applicability (Mitchell, 2014), the persistent dominance of linear regression as a standard for training QSAR models is quite surprising. There seem to be two primary reasons for this preeminence: as a research concept, QSAR predates the formulation of most artificial intelligence algorithms (thus lending the strength of tradition to linear regression), and the interpretive simplicity of a regression model confers a major advantage for elucidating practical compound redesign prospects.

Ultimately, as greater computational literacy is conferred on subsequent generations of scientists, it is unlikely that either of these arguments will continue to sway the masses. Open source software such as Weka (Hall et al., 2009) is likely to facilitate the migration of scientists away from the old linear regression default, and instead facilitate experimentation with a diverse range of model-training tools implemented conveniently within a single environment such as the Weka Data Explorer. The ease with which different models can be trained, refined, and rigorously validated should typically enable the discovery of QSAR models that are not only locally more accurate than the best performing linear regression models, but also encompass broader applicability domains.

It is true that models with the best predictivity and generality often tend to embrace complex SARs, but to some extent such complexities may entail interpretive wisdom rather than obstacles. In our earlier thought experiment regarding the prospective influence of molecular volume on activity, a well-trained model might identify, for small heterocycles, a nonlinear relationship whose predicted receptor affinity peaks for molecules with a certain midlevel volumetric profile, but the model may concurrently exhibit a completely distinct dependency for linear peptide-like quantities. Given careful scrutiny, many machine-learned models may be rationally parsed in order to distinguish sensible relationships.

Even if the model is too complex for rational deconvolution, it may have semiintuitive analytical value. A reasonably predictive model with good generality can be used as a trial-and-error sand box within which to conceive of and test possible structural variations. Rather than rely strictly on logic, the medicinal chemist can build up a set of potentially interesting analogs simply by proposing a variety of different synthetic variations and then seeing which are viewed most favorably by the model.

RELIABLE STRUCTURE-BASED DESIGN

Amenable to either qualitative intuition from eyeballing crystal structures or more rigorously employed from a molecular modeling perspective via molecular docking or molecular dynamics simulations, structure-based design is utilized even more than QSAR as a tool for lead optimization. Superficially, the paradigm appears to provide compelling rationalization for modifications to hit structures, using prospective ligand-receptor hydrogen bonds, lipophilic surface contacts, and steric limits as optimization criteria. Given our detailed knowledge of the standard geometrical configuration of favorable H-bonds and nonpolar functional group overlap, one would expect such a strategy to more than justify the effort and cost associated with crystallographic and NMR structural resolution, and produce major conceptual breakthroughs on the road to high potency and high selectivity therapeutics.

The truth, however, is that while a ligand-receptor structural resolution is frequently relied upon for detailed postfacto rationalization of observed activities, and is sometimes the source of useful optimization insight, the practice of structure-based drug design trends toward disappointment (Yuriev and Ramsland, 2013). While to the naive eye, a three-dimensional PDB structure looks like a clear, informative, and definitive rendition of a receptor target or a receptor-ligand complex, there are numerous sources of error that include (but are not limited to):

- The conditions under which many structures are resolved are at best only rough approximations to the real physiological scenario. For example, the crystallization temperature and dielectric environment may be unrealistic.
- Intermolecular interactions are often inappropriate: physiologically important partners are often sacrificed in order to achieve structural resolution in crystallographic terms, and each unit is frequently instead presented in unphysically close proximity to copies of itself.
- Finally, real-life ligand-induced receptor fit effects may be substantial: the receptor conformation that corresponds to the physiological scenario for your chemotype of interest may vary significantly from any structures resolved in the presence of distinct ligands.

In the past decade, molecular docking simulation techniques have been in a state of continual improvement, both in terms of their prospects for correctly reproducing the bound conformation of ligands capable of complexing with a given receptor and (albeit more gradually and haltingly) in their ability to accurately rank the ultimate binding affinity of different ligands. Key contributions to this improvement have come from more reasonable and sophisticated schemes for approximating solvation/desolvation effects and receptor flexibility (Elokely and Doerksen, 2013). Despite this progress, a prudent researcher should be aware that any structure-based design inference may fail, but should also keep in mind that there are a number of strategies that one may rely upon to at least partially mitigate the risk of erroneous analysis:

- When choosing a receptor model as a basis for rationalizing the SARs in a target of interest, the most single important selection criteria should always be finding a receptor structure that has been resolved in the presence of a ligand whose ligand-receptor interactions are at least plausibly analogous to the chemotype that one is most interested in.
- When choosing a ligand pose to represent your ligand of interest, it is generally better to rely on preconceptions (especially if dictated by experimentally resolved insight involving ligands and receptors similar to yours) than on the docking scores generated by docking software.
- If you have no preconceived notion of the binding mode, it is better to rely on pose clustering to select your more plausible docked conformer (i.e., choose the highest-scoring poses from within a well-populated family of similar poses) than on the single highest-scoring pose, especially if the manifold of docked structures has few other poses similar to the top scoring mode.

The above recommendations consistently dissuade researchers from placing major decision-making emphasis on the computed scores of specific poses. In one sense, this may seem unfair because computed docking scores generally correlate significantly (i.e., better than random by a statistically demonstrable margin) with true experimental bioactivities when one averages performance over a broad selection of receptors and a comparably broad array of real binding ligands. Unfortunately, the margin of error in score-based ranking is still unacceptable for important tasks such as reliably prioritizing structurally similar ligands according to their prospective binding kinetics and for confidently deciding on one particular pose as a basis for structure-based design.

If one is engaged in a lead optimization project that is blessed with both a reasonable basis of bioactivity data across a manifold of ligands with comparable mechanism of action, coupled with a plausible structural model for that specific mechanism of action, it is possible to apply chemical informatics to achieve a powerful degree of synergy between QSAR and structural information. This synergy, availed by a technique known as comparative binding energy (COMBINE) analysis (Wang and Wade, 2002) can help one to at least partially overcome many of the limitations associated with the component modeling techniques (Lushington et al., 2007).

COMBINE modeling can be classified as a structure-based QSAR technique in which a structure-activity model is trained for a collection of ligands based on a manifold of descriptors derived from electrostatic and van der Waals interactions between each ligand and each receptor amino acid within a certain cutoff radius. In training a QSAR model from such a descriptor basis, the machine learning process evaluates each structure-based parameter

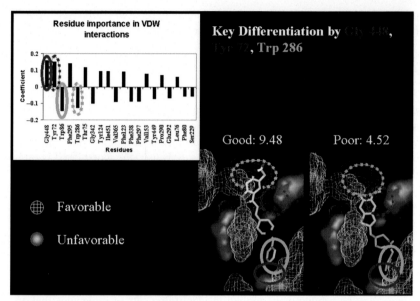

FIGURE 10.3 Key amino acids influencing the van der Waals interactions between noncovalent ligands and the acetylcholinesterase active site. Coefficient plot (upper left) indicates the relative magnitude of amino acid coefficients, where positive coefficients reflect amino acids with unfavorable van der Waals surfaces, while negative coefficients indicate favorability. Key features are shown spatially (lower right) in the context of a high potency ligand ($-$pIC50 = 9.48) displaying excellent overlaps with favorable residues, and a much weaker analog ($-$pIC50 = 4.52) with close contacts to unfavorable surfaces.

according to its capacity for effectively reproducing activity trends. As is represented in Fig. 10.3 for van der Waals interactions in noncovalent complexes with acetylcholinesterase (based on data reported by Guo et al. (2004)), model coefficients thus tend to emphasize or de-emphasize specific interaction terms in a way that conceptually corrects for limitations in the purely structural model. For example, if dynamic extropy present in a given amino acid side chain tends, for the ligands of interest, to produce interactions that are generally more favorable than what one might guess from a static docking score alone, that should be reflected in a well-trained model. Similarly, if induced-fit produces a receptor relaxation that, physiologically, enables a specific receptor pocket to support sterically favorable interactions, that should also be evinced by a good model, even if the original receptor conformation was unrealistically constrained in the pocket of interest. Coefficients for the specific amino acids also provide an intuitive framework for perceiving specific aspects of the ligands that are ripe for strategic refinement in the pursuit of optimal affinity. Finally, reverse-optimization is possible when refining ligands for selectivity against a competing receptor (e.g., as one might wish when selecting against a given side effect profile) using precisely the same COMBINE methodology, except with opposite criteria (i.e., looking to amplify interactions that the model judges to be unfavorable).

ACHIEVING TARGET SPECIFICITY

Just as COMBINE analysis can be a useful tool for optimizing a given lead for selective modulation of the therapeutically intended target, the other aforementioned informatics strategies discussed in this chapter may be of value in selecting against the modulation of undesired biomolecules. When it comes to collateral toxicity and side effects, however, the worst devil is often the one you don't recognize. In other words, for a novel therapeutic candidate, there may be unforeseen deleterious effects arising due to interactions with unexpected biomolecules.

While no method is likely to prove foolproof in circumventing side effect risks, the most useful resource may prove to be the same type of protocol discussed earlier in the context of focusing screening sets toward prospective efficacy toward the target of interest. This same combination of chemical biology data and informatics methods for assessing prospective chemical relevance may be productively applied in identifying sets of molecules that are deselected against all target classes except the one of interest. In truth, the depth and expanse of chemical biology knowledge is nowhere near to the comprehensive level likely required to make such negative assessments with high degrees of confidence, however, the current basis should at least help to slant the odds toward finding suitably selective lead candidates.

One critical factor to recognize in the pursuit of target specificity is that the compound one designs and administers may not be the compound (or the "only" compound) that exerts a resulting biochemical influence. When attempting to predict the biochemical outcome of compounds, it is critical to examine not only the parent chemical, but to also identify and evaluate potentially multiple prospective metabolic products of that compound (Kalgutkar and Dalvie, 2014), where each compound is gauged according to whether it is likely to produce undesirable or potentially toxic biochemical effects (Kellici et al., 2015).

ACCURATE TOXICITY PREDICTION

Side effect prediction, as described in the previous paragraph, is a key component of drug toxicology, but the methods described therein are by no means a full basis for comprehensive toxicity prediction. The reason for this is obvious—the resources and techniques described earlier are geared toward a combination of chemical biology understanding and the productive exploitation thereof for therapeutic purposes. Toxic responses, however, range from the highly target-specific modulations that underlie most drug mechanisms, all the way to highly general effects that might compromise the function of dozens or hundreds of different cell types, and further include a broad swath of possible effects situated somewhere in between these extremes.

Accurate toxicology assessment is an objective that spans multiple fields of major commercial value, including manufacturing and agriculture, as well as the pharmaceutical industry. The sheer number of distinct modes of toxic manifestation render the task of reliable de novo predictions very challenging, but pragmatic computational methods are evolving to address the requirement through similarity and analogy.

To understand the underlying basis for toxicology assessment, it helps to visualize the different mechanisms of a toxic effect. At one end of the spectrum, one has the equivalent of an undesired pharmacological effect—a chemical that interacts with fair specificity toward a specific biomolecule, with the distinct caveat that the interaction is undesirable and potentially deleterious. Computational prediction of such effects proceeds in the same manner as one might choose for assessing the prospective target profiles of specific compounds. We need not elaborate further on this since it has been discussed previously in this chapter.

Other toxicity instances arise from much more general phenomena. Some compounds have chemically reactive subgroups that are prone to coupling with a broad range of different proteins in ways that might impact their function. Others may inherently disrupt nucleic acids through intercalation (in the case of DNA) or covalent complexation (both DNA and RNA). Still others might couple with lipids in ways that compromise many types of cell membranes. In these cases, the molecular properties that dictate toxicity (i.e., special reactive chemical groups in the former case; distinct amphiphilicities in the latter) differ substantially from target-specific toxins; however, the structure-activity profile is typically much easier to predict.

A major practical challenge encountered in de novo toxicity prediction for a given compound entails not only the process of using a model to predict a toxic effect, but also needing to identify which, out of multiple possible models, is actually the most appropriate for assessing that compound. This issue is starting to be addressed by open-data resources such as the TEST suite of online toxicity prediction models (http://www.epa.gov/nrmrl/std/qsar/qsar.html). In the TEST paradigm, a researcher enters a structural representation of a compound of interest into the user interface, and the front-end processor within the utility examines the compound to see, within default constraints, whether it falls within the applicability domain (Sushko et al., 2010) of any of its multiple models. If the compound is plausibly represented by any of the phenotypically specific toxicological mechanisms, TEST reports a toxicity prediction for the compound for all suitable virtual assays, and typically offers contextual information including details about the training set and the reliability level of the model. Within the current representation, compounds that have a structural predisposition toward well-understood toxicity mechanisms will often be assessed fairly accurately, but relatively unusual compounds (or species with somewhat aberrant toxicity profiles) may be predicted with poor accuracy or be ignored entirely.

PHARMACOGNOSY

For thousands of years, humanity's greatest source of therapeutics was the natural world around us—unusual chemicals synthesized by microorganisms, plants and animals that tend to have effects on other life forms, including pathogens that threaten our health, as well as modulating various of our own cells that are not behaving in physiologically productive ways. The fact the such chemicals frequently exhibit pharmacological effects is not surprising, given that many have arisen courtesy of environmental or evolutionary pressures that in some way may mirror our own challenges. The chemical diversity inherent in available natural product space is comparable to what one encounters within the screening decks that comprise conventional drug discovery projects. This similarity tends to point toward a prospect of providing informatics-guidance to pharmacognosy-based drug discovery, but in practice we are faced with two related complications that alter the informational landscape. This first confounding factor is that natural product extracts are often presented in crude form as solubilized organic matter, obtained from a source organism but not rigorously separated into recognizable distinct chemical compounds. The second source of tantalizing frustration is the fact that, even when the chemical identities of mixture components can be resolved, the therapeutic effect of the mixture may exhibit complex, nonlinear dependence on the components, perhaps reflecting some convoluted biochemical complementarity—a natural drug cocktail whose optimal component ratio is unknown and whose minimally requisite components may be unclear.

In the face of informational ambiguities and imperfect characterization, is it possible to productively apply artificial intelligence techniques to parse the informational haystack and arrive at an adequate basis of tangible needles from which to embark on plausible optimization?

Let us begin with a scenario that, although distinct from canonical lead optimization, bears it at least some passing resemblance. Specifically, let us suppose that from extract screening, we have identified one particular extract fraction that demonstrates promising activity toward our phenotype of interest, and we have subjected this fraction to rigorous analytical characterization, such that we have reasonable confidence in the assignment of chemical identities to key components of the mixture. What we may not be immediately certain of is which components ultimately affect the observed physiological effect and, if more than one component is important, how might the multiple players couple to deliver the observed outcome?

Under these circumstances, there are two different strategies that may be applied (alone or in combination) to shed light on bioactive components and prospective interdependencies. The first tactic once again entails a reliance on the gradual accrual of massive screening data compendia, spanning both a broad array of chemotypes (including a large span of natural-product-like chemicals) and their effects on numerous different assays of both target-specific and phenotypic natures.

A first pass evaluation of known components of a screened extract may wish to prioritize chemicals simply by how much prior evidence there is for at least some measurable degree of activity against any biological screen for the observed compound or for chemical analogs thereof. This will likely not prove to be a definitive discriminant of active versus inactive components in your extract of interest, but it provides a degree of tangible evidence, since the confidence of a compound being active in one screen is immediately elevated by knowledge that the compound has been demonstrably active in any other screen. Conversely, many (though not all) compounds that have been found inactive in all tested screens to date have been recorded as such for fundamental reasons—the compound may distribute poorly, might be unstable in polar media, or may simply possess a chemical functionality that is consistently unfavorable for effecting biochemical modulation.

If one has the informational basis to go beyond the simple "global bioactivity" evidence, then one should do so. Specifically, if one knows the identity of the target being screened, then it is particularly helpful to focus on prior screening results for that precise target or for homologous biochemicals. Analogously, if the screen of interest is phenotypic, then the greatest informational value is found in data from phenotypes that are identical or similar to the one of interest. Both of these forms of comparative reasoning are of a nature similar to strategies discussed earlier for side effect perception, and thus are well-established informatics concepts that can aid in the rationalization of pharmacognosy data.

If one is able to rationalize, based on informatics comparisons with prior screening, a plausible set of bioactive compounds within a given active extract fraction, it is often useful to look for bioactivity trends when sampling over other extract fractions that may have some of the same constituent compounds, but perhaps in differing ratios. This can serve to begin verifying whether specific compounds truly do seem to impart biochemical modulation (e.g., if fractions that contain a given compound tend to be disproportionately active and fractions lacking the compound tend to be inactive, then the individual activity of that compound can be qualitatively inferred). When fractions are collected from an extract, however, there is no guarantee that enough distinct fractions containing a given compound will be available to give a statistically significantly assessment of that compound's individual activity. In such cases, it may prove valuable to enlist the support of experimentalists in generating a more diverse fraction basis. In other words, by varying the fraction collection protocol (e.g., by experimenting with different solvent mixtures or alternating the fraction partitioning parameters), one may produce a more comprehensive sampling from which the resultant screening can produce a greater perception of the relative importance of different components.

While general statistical sampling techniques provide a simple mechanism for probing the individual significance of an extract component toward the observed bioactivity, a good data set spanning a diverse array of different fractional compositions can lead one to greater insight in terms of how activity may be enhanced by optimizing mixtures of multiple component compounds. By treating relative quantities of specific compounds within a fraction as a basis of features, one may apply any of numerous machine learning techniques to perceive specific combinations of compounds that, when acting in concert or in mutual exclusion, tend to have critical effects on bioactivity.

Many forms of natural product extract contain so much intrinsic chemical diversity that even separation methods may produce mixtures that are too complex for detailed chemical characterization. Analogously, one may encounter scenarios in which many protocols for partitioning the extract into fractions severely compromise the bioactivity observed for the crudest extract form. In such cases, it is still possible to apply informatics methods toward knowledge elucidation and sample refinement, although the relationships that one may arrive at are more abstract and further removed from the intuitive detail one may achieve in pharmacologically simpler cases.

Specifically even if one cannot definitively identify the chemical identity of specific compounds, it may be possible to optimize fraction collection by at least keying on specific mass peak intensities evident in mass spectrometric distributions. The relative preponderances of specific peaks or combinations of peaks that correspond to a predisposition toward greater activity of comprising fractions might thus reflect individual compounds with the desired bioactivity effect, or else advantageous combinations of compounds that yield synergistically beneficial outcomes. This framework, within which the mass spectrometry peak abundances are the primary descriptor basis for model training, may enable the development of an optimization engine that is useful, even if it doesn't perceive the true chemical identities of the fractions that are being optimized.

If one is never able to definitely report the chemical identity of key fractional components, one is ultimately shutting the door on future QSAR or structure-based design efforts aimed at efficacy or selectivity refinement. However, it still can be possible to produce a viable, marketable therapeutic without ever pursuing this subsequent refinement.

CONCLUSIONS

The pharmaceutical industry, which has spent many years languishing in the doldrums of paltry therapeutic discovery, has been entering a state of revolution as it revamps many aspects of its philosophy and practices. Greater acceptance of natural product extracts as a key (if complex) source of novel chemistries, as well as increased appreciation for holistic approaches in therapeutic optimization, offers critical avenues for growing the pipeline of new candidate prospects, and achieving more systematic guidance regarding the most important optimization criteria for safe, effective medicines.

Many aspects of the paradigm shift rely extensively on the availability, and reliable processing, of high-volume data. The practical applicability of such information is expanding explosively, yet old numerical practices are proving to be largely inept for extracting useful knowledge from the voluminous raw numbers. Fortunately, from an informatics perspective, exciting new methods available for addressing the greater computational challenges in these new drug discovery pipelines are emerging rapidly.

Based on a clear need for new informatics tools, as well as a community of methods developers who are increasingly sensitive to the real needs of large-scale data mining and pattern recognition, the field of chemical informatics is truly now rising to the occasion. The survey of concepts and paradigms reported in this chapter, itself representing but a few snapshots of a dynamic and evolving field, show great promise toward alleviating the disappointing prior performance of modeling studies. New techniques and resources, grounded in sound scientific reasoning and rational well-validated approaches that exploit a growing volume of publically available data, stand to become cornerstones of the new pharmaceutics arena.

REFERENCES

Aaron Smalter-Hall, A., Lushington, G.H., 2012. Discovering mechanisms of action in chemical structure-activity data sets. Recent Adv. Biol. Biomed. Ser. 1, 47–53.

Coleman, R.G., Sharp, K.A., 2010. Protein pockets: inventory, shape, and comparison. J. Chem. Inf. Model. 50, 589–603.

Drakakis, G., Koutsoukas, A., Brewerton, S.C., Bodkin, M.J., Evans, D.A., Bender, A., 2015. Comparing global and local likelihood score thresholds in multiclass laplacian-modified naïve bayes protein target prediction. Comb. Chem. High. Throughput. Screen. 18 (3), 323–330.

Elokely, K.M., Doerksen, R.J., 2013. Docking challenge: protein sampling and molecular docking performance. J. Chem. Inf. Model. 53, 1934–1945.

Filimonov, D.A., Lagunin, A.A., Gloriozova, T.A., Rudik, A.V., Druzhilovskii, D.S., Pogodin, P.V., et al., 2014. Prediction of the biological activity spectra of organic compounds using the pass online web resource. Chem. Heterocycl. Comp. 50, 444–457.

Guo, J., Hurley, M.M., Wright, J.B., Lushington, G.H., 2004. A docking score function for estimating ligand-protein interactions: applications to acetylcholinesterase inhibition. J. Med. Chem. 47, 5492.

Hall, M., Frank, E., Holmes, G., Pfahringer, B., Reutemann, P., Witten, I.H., 2009. The WEKA data mining software: an update. SIGKDD Explor. 11 (1), 10–18.

Irwin, J.J., Shoichet, B.K., Mysinger, M.M., Huang, N., Colizzi, F., Wassam, P., et al., 2009. Automated docking screens: a feasibility study. J. Med. Chem. 52, 5712–5720.

Jogalekar, A., 2013. Drugable.com "ranks billions of drug interactions"? Hold your horses. The Curious Wavefunction. <http://wavefunction.fieldofscience.com/2013/12/drugablecom-ranks-billions-of-drug.html>.

Kalgutkar, A.S., Dalvie, D., 2014. Predicting toxicities of reactive metabolite−positive drug candidates. Annu. Rev. Pharmacol. Toxicol. 55, 35−54.

Kellici, T., Dimitrios Ntountaniotis, D., Vrontaki, E., Liapakis, G., Moutevelis-Minakakis, P., Kokotos, G., et al., 2015. Rational drug design paradigms: the odyssey for designing better drugs. Comb. Chem. High. Throughput. Screen. 18 (3), 238−256.

Kuhn, M., Szklarczyk, D., Pletscher-Frankild, S., Blicher, T.H., von Mering, C., Jensen, L.J., et al., 2014. STITCH 4: integration of protein-chemical interactions with user data. Nucl. Acids Res. 42, D401−D407.

Lushington, G., Chaguturu, R., 2014. To screen or not to screen: an impassioned plea for smarter chemical libraries to improve drug lead finding. Future Med. Chem. 6, 497−502.

Lushington, G.H., Guo, J.-X., Wang, J.L., 2007. Whither COMBINE? New opportunities for receptor-based QSAR. Curr. Med. Chem 14(17), 1863−1877.

Mannhold, R., Poda, G.I., Ostermann, C., Tetko, I.V., 2008. Calculation of molecular lipophilicity: state-of-the-art and comparison of log p methods on more than 96,000 compounds. J. Pharm. Sci. 98, 861−893.

Martini, C., Olofsen, E., Yassen, A., Aarts, L., Dahan, A., 2011. Pharmacokinetic-pharmacodynamic modeling in acute and chronic pain: an overview of the recent literature. Exp. Rev. Clin. Pharmacol. 4, 719−728.

Mitchell, J.B.O., 2014. Machine learning methods in chemoinformatics. WIREs Comput. Mol. Sci. 4, 468−481.

Oprea, T.I., 2005. Chemoinformatics in Drug Discovery. Wiley-VCH, Weinheim, Germany.

Schenone, M., Dančík, V., Wagner, B.K., Clemons, P.A., 2013. Target identification and mechanism of action in chemical biology and drug discovery. Nat. Chem. Biol. 9, 232−240.

Sushko, I., Novotarskyi, S., Körner, R., Pandey, A.K., Cherkasov, A., Li, J., et al., 2010. Applicability domains for classification problems: benchmarking of distance to models for AMES mutagenicity set. J. Chem. Inf. Model. 50, 2094−2111.

Wang, T., Wade, R.C., 2002. Comparative binding energy (COMBINE) analysis of OppA-peptide complexes to relate structure to binding thermodynamics. J. Med. Chem. 45, 4828−4837.

Wang, W., 2014. Potency Testing of Biopharmaceutical Products. American Pharmaceutical Review. <http://www.americanpharmaceuticalreview.com/Featured-Articles/169473-Potency-Testing-of-Biopharmaceutical-Products/>.

Yuriev, E., Ramsland, P.A., 2013. Latest developments in molecular docking: 2010−2011 in review. J. Mol. Recognit. 26, 215−239.

Zhang, J., Lushington, G.H., Huan, J., 2011. Characterizing the diversity and biological relevance of the MLPCN assay manifold and screening set. J. Chem. Inf. Model. 51, 1205−1215.

Chapter 11

Vaccines and Immunodrugs Discovery

Manish Gautam[1], Bhushan Patwardhan[2], Sunil Gairola[1] and Suresh Jadhav[1]

[1]*Serum Institute of India Private Limited, Pune, Maharashtra, India,* [2]*University of Pune, Pune, Maharashtra, India*

INTRODUCTION

The current decade, from 2010–20, has been declared the decade of vaccines. Vaccines contribute enormously in reducing the global healthcare burden presented by infectious diseases. Vaccine development is technology-intensive. Global efforts are committed toward the discovery, development, and delivery of life-saving vaccines. A number of vaccines including *Haemophilus influenzae* type b (Hib), pneumococcus, meningococcus, combination vaccines, and subunit vaccines such as acellular pertussis vaccines were developed and introduced at a relatively faster pace. The scope of vaccines has widened in the 21st century, and vaccines are now envisaged against noninfectious disorders such as e.g., cancer, autoimmune, and neurodegenerative diseases. In addition to these major achievements, challenges, and failures in the development of vaccines against some complex pathogens such HIV, TB, and HCV still remain. Optimal strategies eliciting protective immune responses against antigens remain elusive, and this challenge becomes bigger in the absence of safe and effective immunomodulatory adjuvants. Further, emerging pathogens (SARS, Ebola, and Zika viruses) pose a major threat to human life. These obstacles and challenges highlight the need to move beyond the classical vaccinology paradigm of "isolate, inactivate, and inject." Technological advances in genomics, proteomics, immunology, synthetic biology, and bioinformatics coupled with reverse vaccinology and systems-based approaches present significant opportunities to address these challenges. These tools and approaches permit the exploration of molecular mechanisms of protective immunity. As a consequence, novel immune targets for vaccine and adjuvants are being discovered (Plotkin, 2014). Targets for adjuvants and delivery systems such as the toll-like

Innovative Approaches in Drug Discovery. DOI: http://dx.doi.org/10.1016/B978-0-12-801814-9.00011-8

receptor (TLR) and Th-1/Th-2 immunity appear promising, and small-molecule immunodrugs are being researched for efficient modulation of these targets. The chemical diversity offered by botanical immunodrugs will prove attractive for such discoveries (Poland, 2012; Delany et al., 2014).

DISCOVERY APPROACHES FOR VACCINES

Empirical Approaches

In the early 19th century, microbes were discovered as causative agents for diseases. Louis Pasteur established basic rules of vaccinology. To date, most vaccines have been developed based on Pasteur's principles of "isolate, inactivate, and inject" as the causative agents of disease. These approaches are considered empirical, even though vaccines are developed with little or no understanding of the complex immunological mechanisms by which they induce protective immunity. The empirical approach is based on a unifying rationale that reducing the virulence of the disease-causing organism (killing, inactivation, and attenuation) reduces or inhibits the pathogenicity while preserving their immunogenicity. Vaccines for trabies and anthrax were the first to be developed using attenuation. Inactivating microorganisms was another successful approach wherein whole organisms could be killed without losing immunogenicity. Vaccines for typhoid, cholera, pertussis, influenza, and hepatitis A were derived using the inactivation approach. Other approaches consisted of isolating virulent factors from microorganisms such as toxins or capsular polysaccharides. Tetanus and diphtheria vaccines represent formalin-inactivated toxins. Hib, meningococcal and pneumococcal vaccines represent examples of capsular polysaccharides. However, capsular polysaccharides as immunogens show limitations in induction of T cell−dependent immunity in infants and elderly populations. These limitations led to the development of glyco-conjugation technology, wherein a covalent linking of capsular polysaccharide to a protein carrier results in the induction of T cell−dependent memory and thereby significantly improves the vaccine efficacy in all the age groups. Glyco-conjugate vaccines for Hib, meningococcal, and pneumococcal serotypes currently play an important role in control of these infectious diseases.

Although many vaccines have proved successful, empirical approaches show the limitations of discovering vaccines against complex and variable pathogens. The following limitations of empirical approaches are highlighted:

- Suits well to microorganisms that can be cultured in vitro.
- Focuses and allows targeting of only predominant components. Have challenges with pathogens which do not have identifiable immunogenic regions. The identifiable antigen may be a poorly immunogenic, for example, the polysaccharide capsule for Meningococcal type B.

- Needs facilities and safety procedures for handling of pathogenic microorganisms. This will be further challenging for complex pathogens such as HIV, TB, malaria, SARS, and Ebola.
- Risks involved because of incomplete activation or attenuation of pathogenic organism. Challenges for quality control and assurance to control the inherent variability and complexity.
- Most importantly, there's time: it may take decades to develop newer vaccines.

These limitations led to a rethink on vaccine discovery approaches globally, and as a result, more rational design of vaccines have been envisaged. A rational design of vaccines would involve an optimum selection of antigen, adjuvant, and delivery system to elicit predictable protective immune responses against known specific epitopes to protect against the pathogen. There are no universally accepted strategies and tools to rationally design such vaccines.

RATIONAL APPROACH TO DISCOVERY

Change in paradigm from isolate-inactivate-inject to discover-validate-characterize-inject based approaches.

GENOMIC APPROACHES FOR DISCOVERY OF ANTIGENS

With the advent of whole-genome sequencing and advances in bioinformatics, the vaccinology field has radically changed, providing the opportunity for developing novel and improved vaccines. The availability of the complete genome sequence of a free-living organism *H. influenzae* in 1995 marked the beginning of a "genomic era," which allowed scientists to employ new approaches for vaccine design. Knowledge of the complete genome for pathogens can now be used for identifying antigenic targets by using the approach known as Reverse Vaccinology Approach. The best example is that of discovery of vaccine against serogroup B *Neisseria meningitidis*. The classic approach to developing a vaccine against meningitis B failed due to the homology of the proteins to humans. A recombinant approach also failed due to antigenic variations observed in circulating Men-B strains. The problem was solved, however, through a rational selection of candidate antigens based on genomic information (Delany et al., 2014). The whole genome of *N. meningitidis* was computationally analyzed, and the specific sequences of surface proteins or surface-associated lipoproteins as vaccine candidates were identified. More than 600 potential antigens were identified and tested for antigenicity. The candidate sequences were expressed in *Escherichia coli* and were tested in animals. Sera analysis resulted in 90 previously unknown surface located proteins and that 29 of them were found bactericidal. The merits of this approach were noted: it resulted in the identification of four or five new surface proteins with bactericidal activities. The antigen with the broadest bactericidal activity against circulating Men-B strains was selected. This was followed by successful preclinical and clinical studies, which led to the development of a licensed vaccine. Reverse vaccinology is now used for many bacterial, viral, and eukaryotic pathogens and has been successful in all cases in providing novel antigens for the design of new vaccines. The approach is widely applicable, as there are many genome sequences available publicly. In the last decade, sequencing of 1129 bacterial genomes has been completed, and 2893 are currently in progress. Recent advancements in genome sequencing technologies and the approaches used to screen the genome and proteome of a bacterial pathogen have greatly improved the efficiency and time needed for antigen discovery. These advancements have also improved antigen discovery and characterization for eukaryotic pathogens, which often encode >10,000 genes (Sette, 2010).

Proteomics-Based Approaches

Proteomics is an important tool for studying the entire complement of proteins expressed by cells. Technology advancements in chromatography, mass spectrometry and protein arrays have enabled us to identify vaccine targets and proteins of interest. Proteome databases of diverse microrganisms such as *Salmonella typhimurium*, *Chlamydophila Pneumoniae*, *Mycobacterium tuberculosis*, *Bacillus anthracis* are available presently. These databases will be important for strategies aimed at comparing proteomes of virulent and a virulent strains, clinical isolates, which can lead to fast identification of potential candidates (Jagusztyn-Krynicka et al., 2009).

Other Technologies

Among newer technologies, structural vaccinology and synthetic biology represent considerable potential. Structural vaccinology-based research led to the discovery of peptide epitope of RSV, which was shown to be a protective correlate of functional neutralizing antibodies in preclinical models. Synthetic biology has led to capabilities to make a completely synthetic RNA vaccine of pandemic H7N9 virus, which was shown to induce protective antibody titers in preclinical models (Finco and Rappuoli, 2014). In addition, formulation of selected antigens with appropriate adjuvants may also expand the protection provided against variable pathogens (Seib et al., 2012).

Newer approaches to antigen discovery including reverse vaccinology, proteomics, structural vaccinology, and synthetic biology hold significant potential for identification of potential antigens. However, their scope remains limited with respect to prediction of protective antigens.

Another approach, also based on reverse engineering of vaccines, is currently being applied for discovery of antigens against HIV, influenza, etc. as variable pathogens. This approach is based on the interrogation of the antibody repertoire from subjects infected with the pathogen. This approach is based on technological advances in isolation and development of monoclonal antibodies, sequencing, computational, and protein crystallography based techniques. The steps include (1) identification of subjects with broadly neutralizing serum responses, (2) identification of broadly neutralizing monoclonal antibodies from such subjects and cloning them using vectors, (3) determination of structure of binding sites of such monoclonal antibodies using crystallographic techniques, and finally (4) use of binding sites to design immunogens and protein scaffolds to elicit such bnAbs. The first proof-of-concept for reverse engineering of vaccines has now been achieved for respiratory syncytial virus (RSV), where computationally designed immunogens mimicking the binding site for an RSV neutralizing monoclonal antibody have successfully elicited RSV specific neutralizing antibodies in monkeys (Koff et al., 2013).

Such advances in antigen identification have also influenced the development of therapeutic vaccines against cancer. The therapeutic use of vaccination based on specific antigens associated with the disease has not had equal success despite many attempts to cure chronic infections and cancer. However, in 2010, the FDA approved Sipuleucel-T, the first therapeutic vaccine for prostate cancer. Sipuleucel-T represents a milestone and may pave the way for a wider use of cancer vaccine immunotherapy based on innovative technologies that allow for simpler immunization methods. Several cancer vaccine candidates, based on recombinant antigens or viral vectors, are in advanced development with promising phase II results. If they confirm their partial efficacy in larger phase III trials, the next step will be to combine cancer vaccines with additional immunotherapies such as monoclonal antibodies acting on negative regulators of the immune response (e.g., CTLA-4 and PD-1). Recognizing these efforts in 2013, cancer immunotherapy was picked by *Science* as an outstanding scientific achievement as the "breakthrough of the year" (Coontz, 2013).

Finally, novel adjuvants hold the potential for newer, efficacious vaccines. The only adjuvants licensed for human use were hydroxide and phosphate salts of aluminum (alum). The potential of developing novel adjuvants has increased exponentially with the discovery of innate immune receptors such as TLRs and nucleotide-binding oligomerization domain-like receptors (NLRs). The licensure of the new adjuvant such as MF59 led to the improved effectiveness of seasonal influenza vaccines in the elderly and the development of vaccines against pandemic influenza strains such as H5N1 or H7N9. Other adjuvants recently licensed for human use are ASO3 and ASO4 for influenza and HPV respectively. Different adjuvants can synergize if combined in the same formulation. For example, AS01 is a mix

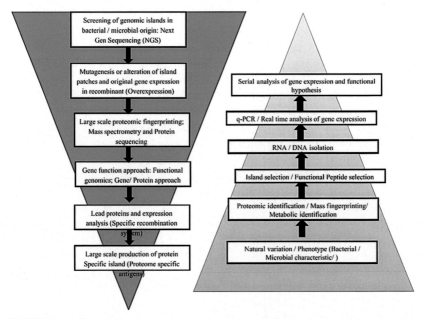

FIGURE 11.1   Gives a comparative account of reverse vaccinology and conventional approaches used for discovery of antigens.

of liposome, saponin, and monophosphoryl lipid A. It was used to enhance the efficacy in the RTS, S malaria vaccine. In a phase II study, RTS,S/AS01 showed 53% efficacy against first episodes of malaria in children (O'Hagan and Fox, 2015). These developments highlight an important paradigm shift from empirical to rational design approach, resulting in safer, efficacious, and better-characterized vaccines as compared to earlier empirical approach towards vaccine development. Fig. 11.1 gives a comparative assessment of approaches used for discovery of antigens.

In the following sections, two case studies of vaccine discovery against complex pathogens are presented. The case studies clearly depict trends on how the advanced technologies and approaches are guiding the development of vaccines against complex pathogens.

VACCINES AGAINST COMPLEX PATHOGENS

Vaccine discovery against highly complex, variable, and challenging pathogens like HIV and malaria face many challenges.

CASE STUDY 1: HIV/AIDS VACCINE

AIDS is an infectious disease that continues to spread, and since its discovery in 1983, more than 25 million people have died from it. Approximately

35 million people are estimated to be living with HIV/AIDS; the majority do not have access to HIV prevention, care, and treatment. The current highly active antiretroviral therapy allows viral replication to be controlled; however, it does not affect latently infected resting memory CD4 + T cells. Therefore, an HIV cure is not possible until this reservoir (infected resting CD4 + T cells) is purged or targeted (Whitescarver, 2016). The development of a safe and effective prophylactic HIV-1 vaccine would be the best approach for its control and elimination.

WHY HIV VIRUS IS CHALLENGING

1. A higher mutation rate gives rise to multiple HIV subtypes that circulate around the globe, allowing the virus to escape the responses that human immune systems mount against it. This limits the approach of using attenuated or killed versions of the pathogens for immunization.
2. Quickly following transmission, the virus disseminates and establishes a persistent infection and hidden reservoirs from which it can strike again at any time. The opportunity for a vaccine-induced response to prevent infection or to control the initial, limited infection is thus short-lived.
3. Limited knowledge on the correlates of protection for durable and specific immune responses against HIV (Koff, 2015).

Table 11.1 lists the major clinical studies carried over the years for HIV vaccine development. In early 1980, driving on the success of the hepatitis B vaccine led to the belief that a recombinant subunit of viral envelope would be the best approach for an HIV vaccine. Unfortunately, this did not work. The subunit vaccines based on the HIV envelope were tested in several phase I and II studies. The studies clearly showed that antibodies induced to subunit vaccines do not demonstrate a cross protection against divergent or primary viruses. Two important trials were undertaken: one with VaxGen, using a vaccine composed of a mixture of the recombinant subunits from two clade B viruses adjuvanted with alum; and AIDSVAX, using a mixture of clade B and clade E envelopes (AIDSVAX B/E). These failures also led the scientific community to look at the role of cellular immunity (T cell) in HIV infection.

T cell–based vaccines led to the design of the STEP trial, an efficacy study wherein immunization with a nonreplicating adenovirus 5 (MRKAd5 HIV-1) expressing Gag/Pol/Nef or placebo was studied. The vaccine failed to prevent infection or to control viral load. Among all these failures, RV 144 trial in the year 2009, showed some promise. RV 144 trial was based on a prime-boost regime: priming with a canarypox expressing the subtype B HIV Gag, Pro and the subtype E gp120 (ALVAC-HIV) and boosting with the alum adjuvanted mix of gp120 AIDSVAX B/E. Conducted in 16,000 heterosexuals in Thailand, this trial yielded a modest 31.2% prevention of HIV infection. This trial brought the focus on prime-boost strategies and

TABLE 11.1 Major Successes and Failures of HIV Vaccine Development

Year	Details of Study	Target/Focus	Outcome
1986–96	First human trial in Congo (Year 1986) and trials thereafter	Monomeric HIV-1 Env gp120 protein. Env-specific humoral immune responses as target	Antigens failed to induce broadly neutralizing antibodies (bNAbs)
Based on above findings, a global rethink on approach occurred. Vaccine strategies for targeting of cellular immune response were-considered			
Studies in rhesus monkeys	Virus specific T-lymphocytes as target	Prolonged survival of SIV- challenged rhesus monkeys was observed. The increased survival correlated with a lower viral set point	Virus specific T-lymphocyte responses seemed to play a critical role in controlling SIV replication
			T cell immunity proposed as important target in HIV vaccine
Year 2007 STEP Trial NIH & Merck	The most famous HIV-1 vaccine focused on T cell immunity is HIV vaccine trials network (HVTN) 502, also known as the "STEP" trial	The vaccine candidate was formulated as a trivalent mixture of rAd5 vectors expressing HIV-1 clade B Gag, Pol, and Nef, respectively	STEP trial was terminated in year 2007
			The vaccine could neither prevent infection nor decrease early plasma virus levels in those who received the vaccine
	Preclinical and animal studies suggested a significant potential of the approach and the results were very encouraging		Moreover, a completely unexpected observation emerged in the STEP trial, in which a greater number of vaccine recipients got infected

Year 2009 RV 144 Trial (only successful study in humans)	The trial used a "prime-boost" combination of two vaccines including vCP1521 canarypox vectored vaccine, which was manufactured by Sanofi Pasteur, and AIDSVAX B/E gp120 subunit vaccine, which were previously tested in the VAX003 and VAX004 trial	Thai trial demonstrated a 31.2% efficacy in preventing HIV-1 infection, which was the first vaccine showing a modest protection The data failed to identify a neutralization antibody as a potential correlate, but, surprisingly, the nonneutralizing antibodies, especially those involved in mediating antibody-dependent cell-mediated cytotoxicity (ADCC), may play a role in the protection
Year 2013 HVTN trial		In 2013, vaccinations were terminated in the HVTN 505 trial, which tested a different Ad5 candidate in a prime/boost combination with a DNA-based vaccine The candidate vaccine failed to prevent HIV infection or blunt the disease's course in those who became infected
Year 2016 (future studies)		New trials are designed to evaluate modifications to the vaccine candidates and regimen, including testing: – Related HIV immunogens – Different adjuvants, and new immunization schedules with additional booster shots intended to improve both strength and durability of immune responses

new efficacy trials are now being planned. If successful, these new efforts could provide licensable vaccines within this decade. In the meantime, an expanded phase II trial based on a multiclade DNA priming and adenovirus five boost is also being conducted by the NIH Vaccine Research Center. Overall, the results of these studies suggest that antibodies alone or CD81 T cells alone are not effective, and that a combination of both antibodies and T cells offers marginal protection against disease. Because no protective vaccines exist for HIV, it is not currently possible to define correlates of protection. Systems-based approaches will be key to better understand the protective correlates of HIV disease (Rappuoli and Aderem, 2011).

CURRENT APPROACHES FOR HIV VACCINE

Three scientific paradigms are proposed as the way forward for HIV development:

1. *Induction of neutralizing antibodies*: A vaccine should elicit a number of antibodies capable of neutralizing many genetically different strains. However, the virus develops resistance to these antibodies and thrives in the host superseding the humoral and cellular immune responses. Notable exceptions to this are nonconventional bnAbs, which are observed in a very small percentage of HIV-infected individuals. Such bnAbs are known to develop during the first three years of natural infection. Therefore, vaccine regimens should focus on inducing useful bnAbs for neutralization of the viral strains. Currently, many neutralizing antibody targets are being researched as potential candidates for inducing bnAbs production. These include receptor binding sites on gp120 for CD4 receptors and CCR5 or CXCR4 coreceptors; variable regions like V1, V2, and V3 on gp120; and binding sites on gp41 molecules such as conserved helices and membrane-proximal external region of gp41 (Rubens et al., 2015).

2. *Induction of CD8 T cell-mediated immunity*: Another broad arm of vaccine development includes eliciting HIV specific CD8 T cell responses. CD8 T cells destroy viruses and infected cells thereby helping in the process of convalescence in any viral infection. Recent studies have focused on some viral vectors for stimulating and sustaining useful CD8 T cell activity. Vaccination with SIV protein-expressing rhesus cytomegalovirus (RhCMV/SIV) vectors offered long-term control over viral load through stimulation of CD8 T cells immune responses.

3. *Combination approaches*: A number of viral vectors and alternative delivery systems are being researched for advanced HIV vaccines. These include vectors such as nonreplicating adenovirus, adeno-associated virus, Venezuelan equine encephalitis virus, Sindbis virus, herpes simplex virus, Measles virus, modified vaccinia virus Ankara, vesicular stomatitis virus, canarypox, Semliki forest virus, DNA vectors, mRNA vectors, and nano-formulations.

CASE STUDY 2: MALARIA VACCINE

Malaria affects about 3.2 billion people, which is nearly half of the world's population. In 2015, there were roughly 214 million malaria cases and estimated 438,000-malaria related deaths. Increased prevention and control measures have led to a 60% reduction in malaria mortality rates globally since 2000. Malaria is caused by five species of Plasmodium that infect humans (*Plasmodium falciparum, Plasmodium vivax, Plasmodium ovale* spp., *Plasmodium malariae,* and *Plasmodium knowlesi*) and is transmitted by the bite of the infected female Anopheline mosquitoes. Progress toward developing malaria vaccines has accelerated in the last decade owing to greater awareness as well as advances in science and vaccine technologies. The goal of the malaria vaccine-development program is to develop and license a first-generation malaria vaccine that has a protective efficacy of more than 50% against the disease, and immunity should last longer than one year. Currently, three types of vaccine are in development:

- Preerythrocytic vaccine
- Blood-stage vaccine
- Transmission-blocking vaccine

Preerythrocytic vaccine candidates: Preerythrocytic vaccine candidates aim to protect against the early stage of malaria infection—the stage at which the parasite enters or matures in an infected person's liver cells. These vaccines would elicit an immune response that would either prevent infection or attack the infected liver cell if infection does occur. These candidates include:

1. Recombinant or genetically engineered proteins antigens from the surface of the parasite or from the infected liver cell.
2. DNA vaccines programmed for producing the vaccine antigen in the vaccine recipient.
3. Live, attenuated vaccines that consist of a weakened form of the whole parasite (the sporozoite) as the vaccine's main component.

Blood-stage vaccine candidates: Blood-stage vaccine candidates target the malaria parasite at its most destructive stage—the rapid replication of the organism in human red blood cells. The goal of a vaccine that contains antigens or proteins from the surface of the blood-stage parasite (the merozoite) would be to allow the body to develop that natural immunity with much less risk of getting ill.

Transmission-blocking vaccine candidates: Transmission-blocking vaccine candidates seek to interrupt the life cycle of the parasite by inducing antibodies that prevent the parasite from maturing in the mosquito after it takes a blood meal from a vaccinated person. These vaccines would not prevent a person from getting malaria, nor would they lessen the symptoms of the disease (Fact Sheet on malaria vaccine development).

FIRST SUCCESSFUL MALARIA VACCINE

Novel adjuvant played an important role in vaccine efficacy, which resulted in the first success with malaria. Purified or subunit antigens based on irradiated sporozoites were not able to replicate the characteristics of natural infection for malaria vaccines. The best results were achieved by using the circumsporozoite (CS) protein, the most abundant antigen on the surface of the sporozoites. The active substance in candidate malaria vaccine is a recombinant antigen expressed in *Saccharomyces cerevisiae* coded RTS,S. RTS is a hybrid polypeptide consisting of a portion of the CS protein, a sporozoite surface antigen of the malaria parasite *P. falciparum* strain NF54, fused to the amino-terminal end of the hepatitis B virus S protein. S designates the surface antigen of Hepatitis B virus (RTS, 2009).

The vaccine was studied with different novel adjuvants based on oil in a water-emulsion platform. GSK Proprietary AS01 Adjuvant System consists of a liquid suspension of liposomes with two immunostimulant components: 3'-*O*-desacyl-4'-monophosphoryl lipid A (MPL) and *Quillaja saponaria* 21 (QS21). The first human antiparasite vaccine RTS,S/AS01E got regulatory approval from EMEA in 2015. This product was developed through a partnership between GSK and PATH Malaria Vaccine Initiative, with funds from the Gates Foundation to MVI. This is by far the most successful malaria vaccine to demonstrate efficacy in reducing the rate of all episodes of clinical malaria. RTS,S/AS01 prevented a substantial number of cases of clinical malaria over a three-to-four-year period in young infants and children when administered with or without a booster dose. The vaccine used a novel adjuvant AS-01, which played an important role in the efficacy of the vaccine. Immunologic analyses indicate that high titer anti-CS IgG are most strongly associated with RTS,S-mediated protection, with an important additive component from CS-specific Th1 cells. Efficacy was enhanced by the administration of a booster dose in both age categories.

Interestingly, no relevant differences in antibody titers or T cell immunity were observed between the protected group and the nonprotected groups, indicating that the quality rather than the quantity of B and T cells was the key for protection. Thus, the vaccine has the potential to make a substantial contribution to malaria control when used in combination with other effective control measures, especially in areas of high transmission (Neafsey et al., 2015).

Systems biology is an ideal approach to look for nonobvious differences between protective and nonprotective immunity. The availability of a well-validated human challenge model where complex vaccines based on sporozoites will induce protection only if the sporozoites are irradiated but still alive. The availability of a simple vaccine like RTS,S that can only induce protection when combined with a particular adjuvant such as AS02, represents a unique resource to look for network signatures that may distinguish a protective immune response from a nonprotective one.

CHALLENGES TO DEVELOPING MALARIA VACCINES

Even with recent progress, accelerating the development of malaria vaccines remains as complex as ever. Developers face myriad challenges:

- *P. falciparum* is a highly immuno-evasive, multistage protozoal parasite with several antigenically distinct mosquito vector and human stages. Despite the success of the *P. falciparum, Anopheles gambiae* and human genome projects, there has been little translation of antigenic targets from postgenomic antigen discovery to clinical evaluation, partly because of the problems of selecting appropriate targets, and the lack of robust and reliable predictive animal models.
- There are no known correlates of immunity for malaria vaccines; therefore, vaccine candidates can only be shown to work (or not work) by going through clinical trials.

SYSTEMS APPROACH TO VACCINOLOGY

Systems-based approaches aim to generate data through high-throughput measurements in the context of vaccination to characterize the interactions between individual components of immune system to predict the behavior of immune system as a whole in response to vaccination. This includes analysis of transcriptional, signaling, and metabolic pathways whose activity is perturbed in the various cells of immune systems in response to vaccination as well as in the identification of molecular signatures that are predictive of protection from the infection. Such approaches also allow correlations to current large-scale profiling technologies, multiplexing platforms spanning flow cytometry, and multiplex serum protein assays, to explore unbiased information at cellular/subcellular and single-cell level (Porichis et al., 2014). The complexity of protective immunity is best characterized by unbiased, hypothesis-free, "holistic" analyses. These include biomics studies of the protein, transcript, or metabolite content of relevant compartments in the human body following vaccination. In most cases, samples from vaccinated subjects (naturally infected individuals) are collected from the peripheral blood and genome-wide transcriptomics (analysis of global gene expression profiles), using mostly RNA from whole blood or isolated blood leukocytes (Kaufmann et al., 2015) are carried out. The knowledge obtained through these analyses can aid in the rational design of newer vaccines that generate long lasting protection and induce improved responses in populations with immunocompromised status such as the elderly (Pulendran, 2014; Buonaguro and Pulendran, 2011). The vaccine development against diseases like HIV, malaria, tuberculosis, and dengue fever has challenges in identifying the protective correlates of vaccine efficacy, and systems approaches are currently being followed for the determination of such correlates. Vaccines are expected to contain at minimum two antigenic epitopes: one to induce specific B cell or cytotoxic T cell responses, and one to provide T cell help. Broadly protective vaccines require cocktails of target antigens or epitopes in addition to immunomodulatory components (adjuvants and enhancers) that would enable desired immune responses.

EXAMPLES OF SYSTEMS APPROACH

Yellow fever vaccine (YF-17D): The understanding of an entire immune response induced by YF-17D was well studied using live attenuated yellow fever vaccine. Postinduction, using YF-17D vaccine, a significant enhancement of early antiviral gene expression signatures occurred characterized by type I interferon activation in consortium with a complement pathway, inflammasome, and innate immune sensing in peripheral blood mononuclear cells (Querec et al., 2009).

Another example comes from neonatal Bacille Calmette–Guerin (BCG), the live attenuated strain of *Mycobacterium bovis*. The animal studies suggested that vaccine afforded immunity through CD4 + T cells and IFN-gamma. However, such findings did not find confirmation with human infant models. Systems biology-based approaches revealed that that BCG induces nonspecific or heterologous expression via epigenetic reprogramming of monocytes and natural killer cells such that innate immunity is enhanced. Such mechanistic insights will be important for redefining the suboptimal immune response to existing and newer vaccine designs (Netea and Van Crevel, 2014).

A similar approach using reverse genomics and systems approach was applied to decipher the mechanistic differences between inactivated and live, attenuated influenza vaccine. Live, attenuated vaccine was found to induce a robust interferon response as compared to inactivated vaccines that induced largely B-cell response signatures. The outcome of such studies support the potential of systems vaccinology approach to characterize and validate the interactions of vaccines with immune systems.

In a recent report, NGS approaches were used to decipher B-cell receptor repertoire following vaccination as a new measure of immunogenicity. In another study on tetanus toxoid vaccine, integration of NGS and mass-spectrometry proteomic analyses were used to generate specific B-cell repertoire patterns associated with serum tetanus IgG responses.

Genome-wide association studies in vaccines using microarrays identified genetic variants associated with various human traits, including vaccine immunogenicity. For example, a variant proximal to HLA-DPB1 was found associated with responses to hepatitis B vaccine; this variant has also been associated with chronicity of hepatitis B infection, suggesting that a genetically determined inability to produce antibodies to hepatitis B surface antigen predisposes individuals to chronic hepatitis B infection. Similarly, genetic variants associated with interferon-stimulated gene (IFI44L) and the

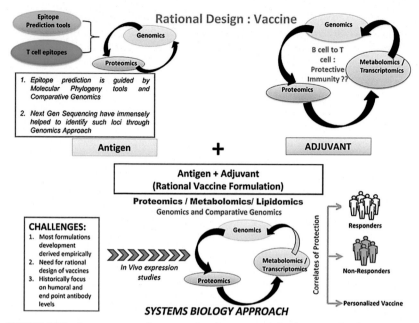

FIGURE 11.2   Systems approaches to vaccine discovery and development. The figure depicts applications of omics technologies in the discovery of antigen, adjuvant and vaccine formulations. Such approaches also offer opportunities for identifying the genetic basis for response to vaccines.

measles receptors (CD46) were found to be associated with febrile seizures following measles-mumps-rubella vaccination. Such approaches focused on understanding the genetic basis of immunogenicity and reactogenicity will further reveal the molecular pathways underlying vaccine outcomes, and this therefore highlights the importance of large-scale GWASs in vaccinology (Blohmke et al., 2015).

Fig. 11.2 gives an account of systems approach to vaccine discovery. It also depicts the role of technologies in the rational design of vaccines.

VACCINE ADJUVANTS

The term adjuvant means to assist or aid, and its use can be traced to the early 17th century. From a medical perspective, "An adjuvant is a substance that, when added to a prescription, assists the action of the principal ingredient or base." From a vaccinology perspective, adjuvants are chemical substances of various types that, when added to vaccines, typically augment or modify any concomitant immune response, thus inducing protection. Adjuvants in vaccines can either act as an immunomodulator or as immune potentiators (Flower and Perrie, 2013) and exhibit their immune effects through a broad variety of molecular and cellular mechanisms.

Vaccine adjuvant's major functions are dose sparing of administered antigen and secondly, to augment, hasten, and lengthen specific immune responses made to vaccine antigens and thus provide a better and longer-lasting protection against target pathogens. Thus, the adjuvant is any substance, compound or even strategy, which results in the enhancement of adaptive immune responses when delivered together with the antigen.

Currently, the pharmaceutical industry largely relies on the use of aluminum-based mineral salts (alum) as adjuvants owing to their successful track record of safety, efficacy with vaccines, including diphtheria-tetanus-pertussis, human papillomavirus, influenza, and hepatitis vaccines. Notably in recent times, limitations of alum in the induction of cytotoxic T cell immunity and T helper (Th) type 1 immune responses are reported. Several hundred adjuvants have been tested for their ability to exacerbate immunity in the last decade. Such adjuvants include those derived from microorganisms, nucleic acids, proteins such as cytokines and polysaccharides, amongst many others. Very few of such adjuvants proved successful, with limitations such as a lack of efficacy, cost, toxicity, and ease of manufacture, poor adsorption, or poor stability. However, a few immunopotentiatory adjuvants (MF59, AS03, and AS04) containing vaccines were approved for human use. Thus, there remains an imperative need for new substances that can act as adjuvants. Until the recent past, adjuvant development was largely empirical; however, the increased understanding of the immune systems and its interactions have made discovery, optimization, and formulation of adjuvants more rational.

IMMUNE TARGETS FOR ADJUVANT DISCOVERY

Vaccine development is transitioning from a process of empirical experimentation to rational design of vaccines. Rational vaccine design involves well-defined antigenic units formulated with tailored adjuvants and/or delivery systems to induce optimum protective immune responses. Such approaches require in-depth understanding of disease, correlates of protection, immunological interactions and the intended role of adjuvants in the formulation. It is becoming increasingly clear that the innate immune response regulates the quality of adaptive immune response and adjuvants can play an important role in governing the ability of vaccine to induce Th-1 or Th-2 responses, Ab responses of broad breadth or affinity, and memory development or cellular immune responses.

A simplistic functional classification of adjuvant activity reported by O'Hagan (10) stills hold true which suggested that an adjuvant can influence any or all of following signals necessary for a successful immune response to a vaccine antigen:

Signal 0 — Activation of the innate immune response
Signal 1 — Antigen

Signal 2 — Costimulation of immune cells, including antigen-presenting cells (APCs)

Signal 3 — Immune modulation.

Signal 0 relates to the activation of innate immunity. Innate immune responses are governed by a recognition of conserved pathogen—associated molecular patterns expressed by various cells of immune systems. Several families of PRRs have been characterized, with TLRs being the most relevant to adjuvant activity, owing to their roles in the activation of adaptive immune responses. Various synthetic TLR agonists have been tested in clinical trials as adjuvants. The inclusion of specific TLR agonists or combinations in the vaccine formulation can direct the type of vaccine immune response.

Signal 1 facilitates adjuvants beneficially modify antigen-associated characteristics such as antigen residence time, the spatio—temporal behavior of the antigen (antigen geography) and the amount of the antigen that eventually reaches the adaptive immune cell receptors, for instance, antigen-specific receptors on T- and B-lymphocytes. Examples include aluminum salts, antigen-loaded micro- or nanoparticles or gels. Adjuvants may exert their effects through different mechanisms. Some adjuvants, such as alum and emulsions (e.g., MF59®), function by generating depots that enhance the antigen persistence at the injection site and increase recruitment and activation of APCs. Particulate adjuvants (e.g., alum) have the capability to bind antigens to form multimolecular aggregates, which encourages uptake by APCs. Signal-1 facilitators such as alum promote Th-2 responses by modulating dendritic cells and granulocytes signaling.

Signal 2 facilitates target cells of the innate immune system including macrophages, DCs, neutrophils, eosinophils, mast cells, NK cells, NK T cells, etc. These cells express various cell-type-related receptors such as TLRs, NLRs, RIG-I-like receptors (RLRs), and C-type lectin receptors (CLRs). TLR ligands, especially TLRs 2, 3, 4, 7/8, and 9, have shown promising results as vaccine adjuvants. Various preclinical and clinical studies on antigens such as lyme, malaria, HIV, hepatitis B have supported their potential as adjuvants with vaccines containing such ligands already licensed in the US, Europe, and Argentina (Steinhagen et al., 2011). There are adjuvants that facilitate both signal 1 and 2 and act synergistically. A prototype example is the immunostimulating complex (ISCOM), which is both an antigen-delivery system and exhibits immunostimulating activity. In addition, AS04 adjuvant may belong to the signal 1 and 2 providing combination adjuvants. Recombinant cytokines, such as IL-12, may also be categorized as signal 2—facilitating adjuvants.

Signal 3 is required to modulate a selective (Th) cell—type response, which enables the activation of distinct adaptive defense pathways resulting in the proper immune-effector elements. For example, the predominance of a Th1-type response, supporting the generation of CD8 + cytotoxic T-lymphocytes

(CTLs) is believed to be crucial for intracellular microorganisms and for tumors. Or alternatively, the predominance of Th-2–type response will support the generation of humoral responses driven by CD4 + T-lymphocytes, which will be crucial for extracellular threats. The nature of signal 2 eventually mediates signal 3. For instance, adjuvants such as MF59 and ISCOMs and TLR 2 and 5 ligands boost T cell and antibody responses without polarization of Th1/Th2 responses against antigens. In contrast, adjuvants such as ligands of TLRs 3, 4, 7, 8, and 9, complete Freund's adjuvants and polarize the antigen responses to T cells towards Th1 and Th17 responses. Thus, the adjuvant not only compensates for poor immunogenicity of recombinant, or synthetic vaccine antigen candidates, but also evokes the desired type of immune-effector response. Most traditional infectious disease vaccines are based on antibody responses for which pathways are well understood. The challenges lie in developing approaches or adjuvants that will generate protective CD8 + T cell responses to soluble proteins. An ideal Th-1 adjuvant is envisaged to trigger dendritic cell (DC) activation, induce type I interferon (IFN) production, and promote differentiation of functional CD8 + T cells through MHC class I processing pathway. Such adjuvants hold the key for vaccines against HIV/AIDS, malaria, and generating T cell responses in patients who respond poorly to the relevant tumor or viral antigens because of biased Th1/Th2 immunity. Consequently, novel adjuvants are being explored and tested (Schijns and Lavelle, 2011; Coffman et al., 2010).

TRENDS IN ADJUVANTS AND IMMUNOMODULATORS

Aluminum salts are the most widely used adjuvants, and have been used successfully for 80 years for induction of Ab responses. Toxoid-based vaccines such as DPT or DTaP are good example of vaccines that contain alum. The poor immunogenicity of toxoids was improved by their formulation with alum salts as adjuvants. Alum salts offers an excellent safety profile, they are easy to formulate, and most importantly, they are cost effective. There are generally three types of alum-containing adjuvants used in industry: aluminum hydroxide, aluminum phosphate, and potassium aluminum sulphate (alum). Alum salts induce Th-2 dominant responses and are reportedly to have limitations in modulating or boosting cellular responses required for immunity against intracellular infections and cancer. For example, the most advanced malaria vaccine candidate (RTS, S) did not produce protection when it was formulated with alum but induced moderate protection when formulated with adjuvants such as AS02 and AS03. The other category of successful vaccine adjuvants is oil-in-water emulsions. The adjuvant MF59 developed by Novartis and AS03 by GSK are squalene-based oil in water-based adjuvants licensed for seasonal influenza vaccine (Fluad) with good results. These adjuvants also resulted in significant amount of dose sparing, which is critical during a pandemic. These developments led to increased research into possible targets for adjuvant activity. Several families of PRRs have been characterized and have resulted in the development of synthetic TLR agonists. The inclusions of specific TKR agonists or combinations thereof in vaccine formulations can direct the type of immune responses. For example, TLR5 agonist's flagellin can promote T cell immunity but does not alter Th1/Th2 balance, whereas TLR3, 4, 7/8, and 9 agonists polarize the response towards a Th-1 bias.

The current trend in vaccine development is to formulate vaccines with multiple adjuvants to improve their efficacy. The rationale for this approach lies on the assumption that such vaccines would engage multiple signaling pathways and elicit distinct and ultimately synergistic immune outcomes. Such trends have also resulted in considerable interest in approaches of combining immunostimulatory adjuvants and delivery systems wherein immunostimulatory adjuvant increases specific responses by direct stimulation of the immune system, whereas delivery systems carry the antigens to the immune cells. Additionally, the delivery system allows the coadministration of multiple immunostimulants and antigens into the same system. These trends have created newer avenues for immunopotentiators in adjuvant discovery, and many agents derived from bacteria, viruses and plant sources, which directly activate immune cells, are under investigations.

SMALL-MOLECULE IMMUNODRUGS

As presented in previous sections, licensed adjuvants are represented by alum-based substances, squalene oil-in-water emulsions, and MPL based. These classes of adjuvant per se act by their (1) physical form and (2) by securing temporal stability of antigen while presenting it to APCs. There is another often-neglected class of adjuvants, which are small molecules, and they act by direct stimulation or engagement of immune targets resulting in stimulation of responses against antigens. The targets such as TLRs, C-lectins, and regulatory T cells are emerging as important targets for small-molecule extant adjuvants. The successful examples of such an approach to vaccine adjuvant discovery include imidazoquinolines, variety of natural products, such as QS21 or MPL, Bestatin, levamisole, (4-methoxyphenyl)-N-methylethanamine, etc.

Interestingly, the reported adjuvant activity of these molecules is incidental to their original discovery. Therefore, attempts for systematic discovery of small molecule and or natural products as vaccines adjuvants are missing. With recent discoveries of TLR receptors and TLR agonists as vaccine adjuvants, there is an impetus to undertake systematic research towards exploring the use of small molecules as vaccine adjuvants. Such small-molecule adjuvants can be discovered using either synthetic route or are discovered by bioprospecting of natural products. Natural products offer chemical, structural, and chiral diversity, but present challenges in developing successful synthetic routes. The computational approaches coupled with advances in immunology, allows discovering novel small molecules that can act in vivo as adjuvants.

BOTANICALS FOR VACCINE ADJUVANTS

Plants are known to possess substances that stimulate or regulate immunity. A group of compounds that has in recent years garnered much interest in the field of adjuvants are terpenoids (QS-21) and polysaccharides. Several plant molecules were found to influence important targets of adjuvant activities such as dendritic cells, B-lymphocytes, and Th1/Th2 modulatory activities (Licciardi and Underwood, 2011). For instance, polysaccharides derived from *Astragalus* species were shown to up-regulate murine DC expression of CD11c and MHC class II in vitro, suggesting enhanced DC antigen presentation capacity. Further, a flavonoid-rich fraction from *Alchornea cordifolia* was reported to be associated with increased HLA-DR, CD40, CD80, and CD86 expression on human and murine DCs. Botanicals are also reported to induce B cell and T cell functions. A combination of saponins from *Polygala tenuifolia* and DPT vaccine elevated anti-DT, anti-TT, and anti-PT IgG titer responses significantly. Another plant component, Taxol from *Taxus brevifolia* is an alkaloid recognized by human TLR4. The scope of plant based immunomodulators as adjuvants in mucosal delivery of vaccines has also been studied. The bioactive plant compound pinellic acid was shown to enhance serum antiinfluenza HI titers on oral administration. The increased titers were observed in mucosal secretions including bronchoalveolar lavage and nasal washes. In another report, a significant increase in mucosal responses was observed with intranasal influenza vaccine when administered with saponins derived from *Paeonia tenufolia*. Elevated mucosal responses have also been reported for cholera toxin when combined with saponins from *Chenopodium*. Botanicals modulating T-lymphocyte functions are also important candidates for adjuvant discovery. The botanicals with modulatory effects on CD4 and CD8 immunity are reported and have shown interesting vaccine adjuvant activities.

SAPONINS AS VACCINE ADJUVANTS

Saponins are a chemically heterogeneous group of steroid and triterpenoid glycosides present in a wide range of plant species. Notably, saponins can activate the mammalian immune system, which has led to a significant interest in their potential as vaccine adjuvants. The lead candidate saponin adjuvants are Quil A and its derivative, QS-21. The unique capacity of Quil A and QS-21 to stimulate Th1 immune responses against exogenous antigens makes them ideal for use in vaccines against intracellular pathogens such as RSV cytomegalovirus *Toxoplasma gondii*, and visceral leishmaniasis and therapeutic vaccines such as cancer. i QS saponins were also reported to have limitations such as high toxicity, undesirable hemolytic effect and instability in aqueous phase, which limits their use as adjuvants in human vaccination. Therefore, many saponins from other botanicals are being studied for their potential as vaccine adjuvants. Notably, saponins represented by genin-senosides, notoginsenosides, and gypenosides were shown to display a slight hemolytic effect and enhance significantly a specific antibody and cellular immune response against OVA in mice.

Adjuvant activity of *Panax notoginseng* saponin, ginsenoside was reported to increase an antigen-specific antibody and cellular response and elicit a Th1 and Th2 immune response by regulating production and gene expression of Th1 cytokines and Th2 cytokines. The saponins from the root extract of *Pelargonium grandiflorum* increased specific antibody and cellular response against OVA in mice, and could be a promising balance between Th1- and Th2-directing immunological adjuvants. Further purification of this extract afforded four adjuvant-active saponins, platycodin D, D2, D3, and platycoside E Platycodin D and D2 have recently proved to possess the adjuvant activities on recombinant hepatitis B surface antigen, Newcastle disease virus-based live attenuated vaccine, and fowlpox virus expressing the avian influenza virus H5 gene.

In a recent study, a saponin rich extract of an Indian medicinal plant, *Asparagus racemosus*, significantly modulated the immune response to DPT-based vaccines, and also enhanced the mucosal responses of the tetanus toxoid vaccine when formulated with chitosan-based nanoparticles. Among the hot water extracts from 267 different types of Chinese and Japanese medicinal plants screened for the adjuvant activity, the root of *P. tenuifolia* contained the most potent adjuvants when combined with nasal influenza or diphtheria−pertussis−tetanus (DPT) vaccine, and its active substances were identified as onjisaponins A, E−G. These four onjisaponins provided safe and potent adjuvants for intranasal inoculation of influenza HA and DPT vaccines (Nagai et al., 2001).

BOTANICALLY DERIVED POLYSACCHARIDES AS VACCINE ADJUVANTS

Carbohydrate structures play critical roles in immune system function and carbohydrates also have the virtue of a strong safety and tolerability record. A number of carbohydrate compounds from plant, bacterial, yeast, and synthetic sources have emerged as promising vaccine adjuvant candidates. One of the first polysaccharides recognized to have immunological effects was β-D-(2-1) poly (fructo-furanosyl) β-D-glucose, more commonly known as inulin, a natural, plant-derived storage carbohydrate of various plants that is also produced by Aspergillus family microorganisms and *Streptococcus mutatis*.

Inulin is a polymer comprising linear chains of fructosyl groups linked by β(2-1) glycosidic bonds terminated at the reducing end by an α-D- (1−2)-glucopyranoside ring group. Inulin's immune activity was first identified to activate complement proteins through a nonclassical pathway. Gamma inulin is nontoxic in several species including humans and is nonpyrogenic. Its primary chemical structure is completely known, and it is inexpensive, readily available, and easy to handle and manufacture. The combination of Alum and gamma-IN is also registered as Algammulin, and are potent enhancers of the Th1 immune response pathway, boosting seroconversion rates and immunological memory in protective Ab classes and enhancing cell-mediated immunity. Their primary targets in vivo are probably lymphocytes rather than macrophages. Gamma inulin-based adjuvants therefore comprise new, safe, potent, and attractive candidates for enhancing responses to human and veterinary vaccines, especially those requiring cell-mediated defenses. Such reports also generated interest in botanical polysaccharides, as botanical and microbial polysaccharides bind to common surface receptors and induce similar immunomodulatory responses in macrophages, suggesting that evolutionarily conserved polysaccharide structural features are shared between these organisms (Schepetkin and Quinn, 2006). Thus, the evaluation of botanical polysaccharides provides a unique opportunity for the discovery of novel therapeutic agents and adjuvants that exhibit beneficial immunomodulatory properties.

Studies on popular immuomodulatory botanicals have shown that polysaccharides are one of key constituents responsible for immmunomodulatory activity. Astragalus polysaccharides (APS) extracted from *Astragalus membranaceus* was found to stimulate proliferation of T cells and promote the expression of surface antigens on lymphocytes (Shao et al., 2004). Xu et al. investigated the effects of APS on the phagocytosis of *M. tuberculosis* by macrophages. Their results suggested that APS not only enhanced the phagocytotic activity of macrophages to *M. tuberculosis*, but also increased the secretion of cytokine IL-1, IL-6, and TNF-α (Xu et al., 2007). Shao et al. reported that macrophages from C3H/HeJ mice (TLR4 mutation mice) are unable to respond to APS stimulation, suggesting the positive involvement of TLR4 in APS-mediated macrophage activation. Monoclonal antibodies against mouse TLR4 partially inhibit APS binding with macrophages, implying that there is a direct interaction of APS and TLR4 on the cell surface. They also discovered that APS could activate mice B-lymphocyte and macrophage (Shao et al., 2004).

Radix glycyrrhizae polysaccharides (GPS), one of the main active ingredients of *R. glycyrrhizae*, are attributed to many healing properties of the herb. It is composed of rhamnose, glucose, arabinose, and galactose. Of all the monosaccharide compositions, glucose is identified as the largest chemical component in the polysaccharides. In another study, treatment of DCs with GPS resulted in the enhanced expression of cell surface molecules CD80, CD86, and MHC I-A/I-E. Furthermore, using TLR4, NF-κB, p38 MAPK, and JNK inhibitors partly inhibited the effect of GPS to DCs. These results suggested that GPS induced maturation and function of DCs in vitro, which were partly regulated via the TLR4 related signaling pathway.

Ginseng polysaccharides have been shown to have multiple immunomodulatory biological activities. Studies demonstrated that Ginsan, an immunomodulatory polysaccharide from *Panax ginseng*, induced DCs maturation increased the production of cytokines by macrophages, elevated the number of bone marrow cells and enhanced humoral antibody response.

DISCOVERY APPROACHES

Two major approaches are followed for selection of botanicals for adjuvant discovery. First, there's the classical method that relies on phytochemical factors, serendipity, and random screening approaches. QS-21 is the best example in this category. The second approach uses traditional knowledge and relies on observations, experiential, traditional knowledge, and practices. This is also known as ethnopharmacology approach. Traditional medicine systems such as Chinese medicine, Japanese Kampo, and Indian Ayurveda are important sources for discoveries based on ethnopharmacology approaches. Well-standardized extracts from traditional medicine systems including Astragalus, Triterpygium, *Angelica sinesis, Uncaria tomentosa, Echniacea purpurea, Glycrrhiza glabra, Picorrihiza kurroa, Actinidia eriantha*, and Sho-saiko have shown potential as sources for discovery of immunopotentiatory adjuvants. For example, *Withania somnifera*, an herb used in Ayurveda for immunomodulation, inflammatory symptoms, and various disorders for more than 3000 years, was found to contain steroidal lactones, withanolides with T cell regulatory activities, which are presently under evaluation as vaccine adjuvants. Such bioprospecting has also resulted in identification of important molecules such as psoralens, picrosides, phyllanthins, curcumines and many other steroidal lactones and glycosides, which are candidates for immunomodulatory activities.

The next stage after selection of an herb includes the preparation and characterization of extracts with respect to its constituents and its effects on innate and adaptive immunity functions. Newer technologies such as supercritical carbon dioxide—extraction technology, membrane separation technology, molecular distillation technology, are being currently followed for extractions. The well-standardized extracts are then studied for their immunomodulatory activities.

Based on extract immunomodulatory activity profiles, the vaccines or antigens are selected for adjuvant studies. The candidate extract showing desired adjuvant activity is taken up for further studies. Bioassay-guided fractionation has proven successful as a well-established platform to isolate and characterize active constituents present in extracts. Recent technological improvements in the area of microfractionation approaches based on advanced high-performance liquid chromatography techniques are now enabling the systematic separation of complex plant extracts.

The efficacy of botanical extracts is based on interaction of multitude of phytochemicals with a plethora of targets, and represents a challenge for activity monitoring and screening. For instance, clinical studies on standardized elderberry extract showed its potential in the reduction of influenza symptoms during an outbreak of influenza B/Panama in southern Israel. The subsequent studies attributed immunomodulatory (Th-1) and virus (HINI) binding activities in extracts. Subsequently, two flavonoid compounds (5,7,3ʹ4ʹ-tetra-Omethylquercetin and 5,7-dihydroxy-4-oxo-2-(3,4,5-trihydroxy-phenyl) chroman-3-yl-3, 4,5-trihydroxycyclohexanecarboxylate) were identified as H1N1-binding molecules (Roschek et al., 2009). Constituents responsible for observed Th-1 activity in extracts are yet to be identified. In another case, Benson et al. reported that the fate of functions of dendritic cells is differentially affected when exposed to various *Echinacea pursuer* extracts. These trends were observed in both human as well as mouse dendritic cell populations (Benson et al., 2010). Further studies on extracts deciphered that this was due to the presence of polysaccharides and alkylamides in extracts. Alkylamides were found to be agonists of cannabinoid receptors, which is expressed by immune cells including dendritic cells and agonist activity leads to downregulation of cytokines while polysaccharides especially glucitol acetate and mannitol acetate acted on DCs in a stimulatory manner (Yin et al., 2010).

There is an ongoing debate between the merits and demerits of reductionist approaches vis-à-vis holistic multitargeting and systems approaches for activity screening. Transcriptome analysis in combination with pathway-focused bioassays would be a useful approach for mechanistic studies on extracts showing adjuvant potential.

The rapid identification of known natural products, a process known as dereplication, is important for targeting isolation of bioactive compounds of interest from natural resources. The most common dereplication methods, LC-UV and LC-MS and have been increasingly used in the dereplication of natural products (Qiu et al., 2012). The isolation of active ingredients from herbal medicines should be based on feasibility studies on the concentration of the bioactive component(s) in the herb or plant, the degree of difficulty in purification, and primarily on the availability of the herb or plant. The most characterized plant constituent from adjuvant perspective is QS-21. Extensive studies on characterization and molecular studies have led to creation of range of chemically modified variants of QS-21. GPI-0100 is QS-21 variant with incorporation of a C-12 alkyl chain at glucuronic acid residue of de-acylated saponin, which resulted in 20 times reduction of toxicity as observed with QS-21. Additionally, GPI-0100 showed selective stimulation of Th-2 immune responses as against the characteristic selective Th-1−like stimulation observed with QS-21.

SUMMARY AND CONCLUSION

Many important human pathogens continue to undergo genetic evolution. Additionally, we are witnessing threats from newer and remerging pathogens. Increasing the breadth of protection of existing vaccines and development of newer vaccines is a key agenda in the next decade of vaccines. The continual advancements in genome sequencing and proteomics have significantly improved the discovery and characterization of antigens. The comprehensive analysis at systems level of immune response to vaccines and immunotherapies (vaccinomics or systems vaccinology) is providing valuable knowledge in understanding the molecular mechanisms (genes, immune pathways) responsible for protective immunity, which is guiding the optimum selection of antigen, adjuvants, and delivery systems for vaccine formulations. Systems-based approaches are also establishing the genetic basis of immune responses and thus will be helpful in understanding the impact of genetic variations on the vaccine responses. Moreover, it will greatly facilitate screening for responsiveness to vaccines or immunotherapies and the understanding eventual failures in individuals enrolled in clinical trials. Indeed, the identification of gene transcriptional profiles or gene polymorphisms closely associated with immune response to such immunological strategies shows the relevance of such comprehensive analysis in the personalization of treatment to obtain the best clinical outcomes. The future success of such approaches will be largely dependent on our ability to interpret and analyze large data sets leading to newer insights into the correlates of protection or signatures of immunogenicity.

The systems biology in vaccinology will have to go through several steps before becoming a widely used approach. Moreover, validation studies in larger settings of different genetic background will be required to distinguish between natural and immune response related genetic-gene expression or polymorphism-modifications. Nevertheless, regardless of the technical, cultural, and financial challenges, systems biology applied to vaccinology represents a primary way to go in order to develop novel vaccines and to redevelop established vaccines, switching from the "empirical" to the "knowledge-based" age of vaccinology. This should enable the development of even more successful vaccines for preventive as well as therapeutic intervention strategies for human diseases according to individual- or group-personalized strategies.

The immunopotentiatory adjuvants that induce protective responses increase antibodies with greater avidity with the potential for neutralization, and the ability to modulate Th1 and Th2 responses will be important for optimizing a protective immune response against the vaccines. Newer technologies such as transcriptomics and proteomics offer prospects of unraveling the adjuvant mechanism of action during nonclinical studies. Such studies will help to generate a hypothesis regarding efficacy and toxicity and they will also be helpful in addressing safety considerations during the later stages of adjuvant development.

Immunmodulators derived from botanicals, viral, and bacterial sources can offer opportunities as sources for discovery of small-molecule immunopotentiators and combination adjuvants. It is clear that delivery systems will be required for vaccine delivery to ensure that the antigen and adjuvant combination is delivered preferentially to key immune cells. A major challenge for the next decade will be to translate these findings into protective human vaccines that have an acceptable safety profile.

REFERENCES

Benson, J.M., Pokorny, A.J., Rhule, A., Wenner, C.A., Kandhi, V., Cech, N.B., et al., 2010. *Echinacea purpurea* extracts modulate murine dendritic cell fate and function. Food Chem. Toxicol. 48 (5), 1170–1177.

Blohmke, C.J., O'Connor, D., Pollard, A.J., 2015. The use of systems biology and immunological big data to guide vaccine development. Genome Med. 7 (1), 114.

Buonaguro, L., Pulendran, B., 2011. Immunogenomics and systems biology of vaccines. Immunol. Rev. 239 (1), 197–208.

Coffman, R.L., Sher, A., Seder, R.A., 2010. Vaccine adjuvants: putting innate immunity to work. Immunity. 492–503.

Coontz, R., 2013. Science's top 10 breakthroughs of 2013. Science.

Delany, I., Rappuoli, R., De Gregorio, E., 2014. Vaccines for the 21st century. EMBO Mol. Med. 708–720.

Fact Sheet on malaria vaccine development. [Internet]. Available from: http://www.malariavaccine.org/malaria-and-vaccines/vaccine-development (accessed 28.02.2016).

Finco, O., Rappuoli, R., 2014. Designing vaccines for the twenty-first century society. Front. Immunol.

Flower, D.R., Perrie, Y. (Eds.), 2013. Immunomic Discovery of Adjuvants and Candidate Subunit Vaccines, first ed., X. Springer-Verlag, New York, NY, p. x,314.

Jagusztyn-Krynicka, E.K., Dadlez, M.M.I., Grabowska, A., Roszczenko, P., Jagusztyn-Krynicka, E.K., Roszczenko, P., 2009. Proteomic technology in the design of new effective antibacterial vaccines. Expert Rev. Proteomics 6.3 (3), 315.

Kaufmann, S.H.E., Fletcher, H.A., Guzmán, C.A., Ottenhoff, T.H.M., 2015. Big data in vaccinology: introduction and section summaries. Vaccine 33 (40), 5237–5240.

Koff, W.C., 2015. Defeating the virus. Scientist.

Koff, W.C., Burton, D.R., Johnson, P.R., Walker, B.D., King, C.R., Nabel, G.J., et al., 2013. Accelerating next-generation vaccine development for global disease prevention. Science 340 (6136), 1232910.

Licciardi, P.V., Underwood, J.R., 2011. Plant-derived medicines: a novel class of immunological adjuvants. Int. Immunopharmacol. 390–398.

Nagai, T., Suzuki, Y., Kiyohara, H., Susa, E., Kato, T., Nagamine, T., et al., 2001. Onjisaponins, from the root of *Polygala tenuifolia* Willdenow, as effective adjuvants for nasal influenza and diphtheria–pertussis–tetanus vaccines. Vaccine 19 (32), 4824–4834.

Neafsey, D.E., Juraska, M., Bedford, T., Benkeser, D., Valim, C., Griggs, A., et al., 2015. Genetic diversity and protective efficacy of the RTS,S/AS01 Malaria Vaccine. N. Engl. J. Med. 373 (21), 2025–2037.

Netea, M.G., Van Crevel, R., 2014. BCG-induced protection: effects on innate immune memory. Semin. Immunol. 512−517.

O'Hagan, D.T., Fox, C.B., 2015. New generation adjuvants-from empiricism to rational design. Vaccine. B14−B20.

Plotkin, S., 2014. History of vaccination. Proc. Natl. Acad. Sci. U. S. A. 111 (34), 12283−12287.

Poland, G.A., 2012. Systems biology approaches to new vaccine development. Curr. Opin. Immunol. 23 (3), 436−443.

Porichis, F., Hart, M.G., Griesbeck, M., Everett, H.L., Hassan, M., Baxter, A.E., et al., 2014. High throughput detection of miRNAs and gene-specific mRNA at the single-cell level by flow cytometry. Nat. Commun. 5, 5641.

Pulendran, B., 2014. Systems vaccinology: probing humanity's diverse immune systems with vaccines. Proc. Natl. Acad. Sci. U. S. A. 111 (34), 12300−12306.

Qiu, F., Imai, A., McAlpine, J.B., Lankin, D.C., Burton, I., Karakach, T., et al., 2012. Dereplication, residual complexity, and rational naming: the case of the actaea triterpenes. J. Nat. Prod. 75 (3), 432−443.

Querec, T.D., Akondy, R.S., Lee, E.K., Cao, W., Nakaya, H.I., Teuwen, D., et al., 2009. Systems biology approach predicts immunogenicity of the yellow fever vaccine in humans. Nat. Immunol. 10 (1), 116−125.

Rappuoli, R., Aderem, A., 2011. A 2020 vision for vaccines against HIV, tuberculosis and malaria. Nature 473 (7348), 463−469.

Roschek, B., Fink, R.C., McMichael, M.D., Li, D., Alberte, R.S., 2009. Elderberry flavonoids bind to and prevent H1N1 infection in vitro. Phytochemistry 70 (10), 1255−1261.

RTS,S/AS01 Candidate Malaria vaccine. RTS,S/AS01 Candidate Malar vaccine. 2009;(October 2009):1−14.

Rubens, M., Ramamoorthy, V., Saxena, A., Shehadeh, N., Appunni, S., 2015. HIV vaccine: recent advances, current roadblocks, and future directions. J. Immunol. Res.

Schepetkin, I.A., Quinn, M.T., 2006. Botanical polysaccharides: macrophage immunomodulation and therapeutic potential. Int. Immunopharmacol. 6 (3), 317−333.

Schijns, V.E.J.C., Lavelle, E.C., 2011. Trends in vaccine adjuvants. Expert Rev. Vaccines 10 (4), 539−550.

Seib, K.L., Zhao, X., Rappuoli, R., 2012. Developing vaccines in the era of genomics: a decade of reverse vaccinology. Clin. Microbiol. Inf. 109−116.

Sette, A., 2010. Reverse vaccinology: developing vaccines in the era of genomics. Immunity 33 (4), 530−541.

Shao, B.-M., Xu, W., Dai, H., Tu, P., Li, Z., Gao, X.-M., 2004. A study on the immune receptors for polysaccharides from the roots of *Astragalus membranaceus*, a Chinese medicinal herb. Biochem. Biophys. Res. Commun. 320 (4), 1103−1111.

Steinhagen, F., Kinjo, T., Bode, C., Klinman, D.M., 2011. TLR-based immune adjuvants. Vaccine 3341−3355.

Whitescarver, J., 2016. Trans-NIH Plan for HIV-Related Research. National Institutes of Health.

Xu, H.-D., You, C.-G., Zhang, R.-L., Gao, P., Wang, Z.-R., 2007. Effects of *Astragalus* polysaccharides and astragalosides on the phagocytosis of *Mycobacterium tuberculosis* by macrophages. J. Int. Med. Res. 35, 84−90.

Yin, S.-Y., Wang, W.-H., Wang, B.-X., Aravindaram, K., Hwang, P.-I., Wu, H.-M., et al., 2010. Stimulatory effect of *Echinacea purpurea* extract on the trafficking activity of mouse dendritic cells: revealed by genomic and proteomic analyses. BMC Genomics. 11 (1), 612.

Chapter 12

Curcumin, the Holistic Avant-Garde

Subash C. Gupta[1], Ajaikumar B. Kunnumakkara[2] and Bharat B. Aggarwal[3]

[1]*Banaras Hindu University, Varanasi, Uttar Pradesh, India,* [2]*Indian Institute of Technology, Guwahati, Assam, India,* [3]*Anti-inflammation Research Institute, San Diego, CA, United States*

Turmeric (*Curcuma longa*) is a rhizomatous herbaceous plant that has been used in Ayurveda and in traditional Chinese medicine for a wide variety of human ailments including inflammatory conditions, hepatic disorders, gastric problems, gynecological problems, asthma, infectious diseases, boils, sprains, cough, and cold. More than 200 active constituents have been identified from this plant, the major of which is curcumin. Curcumin is a highly pleiotropic polyphenol that was discovered around two centuries ago as "yellow-coloring matter" (Vogel and Pelletier, 1815).

The pleiotropic activities of curcumin originate from its ability to modulate multiple cell-signaling pathways (Table 12.1). Depending on the target and the cellular context, curcumin may lead to upregulation or downregulation of signaling pathways. Curcumin can modulate signaling pathways either by direct binding to molecules or in an indirect manner. The indirect targets of curcumin include transcription factors, inflammatory mediators, protein kinases, drug-resistant proteins, adhesion molecules, growth factors, cell-survival proteins, cell-cycle regulatory proteins, receptors, enzymes, chemokines, and chemokine receptors. Curcumin can also bind to several targets in a direct manner such as cell-survival proteins, protein kinases, protein reductases, inflammatory molecules, histone acetyltransferase, histone deacetylase, DNA methyltransferase 1, FtsZ protofilaments, carrier proteins, xanthine oxidase, proteasomes, sarco/endoplasmic reticulum Ca2 + ATPase, HIV1 integrase, HIV1 protease, and glyoxalase I (Goel et al., 2008; Gupta et al., 2011). The proinflammatory transcription factors, such as NF-kB, activator protein-1, and signal transducer and activator of transcription (STAT) proteins, are the most important targets of curcumin (Shishodia et al., 2007). These transcription factors regulate the expression of tumorigenic genes, and curcumin can negatively regulate these transcription factors (Shishodia et al., 2007). For a complete list of signaling molecules modulated by curcumin,

Innovative Approaches in Drug Discovery. DOI: http://dx.doi.org/10.1016/B978-0-12-801814-9.00012-X

TABLE 12.1 Molecular Targets of Curcumin

Adhesion molecules
- Endothelial leukocyte adhesion molecule-1
- Intracellular adhesion molecule-1
- Vascular cell adhesion molecule-1

Cell-survival proteins
- B-cell lymphoma protein 2
- Bcl-xL
- Inhibitory apoptosis protein-1

Enzymes
- Arylamine N-acetyltransferases-1
- ATPase
- Cyclooxygenase-2
- Desaturase
- DNA polymerase
- Farnesyl protein transferase
- Gluthathione-S-transferase
- Glutamyl cysteine ligase
- Hemeoxygenase-1
- Inducible nitric oxide synthase
- Lipoxygenase
- Matrix metalloproteinase
- NAD(P)H:quinoneoxidoreductase
- Ornithine decarboxylase
- Phospholipase D
- Telomerase
- Tissue inhibitor of metalloproteinase-3

Growth factors
- Connective tissue growth factor
- Epidermal growth factor
- Fibroblast growth factor
- Hepatocyte growth factor
- Nerve growth factor
- Platelet derived growth factor
- Tissue factor
- Transforming growth factor-β1
- Vascular endothelial growth factor

Inflammatory molecules
- Interleukins (-1, -2, -5, -6, -8, -12, -18)
- Monocyte chemoattractant protein
- Migration inhibition protein
- Macrophage inflammatory protein
- Tumor necrosis factor alpha

Kinases
- Autophosphorylation-activated protein kinase
- Ca^{2+}-dependent protein kinase
- EGF receptor kinase
- Extracellular receptor kinase
- Focal adhesion kinase
- Interleukin-1 receptor-associated kinase
- Janus kinase
- c-jun N-terminal kinase
- Mitogen-activated protein kinase
- Phosphorylase kinase
- Protamine kinase
- Protein kinase A
- Protein kinase B
- Protein kinase C
- pp60c-src tyrosine kinase
- Protein tyrosine kinase

Receptors
- Androgen receptor
- Aryl hydrocarbon receptor
- Chemokine (C-X-C motif) receptor 4
- Death receptor-5
- Epidermal growth factor receptor
- Endothelial protein C-receptor
- Estrogen receptor-alpha
- Fas receptor
- Histamine (2)-receptor
- Human epidermal growth factor receptor-2
- Interleukin 8-receptor
- Inositol 1,4,5-triphosphate receptor
- Integrin receptor
- Low density lipoprotein-rceptor

Transcriptional factors
- Activating protein-1
- β-Catenin
- CREB-binding protein
- Early growth response gene 1
- Electrophile response element
- Hypoxia inducible factor-1
- Notch-1
- Nuclear factor-kappa B
- Nuclear factor 2-related factor
- Peroxisome preoliferator-activated receptor-gamma
- Signal transducers and activators of transcription-1
- Signal transducers and activators of transcription-3
- Signal transducers and activators of transcription-4
- Signal transducers and activators of transcription-5
- Wilms' tumor gene 1

Miscellaneous
- Cyclin D1
- Heat-shock protein 70
- Multidrug resistance protein
- Urokinase-type plasminogen activator

readers should consult reviews from our laboratory (Goel et al., 2008; Gupta et al., 2011; Kunnumakkara et al., 2008). Through modulation of signaling molecules, curcumin can exhibit multiple activities such as antiinflammatory, antinociceptive, antiparasitic, schistosomicidal, antioxidant, antimalarial, nematocidal, antiproliferative, antimicrobial, wound healing, and proapoptotic activities. Cucrcumin can also sensitize tumor cells to chemotherapy and radiotherapy (Shishodia et al., 2007).

Multiple studies have indicated the safety and efficacy of curcumin in animals including rodents, monkeys, horses, rabbits, and cats (Gupta et al., 2013a). In animal models, curcumin has exhibited efficacy against inflammatory conditions, cancer, diabetes, psychiatric disorders, obesity, eye disorders, neurological disorders, lung disorders, gastrointestinal disorders, renal disorders, cardiovascular disorders, fibrosis, wound healing, aging, and many other conditions (Gupta et al., 2013a). For example, in a streptozotocin-induced diabetic mouse model, curcumin exhibited antidiabetic activities and maintained the normal structure of the kidney (Sawatpanich et al., 2010). Similarly, in a rat model of type 2 diabetes mellitus (T2DM), curcumin showed an antihyperglycemic effect and improved insulin sensitivity (El-Moselhy et al., 2011). These actions were attributed in part to its antiinflammatory properties and antilipolytic effects. Interestingly, in T2DM mice, curcumin was found to be a potent glucose-lowering agent without any effect in nondiabetic mice (Seo et al., 2008). Dietary curcumin has been shown to prevent obesity in an obese mouse model (Ejaz et al., 2009). More specifically, curcumin reduced body weight gain, adiposity, and microvessel density in adipose tissue. These changes were correlated with reduced expression of vascular endothelial growth factor and its receptor-2, peroxisome proliferator-activated receptor-γ, and CCAAT/ enhancer-binding protein-α. In animal models, curcumin has also shown activities against neurological diseases. The commonly studied neurological diseases where curcumin has exhibited activities include Alzheimer's, Parkinson's, epilepsy, brain ischemia, encephalomyelitis, diabetic encephalopathy, spinal cord injury, intracerebral hemorrhage, convulsions, and cerebral malaria (Gupta et al., 2012). The activity of curcumin as a chemopreventive and chemotherapeutic agent is well established in rodent models of cancer. The most common cancer against which curcumin has been studied include colon cancer, pancreatic, brain, esophageal, lung, mouth, kidney, breast, liver, bladder, small intestine, stomach, leukemia, skin, and prostate cancers (Gupta et al., 2012). Curcumin has shown potential activity against numerous other disorders and diseases, including disorders of the gastrointestinal system, cardiovascular system, and those of kidneys, lungs, eyes, and liver. Curcumin's potential against asthma, aging, fibrosis, endometriosis, wound-healing problems, and muscle wasting is also well established in animal models.

The extensive preclinical studies over the past several years have provided a strong basis for measuring the pharmacokinetics, safety, and efficacy of curcumin in humans. The efficacy of curcumin has been observed in humans with a wide range of diseases including cancer, cardiovascular disease, uveitis, Crohn's disease, arthritis, ulcer, irritable bowel disease, acquired immunodeficiency syndrome, diabetes, vitiligo, psoriasis, and other diseases. In clinical trials, curcumin has been used as a single agent and also in combination with other agents. Although curcumin concentration for humans varies from one disease to another, the nutraceutical has been used at doses as high as 12g/d for more than 3 months. Curcumin has been shown to modulate multiple cell-signaling molecules in humans including proinflammatory transcription factors (NF-kB and STAT3), cytokines, prostaglandin E2, cyclooxygenase-2, 5-LOX, transforming growth factor-β, C-reactive protein, adhesion molecules, phosphorylase kinase, and triglyceride (Gupta et al., 2013b). Curcumin has been administered to humans in the form of turmeric and also in other formulations such as capsules, tablets, nanoparticles, emulsions, and liposomal encapsulation. Curcumin's efficacy in humans was first published in 1937 by Oppenheimer (Oppenheimer, 1937), who reported beneficial effects of this polyphenol for human biliary diseases. Since this initial discovery, more than 65 clinical trials have been completed while more than 35 studies are at different phases of clinical trial (Gupta et al., 2013b).

Curcumin has shown efficacy against pancreatic cancer, colorectal cancer (CRC), lung cancer, multiple myeloma, breast cancer, oral cancer, prostate cancer, and head and neck squamous-cell carcinoma in humans. Curcumin's efficacy against CRC is well studied. Familial adenomatous polyposis that is characterized by multiple adenomas is a precursor for CRC. In one study, oral administration of curcumin was associated with a reduction in the number and size of polyps in patients (Cruz-Correa et al., 2006). Curcumin has also been shown to reduce the formation of aberrant crypt foci, the precursor of colorectal polyps in patients (Carroll et al., 2011). Curcumin administration has also been shown to decrease serum TNF-α level, induce apoptosis, and to enhance the expression of p53 in tumor tissue (He et al., 2011).

Curcumin's efficacy against inflammatory bowel disease, a condition of the intestine, has also been investigated. Curcumin administration was associated with a reduction in p38 MAPK activation, level of IL-1β, and an enhancement in IL-10 levels in mucosal biopsies from patients (Epstein et al., 2010). Curcumin has also been found to be well tolerated with no adverse effects and produce an antirheumatic activity in patients with rheumatoid arthritis (Chandran and Goel, 2012). Meriva, a phytosome complex of curcumin with better bioavailability, was found to benefit patients with osteoarthritis (Belcaro et al., 2010). Curcumin has also been proposed to act as a chemopreventive agent against atherosclerosis (Soni and Kuttan, 1992). These are only few of many examples demonstrating the efficacy of curcumin against human diseases. Readers interested in understanding the detailed clinical efficacy of curcumin should consult one of our recent articles (Gupta et al., 2013b).

Although being mostly beneficial to humans, curcumin has its own limitations. For example, poor bioavailability limits the therapeutic efficacy

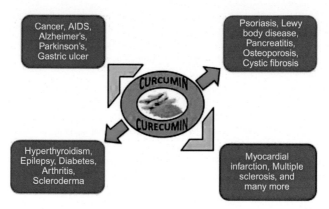

FIGURE 12.1   Diseases that can be cured with curcumin.

of curcumin (Anand et al., 2007). Therefore, several modifications have been made to improve the bioavailability of curcumin. These include use of piperine (Shoba et al., 1998), nanoparticles (Sasaki et al., 2011), liposomes (Gota et al., 2010), phospholipid complexes (Cuomo et al., 2011), and structural analogues (Anand et al., 2007). Some other limitations associated with curcumin use are its ability to (1) inhibit drug-metabolizing enzymes (Thapliyal and Maru, 2001), (2) induce DNA damage in cells (Cao et al., 2006), (3) induce anemia in mice (Jiao et al., 2009), and (4) to produce nausea and diarrhea in human subjects (Sharma et al., 2004).

In summary, curcumin has demonstrated the efficacy at molecular, cellular, animal, and human levels. Considering curcumin's multitargeting nature and its efficacy against multiple human diseases (Fig. 12.1), curcumin appears to represent a holistic approach pointing to the entire human body, unlike the monotargeted approach. Furthermore, advances in modern technologies have provided scientific evidences for the multifaceted effects of curcumin in humans. In fact, the use of turmeric, the source of curcumin, was recorded in Ayurveda and in traditional Chinese medicine since ancient time for a number of human conditions. The United States Food and Drug Administration (USFDA) has approved curcumin as a "generally regarded as safe" agent. However, the nutraceutical has not been approved for human use. Although ongoing studies from several laboratories continue to demonstrate curcumin's efficacy, more efforts are required in bringing this molecule to the forefront of novel therapeutics.

REFERENCES

Anand, P., Kunnumakkara, A.B., Newman, R.A., Aggarwal, B.B., 2007. Bioavailability of curcumin: problems and promises. Mol. Pharm. 4, 807–818.

Belcaro, G., Cesarone, M.R., Dugall, M., Pellegrini, L., Ledda, A., Grossi, M.G., et al., 2010. Product-evaluation registry of Meriva(R), a curcumin-phosphatidylcholine complex, for the complementary management of osteoarthritis. Panminerva. Med. 52, 55–62.

Cao, J., Jia, L., Zhou, H.M., Liu, Y., Zhong, L.F., 2006. Mitochondrial and nuclear DNA damage induced by curcumin in human hepatoma G2 cells. Toxicol. Sci. 91, 476–483.

Carroll, R.E., Benya, R.V., Turgeon, D.K., Vareed, S., Neuman, M., Rodriguez, L., et al., 2011. Phase IIa clinical trial of curcumin for the prevention of colorectal neoplasia. Cancer Prev. Res. (Phila.) 4, 354–364.

Chandran, B., Goel, A., 2012. A randomized, pilot study to assess the efficacy and safety of curcumin in patients with active rheumatoid arthritis. Phytother. Res. 26, 1719–1725.

Cruz-Correa, M., Shoskes, D.A., Sanchez, P., Zhao, R., Hylind, L.M., Wexner, S.D., et al., 2006. Combination treatment with curcumin and quercetin of adenomas in familial adenomatous polyposis. Clin. Gastroenterol. Hepatol. 4, 1035–1038.

Cuomo, J., Appendino, G., Dern, A.S., Schneider, E., McKinnon, T.P., Brown, M.J., et al., 2011. Comparative absorption of a standardized curcuminoid mixture and its lecithin formulation. J. Nat. Prod. 74, 664–669.

Ejaz, A., Wu, D., Kwan, P., Meydani, M., 2009. Curcumin inhibits adipogenesis in 3T3-L1 adipocytes and angiogenesis and obesity in C57/BL mice. J. Nutr. 139, 919–925.

El-Moselhy, M.A., Taye, A., Sharkawi, S.S., El-Sisi, S.F., Ahmed, A.F., 2011. The antihyperglycemic effect of curcumin in high fat diet fed rats. Role of TNF-alpha and free fatty acids. Food Chem. Toxicol. 49, 1129–1140.

Epstein, J., Docena, G., MacDonald, T.T., Sanderson, I.R., 2010. Curcumin suppresses p38 mitogen-activated protein kinase activation, reduces IL-1beta and matrix metalloproteinase-3 and enhances IL-10 in the mucosa of children and adults with inflammatory bowel disease. Br. J. Nutr. 103, 824–832.

Goel, A., Kunnumakkara, A.B., Aggarwal, B.B., 2008. Curcumin as "Curecumin": from kitchen to clinic. Biochem. Pharmacol. 75, 787–809.

Gota, V.S., Maru, G.B., Soni, T.G., Gandhi, T.R., Kochar, N., Agarwal, M.G., 2010. Safety and pharmacokinetics of a solid lipid curcumin particle formulation in osteosarcoma patients and healthy volunteers. J. Agric. Food Chem. 58, 2095–2099.

Gupta, S.C., Kismali, G., Aggarwal, B.B., 2013a. Curcumin, a component of turmeric: from farm to pharmacy. Biofactors 39, 2–13.

Gupta, S.C., Patchva, S., Aggarwal, B.B., 2013b. Therapeutic roles of curcumin: lessons learned from clinical trials. AAPS J. 15, 195–218.

Gupta, S.C., Prasad, S., Kim, J.H., Patchva, S., Webb, L.J., Priyadarsini, I.K., et al., 2011. Multitargeting by curcumin as revealed by molecular interaction studies. Nat. Prod. Rep. 28, 1937–1955.

Gupta, S.C., Patchva, S., Koh, W., Aggarwal, B.B., 2012. Discovery of curcumin, a component of golden spice, and its miraculous biological activities. Clin. Exp. Pharmacol. Physiol. 39, 283–299.

He, Z.Y., Shi, C.B., Wen, H., Li, F.L., Wang, B.L., Wang, J., 2011. Upregulation of p53 expression in patients with colorectal cancer by administration of curcumin. Cancer Invest. 29, 208–213.

Jiao, Y., Wilkinson, J.T., Di, X., Wang, W., Hatcher, H., Kock, N.D., et al., 2009. Curcumin, a cancer chemopreventive and chemotherapeutic agent, is a biologically active iron chelator. Blood 113, 462–469.

Kunnumakkara, A.B., Anand, P., Aggarwal, B.B., 2008. Curcumin inhibits proliferation, invasion, angiogenesis and metastasis of different cancers through interaction with multiple cell signaling proteins. Cancer Lett. 269, 199–225.

Oppenheimer, A., 1937. Turmeric (curcumin) in biliary diseases. Lancet 229, 619–621.

Sasaki, H., Sunagawa, Y., Takahashi, K., Imaizumi, A., Fukuda, H., Hashimoto, T., et al., 2011. Innovative preparation of curcumin for improved oral bioavailability. Biol. Pharm. Bull. 34, 660–665.

Sawatpanich, T., Petpiboolthai, H., Punyarachun, B., Anupunpisit, V., 2010. Effect of curcumin on vascular endothelial growth factor expression in diabetic mice kidney induced by streptozotocin. J. Med. Assoc. Thai. 93 (Suppl. 2), S1–S8.

Seo, K.I., Choi, M.S., Jung, U.J., Kim, H.J., Yeo, J., Jeon, S.M., et al., 2008. Effect of curcumin supplementation on blood glucose, plasma insulin, and glucose homeostasis related enzyme activities in diabetic db/db mice. Mol. Nutr. Food Res. 52, 995–1004.

Sharma, R.A., Euden, S.A., Platton, S.L., Cooke, D.N., Shafayat, A., Hewitt, H.R., et al., 2004. Phase I clinical trial of oral curcumin: biomarkers of systemic activity and compliance. Clin. Cancer Res. 10, 6847–6854.

Shishodia, S., Singh, T., Chaturvedi, M.M., 2007. Modulation of transcription factors by curcumin. Adv. Exp. Med. Biol. 595, 127–148.

Shoba, G., Joy, D., Joseph, T., Majeed, M., Rajendran, R., Srinivas, P.S., 1998. Influence of piperine on the pharmacokinetics of curcumin in animals and human volunteers. Planta Med. 64, 353–356.

Soni, K.B., Kuttan, R., 1992. Effect of oral curcumin administration on serum peroxides and cholesterol levels in human volunteers. Indian. J. Physiol. Pharmacol. 36, 273–275.

Thapliyal, R., Maru, G.B., 2001. Inhibition of cytochrome P450 isozymes by curcumins in vitro and in vivo. Food Chem. Toxicol. 39, 541–547.

Vogel, A., Pelletier, J., 1815. Examen chimique de la racine de Curcuma. J Pharm. 1, 289–300.

Chapter 13

Safety of Traditional Medicines

Dnyaneshwar Warude

Lupin Research Park, Pune, Maharashtra, India

INTRODUCTION

Widespread use and increased demands of botanicals have generated public health challenges globally in terms of quality and safety. There have been concerted efforts by the USFDA; WHO; NIH; ESCOP; Department of Health, UK; Commonwealth of Australia; Department of Indian Systems of Medicine; and the federal government of China to monitor the quality and regulate the growing business of these products. Development of guidelines, monographs and databases, training and education, funding research, and spreading awareness among consumers are some of the efforts undertaken by these regulatory authorities. However, rapidly changing global health demands have posed newer challenges. Increasing world population, rapid urbanization and changing lifestyles, instant availability of information (authentic or spurious) on the web and social media, and constant failures of modern medicine to treat chronic ailments are few of them. Sources of genuine botanical raw materials are shrinking due to the rapid extinction of natural habitats over the past few decades. Lands that are available for mass cultivation are becoming infertile due to uncontrolled usage of organic fertilizers and pesticides. On the other hand, there have been significant advancements in science and technology. We are now close to sequencing the entire genome of an individual for about US$1000 (Hayden, 2014), which, once upon a time, was beyond imagination. Generating blue light through light-emitting diodes (LED), which was thought to be impossible in the last century, has become common through the energy-saving LED lamps that now demonstrate diverse uses in analytical chemistry (Macka et al., 2014). Technological advances can easily provide newer, cost-effective, and complementary ways to judge and monitor the quality and safety of botanicals.

This chapter takes a concise overview of frequently used quality-control methods for botanicals. Newer approaches based upon advanced analytical and genomic techniques are discussed with case studies. Significant advancements have occurred in monitoring the safety of

Innovative Approaches in Drug Discovery. DOI: http://dx.doi.org/10.1016/B978-0-12-801814-9.00013-1

modern medicine. The utility of possibly extending similar approaches is discussed to monitor safety of botanical products.

CONVENTIONAL APPROACHES OF QUALITY CONTROL

National and herbal pharmacopoeias of nations including India, USA, and China, and guidelines provided by agencies such as WHO, describe monographs of several botanicals and a series of methods to assess their quality. Moreover, the publications also provide specifications and standards for the botanicals and limits for the possible contaminants (Warude and Patwardhan, 2005). Examinations to determine sensory, macroscopic, and microscopic characteristics are the first and key steps suggested to establish identity and the degree of purity. It is recommended that these studies should be carried out before any further tests are undertaken. Ash after the ignition of botanicals is a good indicator of its purity. Ash values that include total, acid-insoluble, and water-soluble ash provide additional information about the herb apart from its dry weight. Detection of extractable matter, water, or oil content in the case of aromatic plants, saponification value, tannin content, bitterness value, are some of the other material-specific test parameters recommended by the pharmacopoeias and guidelines. Thin layer chromatography (TLC) is a frequently used method of choice for herbal analysis. This technique underwent a revolution when automated sample applications became possible on uniformly precoated silica gel plates followed by a UV-densitometric detection system. CAMAG (Switzerland) made a significant contribution in this field (WHO, 2011). Moreover, it is cost-effective and fast, as analysis of more than 25 samples can be performed in a single run. These methods can certainly describe the quality of the botanicals, if used judiciously. However, there are few methodical limitations. Availability of trained personnel to test the sensory parameters and suitability for identification of only nonprocessed and to some extent semi-processed botanicals are some of the shortfalls of macro and microscopic tests. Limited scope of staining and detection agents as well as quantitative analysis of marker constituents limits utility of the TLC techniques. Progress in analytical chemistry and genomics can provide newer ways to control the quality of the botanicals.

NEWER APPROACHES FOR QUALITY

Hyphenated Techniques

Subtle separation of the macro and micrometabolites, understanding their exact chemical nature, and, finally, quantification of the unique biomolecules can improve the quality control of botanicals. Recent advancements in analytical chemistry with the aid of sophisticated instrumentation can be wisely used to characterize the complex biomaterials. High Performance Liquid

Chromatography (HPLC) is one of the most widely used methods for analysis of complex mixtures. The technique has also gained popularity in the analysis of botanicals. Ease of operations, requirement of small sample size and increasing commercial availability of pure reference phytoconstituents and recent innovations in the Reversed-Phase (RP) columns that allow characterization of lipophilic molecules are few of the reasons of its increasing utility. Liquorice root is an Ayurvedic medicine popular worldwide for its cough suppressant effects. Along with the known constituents, glycerrhizin and its acids, it contains an array of phenolic compounds (flavonoids, coumarins, and diphenyl ethanones) that might play a role in its therapeutic activity. Due to high structural diversity, low abundance, and coelution with saponins, these phenolic compounds are difficult to separate by conventional chromatography. Qiao and colleagues (Qiao et al., 2015) used the RP technique with its advanced version and characterized the liquorice phenolic compounds and triterpenoid saponins to describe the quality of the botanical raw material. Due to the ease of separation of the compounds with diverse polarity, it is easier now to characterize botanical raw materials and multicomponent formulations using the advanced system (Wei et al., 2013; Wang et al., 2014). HPLC and tandem Mass Spectroscopy (MS) based methods are available for quantitation of shatavarin, a major constituent of asparagus (Patil et al., 2014b), which stimulates immune cell proliferation in dose dependent manner (Pise and Rudra, 2015).

In recent years, Ultra High Pressure Liquid Chromatography (UHPLC) has emerged as a technique that can withstand pressure around 8000 psi and makes it possible to perform high resolution separations of the metabolites with the aid of improved columns bearing solid-phase particles of less than 2 mm in diameter to achieve superior sensitivity and resolution. The results obtained not only showed decreased analysis time but also improved selectivity compared to conventional HPLC analysis as well as RP methods (Bansal et al., 2014). Jaiswal et al. did comparative studies of tissue-specific distribution of secondary metabolites and the major constituents from the asparagus (Jaiswal et al., 2014) and turmeric (Jaiswal et al., 2014), the widely used botanicals common in Ayurveda and Traditional Chinese Medicine (TCM) using UHPLC. They concluded that turmeric rhizomes grown in India and China are qualitatively and quantitatively indistinguishable; asparagus needs careful consideration, however.

Other methods such as Micellar Electrokinetic Capillary Chromatography, High-Speed Counter-Current Chromatography (HSCCC), low-pressure Size-Exclusion Chromatography (SEC), and Strong Anion-Exchange HPLC (SAX-HPLC) can also be used to separate biomolecules from complex mixtures for which markers are not well characterized. For instance, fractionation and purification of alkaloids from botanicals present practical difficulties using the conventional chromatographic techniques because of their alkalinity and structural diversity. HSCCC, a liquid–liquid partition chromatography with a support-free liquid stationary phase can be effectively used to separate and characterize the components from botanicals (Fang et al., 2011). The advancements made in detection systems have also played a key role in increasing the popularity of systems such as HPLC, which, coupled with Evaporative Light Scattering Detection (ELSD), can detect almost all the compounds in the elute that are less volatile than the mobile phase. The response of the ELSD is related to the absolute quantity of the compound and is independent of the analyte's optical properties (Zhang et al., 2008). Wang et al. used the technique aptly to develop fingerprint of European black nightshade (*Solanum nigrum*) grown in different habitats. The results showed significant differences in chemical composition of the botanical constituents grown in different geographical conditions, which is otherwise difficult to detect using conventional analytical techniques. A new, sensitive version of ELSD has been developed recently in which the aerosol particles were not detected by light scattering but instead were given an electrical charge by passing them close to a stream of charged nitrogen. This novel method subsequently commercialized by ESA Biosciences as Corona charged Aerosol Detection, a combination of HPLC and electrical aerosol technology. The advancement can further improve the analysis of natural product analysis.

Coupling of instruments for simultaneous separation, purification, and structural elucidation have made the sample analysis fast, accurate, and unbiased. For example, HPLC can be coupled with Diode Array Detector (DAD) and MS or Nuclear Magnetic Resonance (NMR). With the help of this hyphenation in most cases one could identify the chromatographic peaks directly on-line by comparison with literature data or with standard compounds. This is becoming a powerful tool for rapid identification of phytoconstituents in botanical formulations (Liang et al., 2014).

Gas Chromatography (GC) analysis is by far the most reliable technique for analyzing aromatic and volatile components and fixed oils from botanicals. The technique also underwent revolution when coupling with advanced MS- and NMR-based detection systems became possible. Cox et al. (2012) used the headspace solid-phase microextraction technique couple with GC and MS to detect adulteration of the cannabinoids containing herbal formulations with potent synthetic cannabinoid analogs as including AM-694 having various adverse effects (Bertol et al., 2015). Due to structural similarities with natural cannabinoids and microadulteration, detection is only possible due to the hyphenation.

Capillary electrophoresis (CE) is another technique that has gained importance in the analysis of complex mixtures. Introduced in early 1980s, significant advancements in the instrumentation has happened, which allowed analysis of almost every kind of charged components ranging from simple inorganic ions to nucleic acids. Capillary Zone Electrophoresis, Capillary Gel Electrophoresis, and Capillary Isoelectric Focusing are few of the examples. CE is promising for the separation and analysis of constituents from botanicals and can be used for the analysis of biosamples where HPLC and other techniques face limitations. Decaffeinated coffee accounts for 10% of coffee sales in the world; it is preferred by consumers that do not wish or are sensitive to caffeine effects. Bizzotto et al. (2013) performed analysis of commercial coffee samples with CE and HPLC. They report that CE analyses were 30% faster, the reagent costs were 76.5-fold lower, and the volume of the residues generated was 33-fold lower compared to HPLC analysis.

Phyto-Equivalence Studies

Though it is possible to detect metabolites from botanicals used in the herbal preparations using hyphenated techniques, its pharmacological efficacy is often the sum of effects produced by multiple molecules. Comparative analysis of the chromatographic fingerprints with that of the standard botanical/ formulation thereof, which has a known efficacy, can be an alternative way in describing quality. To determine whether or not a botanical preparation is "not significantly different," or "essentially the same," it is necessary to establish a base value from which variance may be considered. The comparative study is known as phyto-equivalence. Jiang and colleagues developed a HPLC-DAD−MS method to study phyto-equivalence for quality check of a spice *Cistanche deserticola*. They report that *Cistanche salsa* has a high similarity with the standard and can be used as a substitute (Jiang et al., 2009). No single technique can be recommended for developing a profile chromatogram. Considering the nature of the major or significant constituents of the substance, suitable techniques can be selected: e.g., volatile oils in a substance would be better determined by GC than HPLC, whereas TLC may be more appropriate than HPLC for determining sugars in a substance. The interpretation in the profile is done by comparing size, shape, location of the peaks or spots with the reference standard. The Department of Health, Australia (Department of Health Government of Australia, 2011) provides limits for such equivalence analysis of the botanicals. Factors such as the natural variability of the herbal material (in particular the total extractable matter) combined with the solvent system, extraction method and extraction conditions can have a significant impact on the quantity and composition of a herbal extract. A change in any one of these factors is generally reflected in the native extract ratio. Considering these factors, a judicious use of the phyto-equivalence methods can certainly be informative about quality of the botanicals.

DNA Markers

DNA-based molecular markers have proved their utility in fields such as taxonomy, physiology, embryology, and genetics. As the science of plant genetics progressed, researchers have tried to explore these molecular marker techniques for their applications in commercially important plants such as food crops, horticultural plants, and in the pharmacognostic characterization of botanicals (Joshi et al., 2004). It has been well documented that geographical conditions affect the active constituents of the medicinal plant and hence their activity profiles (Oleszek et al., 2002). Many researchers have studied geographical variations at the genetic level. Random Aplified Polymeric DNA (RAPD)−based molecular markers are useful in differentiating different accessions of *Taxus wallichiana* (Shasany et al., 1999), neem (Farooqui et al., 1998), *Juniperus communis* L. Adams et al. (2002), *Codonopsis pilosula* (Fu et al., 1999), *Allium schoenoprasum* L. Friesen and Blattner (1999), *Morinda officinalis* (Ding et al., 2006), *Tinospora cordifolia* (Willd.) Miers (Rout, 2006) collected from different geographical regions. The technique also can be effectively used for the detection of adulterants or substituents for the authentic botanicals. *Panax ginseng* is often substituted by *Panax quinquefolius* (American ginseng). DNA markers as Sequence Characterized Amplified Region (SCAR), RAPD and Restriction Fragment Length Polymorphism have been successfully applied for differentiation and for detecting substitution by other closely related species (Shaw and But, 1995). DNA fingerprinting and polymorphism in the Chinese drug "Ku-Di-Dan" (Herba elephantopi) and its substitutes were studied using RAPD. The results are used for authentication of "Ku-Di-Dan" (Cao et al., 1996). Our group is also instrumental in the development of DNA markers for standardization and quality control of Ayurvedic botanicals.

Case Studies

Phyllanthus emblica (amla) fruit is one of the top-selling botanicals having numerous applications in the healthcare, food, and cosmetics industries. It is a main component of the popular multicomponent Ayurvedic formulations; Triphala churna, and Chavanprash. Tannin-based chemical markers are often used to check the quality of botanical and products thereof. However, these markers can only compare the integrated sameness and/or difference of the chemical constituents that may not reflect the therapeutic effect of the botanical as described above. Further, many factors may affect the ultimate chemical profile of any botanical. Intrinsic factors such as genetics, and extrinsic factors such as cultivation, harvesting, drying, and storage conditions are few examples. Understanding these limitations, we developed an RAPD-SCAR−based DNA marker for amla and used it for identification of the botanical in semiprocessed and processed formulations. Due to high tannin contents and its acidic nature, DNA isolation from amla tissues was challenging. We developed a Cetyl Trimethyl Ammonium Bromide−based method of DNA isolation from fresh and dry amla tissues as well as its semiprocessed formulations (Warude et al., 2003). A RAPD marker (DNA

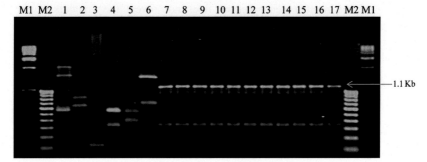

M1 M2 1   2   3   4   5   6   7   8   9   10 11 12 13 14 15 16 17 M2 M1

—1.1 Kb

FIGURE 13.1   RAPD profiles of different *Phyllanthus* species (Lane 1−7) and *P. emblica* cultivars (Lane 7−17) amplified with OPA-16 on 1.5% agarose gel. M1: Mole wt. marker (1 kb), M2: Mole wt. marker (100 bp), Lane 1: *P. destichus*, Lane 2: *P. urinaria*, Lane 3: *P. reticulatus*, Lane 4: *P. niruri*, Lane 5: *P. simplex*, Lane 6: *P. indofischeri*, 7: NA-06, 8: NA-07, 9: NA-10, 10: Kanchan, 11: Chakaiya, 12: Francis, 13: Banarasi, 14: Hathizool, 15: Dongri, 16: Bansired, and 17: Anand-01.

fragment of 1.1 kb) specific for the commercially available 11 cultivars of amla was identified. This marker is unique for amla and could not be detected in any other tested *Phyllanthus* species (Fig. 13.1). However, the RAPD analysis is not foolproof. It may lack specificity as the primers used are short and random. Sensitivity of the RAPD reaction to a number of reaction parameters at a low annealing temperature has failed to generate consistent profiles even under the same laboratory conditions. To overcome these limitations, we developed a SCAR marker by cloning and sequencing the RAPD DNA amplicon. The SCAR marker is highly specific for amla, which can be used for identification of the botanical in the Ayurvedic formulation like Triphala (Warude et al., 2006).

A similar approach was used to develop and apply the RAPD-SCAR marker for authentication of ginger (*Zingiber officinale*), a well-known Ayurvedic drug and commonly used spice. *Zingiber cassumunar* and *Zingiber zerumbet* rhizomes, being morphologically similar to that of *Z. officinale*, are known adulterants of the official species. We identified and developed a SCAR marker from a selected RAPD amplicon that can be amplified in more than 30 ginger samples collected from different regions of India and not in tested possible adulterants or substitutes (Chavan et al., 2008).

Although DNA markers are considered to be useful, they have certain limitations. To establish a marker for identifiying a particular species, DNA analysis of large number of related species and/or varieties and common botanical contaminants and adulterants is necessary, which is a costly and time-consuming process. Isolation of good-quality DNA suitable for analysis from semi-processed or processed botanicals is also a challenge. Further, a DNA fingerprint will remain the same irrespective of the plant part used, while the phytochemical content will vary. DNA fingerprinting ensures presence of the correct genotype but does not reveal the contents of the active principle or chemical constituents. Hence, DNA analysis and pharmacognostic techniques for chemoprofiling will have to be used hand in hand rather than in isolation for optimum characterization of botanicals. For quantitative analysis, molecular techniques such as real time PCR could be tried along with chemoprofiling.

APPROACHES IN SAFETY

The safety of botanicals is always debated among consumers, health care providers, and regulatory agencies. Botanical drugs with "therapeutic claims" that are about to enter the markets have to follow the routine drug development process that include the toxicity and safety studies as recommended by the US Food and Drug Administration (USFDA). There are many safety concerns regarding botanical products that are already in the public and used as food and/or dietary supplements. The general belief that "natural is safe" in society poses serious health concerns. A recent report from The New England Journal of Medicine highlights the gravity of the safety issue. Between 2003 and 2013, there were 23,000 hospital emergency department visits in the United States every year attributed to adverse events related to dietary supplements. Such visits commonly involve cardiovascular manifestations from weight-loss or energy products among young adults, and swallowing problems, often associated with micronutrients, among older adults (Geller et al., 2015). Though all of the adverse effects may not be directly linked to consumption of dietary supplements containing botanicals, it creates confusion. Safety assessment of the botanicals using systemic pharmacological approach under regulated conditions has therefore become essential. The safety pharmacology is often confused with toxicology. Safety studies use the basic principles of pharmacology in a regulatory-driven atmosphere to generate data to inform a risk/benefit assessment. The aim of safety pharmacology is to characterize the pharmacodynamic/pharmacokinetic (PK/PD) relationship of a drug's adverse effects (Pugsley et al., 2008). In contrast, objective toxicological studies define the maximum tolerated dose of a drug in single and in repeat regimens. Unlike toxicology, safety pharmacology includes a regulatory requirement to predict the risk of possible lethal events (Broichhausen et al., 2014). This gives safety pharmacology its unique character. Most of marketed botanical products, including the dietary supplements and products with therapeutic claims in certain countries, are formulated empirically and have not been thoroughly tested for their pharmacology and toxicity. Moreover, the quality of these products is often a question due to their complex nature, differential processing, and the possibility of adulteration or substitution, as discussed earlier. Therefore, detection of adverse effect liability, deciding safety margins, and clinical safety monitoring of the botanicals are essential. Evolving knowledge of pharmacogenomics and pharmacovigilance can be effectively used to cater to needs. Moreover, to get a maximum and quick effect, patients often tend to coadminister the botanical preparations with conventional/modern drugs. Systematic studies of the herb—drug interactions are also warranted for the patient's safety.

Pharmacogenomics

Variations in the human genome could affect the quality of drug disposition and safety. Several reports are emerging with polymorphism in the genes relevant to PK, pathways responsible for pharmacological effects, genes that are predisposed to toxicity as immune reactions, and genes that influence disease susceptibility or progression. We reported polymorphism among the Indians in folate-metabolizing genes which are also known to metabolize the antiarthritic drug methotrexate (Godke et al., 2011). This can explain altered pharmacokinetics of the drug in different populations. Such approaches can be effectively used to study the differential effects of the botanicals in patients. Ma et al. (2014) studied gene polymorphism in patients with liver injury induced by *Polygonum multiflorum*, a known antiaging botanical from the TCM. It was shown that the injury is associated with frequency of the *CYP1A2**1C (a liver microsomal enzyme) allele. *Ginkgo biloba*, a known memory enhancer botanical, has been shown to induce enzymatic activity of CYP2C19, the cytochrome isozyme involved in voriconazole metabolism. Based on the genetic polymorphism of the liver enzyme, people can be divided into slow and extensive metabolizers of voriconazole. It was predicted that *G. biloba* can affect metabolism of antifungal drugs. However, such alteration in the metabolism was not detected in a study done with two other distinct health volunteer groups (Lei et al., 2009).

Genomic variations in individuals can show differential pharmacological activity of the botanicals or phyto-constituents. Serotonin (5-hydroxytryptamine, 5-HT) is implicated in the pathogenesis of multiple neuropsychiatric disorders. Berberine and evodiamine are alkaloids found in the botanicals families Berberis and Evodia, respectively. The compounds, alone and in combination, increases serotonin transporter mRNA and protein expression significantly across the various alleles of the gene and there by affecting the 5-HT levels and alter the behavior (Hu et al., 2012). More of such studies are needed to access safety of the botanicals.

This relatively new field of pharmacogenomics combines pharmacology and genomics and can help in the development of effective, safe medications and doses that will be tailored to a person's genetic makeup. Traditional medicines like Ayurveda recognized the inter-individual variations ages ago. The practice is largely based on personalized medicine. It classifies human population in three basic constitution types (Vata, Pitta, and Kapha) defined as "Prakriti." Some drugs can have a differential effect in individuals having different Prakriti, and the concept also holds true for modern medicines. For instance, Vata-Pitta Prakriti individuals respond better to a lower dose of aspirin for its platelet aggregation activity than others (Bhalerao et al., 2012). We have shown that the Ayurvedic Prakriti concept has a genetic basis (Govindaraj et al., 2015) and can be used to study drug disposition (Ghodke et al., 2011). The ancient knowledge of Prakriti and evolving knowledge of genomics, collectively referred as Prakritigenomics, can help in the rational and safe use of botanicals as well as conventional medicines.

Pharmacovigilance

Monitoring effects of marketed medical products under the practical conditions of clinical usage in larger populations is referred as pharmacovigilance. The objective is to extend safety monitoring and detect drug adverse events that have previously been unrecognized despite evaluation in controlled clinical trials. The pharmacovigilance methods developed for monitoring modern medicine can effectively be used for botanicals. Spontaneous reports and prescription event monitoring (PEM) are the commonly used methods to access safety. Spontaneous reports include the reports of "suspected" adverse reactions. The reporter is not obliged to confirm the association between drug and effects. Statistical methods are used to identify proportionate reporting rates that help to develop safety "signals". Most countries have their own systems to report such adverse events. USFDA developed the MedWatch system (MedWatch), while UK has the Yellow Card Scheme (YellowCard). The Indian Pharmacopoeia Commission developed the Pharmacovigilance Program of India (PvPI). Individuals can report any adverse event associated with use of botanical or modern medicines. Data of adverse events related to botanical preparations have started appearing in these systems. In an analysis of adverse events related to natural products from 2011 to 2013, scientists from PvPI reported 39 cases. Sixteen of them were classified as serious, 12 were not serious, and 11 were not assessable (Kalaiselven et al., 2015).

PEM is another hypothesis-generating, noninterventional method of safety assessment. This is best suited for prescription drugs used under controlled clinical conditions. Most of the botanical preparations are over-the-counter products and in some countries they are referred to and used as dietary supplements. In such cases, this method has limitations. However, countries such as India have a large pool and network of registered Ayurvedic practitioners who routinely prescribe fixed dose combinations of the botanicals. Moreover, there are several Ayurvedic drug manufacturing companies that provide quality products. Himalaya, Dabar, Zandu are few of the names. Pharmacovigilance methods such as PEM, which is well validated for modern medicine, can be efficiently used with deeper involvement of the botanical medicine practitioners industry along with regulatory agencies.

Herb—Drug Interactions

Administration of drugs, either from a synthetic or botanical origin, follow the same path of absorption (in case of oral): distribution, metabolism, and elimination using the body systems. Moreover, if they are directed towards the same therapeutic indication, there are chances that they can engage common molecular targets and may cause potentiation or reduction in the net pharmacodynamic effect. Due to partial responses or adverse effects of modern drugs, patients often tend to use herbals concomitantly. It is therefore necessary to monitor their interactions and the resulting net pharmacological effect for the safety of the patients. Pharmacovigilance tools can be effectively used to assess such interactions. Moreover, systematic experimental evidences need to be generated to prove the beneficial or harmful effects of the coadministrations. Pharmacokinetic interactions mediated by drug-metabolizing enzymes or transporters are involved in many herb—drug interactions. Calitz et al. reported effect of selected polyherbal preparations in the absorption and metabolism of indinavir; a known antiretroviral drug. In Caco2 cell-based in vitro absorption model, secretory transport of indinavir increased in a concentration dependent manner in the presence of the herbal preparations while metabolism was significantly inhibited in the LS180 liver cells. The study of such interactions become more important when the botanicals are coadministered with conventional drugs having narrow therapeutic indices. The liver microsomal enzymes, especially CYP3A4, CYP2C9, and CYP2D6 are known to metabolize more than 60% of the marketed drugs. Our group studied the effect of three Ayurvedic "Rasayana" drugs on the modulation of CYP3A4. We found that Guduchi (*T. cordifolia*) and fractionated compounds are potent inhibitors of the cytochrome enzyme, while other two botanicals viz., Ashwagandha (*Withania somnifera*) and the Shatavari (*Asparegus* racemosus), do not show such activity (Patil et al., 2014a). Coadministration of the drugs that are predominantly metabolized by CYP3A4 and have narrow therapeutic indices, including most of the anticancer agents (cyclophosphamide, vinca alkaloids) and antipsychotic agents such as haloperidol with guduchi, can affect the drug disposition and hence may raise safety concerns. Concomitant administration of *Commiphora mukul* (gugulesterons) with propranolol and diltiazem, an antihypertensive drug, in healthy volunteers showed significant reduction in AUC and C_{max}. Dalvi et al. (1994). Administration of sertraline, a known selective serotonin reuptake inhibitor, with Ayurvedic polyherbal formulation containing *Commiphora wighteii* and *Terminalia chebula* showed pharmacokinetic interaction decreases therapeutic efficacy of sertraline leading to the relapses of depression (Prasad et al., 2009). Cyclosporine is another clinically used immunosupressant with a narrow therapeutic index. Concomitant intake of ginger significantly interferes with absorption of cyclosporine, decreasing C_{max} by 71% and AUC by 63% in rats (Chiang et al., 2006). More well-planned studies with selected drugs and the herbal preparations relevant to the clinical situation can help in understanding the interactions.

CONCLUSION

The quality control of botanicals is not mere a technical operation. It requires a deeper understanding of the nature and fate of the botanical raw materials, extracts, and their combinations. The nature of the material includes physical and gross biochemical compositions. Growth conditions, collection, processing and handling, methods used in formulating these products affect quality. Guidelines for good agricultural and collection practices as well as good manufacturing practices have helped to improve the quality of the herbal medicines (Mukherjee, 2002). Unlike the synthetic drugs, the biomaterials are highly complex in their composition. Therapeutic effects produced by them cannot be attributed to one or more phytochemicals. The proposed approaches can certainly improve the quality-control operations. A recent example of DNA barcoding and the barcode library to detect contamination and substitution in North American herbal products (Newmaster et al., 2013) can serve as a prototype. Efforts are already underway to use DNA barcodes on product labels to help in the pharmacovigilance of natural products (de Boer et al., 2015). None of these methods can lead to a complete safe and efficacious use of biomaterials, but common sense and good pharmaceutical practices should be applied while selecting an appropriate methodology.

REFERENCES

Adams, R., Pandey, R., Leverenz, J., Digdard, N., Hoegh, K., Thorfinnsson, T., 2002. Pan-arctic variation on *Juniperus communis*: historical biogeography based on DNA fingerprinting. Sci. Hortic. (Amsterdam). 96, 303–312.

Bansal, A., Chhabra, V., Sarma, G., Rawal, R., 2014. Chemometrics: a new scenario in herbal drug standardization. J. Pharm. Anal. 4, 223–233.

Bertol, E., Vaiano, F., Milia, M., Mari, F., 2015. In vivo detection of the new psychoactive substance AM-694 and its metabolites. Forensic Sci. Int. 256, 21–27.

Bhalerao, S., Deshpande, T., Thatte, U., 2012. Prakriti (Ayurvedic concept of constitution) and variations in platelet aggregation. BMC Complement. Altern. Med. 10, 248.

Bizzotto, C., Meinhart, A., Ballus, C., Poloni, R.A., Sobrinho, M., Cerro-Quintana, R., et al., 2013. Comparison of capillary electrophoresis and high performance liquid chromatography methods for caffeine determination in decaffeinated coffee. Food Sci. Technol. 33, 186–191.

Broichhausen, C., Riquelme, P., Ahrens, N., Wege, A., Koehl, G., Schlitt, H., et al., 2014. In question: the scientific value of preclinical safety pharmacology and toxicology with cell based therapies. Mol. Ther. Methods Clin. Dev. 1, 14026.

Cao, H., But, P., Shaw, P., 1996. Authentication of the Chinese drug "ku-di-dan" (herba elephantopi) and its substitutes using random-primed polymerase chain reaction (PCR). Yao Xue Xue Bao 31, 543–553.

Chavan, P., Warude, D., Joshi, K., Patwardhan, B., 2008. Development of SCAR (sequence-characterized amplified region) markers as a complementary tool for identification of ginger (*Zingiber officinale* Roscoe) from crude drugs and multicomponent formulations. Biotech. Appl. Biochem. 50, 61–69.

Chiang, H., Chao, P., Hsiu, S., Wen, K., Tsai, S., Hou, Y., 2006. Ginger significantly decreased the oral bioavailability of cyclosporine in rats. Am. J. Chin. Med. 34, 845−855.

Cox, A., Daw, R., Mason, M., Grabenauer, M., Pande, P., Davis, K., et al., 2012. Use of SPME-HS-GC-MS for the analysis of herbal products containing synthetic cannabinoids. J. Anal. Toxicol. 36, 293−302.

Dalvi, S., Nayak, V., Pohujani, S., 1994. Effect of gugulipid on bioavailability of diltiazem and propranolol. J. Assoc. Physicians India 42, 454−455.

de Boer, H., Ichim, M., Newmaster, S., 2015. DNA barcoding and pharmacovigilance of herbal medicines. Drug Saf. 38, 611−620.

Department of Health and Ageing, Therapeutic Goods administration. Australian Government, 2011. Guidance on equivalence of herbal extracts in complementary medicines, Version 1.0, pp. 1−16.

Ding, P., Xu, J., Chu, T., 2006. RAPD analysis on germplasm resources of different farm races of *Morinda officinalis*. Zhong Yao Cai 29, 1−3.

Fang, L., Liu, Y., Yang, B., Wang, X., Huang, L., 2011. Separation of alkaloids from herbs using high-speed counter-current chromatography. J. Sep. Sci. 34, 2545−2558.

Farooqui, N., Ranade, S.A., Sane, P., 1998. RAPD profile variation among provinces of neem. Biochem. Mol. Biol. Int. 45, 931−939.

Friesen, N., Blattner, F., 1999. RAPD analysis reveals geographic differentiations within *Allium Schoenoprasum* L. (Alliaceae). Planta Med. 65, 157−160.

Fu, R., Wang, J., Zhang, Y., Wang, Z., But, P., Li, N., et al., 1999. Differentiation of medicinal Codonopsis species from adulterants by polymerase chain reaction-restriction fragment length polymorphism. Planta Med. 65, 648−650.

Geller, A., Shehab, N., Weidle, N., Lovegrove, M., Wolpert, B., Timbo, B., et al., 2015. Emergency department visits for adverse events related to dietary supplements. N. Engl. J. Med. 373, 1531−1540.

Ghodke, Y., Joshi, K., Patwardhan, B., 2011. Traditional medicine to modern pharmacogenomics: Ayurveda Prakriti type and CYP2C19 gene polymorphism associated with the metabolic variability. Evid. Based Complement. Altern Med. 2011, 249528.

Godke, Y., Chopra, A., Shintre, P., Puranik, A., Joshi, K., Patwardhan, B., 2011. Profiling single nucleotide polymorphisms (SNPs) across intracellular folate metabolic pathway in healthy Indians. Indian J. Med. Res. 133, 274−279.

Govindaraj, P., Nizamuddin, S., Sharath, A., Jyothi, V., Rotti, H., Raval, R., et al., 2015. Genome-wide analysis correlates Ayurveda Prakriti. Sci. Rep. 5, 15786.

Hayden, E., 2014. The $1000 genome. Nature 507, 294−295.

Hu, Y., Ehli, E., Hudziak, J., Davies, G., 2012. Berberine and evodiamine influence serotonin transporter (5-HTT) expression via the 5-HTT-linked polymorphic region. Pharmacogenomics J. 12, 372−378.

Jaiswal, Y., Liang, Z., et al., 2014. A comparative tissue-specific metabolite analysis and determination of protodioscin content in Asparagus species used in traditional Chinese medicine and Ayurveda by use of laser microdissection, UHPLC−QTOF/MS and LC−MS/MS. Phytochem. Anal. 25, 514−528.

Jaiswal, Y., Liang, Z., Ho, A., Chen, H., Zhao, Z., 2014. Tissue-specific metabolite profiling of Turmeric by using laser micro-dissection, ultra-high performance liquid chromatography-quadrupole time of fight-mass spectrometry and liquid chromatography-tandem mass spectrometry. Eur. J. Mass Spectom. 20, 383−393.

Jiang, Y., Li, S., Wang, Y., Chen, X., Tu, P., 2009. Differentiation of Herba Cistanches by fingerprint with high-performance liquid chromatography-diode array detection−mass spectrometry. J. Chromatogr. A 1216, 2156−2162.

Joshi, K., Chavan, P., Warude, D., Patwardhan, B., 2004. Molecular markers in herbal drug technology. Curr. Sci.159–165.

Kalaiselven, V., Saurabh, A., Singh, G., 2015. Adverse reactions to herbal products: an analysis of spontaneous reports in the database of the pharmacovigilance programme of India. J. Hebal Med. 5, 48–54.

Lei, H., Wang, G., Wang, L., Ou-yang, D., Chen, H., Li, Q., et al., 2009. Lack of effect of *Ginkgo biloba* on voriconazole pharmacokinetics in Chinese volunteers identified as CYP2C19 poor and extensive metabolizers. Ann. Pharmacother 43, 726–731.

Liang, J., Gao, H., Chen, L., Xiao, W., Wang, Z., Wang, Y., et al., 2014. Chemical profiling of an antimigraine herbal preparation, tianshu capsule, based on the combination of HPLC, LC-DAD-MSn, and LC-DAD-ESI-IT-TOF/MS analyses. Evid. Based Complement. Altern. Med. 2014, 580745.

Ma, K., Zhang, X., Jia, H., 2014. CYP1A2 polymorphism in Chinese patients with acute liver injury induced by *Polygonum multiflorum*. Genet. Mol. Res. 13, 5637–5643.

Macka, M., Piasecki, T., Dasgupta, P., 2014. Light-emitting diodes for analytical chemistry. Annu. Rev. Anal. Chem. 7, 183–207.

MedWatch: The FDA Safety Information and Adverse Event Reporting Program. Available at http://www.fda.gov/Safety/MedWatch/.

Mukherjee, P.K., 2002. Problems and prospects for good manufacturing practice for herbal drugs in Indian systems of medicine. Drug Inf. J. 36 (3), 635–644.

Newmaster, S., Grguric, M., Shanmughanandhan, D., Ramalingam, S., Ragupathy, S., 2013. DNA barcoding detects contamination and substitution in North American herbal products. BMC Med. 11, 222.

Oleszek, W., Stochmal, A., Karolewski, P., Simonet, A., Macias, F., Tava, A., 2002. Flavonoids from *Pinus sylvestris* needles and their variation in trees of different origin grown for nearly a century at the same area. Biochem. Syst. Ecol. 30, 1011–1022.

Patil, D., Gautam, M., Gairola, S., Jadhav, S., Patwardhan, B., 2014a. Effect of botanical immunomodulators on human CYP3A4 inhibition: implications for concurrent use as adjuvants in cancer therapy. Integr. Cancer Ther. 13 (2), 167–175.

Patil, D., Gautam, M., Gairola, S., Jadhav, S., Patwardhan, B., 2014b. HPLC/tandem mass spectrometric studies on steroidal saponins: an example of quantitative determination of Shatavarin IV from dietary supplements containing *Asparagus racemosus*. J. AOAC Int. 97, 1497–1502.

Pharmacovigilance Program of India (PvPI). National Coordination Centre, Indian Pharmacopoeia Commission, Ghaziabad. Available at < http://www.ipc.gov.in/PvPI/pv_home.html >.

Pise, M., Rudra, J., 2015. Immunomodulatory potential of shatavarins produced from *Asparagus racemosus* tissue cultures. J. Nat. Sci. Biol. Med. 6, 415–420.

Prasad, K., Tharangani, P.G., Samaranayake, C., 2009. Recurrent relapses of depression in a patient established on sertraline after taking herbal medicinal mixtures--a herb-drug interaction? J. Psychopharmacol. 23, 216–219.

Pugsley, M., Authier, S., Curtis, M., 2008. Principles of safety pharmacology. Br. J. Pharmacol. 154, 1382–1399.

Qiao, X., Song, W., Ji, S., Wang, Q., Guo, D., Ye, M., 2015. Separation and characterization of phenolic compounds and triterpenoid saponins in licorice (*Glycyrrhiza uralensis*) using mobile phase-dependent reversed-phase × reversed-phase comprehensive two-dimensional liquid chromatography coupled with mass spectro. J. Chomatogr. A 1402, 36–45.

Rout, G., 2006. Identification of *Tinospora cordifolia* (Willd.) Miers ex Hook F & Thomas using RAPD markers. Z Naturforsch. 61, 118–122.

Shasany, A., Kukreja, A., Saikia, D., Darokar, M., Khanuja, S., Kumar, S., 1999. Assessment of diversity among *Taxus wallichiana* accessions from northeast India using RAPD analysis. PGR Newsl. 121, 27–31.

Shaw, P., But, P., 1995. Authentication of Panax species and their adulterants by random primed polymerase chain reaction. Planta Med. 61, 466–469.

Wang, X., Ma, X., Li, W., Chu, Y., Guo, J., Zhou, S., et al., 2014. Simultaneous quantitative determination of six active components in traditional Chinese medicinal preparation Cerebralcare Granule by RP-HPLC coupled with diode array detection for quality control. J. Chromatogr. Sci. 52, 814–817.

Warude, D., Chavan, P., Joshi, K., Patwardhan, B., 2003. DNA isolation from fresh and dry plant samples with highly acidic tissue extracts. Plant Mol. Biol. Rep. 21, 467a–467f.

Warude, D., Chavan, P., Joshi, K., Patwardhan, B., 2006. Development and application of RAPD-SCAR marker for identification of *Phyllanthus emblica* Linn. Biol. Pharm. Bull. 29, 2313–2316.

Warude, D., Patwardhan, B., 2005. Botanicals: quality and regulatory issues. J. Sci. Ind. Res.83–92.

Wei, M., Yang, Y., Chiu, H., Hong, S., 2013. Development of a hyphenated procedure of heat-reflux and ultrasound-assisted extraction followed by RP-HPLC separation for the determination of three flavonoids content in *Scutellaria barbata* D. Don. J. Chromatogr. B Anal. Technol. Biomed. Life Sci. 940, 126–134.

WHO, 2011. Quality control methods for herbal materials. Updated edition of quality control methods for medical plant materials, 1998.

Yellow Card Scheme. Reporting site. Medicines and Healthcare products Regulatory Agency. Available at https://yellowcard.mhra.gov.uk/.

Zhang, B., Li, X., Yan, B., 2008. Advances in HPLC detection--towards universal detection. Anal. Bioanal. Chem. 390, 299–301.

Chapter 14

Holistic Lifestyle

Girish Tillu[1] and Bhushan Patwardhan[2]

[1]Trans Disciplinary University, Bangalore, Karnataka, India, [2]Savitribai Phule Pune University, Pune, Maharashtra, India

The global scenario for health has remained a persistent concern even after four decades when the World Health Organization declared the goal "health for all" in 1978. Despite the progress of medicine, the goal seems nowhere within reach. On the contrary, the last four decades have witnessed a remarkable negative shift in the health status of people leading presently to a sick planet. The healthcare challenge shift, from communicable to noncommunicable diseases (NCD), has increased longevity but has posed newer challenges of degenerative psychological and diseases as important global concerns. The world is witnessing an epidemic of NCD such as heart disease, cancer, diabetes, chronic lung diseases, high blood pressure, obesity, and Alzheimer's disease. The developing world is carrying a double burden of emerging noncommunicable and reemerging communicable diseases. The developed world also remains far from optimum health. In 2012, almost half of US adults had one or more chronic health conditions (Ward et al., 2014). More than one third of US adults are obese and 50% of deaths are due to heart disease or cancer. NCDs have become a global threat irrespective of developing or developed countries. Every year 38 million people die from NCDs, of which about 28 million are from developing countries. Nearly 16 million of these die prematurely before the age of 70. Since the beginning of the new millennium, the number of deaths due to NCD has increased worldwide. The four main killer diseases are diabetes, cardiovascular disease, cancer, and chronic lung disease. Cardiovascular diseases (CVD) contribute to one third of the deaths. Communicable diseases, prenatal and neonatal care, and malnutrition are responsible for one fourth of the deaths. Worldwide, more than 38 million people die from NCDs every year.

Most of the NCDs are termed as lifestyle diseases. They share common causes including improper diet, sedentary lifestyle, stress, occupational hazards, and other challenges of modern living. Generally, the management of communicable diseases include the use of antibiotics, improving nutrition, and prevention from risk factors. The management of lifestyle diseases is

Innovative Approaches in Drug Discovery. DOI: http://dx.doi.org/10.1016/B978-0-12-801814-9.00014-3

367

more challenging because of their diversity, chronicity, presence of comorbidities, and risks of complications. NCDs require highly individualized and specialized management. Although many potent drugs exist for their management, the root causes of these diseases need to be addressed. The causes and risk factors of diseases are related to determinants of health. Most of the risk factors of NCDs are modifiable. Besides genes, other determinants like environment, diet, and lifestyle are within the control of people. But for this people need to take control of their own health. Present health system focuses more on pharmaceutical drugs because people are dependent on doctors not just for disease treatment but also for health. In reality, patient awareness and counseling for diet and lifestyle modifications are hardly addressed by doctors and clinics. Now, even modern medicine has realized the importance of whole-system management of disease, which comprises diet and lifestyle modifications. Earlier, medical textbooks used to advise diet and lifestyle modifications as the primary means of managing type II diabetes before prescribing oral antihyperglycemic drugs (Sainani, 2001). However, over the years the practice of medicine has become reductionist and based more on pathology reports and aggressive use of pharmaceutical prescription drugs.

Commercialization of healthcare begins with diagnosis. A series of diagnostic tests are done on patients, but many times the indications and frequencies of such tests remains debatable. The pharmaceutical and diagnostic companies influence health policies and professional organizations of clinicians. Government healthcare of most of the developing countries is in a poor state because they are not geared to handling lifestyle diseases. The private players get tied up with insurance companies, which makes healthcare costlier and beyond the capacity of common people. This commodification of health care leads to the medicalization of society. However, manipulating diagnostic ranges and aggressively treating patients has reached worrisome levels. A study on diabetic patients' cohort has revealed U-shaped curve of association of plasma insulin and mortality, which suggests overtreatment is as harmful as poor glycemic control (Pyörälä et al., 2000).

Our present healthcare system is overdependent on pharmaceutical drugs. We need medicines when health is lost, but most public health programs have become activities for the mass distribution of medicines. The discovery and development of modern medicines involves highly potent and targeted therapy for specific diseases. The "fire and forget" approach of modern medicine has created lot of undesired consequences that have lead to adverse drug events. An overreliance on medicines has converted healthcare into an industry and, more so, as a commodity. The patients want a quick fix, doctors are influenced by the industry, and the industry is driven by profits. More and more prescriptions of drugs generate profits. Many times drug development is driven by markets and not by societal needs. The present medical management of lifestyle diseases has several limitations. Most of these diseases are polygenic where there is a web of causation. Undermining the biological complexities involved in the whole-body metabolism, can lead to drug-induced disorders. For example, statins used for management of obesity and dyslipidaemia have shown to increase incidence of new-onset type 2 diabetes mellitus (Maki et al., 2015). Diabetic patients are prescribed low dose aspirin and other platelet inhibitors, which can cause cerebrovascular events. NCDs, chronic, and lifestyle diseases need long term treatments where a patient's health is compromised. While scientific research and publications are on the increase, the quality of life and patients' satisfaction is rapidly eroding. For many common conditions like hypertension and diabetes, doctors many times prescribe medicines for a lifetime without sufficient evidence for doing so. As a result, lifestyle-disease management becomes frustrating where the patients become stressful and the doctors remain helpless. The present scenario of NCD therapeutics calls for innovative approaches, not just for discovering material drugs but for behavioral modifications for health protection and disease management.

These approaches will have to integrate nutrition, diet, lifestyle, exercise, meditation, and not just medication.

LIFESTYLE AND BEHAVIORAL INTERVENTIONS

Early signs of many NCDs are due to the modern sedentary lifestyle. Interestingly, this was shown more than 200 years ago in a landmark article by J. Warren on angina pectoris in the first issue of New England Journal of Medicine (Warren, 1812). Consistent rise in deaths due to CVD was observed at the beginning of last century. Systematic studies on CVD were needed to study causation and preventive approaches. Therefore, in 1948 the National Heart Institute of United States instituted the Framingham Heart Study. This ambitious program was aimed at exploring causative factors for CVDs in a population. This cohort study clearly identified blood pressure, diabetes, lipids, obesity, smoking, and sedentary lifestyle as causative and risk factors for CVDs. Over these years, Framingham Study has generated huge data consisting of more than 3000 research papers, several guidelines, and risk calculators for CVDs.

In 1983, an American physician Dean Ornish published a trial of ischemic heart disease patients who underwent stress management and dietary modifications. Results of this trial indicated that in a short period of 24 days there were improvements in left ventricular ejection fraction, reduction in cholesterol levels, and angina episodes (Ornish et al., 1983). Many other trials have shown effects of diet and lifestyle modifications for reduction of coronary artery stenosis and cardiac events. The lifestyle modifications in these studies included dietary changes with low fat vegetarian diet, aerobic exercise, stress management, group psychosocial support, and smoking cessation (Ornish et al., 1990, 1998). Ornish's research positioned lifestyle as an effective intervention for prevention and actually reversing the heart diseases. Lifestyle changes can also have positive effect on longevity in cancer patients. A study conducted by Dean Ornish and Nobel laureate Elizabeth Blackburn has shown beneficial effects of diet, physical activity, stress management, and social support in prostate cancer patients resulting in increased telomerase activity (Ornish et al., 2013).

Such studies have liberated drug-centered therapeutics to lifestyle and behavioral medicine. American college of preventive medicine defines lifestyle medicine as "scientific approach to decreasing disease risk and illness burden by utilizing lifestyle interventions such as nutrition, physical activity, stress reduction, rest, smoking cessation, and avoidance of alcohol abuse" (American College of Preventive Medicine [Internet]). According to the Society of Behavioral Medicine, the concept of behavioral medicine mainly deals with behavioral, psychosocial, and biomedical inputs for understanding of health and illness in the context of prevention, diagnosis, treatment and rehabilitation (Society of Behavioural Medicine [Internet]). Lifestyle and behavioral medicine is emerging as an interdisciplinary field comprising behavioral, sociocultural, psychosocial, and biomedical knowledge domains. The Academy of Behavioral Medicine Research and The Society of Behavioral Medicine were established for interdisciplinary studies on the interactions of behavior with biology and the environment to improve health and wellbeing.

The scientometrics data shows a trend in increasing publications on therapeutic effects of lifestyle interventions. Lifestyle and behavioral approaches have a potential role in managing NCDs. Many meta-analysis and systematic reviews have successfully synthesized evidence from available research data. Cochrane library has about 100 systematic reviews on lifestyle interventions (Cochrane Library). Table 14.1 describes clinical trials and systematic reviews in respective clinical areas.

Despite several clinical trials and increased use in clinical practice, awareness about lifestyle research is negligible. Knowledge and information generated from trials need to be sharpened through careful analysis for its translation into practice. It is possible that clinical trials using similar interventions may not produce similar results. This could be due to variations in methods, risks of bias, or errors in analysis. One of the ways of scientific scrutiny of trial data is meta-analysis based systematic reviews. The Cochrane collaboration promotes research synthesis through such reviews. The Cochrane approach aims to have a critical study of a trial's data on risk of bias, trial quality, transparency in reporting, and outcome analysis. Meta-analysis has many benefits, as it pulls data of similar studies and provides estimates of net effects on larger group of trial participants. The outcomes of these reviews are written for lay practitioners and policy makers who then facilitate the translation of these research findings. A large number of Cochrane reviews have suggested the potential benefits of lifestyle modifications in several diseases.

TABLE 14.1 Research Literature on Lifestyle Interventions

Disease	Clinical Trials	Systematic Reviews
Obesity	1558	12
Cardiovascular diseases	1348	28
Diabetes	1346	35
Hypertension	553	14
Cancer	468	1
Mental stress	393	67
Hyperlipidemia	204	60
Dementia	44	1
Polycystic ovary syndrome	37	4
Alzheimer's disease	20	1
Longevity	14	0
HIV/AIDS	6	0
Autism	4	0

PubMed and Cochrane search in February 2016.

The theory of causality suggests that lifestyle diseases can be better managed with a healthy lifestyle. Therapeutic interventions through diet, physical exercise, and lifestyle modifications have emerged as important prevention and treatment strategies.

Research on lifestyle predictors of various diseases has culminated in risk scores for the prediction of disease. The Framingham Heart Study has proposed risk scores for atrial fibrillation, cardiovascular disease, congestive heart failure, coronary heart disease, diabetes, hypertension, intermittent claudication, and stroke. For example, the risk score for diabetes considers family history, age, BMI, status of glucose, HDL cholesterol, triglyceride, and blood pressure. Research on biomarkers has added newer predictive markers such as interleukin-34 (Zorena et al., 2016). Risk prediction algorithms are also developed for various conditions such as heart failure in older persons, cardiovascular events, diabetic polyneuropathy, blindness, and amputation due to diabetes. Lifestyle management can be an effective preventive intervention in case of known risk predictors.

A review of eight trials with 2241 participants on exercise, diet and a standard recommendation arm of 2509 participants has shown reduction in the risk of diabetes. This also has favorable effects like reduction in weight, waist-to-hip ratio, and waist circumference. Exercise and diet interventions have a favorable effect on blood lipids and improved systolic and diastolic blood pressure levels. These interventions are shown to decrease the incidence of type 2 diabetes in high-risk groups (Orozco et al., 2008). Another review has concluded that lifestyle-modification intervention was effective in treating metabolic syndrome and reducing the severity of related abnormalities such as fasting blood glucose, waist circumference, blood pressure, and triglycerides (Yamaoka and Tango, 2012).

Patients of coronary heart disease can substantially benefit from lifestyle-intervention programs. The evidence summarized in meta-analysis of 23 trials and 11085 patients concludes that lifestyle modification programs are much better as compared to routine clinical care given to coronary heart disease patients (Janssen et al., 2013). It is known that plasma homocysteine levels are associated with cardiac disease risk. A study reveals that lifestyle interventions and vitamin B intake may lower homocysteine and reduce the risk of CVDs (DeRose et al., 2000).

Lifestyle interventions are also effective in autoimmune diseases. Aerobic exercise and muscle training can improve functional ability and muscle strength in patients of Rheumatoid arthritis (Hurkmans et al., 2009). Lifestyle is considered as a cause or risk factor for psoriasis and the same can be said for its reversal. Effects of dietary intervention and physical exercise have shown improvement and beneficial outcomes in psoriasis (Naldi et al., 2014).

There is growing evidence that lifestyle modifications can actually reduce or replace prescription drugs. A review of research on walking as lifestyle intervention and use of aspirin is quite interesting. It is known that a sedentary lifestyle is one of the leading causes of CVD. Walking can be an important intervention to prevent cardiovascular events. Many studies suggest walking can lead to longevity and can play a role in the prevention of cardiovascular deaths. It can also be a beneficial therapy for obesity. Taking anorexic drugs or even bariatric surgery may be justified in extreme cases; however, for treating mild-to-moderate obesity lifestyle modification like walking can be a better and safer treatment. In addition to walking, if stress factors are modulated through simple measures of yoga and meditation, the results can be further augmented. A meta-analysis of 32 trials has observed that walking was helpful for reducing blood pressure, waist circumference, weight, body fat, as well as improving aerobic fitness. The analysis suggested walking as an effective measure for primary prevention for cardiovascular diseases. This study has reported dose response relationship between walking and cardiac risk (Murtagh et al., 2010). A cohort study has reported that daily walking can reduce mortality showing a linear trend, where mortality risk declined with increased walking time (Zhao et al., 2015).

Beneficial effects of walking are actually comparable to aspirin, which is popularly used for prevention of cardiovascular diseases (Table 14.2).

TABLE 14.2 Cardiovascular Prevention: Walking and Aspirin

	Aspirin	Walking
Science		
Reduces blood pressure	No data	Yes
Reduces weight and lipids	No data	Yes
Improves aerobic fitness	No data	Yes
Improves stress	No data	Yes
Reduces chronic inflammation	Yes	No data
Reduces platelet aggregation	Yes	No data
Cardiovascular risk reduction	Yes	Yes
Cerebro-vascular risk	Yes	No
Scientometrics		
Cochrane reviews	35	17
Clinical trials (pubmed)	6979	7647
Research papers (pubmed)	57619	58507
Practice		
Inclusion as treatment protocols	Yes	No data
Industry		
Annual market	>2 Bn$	?
Beneficiary	Patients, distributors, doctors, industry…	Patients

Thus, walking as an intervention can replace or reduce the need for aspirin for cardiovascular prevention. However, there is no systematic effort to consider lifestyle interventions in actual medical practice or patient education. Research and translation on lifestyle modifications needs policy support for possible inclusion in public health, clinical practice, and health education.

EMERGING EVIDENCE FROM RESEARCH

During the last decade, many clinical trials on lifestyle and behavioral approaches have been published. Powerful tools like meta-analysis and systematic reviews are being used to synthesize evidence from available research data. A systematic review has concluded that lifestyle-modification intervention was effective in the management of metabolic syndrome—with a reduction in blood pressure, fasting blood glucose, triglycerides, and waist circumference (Yamaoka and Tango, 2012). The lifestyle-modification interventions involved dietary modifications through a Mediterranean-styled or Dietary Approaches to Stop Hypertension—styled healthy diet, and suitable forms of physical activity.

Type 2 diabetes is a typical disease of lifestyle. A review of eight trials involving 2241 participants who were put on a diet and exercise regime showed a reduced risk of diabetes, as compared with standard treatment group of 2509 participants. This study also reported favorable effects of diet and exercise on weight, body mass index, waist circumference, waist-to-hip ratio, blood lipids, and blood pressure. These interventions decreased the incidence of T2D in high-risk groups (Orozco et al., 2008).

Polycystic ovary syndrome (PCOS) is a common condition affecting women. Overweight women can have reduced ovulation frequency, irregular menstrual cycles, and reduced fertility. Increased testosterone is known to cause acne, and excess hair growth on the body and face. PCOS is known to be associated with hyperinsulinemia, insulin resistance, and abnormal choles-terol levels. PCOS affects quality of life, and can cause psychological conditions such as depression and anxiety. A review of six studies on 164 participants with PCOS has indicated that adopting a healthy lifestyle can reduce testosterone levels, improve insulin resistance, and reduce body weight, and abdominal fat. However, healthy lifestyle did not have significant effect on cholesterol or glucose levels (Moran et al., 2011).

Rheumatoid arthritis and asthma are polygenic, immune-pathological, psychosomatic diseases. Diet and lifestyle are considered as one of the causative factors. Suitable modifications might help in the control of these chronic and difficult-to-treat diseases. However, a systematic review of fourteen trials with a total of 837 patients has not shown any conclusive evidence in support of dietary modification in rheumatoid arthritis (Hagen et al., 2009).

A study of 38 patients with chronic asthma has shown that a calorie-controlled diet can be beneficial as an adjuvant to drug therapy, with no serious adverse effects. However, the impact of a calorie-controlled diet in the general asthmatic population has not been established (Cheng et al., 2005).

Patients with coronary heart disease can benefit substantially from lifestyle-intervention programs. The evidence summarized in a meta-analysis of 23 trials and 11,085 patients confirmed that lifestyle modification programs are much better compared to routine clinical care given to coronary heart disease patients (Janssen et al., 2013). It is known that plasma homocysteine levels are associated with cardiac disease risk. A study reveals that lifestyle interventions, and vitamin B intake might lower homocysteine, and reduce the risk of CVDs (DeRose et al., 2000).

Lifestyle interventions that involve a healthy diet and exercise can be much more effective if they are personalized to individual needs. Recent reports indicate that about 37% of adults in the United States have neuropsychiatric symptoms, which are difficult to treat with standard treatments. Researchers have examined the usefulness of mind—body therapies in neuropsychiatric symptoms. This large study on 23,393 adults compared the use of mind—body therapy like yoga, meditation, deep-breathing exercises, biofeedback, energy healing, guided imagery, hypnosis, relaxation therapy, qi-gong, and tai-chi. The study population was suffering from headaches, daytime sleepiness, anxiety, depression, insomnia, memory, and attention deficit. This study concluded that adults with more than one neuropsychiatric symptom tend to use mind—body therapies more frequently (Purohit et al., 2013).

Psychological stress in cancer patients has been identified as a major problem in oncology. Mind—body therapies, including yoga, mindfulness, qigong, and tai chi have shown a potential to reduce stress and improve the quality of life of cancer patients and survivors (Elkins et al., 2013). In a collaborative clinical study was conducted by the University of California and University of Washington on 435 patients with low back pain. The study reported that patients who practiced yoga or meditation and body awareness had better recovery from pain (Mehling et al., 2014).

A meta-analysis of 34 studies from 39 clinical trials involving a total of 2219 participants has shown evidence that mind—body therapies can increase the immune response to vaccination. Mind—body therapies also resulted in a reduction in inflammation markers and improved virus-specific immune responses (Morgan et al., 2014).

Thus, for psychiatric, psychosomatic, and lifestyle diseases, the role of *mind* needs to be given predominance over body and *brain*. The psychological or mental disorder is not only in the brain—it might be the case that the mind is involved. The emergence and wide acceptance of mind—body therapy, mindfulness, and behavioral medicine is a clear indication of the growing awareness about this reality. Modern psychiatry must address this issue seriously, and judiciously balance pharmacological interventions involving drugs, and nonpharmacological interventions involving yoga, meditation, mind—body, and mindfulness practices.

AYURVEDA AND YOGA

Ayurveda and yoga emphasize health protection through a continuous adherence to diet and lifestyle protocols. Detailed contributions of Ayurveda, yoga, and modern medicine have been discussed in the book *Integrative Approaches for Health* (Patwardhan et al., 2015). All these disciplines concur on dietary modifications, sound sleep, exercise, and stress reduction. Ayurveda describes diet, sleep, and behavior as a triad for good health. Exercise is expected as an integral part of daily routine. Yoga concentrates more on the mind. Lifestyle interventions involve healthy diet and exercise customized to individual needs.

Personalized lifestyle interventions and advice is specific to a person's individual constitution, disease types, history, and several host factors. Ayurveda offers detailed advice in terms of avoiding causative factors, diet restrictions, sleep and behavioral change, known as *Swasthavritta*. It gives emphasis on daily and seasonal healthy routines consisting of diet and exercise, and adopting specific therapeutic modalities for health protection.

The Ayurveda concept of behavioral medicine *(Achara rasayana)* gives an individualized prescription for a healthy diet and lifestyle. Yoga also offers a set of protocols of behavioral conduct. Integrating concepts of Ayurveda and yoga can offer a prescription for healthy, happy, and spiritual lifestyle. This covers personal, social behavior, nonviolence, freedom from anger, truth, equality, desire for a global good, and compassion for all living things. This concept respects the power of mind and proposes that we can achieve our health by adopting an appropriate lifestyle that promotes physiological functions and prevent diseases.

A recent understanding of biological functions throws light on the association between the disturbance of circadian rhythms and lifestyle diseases. Studies involving shift-duty workers have shown that an impaired day/night cycle leads to the development of obesity, cancer, hypertension, diabetes, and heart diseases in such workers. Another study has demonstrated cancer mechanisms in the case of a loss of circadian homeostasis (Ando, 2013). The synchrony with circadian rhythm leads to a loss of energy balance, disturbed immune function, and early aging (Fu and Kettner, 2013).

Ayurveda advises fasting and controlled diet for maintaining homeostasis and gut functions. Clinical trials on fasting have successfully convinced its protective effects in obesity, hypertension, asthma, rheumatoid arthritis, and it also delayed the aging process (Longo and Mattson, 2014). The mechanisms of fasting have shown its effects through lipolysis and upregulation of gluconeogenesis by liver in mice. Fasting stimulates gut-derived serotonin upregulation and prevents glucose uptake by hepatocytes (Sumara et al., 2012). Physiological effects of fasting are getting more attention with regard to the epidemic of NCD such as diabetes, cancer, and autoimmune diseases. It is important to know when not to eat to avoid a burden on the digestive system. Intermittent fasting improves lipid profile and decrease inflammatory responses. Gene expression related to inflammatory response is also reported to be altered with intermittent fasting (Azevedo et al., 2013).

Ayurvedic management considers diet restriction as an important step. Therapeutic fasting is suggested for many diseases such as rheumatoid arthritis, diabetes, and obesity. The logic of therapeutic fasting is to regain homeostasis and digestion of toxic waste product metabolisms. Therapeutic fasting also improves and expedites the excretion of toxins, which relieves fever.

A clinical trial published in *The Lancet* provides an interesting clue about the effect of fasting on rheumatoid arthritis. In a controlled clinical trial on patients of RA, the patients were advised to follow a vegetarian diet for one year out of which 4 weeks of controlled fasting were followed. After 4 weeks the diet group showed a significant improvement in number of tender joints, Ritchie's articular index, number of swollen joints, pain score, duration of morning stiffness, grip strength, erythrocyte sedimentation rate, C-reactive protein, white blood cell count, and a health assessment questionnaire score (Kjeldsen-Kragh et al., 1991).

Quality of sleep is known to influence health and immune status. Sound sleep is one of the indicators of health. Sleep nourishes body and mind. It provides strength, growth, complexion, and longevity. It boosts immunity, calms the mind, and recharges senses. It is one of the three pillars of life along with food and behavior. According to modern physiology, sleep prevents neurobehavioral deficits and improves memory. Association of sleep deprivation with diabetes, stress, hypertension, heart diseases, and obesity are reported in literature.

Yoga as therapy has been studied in many diseases. Psychological stress in cancer patients has been identified as a major problem in oncology. Mind–body therapies, including yoga, and mindfulness have shown potential to reduce stress and improve the quality of life of cancer patients and survivors (Elkins et al., 2013). In a collaborative clinical study by the University of California and the University of Washington, conducted on 435 primary care patients with acute low back pain, those who practiced yoga or meditation and body awareness, reported better recovery from pain (Mehling et al., 2014). An analysis of 1193 abstracts involving 58 trials examining effectiveness of therapies for hot flushes indicated that yoga and mindfulness-based behavioral modifications significantly reduced hot flushes and improved cognitive symptoms more than mere exercise (Woods et al., 2014).

The effects of yoga on various diseases are reported in more than 500 clinical trials. For example, its effects on hypertension were demonstrated by more than 30 trials. Apart from cardiovascular diseases, yoga therapy has successfully shown its effects for management of obesity, chronic obstructive pulmonary disease, HIV, stress reduction, anxiety, and chronic fatigue syndrome. It has also been used for managing complications in high-risk pregnancies, reducing pain, and assisted vaginal deliveries. Yoga has opened a new dimension of lifestyle that combines effects on mind and body. Yoga affects muscular, cardiac, immunological aspects, and so it now being implemented in several programs. Major clinics in US such as the Mayo and Cleveland Clinics have started yoga teaching and implemented the same in their practice of integrative medicine departments. In the UK, a study shows that engaging in yoga can reduce the National Health Insurance Scheme's bill associated to just back pain alone by about 1.5 billion pounds. Yoga has clearly emerged as a preventive, promotive, and therapeutic intervention for managing several diseases.

Mind—body therapies have provided an interesting link to the immune system. A meta-analysis of 34 studies from 39 clinical trials involving 2219 participants has shown evidence that mind—body therapies increase immune responses to vaccination. Mind—body therapies also resulted in reduction in inflammation markers and improved virus-specific immune responses (Morgan et al., 2014).

MEDICATION TO MEDITATION

Many times the concept of medicine gets reduced to use of material pharmaceutical drugs mainly for symptomatic management. Typically, a drug is anything that prevents, alleviates, cures, or manages disease with the ultimate goal of reestablishing health. Normally, pharmacological products whether synthetic, biologic, or herbal are considered as drugs. However, medicine need not be restricted to such material drugs. Various ways of lifestyle and behavioral modifications can play an important role in medicine. These are physiologic interventions based on mind—body medicine. Vedic and Buddhist traditions have given much emphasis to the mind. The role of yoga and meditation to enhance self-awareness and consciousness has been well-recognized in the promotion of mental and physical health. It is possible to train our minds to become more flexible and adaptable without losing focus on the goal. Yoga suggests the means of controlling the mind through a detached watchfulness of our thoughts. The health tips from yoga for achieving a sound mind suggest refraining from greed, grief, fear, anger, jealousy, attachment, and malice. Ayurveda also reiterates the same concept, and states that behavioral errors may lead to diseases.

Yoga offers various ways to achieve health, increase wellness, and prevent disease at physical, mental, and spiritual levels. Yoga and meditation techniques are becoming increasingly popular worldwide. Yoga is not a quick fix for health. Yoga can benefit those who are ready to put forth the effort (Morris, 1998). The spiritual and biological effects—together with physical and mental benefits—of yogic practices are also important. There is fair evidence supporting the belief that biomedicine and yoga may complement each other. Yoga practices have been shown to be useful in the prevention of several psychological problems, chronic diseases, and musculoskeletal disorders. Yoga has helped scientists to explore new paradigms for obtaining insights into physiological states, and mind—body interactions (Shannahoff-Khalsa, 2004). The study of yoga and meditation, with the help of PET, has helped to identify neural networks in brain regions that are active in different states of consciousness. Scientists have shown that systematic breathing exercises can alter cerebral hemisphere activity, neuroendocrine, and autonomic functions (Shannahoff-Khalsa et al., 1997).

The mind—body relationship is becoming clear through research on psychoneuroendocrinology aspects. The next step appears to be its extension to a deeper understanding of the concept of spirituality. Although, the word "spirituality" has yet to find a place in the official definition of health, a fairly good number scientific papers suggest a supportive role of meditation and spirituality—especially for cancer patients. A preliminary study published in *JAMA* has indicated benefits of yoga postures in the treatment of carpal tunnel syndrome (Garfinkel et al., 1998). Chanting yoga mantras has been reported to induce psychological and physiological effects (Bernardi et al., 2001). In a randomized controlled study on lymphoma patients, a yoga program was found to be feasible for patients with cancer in addition to significantly improving sleep-related problems (Cohen et al., 2004). Another prospective, randomized trial has suggested that yoga can be complementary to the conventional treatment of pulmonary tuberculosis (Visweswaraiah and Telles, 2004).

While pharmaceutical drugs are thought of as medicines for disease of the body, meditation can be thought of as a tonic for mind. Yoga places much importance on meditation. Meditation is about various practices and techniques designed to promote peace, tranquility, compassion, love, patience, generosity, and forgiveness. Through meditation, the attempt is made toward relaxation, and to strengthen willpower, and internal energy. Meditation can help improve concentration, and mind activity. Meditation can act as a medicine by enhancing the power of the natural healing force (Khalsa and Stauth, 2002).

Yoga breathing techniques and physical postures are very sophisticated exercises, designed for the whole body. In Indian tradition, the sun is given much importance as the source of vital energy. Salutation to the sun is considered a healthy practice. This practice has been cleverly used by sages to create one of the most simple yet effective exercises for all age groups. This is known as the "Sun Salutation" exercise, or *Surya Namaskara*; it packages key postures from complicated yogic processes. It is actually a set of *Yogasana* with coordinated breathing patterns. Every day, twelve or more repetitions according to the stamina of the individual, are recommended as daily exercise. Many studies have concluded that *Surya Namaskara* can be an ideal exercise to keep oneself in optimum level of fitness (Bhutkar et al., 2011). The regular practice of sun salutations as daily exercises is probably the easiest, most convenient, and economical exercise; it can be practiced singly, or in groups, and can help in disease prevention, and health promotion.

Research on *Surya Namaskara* has revealed its efficacy in controlling bronchial asthma (Nagarathna and Nagendra, 1985) and its potential to improve pulmonary functions, muscle strength and endurance, and cardiovascular parameters (Bhavanani et al., 2011). In another study, the practice of *Surya Namaskara* has shown to result in better synchronization of muscular movements with breathing, sympathetic arousal, and muscular exertion (Bhavanani et al., 2013). An integrative practice involving *Surya*

Namaskara, along with *pranayama*, *Yogasana*, and meditation, has shown significant improvement in social adaptation, and intelligence quotient—including that of mentally retarded children (Uma et al., 1989). The speed of *Surya Namaskara* performance, and associated breathing patterns have specific effects. The effects of performing *Surya Namaskara* at a fast pace are similar to aerobic exercises, whereas the slow performance of *Surya Namaskara* is similar to those of yoga training (Bhavanani et al., 2011). *Surya Namaskara* seems to be the most effective, most easily done, and most inexpensive practice for the protection of health.

Studies have demonstrated that even short-term training in techniques such as yoga and exercise programs can influence the sympathetic nervous system and immune system. Healthy volunteers practicing these techniques have shown profound increases in the release of epinephrine, which leads to increased production of antiinflammatory mediators (Kox et al., 2014). Yoga interventions such as performing gentle postures, breathing exercises, and meditation have definitive advantages over other interventions, such as nature walks, and listening to relaxing music. A comparative study with these two interventions showed that yoga and related practices might provide longer-term physiological benefits and health protection (Qu et al., 2013).

Transcendental Meditation (TM) proposed by the late Maharishi Mahesh Yogi has gained popularity in United States and Europe. TM technique aims at silence at the level of mind and experiencing peace and consciousness through easy-to-practice 20-minute sessions. Various trials on TM have demonstrated benefits in lowering blood pressure, anxiety, depression, insomnia, reduction in heart attacks, stroke, and mortality. It has also reduced stress hormones (cortisol) and improved brain functions and cognitive abilities (Pert et al., 1985). TM leads to restful alertness, a state of consciousness that is physiologically different from an ordinary state of awareness. It slows down the respiration rate, heart rate, and induces deep muscle relaxation. Electrophysiological changes due to TM show improved interhemispheric and intrahemispheric EEG synchrony. Research at the University of Chicago on hypertensive patients has shown a decreased need for antihypertensives, tranquillizers, and antianginal drugs.

Mindfulness medicine is based on yoga and meditation practices from Buddhist and Zen philosophy. Mindfulness is maintaining a continuous awareness of thoughts, feelings, sensations, and developing deep insight into the nature of reality. Research on neuroscience and consciousness is unraveling the secrets of the science of mindfulness. Dr. Jon Kabat-Zinn, Professor of Medicine at the University of Massachusetts Medical School, established the Center for Mindfulness in Medicine and launched a program known as mindfulness-based, stress-reduction program. Mindfulness enhanced heart rate recovery as well as breathing rate after stressful training. It also lowered plasma neuropeptide Y concentration and decreased the blood-oxygen-level—dependent signal. It reduced inflammation and aging, and it also improved cell-mediated immunity. Mindfulness has the potential to reduce stress, anxiety, depression, hypertension, cardiovascular diseases, aging, and various lifestyle diseases.

A meta-analysis of 47 trials with 3515 participants indicated that mindfulness meditation programs showed moderate evidence of improved anxiety, depression, and pain, and some benefit to the mental, health-related quality of life. This study concluded that small-to-moderate reductions of psychological stress can be achieved through meditation programs. Researchers suggested that the clinicians should talk to patients about the positive role of meditation in addressing psychological stress (Goyal et al., 2014). Mindfulness meditation is shown to reduce cognitive rigidity because it overcomes the tendency to be "blinded" by experience (Greenberg et al., 2010). Studies have also shown that mindfulness was related to the somatic marker circuit of the brain (Murakami et al., 2012).

Another meditation practice similar to mindfulness meditation practice, known as *Vipassana*, is popular in India, and a few other countries. Based on Buddhist traditions, *Vipassana* is an introspective practice in which the practitioner tries to develop insight into the true nature of reality. *Vipassana* practice includes contemplation, introspection, and the observation of bodily sensations. This technique of analytic meditation necessitates silence with no external communication on the part of the practitioner; this triggers a deep internal dialogue, and introspection about the meaning of changes in selfconcept, ego defense, life, death, and decomposition. A few studies have shown beneficial neurobiological and clinical changes following *Vipassana* meditation (Chiesa, 2010).

Tai chi chuan (TCC) is a Chinese martial art practice, which is also used for health benefits. A systematic review of seven studies involving 391 participants has shown that fibromyalgia symptoms can be improved by tai chi practice (Raman et al., 2014). In another interesting study, compared with controls, TCC practitioners showed a significantly thicker cortex in the precentral gyrusin of the right hemisphere and in the superior temporal gyrus of the left hemisphere (Wei et al., 2013). Thus, many scientific studies are indicating the usefulness of meditation for modulation of emotions and behavior—be it through mindfulness, *Vipassana*, tai chi, Zen, or Yoga.

Sir Charles Darwin had predicted that physiological basis of emotions would be one day understood. Renowned neurobiologist Dr. Candace Pert, who discovered opiate receptors, has made this prediction true (Pert et al., 1985). Through the theory of emotions, she has explained the importance of neuropeptides and immune system cytokines in communication between the brain and the body. She explains that more than 50 neuropeptides, which are known as hormones, gut peptides, or growth factors, can alter behavior and mood states as psychoactive drugs like morphine, Valium, and phencyclidine. She has spotted the neuropeptides receptors primary sensory (pain) inputs, and motivational processes in the striatum (subcortical part of the forebrain) in humans, monkeys, and rats. This research has discovered neuropeptides and their receptors connections with regard to the brain, glands, and immune system. Her research explains the communication between brain and body, suggesting biochemical substrates of emotion. Dr. Candace has authored a book, *Molecules of Emotions*, that explains how healthy communication and emotional expressions can integrate mind and body (Pert, 2003). The understanding of emotions has led to a biological interpretation of several concepts of yoga and Ayurveda. Her research is also important for understanding the holistic nature of the mind–body connection via immunology, endocrinology, psychology, and neuroscience.

The work of Candace Pert leads to proposition of a hypothesis. Modulations of emotions through mindful yoga and meditation techniques can lead to the formation of neuropeptides that heal our mind and body. A biological understanding of meditation reveals its potential to reduce the need for medicine—and it may also replace drugs for certain clinical conditions.

REFERENCES

American College of Preventive Medicine [Internet]. Available from: <http://www.acpm.org/?page = LifestyleMedicine>.

Ando, H., 2013. Circadian clocks and lifestyle-related diseases. Rinsho. Byori. 61 (11), 1044–1050.

Azevedo, F., Ikeoka, D., Caramelli, B., 2013. Effects of intermittent fasting on metabolism in men. Rev. Assoc. Med. Bras. 59 (2), 167–173.

Bernardi, L., Sleight, P., Bandinelli, G., Cencetti, S., Fattorini, L., Wdowczyc-Szulc, J., et al., 2001. Effect of rosary prayer and yoga mantras on autonomic cardiovascular rhythms: comparative study. Br. Med. J. 323, 1446–1449.

Bhavanani, A., Madanmohan, Udupa, K., Ravindra, P., 2011. A comparative study of slow and fast suryanamaskar on physiological function. Int. J. Yoga 71.

Bhavanani, A.B., Ramanathan, M., Balaji, R., Pushpa, D., 2013. Immediate effects of suryanamaskar on reaction time and heart rate in female volunteers. Indian J. Physiol. Pharmacol. 57, 199–204.

Bhutkar, M.V., Bhutkar, P.M., Taware, G.B., Surdi, A.D., 2011. How effective is sun salutation in improving muscle strength, general body endurance and body composition? Asian J. Sports Med. 2, 259–266.

Cheng, J., Pan, T., Ye, G.H., Liu, Q., 2005. Calorie controlled diet for chronic asthma. Cochrane. Database Syst. Rev. CD004674.

Chiesa, A., 2010. Vipassana meditation: systematic review of current evidence. J. Altern. Complement. Med. 16, 37–46.

Cochrane Library. Available from: <http://onlinelibrary.wiley.com/cochranelibrary>.

Cohen, L., Warneke, C., Fouladi, R.T., Rodriguez, M.A., Chaoul-Reich, A., 2004. Psychological adjustment and sleep quality in a randomized trial of the effects of a Tibetan yoga intervention in patients with lymphoma. Cancer 100, 2253–2260.

DeRose, D.J., Charles-Marcel, Z.L., Jamison, J.M., Muscat, J.E., Braman, M.A., McLane, G.D., et al., 2000. Vegan diet-based lifestyle program rapidly lowers homocysteine levels. Prev. Med. (Baltim) 30 (3), 225−233.

Elkins, G., Johnson, A., Fisher, W., Sliwinski, J., 2013. Efficacy of Mind-Body Therapy on Stress Reduction in Cancer Care. Evidence-Based Non-Pharmacological Therapies for Palliative Cancer Care. Springer, The Netherlands, pp. 153−173.

Fu, L., Kettner, N., 2013. The circadian clock in cancer development and therapy. Prog. Mol. Biol. Transl. Sci. 119, 221−282.

Garfinkel, M.S., Singhal, A., Katz, W.A., Allan, D.A., Reshetar, R., Schumacher, H.R., 1998. Yoga-based intervention for carpal tunnel syndrome: a randomized trial. JAMA 280, 1601−1603.

Goyal, M., Singh, S., Sibinga, E.M.S., Gould, N.F., Rowland-Seymour, A., Sharma, R., et al., 2014. Meditation programs for psychological stress and well-being: a systematic review and meta-analysis. JAMA Int. Med. 174, 357−368.

Greenberg, J., Reiner, K., Meiran, N., 2010. "Mind the trap": mindfulness practice reduces cognitive rigidity. PLoS ONE 5.

Hagen, K.B., Byfuglien, M.G., Falzon, L., Olsen, S.U., Smedslund, G., 2009. Dietary interventions for rheumatoid arthritis. Cochrane Database Syst. Rev.(1), CD006400.

Hurkmans, E.J., van der Giesen, F.J., Vliet Vlieland, T.P.M., Schoones, J., Van den Ende, E.C.H.M., 2009. Dynamic exercise programs (aerobic capacity and/or muscle strength training) in patients with rheumatoid arthritis. Cochrane Database Syst. Rev.(4), CD006853.

Janssen, V., De Gucht, V., Dusseldorp, E., Maes, S., 2013. Lifestyle modification programmes for patients with coronary heart disease: a systematic review and meta-analysis of randomized controlled trials. Eur. J. Prev. Cardiol. 20 (4), 620−640.

Khalsa, D.S., Stauth, C., 2002. Meditation as Medicine: Activate the Power of Your Natural Healing Force. Simon and Schuster, New York, NY.

Kjeldsen-Kragh, J., Borchgrevink, C.F., Laerum, E., Haugen, M., Eek, M., Førre, O., et al., 1991. Controlled trial of fasting and one-year vegetarian diet in rheumatoid arthritis. Lancet 338 (8772), 899−902.

Kox, M., van Eijk, L.T., Zwaag, J., van den Wildenberg, J., Sweep, F.C., van der Hoeven, J.G., et al., 2014. Voluntary activation of the sympathetic nervous system and attenuation of the innate immune response in humans. Proc. Natl. Acad. Sci. U. S. A. 111, 7379−7384.

Longo, V.D., Mattson, M.P., 2014. Fasting: molecular mechanisms and clinical applications. Cell. Metab.181−192.

Maki, K.C., Dicklin, M.R., Baum, S.J., 2015. Statins and diabetes. Cardiol. Clin.233−243.

Mehling, W.E., Price, C.J., Daubenmier, J., Mike, A., Bartmess, E., Stewart, A., 2014. Body awareness and the practice of yoga or meditation in 435 primary care patients with past or current low back pain. J. Altern. Complement. Med. 20 (5), A63−A64.

Moran, L.J., Hutchison, S.K., Norman, R.J., Teede, H.J., 2011. Lifestyle changes in women with polycystic ovary syndrome. Cochrane Database Syst. Rev. CD007506.

Morgan, N., Irwin, M.R., Chung, M., Wang, C., 2014. The effects of mind-body therapies on the immune system: meta-analysis. PLoS ONE 9 (7). Available from: http://dx.doi.org/10.1371/journal.pone.0100903.

Morris, K., 1998. Meditating on yogic science. Lancet 1038.

Murakami, H., Nakao, T., Matsunaga, M., Kasuya, Y., Shinoda, J., Yamada, J., et al., 2012. The structure of mindful brain. PLoS ONE 7.

Murtagh, E., Murphy, M., Boone-Heinonen, J., 2010. Walking: the first steps in cardiovascular disease prevention. Curr. Opin. Cardiol. 25 (5), 490−496.

Nagarathna, R., Nagendra, H.R., 1985. Yoga for bronchial asthma: a controlled study. Br. Med. J. (Clin. Res. Ed.) 291 (6502), 1077–1079.

Naldi, L., Conti, A., Cazzaniga, S., Patrizi, A., Pazzaglia, M., Lanzoni, A., et al., 2014. Diet and physical exercise in psoriasis: a randomized controlled trial. Br. J. Dermatol. 170 (3), 634–642.

Ornish, D., Brown, S.E., Billings, J.H., Scherwitz, L.W., Armstrong, W.T., Ports, T.A., et al., 1990. Can lifestyle changes reverse coronary heart disease? The Lifestyle Heart Trial. Lancet 336 (8708), 129–133.

Ornish, D., Lin, J., Chan, J.M., Epel, E., Kemp, C., Weidner, G., et al., 2013. Effect of comprehensive lifestyle changes on telomerase activity and telomere length in men with biopsy-proven low-risk prostate cancer: 5-year follow-up of a descriptive pilot study. Lancet Oncol. 14 (11), 1112–1120.

Ornish, D., Scherwitz, L.W., Doody, R.S., Kesten, D., McLanahan, S.M., Brown, S.E., et al., 1983. Effects of stress management training and dietary changes in treating ischemic heart disease. JAMA 249 (1), 54–59.

Ornish, D., Scherwitz, L.W., Billings, J.H., Brown, S.E., Gould, K.L., Merritt, T.A., et al., 1998. Intensive lifestyle changes for reversal of coronary heart disease. JAMA 280 (23), 2001–2007.

Orozco, L.J., Buchleitner, A.M., Gimenez-Perez, G., Roqué I Figuls, M., Richter, B., Mauricio, D., 2008. Exercise or exercise and diet for preventing type 2 diabetes mellitus. Cochrane Database Syst. Rev. (3), CD003054.

Patwardhan, B., Mutalik, G., Tillu, G., 2015. Integrative Approaches for Health: Biomedical Research, Ayurveda and Yoga, first ed. Academic Presss, Amsterdam, pp. 141–173.

Pert, C., 2003. Molecules of Emotions. Scribner, New York, NY.

Pert, C.B., Ruff, M.R., Weber, R.J., Herkenham, M., 1985. Neuropeptides and their receptors: a psychosomatic network. J. Immunol. 135 (2 Suppl.), 820s–826s.

Purohit, M.P., Wells, R.E., Zafonte, R., Davis, R.B., Yeh, G.Y., Phillips, R.S., 2013. Neuropsychiatric symptoms and the use of mind-body therapies. J. Clin. Psychiatry 74.

Pyörälä, M., Miettinen, H., Laakso, M., Pyörälä, K., 2000. Plasma insulin and all-cause cardiovascular, and noncadiovascular mortality: the 22-year follow-up results of the Helsinki Policemen Study. Diabetes Care 23 (8), 1097–1102.

Qu, S., Olafsrud, S.M., Meza-Zepeda, L.A., Saatcioglu, F., 2013. Rapid gene expression changes in peripheral blood lymphocytes upon practice of a comprehensive yoga program. PLoS ONE 8.

Raman, G., Mudedla, S., Wang, C., 2014. How effective is tai chi mind-body therapy for fibromyalgia: a systematic review and meta-analysis. J. Altern. Complement. Med. 20 (5), A66.

Sainani, S., 2001. Management of Diabetes. API Textbook of Medicine. Association of Physicians of India, Mumbai.

Shannahoff-Khalsa, D.S., 2004. An introduction to Kundalini yoga meditation techniques that are specific for the treatment of psychiatric disorders. J. Altern. Complement. Med. 10, 91–101.

Shannahoff-Khalsa, D.S., Kennedy, B., Yates, F.E., Ziegler, M.G., 1997. Low-frequency ultradian insulin rhythms are coupled to cardiovascular, autonomic, and neuroendocrine rhythms. Am. J. Physiol. 272, R962–R968.

Sharma, V., Saito, Y., Amit, S., 2014. Mind-body medicine and irritable bowel syndrome: a randomized control trial using stress reduction and resiliency training. J. Altern. Complement. Med. 20 (5), A94.

Society of Behavioural Medicine [Internet]. Available from: <http://www.sbm.org/resources/education/behavioral-medicine>.

Sumara, G., Sumara, O., Kim, J.K., Karsenty, G., 2012. Gut-derived serotonin is a multifunctional determinant to fasting adaptation. Cell. Metab. 16 (5), 588−600.

Uma, K., Nagendra, H.R., Nagarathna, R., Vaidehi, S., Seethalakshmi, R., 1989. The integrated approach of yoga: a therapeutic tool for mentally retarded children: a one-year controlled study. J. Ment. Defic. Res. 33 (Pt 5), 415−421.

Visweswaraiah, N.K., Telles, S., 2004. Randomized trial of yoga as a complementary therapy for pulmonary tuberculosis. Respirology 9, 96−101.

Ward, B.W., Schiller, J.S., Goodman, R.A., 2014. Multiple chronic conditions among US adults: a 2012 update. Prev. Chronic. Dis. 11, E62.

Warren, J., 1812. Remarks on angina pectoris. N. Engl. J. Med. 1 (1), 1−11.

Wei, G.X., Xu, T., Fan, F.M., Dong, H.M., Jiang, L.L., Li, H.J., et al., 2013. Can Taichi reshape the brain? A brain morphometry study. PLoS ONE 8.

Woods, N.F., Mitchell, E.S., Schnall, J.G., Cray, L., Ismail, R., Taylor-Swanson, L., et al., 2014. Effects of mind-body therapies on symptom clusters during the menopausal transition. Climacteric 17 (1), 10−22.

Yamaoka, K., Tango, T., 2012. Effects of lifestyle modification on metabolic syndrome: a systematic review and meta-analysis. BMC Med. 10 (38), 1−10.

Zhao, W., Ukawa, S., Kawamura, T., Wakai, K., Ando, M., Tsushita, K., et al., 2015. Health benefits of daily walking on mortality among younger-elderly men with or without major critical diseases in the new integrated suburban seniority investigation project: a prospective cohort study. J. Epidemiol. 25 (10), 609−616.

Zorena, K., Jachimowicz-Duda, O., Wąż, P., 2016. The cut-off value for interleukin 34 as an additional potential inflammatory biomarker for the prediction of the risk of diabetic complications. Biomarkers1−7.

Chapter 15

Collaborative Strategies for Future Drug Discovery

Rathnam Chaguturu[1] and Bhushan Patwardhan[2]

[1]*iDDPartners, Princeton Junction, NJ, United States,* [2]*Savitribai Phule Pune University, Pune, Maharashtra, India*

PROLOGE

Birth and death are the two irrevocable certainties in life. The average life expectancy has been getting longer and better over the last few decades, and almost doubled in the last 150 years. Thanks to medicines, one of the greatest gifts to humanity. The use of antibiotics and prophylactic vaccines, combined with massive public health advances, has eradicated some of the deadly diseases that claimed millions of lives over the centuries. The list of vaccine-preventable diseases, including polio, measles, and smallpox, now stands at a high of 30, and new vaccine modalities for nontraditional diseases are under serious investigation. The concept of drinking clean water, the germ theory of disease, and an improved standard of living has contributed to healthy lives. The prevention of infant mortality has become a global strategic priority. Despite our continued war against human maladies, many old diseases still remain incurable, and new phenotypes are continually emerging. We need to be ever more nimble and agile to combat the never-ending healthcare crises; for that we must dedicate our energies and stay engaged with the transformative policies and technologies with compassion for the poor and the needy. It must be our core principle. Bench-to-bedside innovation is integral in our efforts to be a step ahead of the next healthcare crisis. The following deserves our critical attention:

1. The clinician must use, with honesty and humility, best healthcare practices to nip the disease in its bud;
2. Nations must provide leadership and engage policy makers and administrators to put forth programs for affordable high-quality healthcare delivery and ready access;
3. The academic scientist must engage in cutting-edge biomedical research with an out-of-the-box mindset; and last but not least,

Innovative Approaches in Drug Discovery. DOI: http://dx.doi.org/10.1016/B978-0-12-801814-9.00015-5

4. The pharmaceutical industry must put patients' needs first over its shareholders'.

For all of this to have a successful outcome, the "stake holders" must engage in open innovation during the precompetitive phase and a collaborative enterprise when the clinical candidate looks promising. These two seemingly similar but distinct paradigms are evolving, and have the transformative potential, when nurtured with respect and understanding, to correct endemic and systemic failures of the past.

The biomedical enterprise spans discovery, development, and delivery of drugs in highly complex ways. The current therapeutics paradigm relies on cross-cultural contributions from traditional and alternative medicines, augmented by academic and corporate efforts. Key limitations in the formulation and development of medical strategies emerge from confines in knowledge transfer and cross-disciplinary redress to scientific and practical obstacles. Patients, payers, physicians, and family members crave better health solutions, and question the value of researched interventions that often bankrupt families. This applies especially to high-risk patients with complex, co-occurring illnesses that often suffer from uncoordinated care. Some therapeutic effectiveness is a prerequisite, but drugs must be affordable and readily available to patients. Equity, availability, and affordability represent three key factors that society must address. No solitary reason exists for the global healthcare crisis. Disparate culprits in the research-to-care enterprise include:

1. research systems steeped in irrelevant traditions and regulations;
2. clinical trial designs that limit applicability while disallowing aging, comorbid populations;
3. patients who suffer bitter realities once diagnosed;
4. rising hospital, physician, and drug costs with questionable benefit;
5. reimbursements based on least-common denominators;
6. misaligned incentives for all; and most importantly
7. significant lack of coordinated, collaborative innovation and integration within the biomedical ecosystem.

Coordinated and committed collaborative-innovation holds the key to discover, develop, and deliver medicines to patients.

THE NEED

More than one billion people across the globe lack ready access to healthcare. While reports of the spread of infectious diseases headline the popular press and newscasts, there are ∼36 million deaths worldwide attributable to noncommunicable diseases. Heart diseases represent almost one-third of all deaths, with a majority of these deaths occurring in the developing countries. More than 7.5 million children under the age of five die from diseases that are otherwise preventable. Malaria still causes acute illness in some 225 million people. Timely diagnosis and adequate treatment of infectious diseases such as malaria is as elusive today as it was a decade ago. Misdiagnosis and over-diagnosis, due to lack of adequate training and/or relevant diagnostic tests, often compete for limited healthcare resources in the endemic countries and erodes confidence in the clinician, but most importantly, the patient is dying in the meantime. *So many deaths, and no end in sight.* Factors affecting healthcare quality, access, and costs that affect patients' outcome. Increasing costs limits access.

The global healthcare crisis: it never seems to go away. Today's epidemic, when not addressed appropriately, is tomorrow's pandemic with catastrophic consequences. The crisis almost always starts as a regional problem, but soon becomes a pernicious epidemic and global. Infectious diseases have wiped out hundreds of millions of people over the centuries; pathogens are continually evolving, and the emerging diseases remain our greatest challenge. Cancer-related deaths far exceed than those of malaria, tuberculosis, and AIDS, combined. At the other end of the spectrum is obesity, which is linked to 60 or more chronic diseases. It is now an epidemic, claiming almost three million deaths as a result of being obese and overweight. While food-borne illnesses and infectious diseases plague the world's poor, lifestyle diseases pervade the populace in the industrialized nations. Mental illnesses may perhaps be biological or psychological. The diseases could be systemic, progressive, or refractory. We need effective and timely intervention before the "disease" takes a significant toll on the individual and, subsequently, on the family and eventually the society.

Disease is never restricted to one individual. It affects and touches the lives of family members and friends in unimaginable ways. It affects quality of life, and the economies of nations alike. So, how do we avert the next crisis? Or, for that matter, the current crises? It could be addressed from many fronts, but the following two items are paramount:

- Healthcare quality, access, and affordability
- Drug discovery and development

The cost of healthcare is astronomical worldwide. Diseases, infectious, inherited, or chronic, affect the economic well being of the families and nations alike. The medical bills push well over 100 million people a year into poverty globally. A healthcare crisis thus in effect becomes a financial crisis. Equity, availability, and affordability are three key factors that a nation must address. Healthcare in developing countries is, most often than not, unsafe, fragmented, and misdirected. Health education and gender equality still persist and stagnate.

BIOMEDICAL ECOSYSTEM

The current biomedical ecosystems build patient navigator programs that blithely promote a broken system instead of fixing it, thereby creating quality vacuums while rewarding high volume, thus widening the healthcare gap. The pharmaceutical sector focuses on FDA approvals and Centers for Medicare and Medicaid Services codes with fee-for-service, assured that the market bears any price. This approach produces marginally better/equivalent p values, with worse outcomes in noninferiority designs. Clinical trials still focus on scientific endpoints, instead of the experiences and outcomes of patients. Many "surrogate" markers and laboratory tests don't explain what actually happens to patients. Meanwhile, decreased government funding, tightened pharma/biotech budgets and layoffs, and the inevitable patent cliff conspire toward an innovation crisis.

There are about 7000 diseases that afflict mankind; yet treatments are available only for ~ 200 diseases. The number of US -FDA-approved drugs target less than 0.05% of the human genome, a mere 106 genes and 378 targets. However, there are over 4500 disease-modifying genes in the human genome which include ~ 3000 druggable genes along with another 10,000 genes that are addressable by protein therapeutics. This stresses the need to critically interrogate the druggable human genome to expand the target universe, and to facilitate the discovery of new, novel, and safer drugs with greater selectivity and specificity. Even with the sequence of the human genome in place, the true and exact genetic basis for most diseases is still unknown, especially for inherited diseases. The question remains: When will remarkable progress made in genomics translate to anything meaningful in finding cures? Partly it is nature's trick, but mostly, it is our inability in one form or another. Even though we heralded the completion of the human genome project, we still don't have an accurate count of genes (somewhere between 20,000 and 25,000) and what all the genes are. The 3.2 billion base pairs that comprise the human genome are not standing still: the loss of a base pair here and there, substitution of one with the other, uncontrolled repetitions, hopping of base pair clusters from one region to the other. It may be nature's Boogie Woogie or Samba, but it sets the cell torpedo toward becoming a cancerous one. But not all cancers are alike. Cancers come in a potpourri of sizes, shapes, varieties, etc. masquerading at its best or worst! This is where personalized medicine, a vogue concept that has caught scientists' imagination, comes in to play. But economies of drug development make personalized medicine, a great concept in theory, something that may not so easily be realized. This scenario is not just for cancer, but is universal for all diseases that afflict mankind.

THE NEW ACADEMIA

Academia has evolved in recent years from its traditional role of target identification and validation from a systems biology perspective to probing for tool molecules (probes) against these disease targets to explore their therapeutic relevance. This new focus in academia is a welcome change, but the road ahead is a long and arduous one. Academic scientists view pharma/bio-tech overtures with a mixture of appreciation and apprehension, citing that too much applied industry-sponsored research may compromise the quality of basic science. Ultimately, the corporate and academic communities must both recognize that a careful balance should be sought between esoteric (basic) science and targeted (applied) research. Without support for specula-tive and objective exploration, truly novel therapeutic paradigms might never emerge; but without focused studies, many prospective technologies might wither on the vine. Many discoveries are driven by a focused need, as opposed to curiosity alone. Academia has recently progressed from its tradi-tional systems biology focus on target identification and validation to tool molecules (probes) against disease targets that explore therapeutic relevance. This new focus provides a welcome change, but perseverance is essential on this long, arduous road. The concept of medicinal chemistry as an unbroken continuum of drug discovery, long held in pharma, needs to take hold in aca-demic drug hunters' minds. Drug discovery operations in academia need to adopt pharma/biotech's best practices. New drug discovery paradigms should be based on complementation, not competition, between pharma/biotech and academia. Competition, the defining characteristic of life's existence (and at least capitalism), and its antithesis, symbiotic collaboration, is diametrically opposite but occasionally join forces in unexpected ways. Amalgamation of these divergent factors can lead to more effective collaborative-innovation models. The new drug discovery paradigm should be based on complementa-tion, not competition, between the pharmaceutical industry and academia.

A ROADMAP FOR SUCCESSFUL DRUG DISCOVERY IN ACADEMIA

The stochastic nature of screening for probes is now a recognized discipline in academia. Each of the academic screening centers, with different speciali-zations, has the potential to develop to a level of maturity and robustness to contribute meaningfully toward development of chemical probes in the era of chemical genomics. In the pharmaceutical sector, new lead discovery has transformed over the years from being an art into a robust scientific disci-pline. However, academia's endeavor in the arena of drug discovery is a Mount Everest in the making, and requires careful nurturing to make it a successful reality. The core strength of academia is in basic and mechanistic biology, and the drug discovery efforts need to be built on this solid plat-form. The pharmaceutical industry's best practice of matrix-based multidisci-plinary team approach should be implemented in the public sector. This approach should formulate the project goals and milestones by laying out a critical project management path with industry-experienced project man-agers. It is important to convey the message that the PI is in the driver's seat and seek strong, healthy collaborations. At the very outset, there should be a draft target hypothesis and validation criteria, HTS assay design, validation, readiness and implementation, active-hit-lead definitions, data analysis routines, secondary, and counter screens to address selectivity and pharmaco-kinetic issues, while working toward a collaborative venture. A workstation-based, state-of-the-art screening facility should be established with pharma--trained personnel. Personnel from the PI's lab should be made part of the project team in transferring and validating the bench-top assays into the HTS lab. This is a critical step in the assay transfer process, because the PI's bench-top assay may not be as adequately robust or reproducible enough for the stringency of HTS. Since the success of any HTS campaign in finding a target-specific probe is dependent on the assay design and on the quality of the chemical library, the best possible assay design should be favored over what has been developed at the origination lab, and a high-quality diverse chemical library should be used. Institutional chemistries are equivalent of the corporate crown jewels. Every possible effort should therefore be made to add the institution's own legacy chemistries into the HTS chemical archives by advocating the novelty and uniqueness of these chemistries, ther-apeutic relevance, and the value of serendipity in finding the unexpected. This could be achieved by emphasizing the fact that any intellectual property (IP) that comes out from testing the institutional chemistries lies with the PI who made the compounds. Because of the suspect authenticity and the qual-ity of the cell lines used in the PI's lab, it is strongly advocated that cell lines for use in cell-based assays be purchased from commercial sources. If com-mercial sources are unavailable, it is important to ascertain the imported cell lines are not contaminated, using a quarantine cell-culture lab. An experi-enced medicinal chemist's intuition is critical for the success of any probe discovery endeavor, and a competent medicinal chemist, either from one's own institution or from a collaborating institution, must be recruited early on to carry data mining to ascertain chemical tractability and early SAR by commerce or synthesis. The personnel from the technology transfer and com-mercialization office must be brought into the project as soon as the target hypothesis has been drafted to ensure that the IP rights are adequately clari-fied, protected, and nurtured. For the probe discovery and development initiatives in academia to be successful, the projects need to be actively man-aged to prevent an exercise in futility. New lead discovery against therapeu-tic targets, especially those involving the rare and neglected diseases, is indeed a Mount Everestonian size task and requires diligent implementation of the pharmaceutical industry's best practices for a successful outcome.

CLINICAL MODELS

Developing a drug is not a trivial matter. Medicine is inherently multidisci-plinary, and includes biochemistry, genetics, physiology, chemistry, and even sociology. The current therapeutics paradigm is based on cross-cultural contributions with fundamental origins in traditional/alternative medicines, augmented by combinations of academic and corporate development efforts and by joint academic-corporate initiatives. Key limitations in the formulation and development of medical-response strategies emerge from fundamental limitations in knowledge transfer and cross-disciplinary redress to the scientific and practical obstacles to therapeutic development.

The discovery of a promising drug candidate leads to the eventual selection of a clinical candidate out of the many, and then the clinical trial design and execution phase kicks in. Clinical trials are a mandatory prerequisite to seek and gain regulatory approval for new drugs or old drugs for new indications. They are quite expensive, costing up to a billion dollars or more, and it is the first time the patient gets involved in drug development. Recruitment and retention of patients in clinical trials is a growing problem. Institutional review boards play a crucial role in setting up the clinical trial design strategies. Clinical protocol approval-to-trial activation takes many months to years; these protracted timelines present a totally unacceptable situation in swiftly addressing impending healthcare crises. Predictive murine models are often used in clinical candidate selection, but the question remains as to how well the sedentary, inbred rats and mice mimic the complex human physiology and disease. Cancer research, among others, has benefitted considerably from the use of relevant mouse models, but the scientific literature is replete with examples of drugs that worked well in mice but ineffective in humans, thus costing millions of wasted dollars and time. Nonhuman primate models may be the answer for proof-of principle studies as well as early stage clinical trials, especially in the development of vaccines against communicable diseases, and where relevant murine models simply do not exist. The globalization of clinical trials, a growing trend in recent years, presents enormous challenges to patients, regulators, and the sponsors alike. Combination drug treatment in clinical trials is gaining prominence lately and is a welcome trend. The drug cocktail approach has effectively contained the AIDS epidemic with dramatic outcomes. It is the new norm in cancer clinical trials. *Crop protection industry has employed for decades the practice of mixing pesticides with different mechanisms of action and with products from competing industry partners in eradicating pest or weed infestations. This is not always the case with pharmaceutical clinical trials.* We always see a new drug mixed with an off-patent drug but not two new drugs from two pharmaceutical companies. The pharmaceutical industry needs to put the patients' needs first: cooperate and collaborate for the patients' good.

OPEN SOURCE AND OPEN SCIENCE

Drug discovery and development takes a village of diverse expertise to be effective, and even large companies struggle to have the resources to address questions that arise along this path. Open source and open science, and their hybrids, are new avenues that may foster innovations in biomedical sciences, especially for rare and neglected diseases. Limited market size and lack of R&D investment are two major obstacles that slow down the development of novel therapeutic drugs for the treatment of these diseases. The open source, especially in the precompetitive stage, can be a scientifically and commercially viable strategy for the rapid development of low-cost and high-quality therapeutic drugs for the treatment of neglected diseases. How, we as a culture of scientists from government, academic, and commercial organizations move to this new model of work, with rewards for teamwork and clear boundaries for competition, is the challenge for us to embrace. The benefits are clear.

COORDINATED, COLLABORATIVE INNOVATION

Advances in cellular and molecular biology and the advent of high-throughput technologies related to drug discovery are extending the reach of the human mind in finding cures not only for the rare and neglected diseases but also the hard-to-cure ailments that have been afflicting humans from time immemorial. We are now in the era of Big Data and Easy Data. It took almost 15 years and 3 billion dollars to sequence the first human genome, but now we can do it for under $1000 and in a matter of hours. The reality is that any one person's genome doesn't represent *the* human genome. We need genomic sequences from thousands of people, of different genders, races, and ages, to make an informative atlas of the human genome. Like wise, for any given disease, we need the genome data from hundreds, if not thousands, of patients of different genders, races, ages, and disease stages, and references that "sequence" against the healthy human genome to find a true and realistic genetic blueprint for any given disease, be that cancer, diabetes, or autism. A single scientist or a single institute cannot decipher the available genomic data in a meaningful way. This realization has paved the way for "open innovation" in various forms and shapes. Pharma's funding focus has shifted in recent years from handpicked, curiosity-driven, disease/biology projects to large integrated programs with a strong emphasis on therapy development. Pharmaceutical giants have also initiated regional/global "science hubs" with academia to regain biomedical innovation. The recently formed Academic Drug Discovery Consortium tracks and disseminates pharma/academia collaboration initiatives. If these game changing attitudes take foothold in our thought process and become the new norm, a complete catalog of disease genes and groundbreaking therapies may not be too far away.

Key Examples

One prime example is Eli Lilly's Phenotypic Drug Discovery Initiative (https://pd2.lilly.com/pd2web), in which the compounds synthesized in academia are screened against phenotypic and other relevant assays opti-mized by Eli Lilly. While Lilly provides all evaluations and data free of charge and both the investigator/institution retains IP rights to the molecule, with Lilly seeking first rights for IP licensing and/or refusal. Merck has cre-ated SAGE, an open-access, nonprofit organization to bring academia and pharma together to develop comprehensive human disease biology models, and provides a vast database of highly consistent data about the biology of disease and software tools to use it. The open-innovation strategy was also adopted by GlaxoSmithKline (GSK), which has removed its IP restrictions for promoting research in the area of neglected diseases such as malaria. GSK has made available 13,500 malaria compounds for open research. GSK has also released genomic and protein expression profiling data for more than 300 cancer cell lines via the NCI's Cancer Bioinformatics Grid for academia to mine. GSK's discovery partnerships with academia (DPAc) is another example of a transformative pharma/academia partnership precompe-titive ventures. To fully explore the potential of drug repurposing, a pharma/academia integration effort was launched through CTSA Pharmaceutical Assets Portal. It now includes 350 researchers from a number of pharmaceu-tical companies (Pfizer, Merck, GSK, Novartis, Genentech, Abbott, Eli Lilly, AstraZeneca, etc.) and 45 universities including University of California Davis, Oregon H&S University, University of Washington, University of Pennsylvania, and the University of Chicago, probing 150 disease targets.

Promising Governmental Partnerships

It is with much enthusiasm that we welcome the creation of "Partnerships to Accelerate Therapeutics" by the US President's Council of Advisors on Science and Technology to accelerate the discovery and development of medicines through alliances involving industry, academia, government, and disease foundations. The creation of TransCelerate BioPharma by the pharma giants is in the same vein. Accelerating Medicines Partnership, under the auspice of the foundation for the NIH, is another transformative effort in tackling global healthcare crises. The $230-million-over-five-years partner-ship between NIH, pharmaceutical giants, and nonprofit disease foundations calls for the drug-makers to collaborate, not compete, on drug discovery pro-jects (Alzheimer's, type 2 diabetes, and autoimmune disorders, for now). The partners are to share their research findings with each other and the bio-medical community at-large. This is collaborative innovation at its best. The Patient-Centered Outcomes Research Institute calls for effective methods (e.g., pragmatic trials, clinical effectiveness) that tie clinical trial results to important outcomes for patients, payers, and physicians. Patient-centered care also requires a new mindset and infrastructure for partnerships with patients instead of decisions made without standards. Data-sharing initiatives for research, registries and care help build a learning health system that uses science, informatics, incentives, and culture to continuously improve and innovate. Additional initiatives may gain momentum, holding more promise, e.g., RightCare Alliance and The Accelerated Clinical Trial Agreement. President Obama's BRAIN (Brain Research through Advancing Innovative Neurotechnologies) and "precision medicine" initiatives are other examples of collaborative innovation.

GOVERNMENT–ACADEMIA–INDUSTRY COLLABORATION: CASE FROM INDIA

The Council for Scientific and Industrial Research (CSIR) launched an ambitious project known as The New Millennium Indian Technology Leadership Initiative (NMITLI) to foster public–private partnership designed to promote innovation-led development and achieve global technology leadership position across various select science and technology sectors. Now, NMITLI has emerged as the largest public–private partnership effort within the R&D domain in India. Apart from promoting public–private partnership, NMITLI also aims to fund scientifically and technologically high-risk projects and build "team India" spirit by bringing together the brightest individuals from public institutes, academia, and the private industrial sector. By 2008, the scheme involved 57 projects, which networked between public and private institutions and enterprises in terms of 270 R&D groups, 80 industry partners, and 1700 researchers with a total project investment outlay of more than US$80 million.

NMITLI Herbal Drug Project

The project adopted a traditional knowledge-guided platform approach where base formulation was used followed by an optimization strategy of adding other ingredients to obtain synergistic activity. Following prior art and several rounds of national level consultations with Ayurvedic physicians and scholars, a few potential botanical drugs were shortlisted. These drugs entered a parallel track of open label observational studies by clinicians and in-depth animal pharmacology studies. A multidisciplinary network of research institutions for this project included Interdisciplinary School of Health Sciences of Savitribai Phule Pune University (formerly known as University of Pune); Indian Institute of Integrated Medicine, Jammu (formerly known as RRL–J); National Botanical Research Institute, Lucknow; Agharkar Research Institute and Interactive Research School for Health Affairs, Pune; Swami Prakashananda Ayurveda Research Center and KEM Hospital, Mumbai; Nizam Institute of Medical Sciences, Hyderabad; All India Institute of Medical Sciences, New Delhi; and Center for Rheumatic Diseases, Pune. The project involved industry partners including Arya Vaidya Shala, Kottakal; Arya Vaidya Pharmacy, Coimbatore; and Nicholas Piramal, Dabur, Zandu

Pharmaceuticals and Natural Remedies, Bangalore (Amirkia and Heinrich, 2015; Chaguturu, 2014).

Open Source Drug Discovery

CSIR envisaged that the Open Source model could be applied to the healthcare sector, especially for identifying drug targets for neglected diseases in an affordable manner (Allarakhia, 2014). Open Source Drug Discovery (OSDD) is a consortium conceived and led by CSIR with multiple global partnerships. This consortium was launched in 2008 with a vision to provide affordable healthcare to the developing world. Launched on the three cardinal principals of collaborate, discover and share, OSDD is a community-driven open-innovation global platform for researchers and scientists from multiple streams of sciences such as informatics, chemistry, pharmacy, wet-lab scientists, clinicians, and hospitals to collectively work together and collaborate to discover novel drug targets, biomarkers, and therapeutics for the neglected diseases such as tuberculosis and malaria. At present, OSDD has more than 6700 registered users from more than 130 countries and has emerged as the largest collaborative effort in the field of drug discovery.

Affordability and accessibility remain the core concerns of delivery of drugs for tropical diseases. The underlying concept in launching OSDD is the firm belief that governments and public funded institutions of the countries with a high burden of neglected diseases must actively participate in the discovery and development of drugs for thwarting the next healthcare crisis. The fundamental principle governing the OSDD model is accessible and affordable healthcare to the developing world. OSDD aims to de-risk clinical trials for tropical diseases by investing public funds and involving public institutions in the countries where disease occurs. Drugs developed due to OSDD's efforts will be available to the developing world in an open source, generic mode, without price monopolies. The OSDD approach to drug discovery and development, therefore, is the much desired IP neutrality. Once a drug is approved for use by the regulatory agencies, OSDD will depend on the business model of the generic drug industry that made drugs affordable in the developing countries. OSDD-developed drugs will be available for any industry player with appropriate manufacturing practices to distribute the drugs to the market. The market competition will ensure accessibility and affordability by the patient.

DEPARTMENT OF SCIENCE AND TECHNOLOGY

Recognizing the profound influence of R&D on the prospects and opportunities for the growth of the Indian Drug Industry, the government of India's Department of Science and Technology (DST) mounted the program on drug development promoting collaborative R&D with specific objectives to synergize strengths of publicly funded R&D institutions and the Indian pharmaceutical industry. The government of India established a Drugs and Pharmaceutical Research Program and a Drug Development Promotion Board under the administrative control of DST for supporting R&D projects jointly proposed by industry and academic institutions/laboratories and to extend soft loans for R&D to the pharmaceutical industry. DST has significantly contributed to boost indigenous R&D and innovations in Indian pharmaceutical industry. Since 2004, DST has invested more than INR 650 crores at 70 institutions by way of collaborative grants and soft loans to industries for conducting clinical trials on neglected diseases. More than 300 collaborative research projects and establishments of more than 100 national facilities involving academia and pharmaceutical industry have been supported.

DEPARTMENT OF BIOTECHNOLOGY

SIBRI and BIRAC

In 2005–06, the Department of Biotechnology (DBT) launched the Small Business Innovation Research Initiative (SBIRI) scheme for supporting small- and medium-sized enterprises with a grant or soft loan to support the early phase of product development, including preproof of concept, early stage innovative research, and providing mentorship. DBT has also established the Biotechnology Industry Research Assistance Council (BIRAC) as an autonomous, flexible, and futuristic organization for promoting innovations by facilitating the startups and SMEs. DBT has made a commitment of investing up to 30% of its budget in academia—industry collaborator schemes to promote innovation, preproof-to-concept research, accelerated technology, and product development in biotechnology related to pharmaceuticals, agriculture, human health, the environment, etc. To support high-risk discovery and innovation projects, a new scheme, Biotechnology Industry Partnership Programme, was introduced as a government—industry partnership program for support on a cost-sharing basis. This new scheme is expected to enable mechanisms to promote biotech industry R&D and public—private partnership programmes. Through this scheme, government contributes between 30% and 50% of the cost and in some cases grant-in-aid support for evaluation and validation of technology and products.

INDIAN COUNCIL OF MEDICAL RESEARCH

Indian Council of Medical Research (ICMR) is a conglomeration of 32 national institutes and also functions as an apex body in India for the formulation, coordination and promotion of biomedical research. ICMR also has large extramural funding programs where interdisciplinary collaborative research at national and international levels is encouraged.

The Clinical Trials Registry - India (CTRI) has been established to encourage all clinical trials conducted in India to be prospectively registered before the enrollment of the first participant. ICMR's bio-ethics initiative has developed ethical guidelines for the conduct of trials and for ethics committees. Postmarketing surveillance studies as well as BA/BE trials are also expected to be registered in the CTRI. The CTRI is working with the WHO ICTRP to ensure that results of all trials registered with the CTRI are adequately reported and publicly available. Being a Primary Register of the International Clinical Trials Registry Platform (ICTRP) (http://www.who.int/ictrp/search/en/), registered trials are freely searchable both from the WHO's search portal, the ICTRP, and from the CTRI (www.ctri.nic.in).

AYUSH

This is an acronym consisting of Ayurveda, Yoga and naturopathy, Unani, Siddha, and Homoeopathy (AYUSH). The Indian medical system known as Ayurveda is one of the oldest extant health systems in the world with fundamental principles and theory-based practices. Literally, the Sanskrit meaning of *Ayu* is life and *Veda* is knowledge or science. Therefore, Ayurveda is also generally translated as the Science of Life. India has more than 600,000 registered practitioners of Ayurveda and other traditional medicines. Due to better accessibility and affordability, these systems enjoy wide acceptance among large segments of the population, especially in India. Thus, Ayurveda remains a most comprehensive and practical medical science that receives acceptance and support of the public. The Department of AYUSH lays emphasis on educational standards, quality control and standardization of drugs, improving the availability of medicinal plant material, research and development and awareness generation about the efficacy of the systems, both domestically as well as internationally. The Traditional Knowledge Digital Library is a collaborative project between CSIR and DST and AYUSH, which involves documentation of the knowledge available in the public domain on traditional knowledge from the existing literature related to Ayurveda, Unani, and Siddha in a digitized format searchable in patent databases in English, French, German, Spanish, and Japanese.

DRUGS AND BIOTECH PARKS

In recent years, several Indian companies have started partnering with multinational companies (MNC) to benefit from the R&D (formulation development) and manufacturing capabilities of the Indian partners and the extensive marketing and distribution footprint of the MNCs in emerging markets. There is also an increasing trend among MNCs for partnering in the domestic market, where marketing and distribution footprint of Indian companies and the product portfolio of MNCs is being leveraged upon.

Six biotech parks are functioning in various parts of India under the public—private partnership and the parks are in different stages of development. Several world-class scientific institutions such as the NIPERs, Central Drug Research Institute, Industrial Microbial Technology, National Chemical Laboratory, Indian Institute of Chemical Biology, All Indian Institute of Medical Sciences, Indian Institute of Chemical Technology, National Center for Biological Sciences, National Center for Cell Sciences, the Indian Institute of Science, and the Center for Cellular and Molecular Biology further lend support to the sector. The CSIR actively collaborates with Indian and foreign companies for contracts and collaborative research projects. The Indian government has promoted development of special economic zones (SEZ) for the pharma sector. There are 19 dedicated SEZs in India at various stages of development. Functional pharmaceutical SEZs in India include Jawaharlal Nehru Pharma City in Visakhapatnam (Andhra Pradesh), PHARMEZ (Gujarat), developed by Zydus Infrastructure; and PhaEZ Park (Gujarat), developed by Cadila Pharma. All these developments are expected to give a necessary boost to promote R&D and innovation in drugs and the pharmaceutical sector.

Pharma Courting Academia

Pharma's erstwhile funding focus has shifted in recent years from hand-picked, curiosity-driven, projects to large integrated programs with a strong emphasis on the development of therapies rather than the documentation of disease biology. The academic scientist views this with a mix of appreciation and apprehension, citing that the industry-sponsored research is too applied, and is at the cost of basic science. Science doesn't have to be esoteric or science for the sake of science. It has to provide value, defined as a benefit over cost, either in the short term or in the long term. The modern day academic scientist seems to have not got this "core" principle right. Many great discoveries have seen the light of day only because of a necessity, not necessarily curiosity, such as "war" times: man's race to the moon, global commerce, and the like.

Using the paradigm "a problem shared is a problem solved," open innovation has taken a strong hold within the last few years in reinvigorating the pharmaceutical R&D endeavors. This is a shift from "innovation within the corporate walls" concept to the acquisition of IP from outside the corporate walls to advance its business models, a concept that literally admits as well as advocates the fact that a problem shared is a problem solved. Pharmaceutical companies have traditionally safeguarded their own interests and eliminated competition by stringent IP protection. With the goal of speeding innovative drug discovery by tapping into global wealth of knowledge and expertise, big pharma is opening up information flow to the public domain and is aggressively establishing new R&D structures to foster open-innovation strategies with academia. Such collaborations are advantageous to both academia and industry. Academia receives more research dollars for innovative projects, greater involvement for faculty in drug discovery process as well as a secure path to product development and licensing processes. Pharma gains novel and relevant targets to feed its pipeline as well as new molecular probes for lead optimization processes. Such collaborations include Novartis Institutes for Biomedical Research to discover and develop drugs for a range of inadequately treated diseases; GSK's Centre of Excellence for external drug discovery; Pfizer's Biotherapeutics and Bioinnovation Center; Lilly Melbourne Academic Psychiatry Initiative for advancing mental health research and education in Australia; and a $14 million investment by Pfizer at the University of California (Santa Barbara, CA), Caltech; MIT, University of Massachusetts; and Entelos, a physiological modeling company, to reexamine the regulatory mechanisms of human energy metabolism and hence to expand the understanding of diabetes and obesity pathobiology. Merck has created a virtual department, External Basic Research, to foster partnerships with academic and biotech collaborators to identify and access novel targets, using a shared risk paradigm to deliver preclinical candidates for its pipeline. Burnham is collaborating with J&J on a multiyear assay development and licensing deal by granting exclusive access to its high-throughput assay screening technologies in order to determine potential targets for new drugs against inflammatory diseases, such as arthritis and lupus. J&J has also established two partnership-focused units to ensure the continued nurturing of early academic research (COSAT) and facilitate translational or applied research toward drug development (eRED). Together, J&J and academia have a unique opportunity to create an enduring partnership that will accelerate the introduction of innovative medicines. One of the most impressive open-access drug discovery partnerships was by UK's Wellcome Trust through a 5-year Seeding Drug Discovery Initiative (SDDI) in 2005 to facilitate the discovery and development of drug leads to fill the unmet medical need gap. It has awarded more than $135 million to 30 institutions supporting 30 drug discovery projects, and has resulted in access to recognized experts in the field, a dozen patents, and three candidates in various stages of clinical trials. The partnership complemented the lack of pharmaceutical expertise of the academic investigators by providing project management oversight, and provided enormous cost savings, as there was no need to develop infrastructure for each of the novel drug targets. A recent review of the SDDI program has indicated the academic collaborators' lack of medicinal chemistry experience to be a major gap, thus confirming our assertion that biomedical researchers tend to me more biology-oriented, and that coordinating therapeutic biology with medicinal chemistry in academia requires efficient matchmaking by experienced project coordinators, an industry best practice.

Open Innovations

Some multimillion-dollar investments have been made by pharmaceutical giants at a number of academic institutions (GSK-Harvard: $50 million, Pfizer-University of California: $9.5 million, Pfizer and University of Pennsylvania: $15 million) to further the basic understanding of systems biology pathways related to human diseases. These open-innovation models are a strategic paradigm shift in overcoming pharma's long held NIH, "not invented here" syndrome, the realization that the task at hand is too large for any one institution, and that the collective wisdom of academia and pharma is critical for combatting human diseases and suffering.

Risk Versus Reward

All diseases occupy a position in the discovery/market risk-space that guides the pharmaceutical industry's drug discovery and development endeavors. The balance between risk and reward can determine the investment and priority of a project for a given institution or company. The risk of a drug discovery project can be measured by the likelihood of success, return on investment, or potential for passing clinical trials. The reward for a project is dependent on the impact of the probe against the target, or the size of the affected patient population. The market risk increases with small patient populations and decreasing financial return projections, and the drug discovery risk increases as targets become unconventional and uncertain. Economic considerations constrain pharma to a low-risk territory and focus on proven targets in diseases with large patient populations. The dynamic between these variables and their interplay for public and private domain drug discovery projects presents a continued challenge in meeting the world's healthcare crises head on.

Philanthropic Investments

The new wave of biomedical research dollars is coming from billionaire philanthropists, who are declaring their own individual wars on diseases. These philanthropists are purpose driven, willing to breakdown the traditional barriers, and to make a difference in peoples lives. The funding, however, is primarily diverted toward "prestigious" universities, and the sponsored research may or may not withstand the rigors of scrutiny by their academic peers. The funding may also be directed toward diseases that afflict families of the billionaire philanthropist, and who mostly happen to be the people of North European descent. So the billionaires of the developing world and the Latin Americas need to make note of the economic and racial aspects of this philanthropy, and step forward to address diseases that are endemic to their own societies. If you don't take care of your own people, then who will?

The not-for-profit disease foundations and charities take our hard-earned dollars and use it in either patient advocacy and/or education, and at times fund research in a high-profile academic investigator's laboratory. The latter gives the much-needed publicity for the foundation's vision and mission but not necessarily help in finding cures for the patient that it so proudly represents. Hundreds of charities are professional money machines, and almost 90% of the collected donations go towards funding employees' salaries and fund-raising efforts, with very little going to the stated cause. A diligent and watchful oversight is more important than ever in the present, wired world.

PROTECTION OF INTELLECTUAL PROPERTY

One of the fundamental tenets of academic research is that the results are to further scientific knowledge by publishing in peer-reviewed journals. Until the 1980s, the government owned IP from federally funded research, and this research went into the public domain in the form of publications and presentations without IP rights. This inhibited the industry from immediately transforming the research ideas coming out of academia into marketable products. The passage of the Bayh–Dole Patent and Trademark Act of 1980 was intended to promote commercialization of inventions resulting from federally funded research. This act provided an incentive to the inventors to use patents to protect their IP. Offices of Technology Transfer were soon created widely across academic institutions, followed by an increase in patent applications from federally funded research. Technology transfer offices continue to assist in the commercialization of research results funded primarily by the government for the welfare of the public. Tasks required by this role include the preparation of confidentiality agreements, materials-transfer agreements, licensing out technology, examining IP, and collaborative agreements with industry. The technology transfer from academia to industry entails prediscovery data-sharing, experimental data for testing computational compound prediction, and pharmacological models. An increase in the academic/industry relationship is also reflected in the establishment and success of the Association of University Technology Managers (AUTM). The AUTM reported an increase in scientific patents issued to universities from 890 to 2120 in the post-Bayh–Dole decade. Under the auspices of the National Science Foundation, Kauffman Foundation, University of Illinois and others, the University–Industry Demonstration Partnership (UIDP) program was launched in 2006 to nourish and expand collaborative partnerships between university and industry in the United States. The UIDP has developed Turbo Negotiator, a software tool, to guide both sides to agreement on the nature of a project. India's Academia Industry Interaction Project is along the same vein, and has created a national database to promote and facilitate pharmaceutical research through government–academia–industry partnership. With regards to the results coming out of the academic HTS labs, including those

of the MLSCN/MLPCN, the IP may lie in the use but not in the composition
of matter. This is because the majority of chemical libraries used by academic HTS labs are in the public domain. Even though the MLPCN is
inching more toward a dedicated chemistry-driven effort in following up
with the screen actives with IP potential, the NIH Roadmap initiative man-
dates that the research results of the sponsored research be deposited in the
public domain through PubChem, with at best a 6 month hold on public disclosure. This does not give enough time to fully explore the chemistry
around the putative probe to make it commercially attractive. Furthermore,
most academic technology transfer offices are unable to extract the IP potential of research coming out of the academic labs, and may not have the experience or the necessary tools to prosecute and defend IP rights. Many times,
the academic investigator approaches pharma to gain access to a tool compound for use in his/her research and signs a Material Transfer Agreement
with terminology such as, "recipient hereby grants to the company a non-
exclusive, worldwide, royalty-free, paid-up license, with the right to subli-
cense, under any patent or other IP rights covering any use of any of the
materials or derivatives arising from requester's research therewith." The
academic investigators should be aware of iron-clad clauses like this that
would permanently exclude them from reaping the benefits of their research.
Another classic example of academia's IP inexperience is exemplified by the
COX-2 story. The University of Rochester School of Medicine and Dentistry
published and filed for a patent in 1992 where in it the usefulness of a COX-
2 inhibitor in pain management was claimed. The same year, Merck and
Searle launched COX-2 programs and launched the hugely profitable drugs,
Celebrex and Vioxx, in 1998. The University filed a suit against Searle
(Pfizer) in the year 2000, but eventually lost in the US Supreme Court
"because the inventors here simply failed to take the last critical step of actually isolating a compound, or even developing a process through which one
of skill would be directly led to such a compound, this patent involves 'little
more than a research plan'" the court concluded. This illustrates the fact of
not rushing to patent prematurely, and this requires effective guidance from
a well-experienced technology transfer office. For spin-off and incubator
companies around academic innovations, careful thought must be given at
the outset whether to license a technology or product, or build a company
around it. Given that 95–97% of projects result in no licensable IP, the
technology-transfer offices have great responsibility in navigating academic
research into a profitable enterprise.

FINDING THE COMMON GROUND

Decreased government funding, tightened budgets in pharma, the
inevitable patent cliff, and pharmaceutical layoffs, all of which are conspir-
ing toward an innovation crisis that is spiraling downward uncontrollably.

The pharmaceutical industry spends well over $135 billion on R&D annually, introducing 25−35 new drugs annually, but still experiences a steep innovation crisis as evidenced by long spells of drying pipeline. It takes almost 15 years, and 3−10 billion dollars, including the cost of failures, to find and bring a drug to patients. The cost is too high, the length of time is long, and both are unsustainable. Clearly, we need a better way to discover and deliver effective treatments. Pharma's new business models seem to rely on the acquisition of drug candidates through alliances and mergers with smaller biotechs, and some active partnerships with academia to address key scientific questions. A resurgence of the pharmaceutical industry to its preeminence can be realized only through strategic collaborative innovation in biomedicine. Since the discovery of insulin at the University of Toronto and its subsequent commercialization by Eli Lilly in the 1920s, academia and the pharmaceutical industry have been involved in a relationship that has been at the heart of drug discovery. Other outstanding examples include the discovery of Alimta (Prof. Edward Taylor's laboratory, Princeton University) and Emtriva (Prof. Dennis Liotta's laboratory, Emory University). Fruitful collaborations, however, rarely materialize without commitment by partners. To avert healthcare crises, pharma/biotech and academia must develop common ground and work together. Pharma/biotech is all about teamwork, a concept not readily embraced by academia. Academic scientists and clinicians apply separate logic on how new drugs function. We need physician scientists to work closely with medicinal chemists to materialize their research ideas.

However, most of the collaborations, open or otherwise never materialize because of lack of commitment by the partners involved. For averting the next healthcare crisis, the two driving forces, pharma and academia, must find a common ground to work together. In pharma, it is all "team" work, a concept that is still not wholeheartedly embraced by academic scientists. The academic scientist (PhD) and the clinician (MD) are miles apart in their thinking of what a new drug ought to/would look like. We need physician scientists to work together with the medicinal chemist to materialize their research ideas. It is undeniable that a major factor influencing the pharmaceutical industry's ability to turn today's innovation into tomorrow's lifesaving medicine is the establishment of strong and diverse partnerships in both the public and private sectors. With so many challenges faced in successfully bringing a medicine to market, we need all the members of the biomedical ecosystem to collaborate. This ecosystem includes academia, nonprofit, and for-profit research institutions, government agencies, the pharmaceutical industry, and disease foundations. Given the complexities and the expense of R&D, we can accomplish much more, in a shorter time, and with less cost and minimal or no duplication of effort when the private and public sectors bring their special strengths to bear. Partnerships, no matter how well conceived or structured, are often fraught with tension. The public and private sectors must engage in a partnership wherein the core missions of each institution are recognized, respected, and accommodated, in order to choose the most disease-relevant therapeutic targets and thereby bridge the translational gap.

Collaboration is not mandatory for success. However, collaborative partnership, open or otherwise, between the stakeholders holds the key in overcoming these hurdles. Partnerships must be coordinated for operational excellence and optimal outcome, based on mutual trust and respect in the core missions of each stakeholder. In recent years, Big Pharma has been exiting in droves from expensive preclinical research because of a lack of guarantee for "success." Many governmental initiatives have stepped in to fund disease biology research to fill the void, and have begun transforming academia into drug discovery behemoths. So, how confident can pharma be in pursuing the discoveries made by the academia? Not very, given the fact than many of the landmark findings in the biomedical and life sciences are not reproducible. Scientific misconduct, including data falsification and peer-review scams, now reaching epidemic proportions, is upsetting this applecart. Since the foundation for successful collaboration is based on mutual trust, all partners, especially the academic scientist, must work harder to rebuild and regain this confidence.

The establishment of strong and diverse partnerships in public and private sectors is critical for patient success. To transcend external challenges for developing better medicines, we need a strong, healthy biomedical ecosystem that includes academia, nonprofit/for-profit research institutions, government agencies, pharma/biotechs, and disease-oriented groups. These partnerships can lower the complexities and expense of R&D, while accomplishing much more in less time. Public—private partnerships can overcome common tensions by recognizing, respecting, and accommodating differences in motivations to focus on the most disease-relevant therapeutic targets.

Deborah Collyar, Patient Advocates in Research, advocates vigorously that it is time to refocus the research system on the true meaning of translational research—to transform scientific discoveries into clinical tools that solve real patient problems. There is no more time for systemic tweaking that produces little but frustration. Patients deal with the dilemmas posed by this broken system every day. It is time for all of the players to center the research culture on patients and turn collaboration into the norm.

IT TAKES A VILLAGE

Drug discovery and development takes a village of diverse expertise to develop effective solutions. First, we must stop "Russian roulette" games that follow unsubstantiated guesses on disease causality. Coordinated collaborative partnerships engaged in unraveling disease etiology will pave the path and eventually lead to effective therapeutic innovations. The much-heralded "open source/science" presents new avenues to foster biomedical innovations through precompetitive strategies that can develop lower-cost, targeted therapeutics for all diseases. Changing the culture for all partners is challenging, but new models will build teamwork, clear boundaries for competition, and reward innovators who embrace these changes.

The 18 year-high new drug introductions in 2014 made the rock-bottom approvals experienced over the past decade a distant memory, but it is the changed mindset of the pharmaceutical industry that embraced coordinated, collaborative innovation that made it all possible. While we preach for effective collaborations between pharma and academia, it is equally critical that pharmaceutical players engaged in therapeutics for a given disease join hands together for better outcomes.

It's time to refocus on the true meaning of translational research—to transform scientific discoveries into solutions for real patient problems. Timidly tweaking an existing dysfunctional system has produced little but frustration. The scope of transformation must expand to include proven communication methods that connect all physicians/scientists, while providing more empathetic coordinated care that engages patients and trial participants. The patient—doctor relationship often governs patient outcomes and satisfaction. It is an open secret that associations with better communications, outcomes, and patient satisfaction result in lower hospitalization rates. Evidence-based medicine also agrees that good outcomes include meaningful results for individuals. A focus on patients will allow patients to know how medical teams meet their needs, and their input should be included. Increasing demands for transparency and data sharing should include how studies are designed, conducted, and summarized. Patient representatives can enhance research efforts and healthcare decisions. Efforts to improve pricing transparency could also enhance quality assessments and patient understanding. Financial transparency is currently represented only when patients are driven to bankruptcy by medical debt. The US Affordable Care Act and biosimilars have helped health systems push back against perceived overpricing and demand more "effective" care, but quality care waivers without better standards.

Patients deal with dilemmas posed by this broken healthcare system everyday. It is time to center the research culture on patients and turn collaboration into the norm. An African proverb suggests it takes a village to raise a child. The same is true for discovering, developing, and delivering drugs to patients, and thwarting the next healthcare crisis before it arises. The difference in the latter case is, according to my good friend Hakim Djaballah, ex-CEO of the Institut Pasteur Korea, we never become our villages but merely guests of leisure, called upon in desperation and ignored during the blooming seasons. That is no way to avert an impending healthcare crisis.

FINAL THOUGHTS

This past year has been a transformative one for the public and private sectors engaged in drug discovery and development, and healthcare delivery. On the plus side, the FDA has approved a total of 45 new drugs in 2015. This is a near all-time high. Again, it is the changed mindset of the pharmaceutical industry that embraced coordinated, collaborative innovation that made it all possible! There are well over 7000 drugs that are in development around the world, with three-fourths being first-in class. Cancer death rates keep falling, thanks to new treatment options and medicines. Cancer immunotherapy, exemplified by Bristol-Myers Squibb's Opdivo and Merck's Keytruda, is now a reality. The HIV/AIDS death rate has fallen by 80–90% in the last two decades. We now have a near 90% cure rate in treating Hepatitis C. On the down side, the cost to develop a drug is still in excess of US$3 billion, with only 20% of the marketed drugs yielding revenues that either match or exceed the R&D costs incurred. It takes more than 10 years to develop a drug, with less than 10–12% of drugs entering clinical trials ever getting FDA approvals. The current failure rate of >80% is unsustainable and we need to find better ways to shepherd clinical candidates toward a successful outcome. Coordinated collaborative innovation, with the pharma, academia, government, and disease-focused foundations working together toward a common goal with the patient in mind, is the only way we can ever achieve this lofty goal.

The ever-increasing cost of prescription drugs makes them out of reach for many, especially the ones with limited means. The new business model promoted by Valeant—buy drug-makers, shrink their R&D, cut jobs, raise prices to astronomical levels—is now being embraced by many in the pharma sector, with Martin Shkreli (Turing Pharmaceutical AG) as its new poster boy! This hypocrisy, raising the cost of a drug to help fund further research, is not in the best interests of the pharmaceutical industry, as it tarnishes its image beyond repair. Take the cue from the British, where the pharmacist buys drugs like Plumicort, which retails for $175 in the US, for about US $20 and then dispenses it free-of-charge.

In the current environment of patent cliffs, high R&D costs, and the paucity of innovative drug discovery, a number of new business models have emerged. The common underlying theme of new business approaches is to finance collaborations that bring together global public and private brainpower, their data sets and experience, with the goal of unraveling biology for improving quality and quantity of drugs while still competing on products.

Scientific research that leads to commercial breakthroughs is vital to the long-term wealth of the nation. But more public spending on science should include ways to ensure that the public shares in profits that result from federally financed research. One possibility would be to require recipients of federal grants to pay a portion of subsequent profits to the government. Another would be to establish a federally backed innovation fund that gives the government an equity stake in companies that use the fund.

We have a right to health, and it is a basic human right.

FURTHER READING

Allarakhia, M., 2014. The successes and challenges of open-source biopharmaceutical innovation. Exp. Opin. Drug Discov. 9 (5), 459–465.

Amirkia, V., Heinrich, M., 2015. Natural products and drug discovery: a survey of stakeholders in industry and academia. Front. Pharmacol. 6, 237.

Chaguturu, R., 2014. Collaborative Innovation in Drug Discovery: Strategies for Public and Private Partnerships. Wiley and Sons, New York, NY.

Collyar, D., Chaguturu, R., 2015. A renaissance in biomedical innovation: global villages raise effective therapies. Future Med. Chem. 7 (8), 971–974.

Collyar, D.E., 2000. The value of clinical trials from a patient perspective. Breast J. 6 (5), 310–314.

Dahlin, J.L., Inglese, J., Walters, M.A., 2015. Mitigating risk in academic preclinical drug discovery. Nat. Rev. Drug Discov. 14 (4), 279–294.

de Vrueh, R.L., Awad, W., Stolk, A., Dijcks, F.A., Rijnders, T.W., Janssen, J.W., 2014. Deal watch: roles and strategies for health foundations in public-private partnerships. Nat. Rev. Drug Discov. 13 (6), 406.

Ehrismann, D., Patel, D., 2015. University - industry collaborations: models, drivers and cultures. Swiss. Med. Wkly. 145, w14086.

Hammonds, T., 2015. Academic-pharma drug discovery alliances: seeking ways to eliminate the valley of death. Future Med. Chem. 7 (14), 1891–1899.

Harris, T., Papadopoulos, S., Goldstein, D.B., 2015. Academic-industrial partnerships in drug discovery in the age of genomics. Trends Biotechnol. 33 (6), 320–322.

Huryn, D.M., 2013. Drug discovery in an academic setting: playing to the strengths. ACS Med. Chem. Lett. 4 (3), 313–315.

Karawajczyk, A., Giordanetto, F., Benningshof, J., Hamza, D., Kalliokoski, T., Pouwer, K., et al., 2015. Expansion of chemical space for collaborative lead generation and drug discovery: the European Lead Factory Perspective. Drug Discov. Today 20 (11), 1310–1316.

Lushington, G.H., Chaguturu, R., 2016. Biomedical research: a house of cards? Future Med. Chem. 8 (1), 1–5.

McDonald, P.R., Roy, A., Chaguturu, R., 2011a. The University of Kansas High-Throughput Screening laboratory. Part I: meeting drug-discovery needs in the heartland of America with entrepreneurial flair. Future Med. Chem. 3 (7), 789–795.

McDonald, P.R., Roy, A., Chaguturu, R., 2011b. The University of Kansas High-Throughput Screening Laboratory. Part II: enabling collaborative drug-discovery partnerships through cutting-edge screening technology. Future Med. Chem. 3 (9), 1101–1110.

Nicolaou, K.C., 2014. Academic-industrial partnerships in drug discovery and development. Angew. Chem. Int. Ed. Engl. 53 (19), 4730–4731.

Powers, B.W., Chaguturu, S., Ferris, T.G., 2015. Optimizing high-risk care management. JAMA 313, 795–796.

Rose, D.M., Marshall, R., Surber, M.W., 2015. Pharmaceutical industry, academia and patient advocacy organizations: what is the recipe for synergic (win-win-win) collaborations? Respirology 20 (2), 185–191.

Roy, A., McDonald, P.R., Sittampalam, S., Chaguturu, R., 2010. Open access high throughput drug discovery in the public domain: a Mount Everest in the making. Curr. Pharm. Biotechnol. 11 (7), 764−778.

Said, M., Zerhouni, E., 2014. The role of public-private partnerships in addressing the biomedical innovation challenge. Nat. Rev. Drug Discov. 13 (11), 789−790.

Sanchez-Serrano, I., 2014. Crisis Mundial de los Sistemas de Salud: Desde el Laboratorio de Investigaciones Hasta la Cama del Paciente. Elsevier, New York, NY.

Smith, G., Cagan, R., 2015. Walking between academia and industry to find successful solutions to biomedical challenges: an interview with Geoffrey Smith. Dis. Model. Mech. 8 (10), 1179−1183.

Yan, W., 2015. Starting up and spinning out: the changing nature of partnerships between pharma and academia. Nat. Med. 21 (9), 968−971.

Yu, H.W., 2015. Bridging the translational gap: collaborative drug development and dispelling the stigma of commercialization. Drug Discov. Today 21 (2), 299−305.

Chapter 16

Righting the Ship: The Data Reproducibility Conundrum

Gerald H. Lushington[1] and Rathnam Chaguturu[2]
[1]*LiS Consulting, Lawrence, KS, United States,* [2]*iDDPartners, Princeton Junction, NJ, United States*

NAVIGATING INNOVATION

There is a great need to foster innovation in drug discovery. Despite being one of the most active application areas of both biology, chemistry, and allied sciences, the discovery and development of biomedical therapeutics remains ensconced behind its frontier, such that a disproportionate amount of research progress is localized within well-trafficked outposts—common, privileged chemotype families targeting known drug targets.

This leaves vast tracts of researchable territory untapped. How many uncharacterized druggable targets lie hidden in that wilderness? How many hitherto unconceived chemotypes and mAbs are waiting to be the next sulfa drugs, statins, or Enbrel? Like the seafarers of old, many of us approach the established frontiers and occasionally gaze out toward the great unknown with no idea on what riches or perils lie in wait. Who will be the great explorer, the drug discovery equivalent of Leif Ericson, Bartolomeu Dias, Zheng He, or Meriwether Lewis? Who next will grow tired of stale conventions and follow the lure of the unknown, ready to face the perils in order to glimpse a new treasure?

Within the confines of a book focusing on innovation, many discussions will slant necessarily toward concepts that are somewhat off the beaten path. If one considers stereotypical routes to drug discovery and development such as either a screening-to-optimization-to-formulation rational design, antibody-drug conjugates, or the derivatization of an intriguingly bioactive natural product isolate, then the chapters in this book will steer you through detours in targeting and refinement strategies, with more speculative protocols such as holistic medicine, ethnopharmacology, reverse pharmacology, polypharmacology, and systems biology. Strategies such as these can produce many opportunities for broadening community perspectives, and may well lead us toward novel opportunities that might never have been uncovered through more conventional means.

Innovative Approaches in Drug Discovery. DOI: http://dx.doi.org/10.1016/B978-0-12-801814-9.00016-7
411

Unfortunately, just as the lure of geographical exploration makes a good analogy for the attractiveness of drug discovery innovation, the metaphor works just as well for the risks. For every historical adventurer who lived to reap great fame, there were others whose fate was to perish far from home. With innovative approaches to therapeutic development, one must consider the odds of a concomitant outcome—after a significant investment of capital or human energy, many projects will either fail to produce a viable product or yield a technology that ultimately demonstrates potentially deleterious toxicity or side effects.

If one ascribes to the growing opinion that conventional drug development protocols have fallen into an endemic state of producing a high rate of efficacy failure, then the temptation to embrace innovation is strong. Even if the prospective chance of success are slim, a fair number of researchers may be willing to gamble their time, and investors or funding agencies may be willing to offer a growing portion of the available funding capital for such innovative opportunities on the chance that possible breakthroughs may be especially transformative and perhaps lucrative.

The key activation barrier toward supporting or pursuing truly novel science may thus not be uncertainty regarding the basic chance of success in optimizing for efficacy and practical drug delivery, but rather the specter of most fundamental risks: especially unexpected adverse health outcomes. In either case, an investment in capital warrants a reciprocal investment in *rigor*—scientists who receive support for risky, outside-of-the-box, cutting-edge research should make every effort to mitigate that risk by ensuring that whatever information and opportunities they produce are backed by the confidence that comes with well-implemented protocols using validated materials and equipment, and producing results that are evaluated by the most rigorous available quality assurance standards. Commitment to such endeavors is easier to justify if one knows that perceived successes are likely to stand the tests of validation, and that any evidence of disappointments or dangers will be examined with brutal rigor and exploited to ensure that resources and time are not unduly wasted on wrong turns. *The ship may be rigged, and the crew may be ready to sail, but nobody should leave the port without a compass and sextant.*

HERE BE MONSTERS: REDUCING THE RISKS

How, in a fundamental sense, does innovation increase risk? Let us examine this question in terms of a thought experiment that focuses on available mechanisms for validation.

Conventional approaches, by their very nature, have a well-established and well-documented track record. Standard protocols are also practiced in similar form by a healthy number of distinct, unaffiliated research groups worldwide. The former condition implies a growing basis for understanding the mechanisms by which previous conventionally produced drugs have failed, and the latter suggests that any time one research group reports enthusiastic progress regarding the development of a new therapeutic candidate, the greater the number of impartial skeptics one may find to subject the reports to judicious scrutiny. So, while the most popular strategies for drug discovery may be somewhat short-sighted and self-limiting, at least the risk of a catastrophic down-stream failure is being gradually mitigated by a growing body of experience. But, can we guarantee a similar set of checks and balances on tantalizing innovations?

There is little doubt that greater innovation produces both a chance of greater reward as well as greater risks. On the reward side of the equation lie considerations such as the prospect that identification of a completely new biomolecular target or therapeutic strategy will open the door for not just one, but potentially many new drugs over the years. Similarly, the discovery of a wholly innovative new chemotype may eventually benefit many target applications beyond the one that originally inspired the development. The fact of the matter is that modulating completely new targets may produce side effects that nobody has hitherto anticipated; the development of new treatment protocols run the risk of untold collateral implications, and new chemotypes may have unpredicted toxic effects that may circumvent standard testing regimens. Above and beyond all of these concerns resides the fact, as stated previously, that for any scientific development that breaks new ground, there will be an inevitable dearth in the availability of high-quality reviewers until independent parties have had an opportunity to not only process the theoretical basis for the development, but also actively apply it in order to perceive realistic strengths, weaknesses, limitations, and practical zones of applicability. Consequently, there may be a period of years in which the innovators may have to rely more critically on self-scrutiny in order to consistently produce meaningful and valuable technical progress with their new paradigm.

If the idea of racing ahead with a new subfield of research, unencumbered by the chafing quibbles of skeptical peers sounds like a great (and potentially very lucrative) opportunity to carve out scientific preeminence, one is advised to reconsider. In the past, the incentive system erected for basic biomedical science researchers (i.e., by funding agencies, journal publishers, and academic administrators) may have favored many people who produced findings that were more "interesting" than accurate, but that tide is turning now in the form of a massive recent surge in studies reporting an epidemic of deleterious scientific irreproducibility. Furthermore, if slipshod research has been permitted within academia, it has long been anathema to industry. Conventional wisdom within the commercialization of novel technology holds that (if accomplished quickly) one is far better off to accurately debunk an "interesting" new prospect before huge amounts of capital are invested in it than to formulate a rash of interesting but unproven new leads.

Putting all of these considerations together lead us to the assertion that innovation is critical to technological development but only if the wheat may be readily separated from the chaff. Such a separation, as we learned long ago from the farmers of ancient Sumer, requires a bit of wind. This chapter is intended to augment some of the key types of innovative analysis reported in the rest of the book, in terms of outlining some key pitfalls that innovative pharmaceutical studies must heed, and proposing a number of best practices to consider in evaluating novel technical developments. In this manner, we hope to provide a bit of a breeze to help researchers separate the grain from the chaff and hopefully also swell the sails of those seeking to set sail upon adventurous new waters.

SHIPWRECKS ON THE REPRODUCIBILITY SEAS

In June of 2015, a long-festering problem exploded into the public consciousness in terms of a perspective piece by Freedman et al. (2015) that outlined the arguments to conclude that there was a $28 billion dollar annual penalty to the United States budget incurred by the waste arising from irreproducible preclinical bioscientific research. The recognition of what can now be justifiably considered a "crisis" had been growing for longer than this, however. The smoke (from which one may infer a major fire) really began to color the horizon several years earlier, beginning with the landmark study by Bayer (Prinz et al., 2011) that attributed a growth decline in the approval rate for phase II clinical trial approvals to a preponderance of highly flawed drug target identification studies originated from academia. While Bayer concluded, in preliminary studies, that as few as 25% of publications reported drug target validation results may be reaching valid conclusions, a paper authored the subsequent year by a former Amgen employee described an Amgen survey that reflected even worse success rates among their attempts to reproduce preclinical scientific results (Begley and Ellis, 2012).

In fairness, the true scope and nature of the problem has not been clearly characterized yet. Neither of the above studies entailed a statistical sampling large enough or sufficiently rigorous to definitively establish a simple expectation value for the percentage of irreproducible studies in the biomedical sciences. Furthermore, there are a broad range of variables that should be accounted for. For example, it would be helpful to rigorously pin down how "irreproducible" is defined. Does the classification include papers in which all seminal predictions are incorrect or merely work that includes at least one erroneous conclusion? How much variation is seen across subdisciplines? Are specific types of measurement especially susceptible to misconceived deductions? Do the errors arise from willful overinterpretation, semi-conscious author bias, innocent misuse of statistics, error in experimental control, or material problems with supplies or testing models?

Despite these unresolved questions, however, there is strong, general empirical evidence to suggest one thing: there is a significant problem with the accuracy of peer-reviewed biomedical research reports and, until major steps are taken to curtail research irreproducibility, there will be major negative consequences to effectiveness through which novel therapeutics are conceived and developed. Lest we immerse ourselves in the consolation that problems within the biomedical sciences are part of a greater problem endemic across challenging technical disciplines, it is sobering to note that preliminary surveys tend to suggest that the biological sciences do tend to lag behind the physical sciences in rigor and objectivity (Fanelli, 2010), and that some biomedical disciplines such as oncology (Begley and Ellis, 2012) and neuroscience (Button et al., 2013) are particularly problematic.

Developing effective strategies for reversing the trend require a better understanding of the issues upon which the problem is predicated. These include the following items discussed in the next section.

AVAST YE SWABS!

Tales of Blackbeard and William Kidd may capture the collective imagination, but far more ships were lost on the Spanish Main by capricious winds and rotting hulls than by the gory glamor of piracy. Similarly, scientific misconduct, in the form of fraudulent manipulation or fabrication of research data, has garnered a substantial amount of attention in the press (Lushington and Chaguturu, 2015; Thomas, 2015), but the true damage it wreaks on scientific integrity tends to be overstated. A 2014 opinion piece in the journal *Nature*, Francis Collins and Lawrence Tabak (Collins and Tabak, 2014) took the rather dramatic step of categorically stating, "Let's be clear: with rare exceptions, we have no evidence to suggest that irreproducibility is caused by scientific misconduct."

This declaration may catch many people by surprise, and counterarguments may certainly be formulated, however the statement underlies a very important cautionary message to the biomedical science community as a whole. If a significant percentage of preclinical biology research is deeply flawed and promulgates research findings whose accuracy is questionable, namely, that a tremendous number of happenstance can interfere with the conduct of reliable, accurate, and reproducible science, that can elude researchers who do not intend to do wrong.

This begs several important questions. If there is far more evidence of inaccurate or defensible biomedical research than there is of fraudulent, where are so many studies going wrong, and why do publications in the field of preclinical biology research slant disproportionately toward positive predictions, in comparison with so-called "hard" scientific disciplines such as physics, chemistry, mathematics, and computer science? Some of the more important reasons may be found in subsequent subsections.

SHIPWORMS IN THE HULL: ANIMAL ANOMALIES, CORRUPT CELLS, AND RECKLESS RNAi

One of the most common sources of research irreproducibility is the most conceptually obvious—sloppiness (Casadevall et al., 2014). There are two common forms—either researchers perform protocols in a way that does not correspond directly to a standard (or stated) protocol, or ensuing publications do not report the protocol in a complete or fully accurate manner. The latter is especially common, and it often occurs not because of negligence on the authors' part but rather because full methodological disclosure is frequently not encouraged by journals or for funding proposals. The simplest solution to this (Lushington and Chaguturu, 2016) might be the mandating of some sort of standardized open-access research protocol repository that could be peer-evaluated, independently of publications and proposals.

Unfortunately, even if the originating researchers summarize their protocol perfectly and report it in all the requisite detail, an independent party is not guaranteed to be able to reproduce the work. Several common sources of irreproducibility have come under a fair bit of scrutiny in recent years.

One noteworthy example of a popular analytical technique with pronounced reproducibility problems is the RNAi technology (Fire et al., 1998) that burst onto the scene in the early 2000s and provided the backbone of the 2006 Nobel Prize in Medicine and Physiology. Billed as a technique that could effectively replace the costly and time-consuming process of producing genetic knockout animals for drug target validation, RNAi promised to open up broad new vistas in drug discovery, but unfortunately many of the exciting new prospects raised by the technique have not been confirmed by independent validation (Bhinder and Djaballah, 2013).

Another technique that has taken a large hit in scientific credibility over the past decade has been the use of antibodies that are widely used for a wide variety of biomedical tasks such as disease diagnostics, biomarker characterization, drug response validation, and target identification. On a simplistic level, it has been assumed that organisms produce antibodies for very specific immune responses, and that each antibody has been designed by an organism to bind to a very specific protein—a property that makes the antibody a tempting tool for tracking any physiological process that produces, or depends on, that protein. Unfortunately, recent surveys have found that many antibodies do not bind to the target protein with reasonable specificity, and some antibodies do not bind to the advertised target protein at all (Monya Baker, 2015). Furthermore, the selectivity and specificity of a given antibody may vary substantially from batch to batch, even when provided by the exact same vendor.

In recent years, substantial doubt has been cast on the validity of a large number of biomedical publications because of an emerging crisis in confidence with respect to many phenotypic cell lines (Freedman, 2015) that have formed the basis for numerous drug design lead discovery campaigns. The problems with cell lines are extensive and broad, including a significant number that are contaminated, others that mistakenly represent phenotypes other than what is specified on their labels, many that do not really correspond to any obvious phenotype at all, and numerous ones that are mislabeled according to tissue source, sex, and even organism (Freedman, 2015). Matters have grown so grim that the International Cell Line Authentication Committee has compiled a list of more than 400 cell lines that are known to be mislabeled (http://iclac.org/databases/cross-contaminations/). Journals such as those in the Nature Publishing Group have now issued a decree that all manuscripts reporting results from cell-based assays must clearly report the source of their cells and to pursue due diligence to confirm the integrity and authenticity of the material (No identified author, 2015).

One final issue whose gravity is now emerging are instances of poor animal study replication. In this case, variations in many studies occur based on very subtle differences in the health of the animals themselves or gender itself. Such irreproducibility can arise from minor variations in diet, subtle handling issues, including temperature, light-level, exposure to noise and numerous other stress factors (Reardon, 2016).

What all of these factors produce is a research atmosphere in which researchers sincerely believe that they are performing careful, diligent, reproducible science, but in fact are generating results that range from qualitatively plausible but not quantitatively reproducible all the way down to being blatantly incorrect.

HEADSTRONG HELM: COGNITIVE BIAS

Experimental uncertainties or inaccuracies such as those described in the previous section can lead to a course correction in an experimental plan. With any luck, such a correction may occur before a huge amount of time, resources, and effort are wasted. Frequently, however, the human brain will miss the signs of error inherent in the use of inaccurate techniques or flawed materials, and instead interpret counter-intuitive behavior as a scientifically interesting outcome.

Because some amount of uncertainty exists in any measurement, and because the human brain is trained to look for abstract patterns based on limited evidence (e.g., that swirl of motion in the tall grass may be a dangerous lion; that tufted shape in the snow may be a vulnerable rabbit), virtually any data-intensive research project may prove vulnerable to a major source of research irreproducibility called *cognitive bias* (Sweedler, 2015). Cognitive bias may be loosely defined as an intrinsic human temptation to quickly ascribe to some notion and, over a longer period of time, use that notion to judge and prioritize subsequent observations.

It is not difficult to imagine data analysis scenarios where human strengths such as nonmachine pattern recognition, cross-disciplinary conceptualization, and intuition turn from virtues into vices. In many cases, the vice arises within the human tendency (frequently a necessity) to attempt to make objective decisions about data we have compiled.

While research efforts in the current generation are blessed with the availability of many powerful computer algorithms for prioritizing and classifying data, and identifying patterns therein, the human brain remains the undisputed master for evaluating semi-processed data (i.e., wherein obvious outliers have been computationally filtered out, and perhaps where some plausible trends models have been identified for consideration) and intuitively determining likely patterns. Our cognitive abilities foster intelligent decisions about data that blend qualitative scientific context with quantitative numerical associations. Simply put, the human brain is blessed with an artist's eye toward visual patterns and a bard's appreciation for a good multifaceted story—attributes that may never truly be replicated or exceeded by machines. Unfortunately, our brains are also equipped with the knave's knack for fooling those around us, as well as ourselves.

In practice, there are two main scenarios where cognitive bias may tend to impact an otherwise rigorous scientific study toward false assumptions that, once emotionally internalized, may prove rather difficult to shed. The first arises from imaginative extrapolation, somewhat analogous to ancient shepherds who could stare up into the night sky, see seven stars, and call it a bear. The second is more of an interpolative process, more akin to a child gazing up at the highly complex shape of a cloud formation and seeing a horse-drawn carriage.

In practice, the interpolative bias case involves the formation of a preliminary hypothesis that, contrary to the ideals of Baconian scientific method, becomes a sacred cow to be sustained with veneration, rather than sacrificed with pragmatism. As an example, one may consider the simplistic conceptualization drawn in Fig. 16.1. These plots depict a small (but let's assume "representative") data set with which one might test for a relationship between the results of some model assay (M) and a clinical outcome (Real).

Based on the full data set (left-most box), one would be hard pressed to find any tangible correlative relationship between the two, which would imply a situation where the model is not the least bit predictive of the clinical outcome. However, if one commences the experiment with a very small preliminary study, one may have a greater chance of encountering a preliminary sample that, based on chance rather than scientific causality, does suggest a prospective trend compelling enough to form a subsequent testable hypothesis.

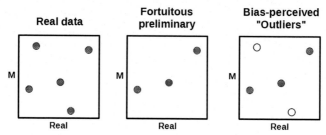

FIGURE 16.1   Cognitive bias as influenced by the order in which data subsets are acquired. Left box represents a complete data set; center reflects a preliminary subset that may bias perception toward a pseudolinear dependency; right box projects our biased treatment of non-corroborative data.

The fate of the future reproducibility of the project hinges on what one does after arriving at the preliminary hypothesis.

We, who have been predisposed to accept the reality of a failed study (i.e., no viable M/Real relationship), would expect the correlation to disappear upon a larger, more comprehensive sampling. But will the researcher who has optimistically formulated a preliminary model based on a fortuitous trend perceive this failure? Might it not be easier to simply find fault with subsequent measurements? Did the reagents degrade in the lag time between initial and confirmatory studies? Was the cell line unstable? Were the animals being treated differently in the later work? Perhaps the laboratory technician performed the experiments in the evening, instead of the morning. If any uncontrolled variables existed by which to contrast the primary and secondary analyses, there is a very human temptation to attribute the non-corroboration to protocol rather than to real biology. Data from the followup study may thus end up being relegated to outlier status, and it is not inconceivable that the researcher will redo the secondary study several times, ostensibly to truly reproduce the original experimental conditions, but perhaps more unconsciously to find another set of secondary data points that confirm the attractive first set.

Whereas the extrapolative cognitive bias trap tends to emerge from starting with too little data, the interpolative case is most likely to manifest in cases when one begins with too much data (MacArthur, 2012).

One common case involves the use of next generation sequencing platforms for target discovery—an analysis in which a great number of prospects may be illuminated, of which some may indeed be targets of legitimate interest, others may hint toward viable targets, and many others may be largely spurious (Gagan and Van Allen, 2015). A second type of experiment that can produce problematic instances of data overload can involve high-throughput chemical screening (Hsieh et al., 2015). In the former case, the most common source of data artifacts involves noisy data produced by the underlying technology, but in the latter case one more frequently encounters a challenging combination of spurious individual data points as well as complex patterns (potentially a blend of both real and ephemeral) that can tempt researchers down various paths of cognitive bias.

In high-throughput chemical screening, it is not uncommon to examine several hundred thousands of compounds screened against a biochemical target or a phenotypic model and potentially arrive at between several hundred and several thousand compounds that (preliminarily) seem to modulate the drug target or model system in a promising manner. It is highly unlikely that any of the compounds emerging from a preliminary screen will ultimately demonstrate the right combination of efficacy, specificity, ADME and favorable toxicology profiles to advance immediately to lead stage, but one generally hopes to be able to identity chemotypes around which one can begin to elaborate promising structure activity relationships that then will foster the formulation of a legitimate lead. The key in this, of course, is to be able to perceive real, meaningful relationships between data points in the screen—a simple-sounding task that is fraught with great ambiguity-related pitfalls.

For any data-intensive experiment, machine-learning algorithms are invaluable tools for attempting to make sense of trends within the raw outputs. Unfortunately, many analyses must at some point give way to human subjectivity. For example, unsupervised clustering calculations may produce multiple possible partitioning scenarios that, from a numerical scoring perspective, all appear to have approximately equivalent strength in describing the data.

If, at this point, human intervention becomes necessary, what is to stop a researcher from choosing a single option that best fits the researcher's preconceived notions about what sort of trends are likely?

As a graphic illustration of this, consider the leftmost square within Fig. 16.2, where the activities (A) of a set of compounds are reported relative to some type of potentially discriminatory molecular property. In order to proceed from this initial study to structure-activity-based lead optimization, it is helpful to parse the data to identify compounds that may represent an analogous mechanism of action. Specifically, within a phenotypic screen,

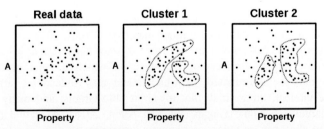

FIGURE 16.2   The clustering dilemma. Left box reports a raw data set; center reflects one clustering scenario in which a larger fraction of data are grouped in a cluster with pseudolinear dependency; right box reflects a second clustering scenario in which only a small fraction of data are grouped in a cluster with pseudolinear dependency.

analogous compounds may predominantly bind to the same molecular target; within a biochemical assay, analogs may exhibit similar pharmacophores. In an ideal case, such groups of chemical analogs should be theoretically evinced by a relationship between bioactivity activity and some key property (or properties) that influence that activity.

From this distribution, an unbiased clustering algorithm might (with minor variations in clustering parameters) arrive at more than one different partitioning schemes with comparable performance in terms of cluster density and contiguity. As seen in the central square of Fig. 16.2, one of these schemes might place a strong plurality of compounds within one central cluster which seems to (rather conveniently) exhibit a near-linear relationship between the observed activity A and a representative (putatively relevant) molecular property. The same level of rigor, however, may produce a rather different partitioning scheme (e.g., right-most box in Fig. 16.2) in which no cluster exhibits a particularly strong relationship between property and activity. If the chosen molecular property truly does have a bearing on the ultimate bioactivity, then it is possible that the large strongly correlating grouping suggested by the middle clustering is a meaningful basis for SAR, and this might seem very cognitively compelling to a researcher. It is also conceivable, however, that the property has little or no true relationship with activity, in which case the weakly pseudolinear (or nonlinear) clusters may be effective evidence of an absence of predictive correlation.

The very different scenarios illustrated by the center box in Fig. 16.2 (property is relevant to activity, and many compounds exhibit strong correlation) versus the right-most clustering (little or no correlation is evident; property relevance is dubious) may come down to a conscious judgment call on the part of a human researcher (an instance of bias blatant enough that most people will not fall for it), or else it will prompt time-consuming confirmatory experiments. The latter may sound like a scientifically rigorous path that most likely will produce reproducible results. However, more often than we realize, the actual strategy ends up being a blend of an *unconscious* judgment call (the researcher decides implicitly that one scenario is more realistic or interesting than the other), and subsequent confirmatory studies are pursued less with a goal of objective validation and more with a subjective intention of producing results that corroborate the predisposed finding.

In other words, the ambiguities posed by having too much data actually end up inviting the same sort of biased human interventions that one might encounter from beginning with too few data.

RIGGING THE SAILS WITH BAD STATISTICS

Conceptually, the cognitive bias scenarios discussed in the prior subsection could be alleviated by placing judgments in the hands of rigorous statistics. Unfortunately, although most biomedical scientists are at least somewhat familiar with good statistical practices, there are many scenarios that are difficult to statistically assess well. Similarly, there are a fair number of circumstances under which it may prove rather easy to statistically assess poorly.

One key source of irreproducibility is the alarming extent to which misleading results may emerge from many experimental methods that are supposedly (and by some measures demonstrably) fairly high in accuracy. A key confounding aspect in this is the "needle in a haystack" effect, whereby experiments produce a strong imbalance between positive and negative outcomes. This scenario is quite common in the drug discovery arena, wherein various experimental surveys (e.g., gene expression profiling for target identification, or high-throughput chemical screening for preliminary hit compounds) are akin to sifting through a great volume of negative instances (the "hay," involving medicinally irrelevant instances), in order to find a small number of positives (the "needles," which are truly relevant to the application).

If we consider an experimental protocol that is 95% accurate in discriminating between negative and positive instances but are conducting an experiment in which 97% of the data points will ultimately prove to be negative (not an outlandish number; many HTS experiments produce a less-than-one-percent hit rate), we encounter significant challenges in arriving at "knowledge" that will be of ultimately reproducible value to our technical objective. This is rendered schematically in Fig. 16.3, where the left-most box depicts the true outcomes that would be determined by an evaluation with 100% accuracy, whereas the middle collection of outcomes shows the more likely scenario of 95% measurement accuracy.

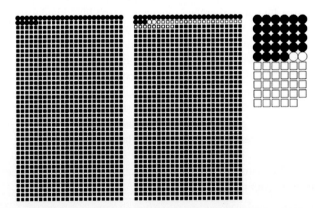

FIGURE 16.3 Experimental outcomes reflecting positive and negative outcomes, as well as correct and incorrect measurements. Leftmost grouping represents real outcomes on 1000 points (black circles are real positives; black squares are real negatives). Center grouping shows experimental assessments (black icons are correctly assessed; white circles are false negatives; white squares are false positives). Rightmost grouping focuses in on the positive determinations (and errors therein) from the center grouping.

Despite the high level of accuracy, the true informational value of the study is distinctly limited. In fact, as we see graphically in the right-most block of Fig. 16.3, the number of false positives (data points that the experiment will misleadingly label as biologically interesting) is actually greater than the number of true positives (data points that are biologically interesting and are correctly recognized as such).

In many biomedical experiments, negative outcomes are largely discarded from future consideration, and it is the positive outcomes that form the informational basis for future work. In such cases, the significant contamination of positives with false positives creates a noisy basis for subsequent studies. Such noise can readily breed misguided conclusions that may be published, cited, and form a foundation for some untold number of future, irreproducible studies.

Nominally, one might expect that the problems associated with low information content in positive/negative imbalanced experiments might be alleviated by carefully validating the experimental technique to ensure better than 95% accuracy for not only the overall predictive performance but also for the positive predictive rate (i.e., false positive rates must be less than 5%).

Such an accuracy target has achieved a wide level of acceptance among data-intensive disciplines as a standard for methodological rigor, as expressed by the standard $p < 0.05$ statistic. Many journals require publications to demonstrate adherence to this standard if they publish conclusions that are based on nonexact determinations (i.e., measurements have a margin of error, or quantification is based on statistical sampling). Unfortunately, a rather alarming number of the studies flagged in the Bayer and Amgen surveys (Prinz et al., 2011; Begley and Ellis, 2012) and in other highly irreproducible disciplines such as psychology use $p < 0.05$ claims with profligacy. How can such a rigorous-seeming standard produce such a volume of irreproducible research?

The answer to this is that many of those studies that justify methodological rigor using $p < 0.05$ criteria actually report a data set that was arrived at in a manner that demonstrates bias not toward a preconceived notion, but rather to an self-consistency that may or may not be representative of data trends in the real world. One example of how such self-consistency bias might be engineered includes a variety of semi-rigorous data point subset selection (random subsets, cluster-based subsets, eliminating "outliers," etc.), that can be applied selectively until one arrives at a subset with an adequate p-value. Another scheme involves shifting the criteria for discriminating between positive and negative outcomes until a favorable positive predictivity can be reported. The final technique for so-called p-hacking is to create a covariate scenario where the outcome depends not on the result of just one measurement but instead on some combination of metrics (Young and Karr, 2011).

In all of these scenarios, researchers might feel justified in claiming that they are not fudging the results, but rather applying deductive reasoning strategies that home in on valuable information. In other words, they may feel that the subset of data points is more accurate and refined in its applicability to the end application than the noisy raw data. Or it may seem that the covariate analysis sheds light on a confluence of factors that jointly influence the underlying biology. The fact of the matter, however, is that in a great many studies, the range of variables that may be selectively tweaked in order to arrive at a favorable p-value is too broad and extensive to support meaningful conclusions. The resulting tweaks are thus more likely to be made in the service of an artificially inflated model performance than they are geared toward honest scientific insight.

Ultimately, although the concept of p-statistics justification has garnered a bad reputation recently, the p-value itself is useful and should theoretically remain as a powerful measure of justifiable persuasion. In order to rehabilitate the concept, it has become critical that a clear record be maintained for just what data the statistic is based on. In this sense, it is not sufficient to report raw quantities for the measurements considered, but rather a study must describe in full detail all preprocessing steps that occurred after raw data was extracted from the source through until the final statistical assessment. All instances whereby data points are dropped from consideration must be explicitly justified, ideally with reference to good data handling practices. In any cases where randomized subsets are selected, it is critical that no final conclusions be based on only one partitioning scheme; the conclusion must be proven to persist in a stable form over multiple orthogonal partitioning instances.

TOWARD CALMER WATERS: RESOURCES AND CONCLUSIONS

Research/data irreproducibility within the biomedical sciences is not a new phenomenon, but what has been emerging recently is a greater understanding of how it can arise, just how much of a problem it poses to medical integrity, and just how much our whole community has to answer for, in terms of letting the problem escalate for so long. While a problem of this nature does not strike us as the sort of situation science would condone, the system of incentives established by our community has not helped the situation. In particular, funding agencies and journals alike have sustained a pronounced bias toward supporting and publishing innovative studies in which the authors report results and conclusions that match (or exceed) their hypotheses.

This status quo has long been implicitly embraced by the broader community. Scientific studies that have ultimately been proven to be irreproducible tend to have been quoted at a statistically significantly higher rate than comparable studies that were later successfully validated (Scientific Electronic Library Online, 2016). This finding is borne out in publications surveyed from among those journals with the highest quartile of impact factor, and the trend is amplified somewhat among publications in journals with the second-highest impact factor quartile. The message inherent in this is that irreproducible research is, on average, valued instinctively in our community, likely as sounding more interesting and being more apt to inspire us than comparatively reliable (perhaps more pedestrian-sounding) studies.

SHAME ON US!

Fortunately, some real teeth are being fixed onto plans and initiatives that may finally have a legitimate impact on the crisis of confidence.

Perhaps the greatest hurdle to overcome on a societal level is the fact that reproducing experiments is costly, time-consuming, and while the US National Institutes of Health has begun making supplement grants available for research groups to support efforts to guarantee replication of their own experiments (No identified author, 2016), even well-intended self-replication is frequently not a close guarantee of independent validation (Aschwanden, 2015). A more promising solution is in early stages in the form of the Reproducibility Initiative (http://www.reproducibilityinitiative.org), which provides a clearinghouse for research groups who would like their work to be independently validated, and other groups who are willing to validate.

The Nature Group, a key leader in the bioscientific publishing industry, aims to transform the culture in which they tacitly facilitated the irreproducibility crisis by taking exploratory steps to foster effective quality control of manuscripts (No identified author, 2014b). Among the changes they are adopting include the commissioning of statistical consultants to evaluate manuscripts in cases where authors or referees request this service. As well, there would be no word count limit in the methods sections of articles, and protocols of even greater detail could be submitted to the open-access protocol repository (http://www.nature.com/protocolexchange). Other services that would aid in research replication (and more generally in scientific advancement) include a *Nature*-affiliated repository for data sets (No identified author, 2014a) and computer code (No identified author, 2014c) produce in conjunction with published studies.

Unfortunately, the resolution promoted by *Nature* falls seriously short of a mindset required to truly necessary to obviate the irreproducibility crisis, in that their efforts do not make any attempt to recognize the scientific value of negative results. Not only does this perpetuate the long-standing scientific tenet that irreproducible advances are more interesting and valuable than honest negative findings, but it also continues to apply the brakes to the mechanism by which science may best advance—a progress through understanding of not only what appears to be, but also by knowing what has already been found not to be.

A variety of informative, online services have emerged for the purpose of disseminating information about the reliability of specific materials and resources that have, in the past, been linked to research irreproducibility. As was mentioned earlier, steps have been taken to publicize the severe problems with cell-line integrity (No identified author, 2015), and a number of services are beginning to watch over the antibody industry, including the independent validation service of Antibodies Online (http://www.antibodies-online.com/independent_validation/) and the compilation of antibody reviews provided by PabMab (http://pabmabs.com/wordpress/).

Our biomedical discipline has entered a state of crisis that reflects an emerging realization of decades worth of questionable science and half-hearted validation. It is perhaps not coincidental that the drug discovery arena has been laboring in a state of technological stagnation for some time. Many experts, when called upon to suggest ways to rise above the discouraging plateau of drug approvals, look at innovation as a means for identifying new pathways, new targets, and new chemotypes to open new physiological and pharmacological horizons. This is a laudable sentiment, but innovation alone is not going to propel our current climate of doldrums. The ship exploring tantalizing new oceans must be sturdy, stable, and water-tight. And as we set foot on new biomedical continents, we must be able to walk accurately and reproducibly before we truly begin to run.

REFERENCES

Aschwanden, C. Science isn't broken. It's just a hell of a lot harder than we give it credit for. Five Thirty Eight. Aug. 19, 2015, <http://fivethirtyeight.com/features/science-isnt-broken/>.

Begley, C.G., Ellis, L.M., 2012. Drug development: raise standards for preclinical cancer research. Nature 483, 531−533.

Bhinder, B., Djaballah, H., 2013. A decade of RNAi screening: too much hay and very few needles. Drug Disc World 14, 31−41.

Button, K.S., Ioannidis, J.P., Mokrysz, C., Nosek, B.A., Flint, J., Robinson, E.S., et al., 2013. Power failure: why small sample size undermines the reliability of neuroscience. Nat. Rev. Neurosci. 14, 365−376.

Casadevall, A., Steen, R.G., Fang, F.C., 2014. Sources of error in the retracted scientific literature. FASEB J. 9, 3847−3855.

Collins, F., Tabak, L., 2014. NIH plans to enhance reproducibility. Nature 505, 612.

Fanelli, D., 2010. Positive results increase down the hierarchy of the sciences. PLoS ONE 5, e10068.

Fire, A., Xu, S., Montgomery, M.K., Kostas, S.A., Driver, S.E., Mello, C.C., 1998. Potent and specific genetic interference by double-stranded RNA in Caenorhabditis elegans. Nature 391, 806−811.

Freedman, L.P., 2015. Know thy cells: improving biomedical research reproducibility. Sci. Transl. Med. 7, 294ed7.

Freedman, L.P., Cockburn, I.M., Simcoe, T.S., 2015. The economics of reproducibility inpreclinical research. PLoS Biol. 13, e1002165.

Gagan, J., Van Allen, E.M., 2015. Next-generation sequencing to guide cancer therapy. Genome Med. 7, 80.

Hsieh, J.H., Sedykh, A., Huang, R., Xia, M., Tice, R.R., 2015. A data analysis pipeline accounting for artifacts in Tox21 quantitative high-throughput screening assays. J. Biomol. Screen. 20, 887–897.

Lushington, G.H., Chaguturu, R., 2015. A systemic malady: the pervasive problem of misconduct in the biomedical sciences. Part I: issues and causes. Drug Discov. World, (spring edition) 79–90, and references therein.

Lushington, G.H., Chaguturu, R., 2016. Biomedical research: a house of cards? Future Med. Chem. 8, 1–5.

MacArthur, D., 2012. Methods: face up to false positives. Nature 487, 427–428.

Monya Baker, M., 2015. Reproducibility crisis: blame it on the antibodies. Nature 521, 274–276.

No identified author. Data-access practices strengthened. Nature, 2014a; 515: 312.

No identified author. Journals unite for reproducibility. Nature, 2014b; 515: 7.

No identified author. Papers in Nature journals should make computer code accessible where possible. Nature, 2014c; 514: 536.

No identified author. Announcement: Time to tackle cells' mistaken identity. Nature, 2015; 520: 7547.

No identified author. Repetitive flaws. Strict guidelines to improve the reproducibility of experiments are a welcome move. Nature, 2016; 529: 256.

Prinz, F., Schlange, T., Asadullah, K., 2011. Believe it or not: how much can we rely on published data on potential drug targets? Nat. Rev. Drug Discov. 10, 712.

Reardon, S., 2016. A mouse's house may ruin experiments. Nature 530, 264.

Scientific Electronic Library Online. Reproducibility of research results: the tip of the iceberg. SciELO in Perspective. [viewed 24 February 2016]. Available from: http://blog.scielo.org/en/2014/02/27/reproducibility-of-research-results-the-tip-of-the-iceberg/.

Sweedler, J.V., 2015. Striving for reproducible science. Anal. Chem. 87, 11603–11604.

Thomas, J.R., 2015. Scientific misconduct: red flags. Scientist <http://www.the-scientist.com/?articles.view/articleNo/44582/title/Scientific-Misconduct--Red-Flags/>.

Young, S., Karr, A., 2011. Deming, data and observational studies. A process out of control and needing fixing. Significance 8, 116–120.

Index

Note: Page numbers followed by "*f*" and "*t*" refer to figures and tables, respectively.

A

Abacavir, 215–216
ABCB1, 209–210
ABCG2, 210
Absorption, distribution, metabolism, excretion, and toxic (ADMET) effects, 127–128, 156, 176–177
Absorption, distribution, metabolism and excretion (ADME) characterization of drugs, 73, 196–197, 281, 420
  role of ADME genes in drug response and adverse drug reactions, 197–198
Academic Drug Discovery Consortium, 394
Accurate toxicology assessment, 308–310
Acetyl-eukaryotic translation initiation factor 5A-1 (acetyl-EIF5A), 284–285
Actinidia eriantha, 337
Activity-based protein profiling, 190
Acyl-CoA dehydrogenase, 282–283
Adenomatous Polyp Prevention on Vioxx (APPROVe) trial, 11–12, 46–47
Adverse drug reactions
  cerivastatin, 26–27
  genetic variability affecting, 214–216
  role of ADME genes in, 197–198
  statins, 26–27
    alteration of muscle cell membrane function, 26–27
    apoptosis, necrosis, and atrophy, 28–29
    cancers, 26–27
    depression, 26–27
    hemorrhagic stroke, 26–27
    liver enzyme elevation, 26–27
    myopathy, 26–27
    myotoxicity, 28
    rhabdomyolysis, 26–27
    type 2 diabetes associated with, 26–27
  thalidomide
    antiangiogenic actions, 50
    damage to embryos, 50
    gene expression profile changes, 50
    induced embryopathy (Phecomelia), 51*f*
  Vioxx (Rofecoxib), 45–46

Aldehyde dehydrogenase-1, 279
Algammulin, 335–336
AlphaScreen technology, 173
Aluminum-based mineral salts (alum), 330
Amplification of intermethylated sites (AIMS), 256–257
Amruta (*Tinospora cordifolia*), 101
Anecdotal drug repurposing, 78
Angelica sinesis, 337
Angiotensin-converting enzyme (ACE) inhibitors, 12–13, 212–213
Anthracycline, 282–283
Antigen identification, 317–320, 320*f*
Apligraft, 16–17
Arg16Gly, 212–213
Arg16/Gly16, 212–213
Arogyavardhini Vati, 100–101
AS01, 319–320
ASO3, 319–320
ASO4, 319–320
Asparegus racemosus (Shatavari), 361
Aspergillus terreus, 25–26
Aspirin, 41–42, 372
  development, 42
  mechanism of action, 42–43
Astragalus, 337
Astragalus polysaccharides (APS), 336
ASTX727, 260
Ataluren (PTC124), 249–250
Atmagupta (*Mucuna pruriens*), 101, 111, 112*f*
Atorvastatin, 25–26, 29–30
ATP binding cassette transporter family (ABC), 209
Aurora kinases, 279
Automated oxidation chemistry for diversified analogues, 108–110
Ayugenomics, 195–196, 222–225
  as a tool for classifying human population, 223
Ayurveda, 91, 93–94, 195–196, 221–222, 225, 337, 353, 375–378. *See also* Triphala
  classical management approach, 113*t*

Ayurveda (*Continued*)
concept of behavioral medicine (*Achara rasayana*), 376
diverse processes during manufacturing, 114
Chausashti pimpali, 114
Piper longum, 114
dosage schedules and dose administrations, 114
fasting and controlled diet, significance of, 376
"Golden Triangle" of, 221–222
hetu-linga-aushadhi (cause-manifestations-management), 100
network ethnopharmacology and, 146
new drug discoveries and, 100–102, 103*t*
panchamahabhuta-tridosha-triguna, 100
pharmacological classification of drugs, 221–222
pharmacotherapeutics in, 113–114
prakriti types, 224
associated with metabolic variability, 223–224
studies, 224–225
product-related attributes, 114
sharir-satva-atman (body-mind-spirit), 100
sleep, quality of, 377
spectrum of ayurvedic drugs, 113*f*
Swasthavritta, 375–376
therapeutics (chikitsa), 112–115
tridosha level (V, P, K) attributes, 221–223
yatha-pinde-tatha-brahmande
(microcosm–macrocosm–continuum), 100
Ayurveda, Unani, Siddha, and homeopathy (AYUSH), 90, 118, 399
Ayurvedic pharmacoepidemiology (AyPE), 96–97
5-Azacytidine, 260

B

Baccosides, 4–5
Bacille Calmette–Guerin (BCG), 328
Bax, 28–29
Bayesian Neural Network (BNN), 170–171
Bayh-Dole Act, 1980, 6
Belinostat, 260–261
Bernard, Claude, 91–92, 91*f*
contributions to modern pharmacology and drug discovery, 92–93
drug discovery paradigm, 93*t*

An Introduction to the Study of Experimental Medicine, 92–93
Beta-blockers, 12–13
BI-2536, 84
Binding database (Binding DB), 142–144
BindingDB database, 301
BiNGO program, 171
Bioactive–target analysis, 133–138
Bioinformatics, 296
Bioinformatic-shRNA/miRNA–validated gene targets, 172–173
BioMarker Identifier (BMI) methodology, 170–171
Biomedical ecosystems, 389–390
Biomedical enterprise, 1
Biotechnology, 5–6
Biotechnology Industry Research Assistance Council (BIRAC), 398
Biotech parks, 400
Black, Sir James, 89
Blood-stage vaccine, 325
Boswellia serrata, 111–112
Botanical medicines, 5
Bushenhuoxue formula, 139–141

C

Calcium channel blockers, 12–13
Camptotheca acuminata, 109–110
Cancer, 282–283
curcumin and, 346
death rates, 1
epigenetic modifications in, 259–260
immunotherapy, 1
statin therapy and, 26–27
triphala and, 149–150
Cancer Bioinformatics Grid™, 394–395
Candidate drug molecules, discovery of, 7
Capillary electrophoresis (CE), 354–355
Capillary gel electrophoresis, 354–355
Capillary isoelectric focusing, 354–355
Capillary zone electrophoresis, 354–355
Carbamazepine (CBZ), 215–216
Carboxymethyl-cofilin-1 (cofilin-1), 284–285
Cc-486, 260
CD4 + T-lymphocytes, 331–332
CD5 molecule-like protein (CD5L), 279
CD8 T cell-mediated immunity, 324
CD8 + cytotoxic T-lymphocytes, 331–332
Celebrex (Celecoxib), 41–42
Celecoxib. *See* Celebrex (Celecoxib)
Cellular thermal shift assay (CETSA), 75–78

Center for Drug Evaluation and Research (CDER), 9−10
Cerivastatin, 25−26
  adverse reactions, 26−27
    induced rhabdomyolysis, 30*f*, 33*f*
  withdrawal of, 26−27
Cetyl Trimethyl Ammonium Bromide−based method of DNA isolation, 356−357
ChemBank database, 300
Chemical genetics, 66*f*, 68−69
Chemical informatics, 296
  for accurate toxicity prediction, 308−310
  for achieving target specificity, 308
  biologically relevant screening sets, 298−302
  challenges in drug discovery, 297−298
  in developing reliable structure-based design, 305−308
  mechanism of action perception, 303
  reliable SAR elaboration analysis, 303−304
  in target identification, 302−303
Chemical investigations center, 105
Chemical libraries, 69−70, 173
ChemMine database, 300−301
Chemotype clusters, 176−177
Chiral switch, 15
Chloroquine, 6
Cholesterol synthesis and membrane excitability, role of statins, 27
  isoprenylation, 27−29
Chromatin immunoprecipitation (ChIP), 257
CIPHER (Correlating protein Interaction network and PHEnotype network to pRedict disease genes), 131
Circumsporozoite (CS) protein, 326
Cistanche deserticola, 355
Cistanche salsa, 355
CK1a, 279
CLARP (caspase-like apoptosis-regulatory protein kinase), 279
Clinical Trials Registry-India (CTRI), 399
Clioquinol, 23−25
Cochrane collaboration, 370
Cognitive bias, 417−421, 419*f*
Collaborative innovation and integration in drug discovery
  academia and, 390−392
  clinical models, 392−393
  culprits in the research-to-care enterprise, 388
  factors considered, 387−388
  government−academia−industry collaboration, 396−397

common ground to work, 404−406
open innovations, 402
pharma courting academia, 400−401
philanthropic investments, 402−403
protection of intellectual property, 403−404
risk and reward, 402
translational research, 407
governmental partnerships, 395−396
need, 388−389
open innovation strategy, 394−396
open source and open science, 393−394
Combination therapy, 81−83
COMBSCORE program, 176−177
Commercialization of healthcare, 368
Commiphora mukul, 361
Commiphora wightii (Guggulu), 101−102, 361
Compactin, 25−27
Comparative binding energy (COMBINE) analysis, 306−308
Comparative Binding Energy (COMBINE) model, 176−177
Comparative Molecular Field Analysis (CoMFA) program, 176−177
Compound collections, screening of, 69−71
Connectivity Map (CMap tool), 145−146, 250
Cordeceps militaris, 106−107
  natural products derived from, 107*f*
CoREST protein, 255−256
Coronin-1A (CORO1A), 279
Council for Scientific and Industrial Research (CSIR), 396
COX-1 and COX-2 enzymes, 42−43
Coxibs, 41−43
  mechanism of, 43, 44*f*
    inhibition of COX-2 mediated pathways, 43
COX inhibitors, 41−42
CP-4200, 260
CRISPR-Cas system, 17−18, 185
Crohn's disease, 73−74, 111−112
Croscarmellose sodium, 43−44
CTSA Pharmaceutical Assets Portal, 394−395
Curcumin, 4−5, 18, 343
  as a chemopreventive agent, 346
  diseases cured with, 347*f*
  limitations associated with usage, 346−347
  modulation of multiple cell-signaling molecules, 345−346
  multiple activities of, 343−345
  multitargeting nature of, 347

Curcumin (*Continued*)
  pleiotropic activities of, 343—345
  safety and efficacy of, 345—346
    against cancers, 346
    against inflammatory bowel disease, 346
  targets of, 343—345, 344*t*
CVDHD database, 142—144
CYP1A2, 201—202
CYP2C9, 195—196, 203, 213
CYP2C19, 202—203
CYP2D6, 204—205
CYP3A4, 205—206
CYP3A5, 205—206
CYP4a inhibitor (HET0016), 48
Cytochrome P450s (CYPs), 287—288
  superfamily of microsomal enzymes, 201
Cytoscape, 145—146, 171

D
D816V, 72
Darwin, Sir Charles, 381—382
Dasatinib, 280
Database relationship network, 145*f*
Decitabine (Dacogen), 260
De novo toxicity prediction, 309—310
Department of Biotechnology (DBT), 398
Department of Science and Technology
  (DST), 397—398
DEREK knowledgebase, 176—177
3'-*O*-Desacyl-4'-monophosphoryl lipid A
  (MPL), 326
Desmin, 282—283
Diabetes mellitus, 286, 368—369. *See also*
  Statin-induced diabetes; Type 2
  diabetes mellitus (T2DM)
Diclofenac, 41—42
Differential methylation hybridization (DMH),
  256—257
1,2-Dihydroxy-3-keto-5-methylthiopentene
  dioxygenase, 284—285
Diode Array Detector (DAD), 354
Discovery space size, 8
Distance—based, mutual-information model
  (DMIM), 132—133
DNA-based antimetabolites, 5
DNA-based molecular markers, 355—358
DNA methylation, 255—258, 260—261
DockBlaster database, 301
Doxorubicin, 282—283
Dragon's blood (DB) tablets, 138—139
Drugable database, 301—302

Drug affinity responsive target stability
  (DARTS) method, 190
DrugBank database, 300
Drug-centered therapeutics, 370
Drug discovery process, 6—8, 167—170.
    See also Genomics-driven drug
    discovery process
  biological approaches, 16—18
  chemical approach, 14—16
  formulation discovery, 18—19
  general path, 168—169
  holistic approaches, 76*f*
    ADME (absorption, distribution,
      metabolism and excretion)
      characterization, 73
    biological redundancy and, 73—75
    combination therapy, 81—83
    drug repositioning, 78—81
    forward and reverse genetics screening
      approaches, 66*f*, 68—69
    high throughput screening (HTS) of
      druggable targets, 69—71
    holistic drug targeting, 75—78
    human genome sequencing, analysis of,
      74
    lead development phase, 73
    multitarget drug discovery approach
      (MTDD), 65—66, 77*f*, 83—85
    rational drug design or virtual HTS
      (vHTS), 71—72
    single target specificity approach, 67
    target identification and validation,
      67—68
  information technology revolution and,
    127—128
  natural products-based new chemical
    entities, 102—108
  need for novel approaches, 13—14
  pharmacognosy-based, 310—312
  pharmacology approaches, 16
  transcriptomics, application of, 248—254,
    249*f*
    herbal drugs, 249—250
    lead optimization, 251—252
  transitions, last 25 years, 8—9
Drug failures, 12—13, 23
Drug hypersensitivity reactions (DHR),
  215—216
  hypersensitivity syndrome, 215—216
  maculopapular eruption, 215—216
  Stevens—Johnson syndrome (SJS), 215—216
  toxic epidermal necrosis (TEN), 215—216

Drug-induced liver injury (DILI), 214–215
Drug lead discovery, 2
Drug metabolizing enzyme (DME), 197–198
  CYP2C19 gene polymorphism model,
    223–224
Drug recalls and withdrawals, 10–12, 23–25
  worldwide, 1950–2015, 24f
Drug repositioning, 78–81
  bioinformatics tools, using, 80–81
  information extraction (IE) methods, 81
  partnerships across academia and industry,
    81
  screening of USFDA approved drug
    collections, 78–80
  systematic literature based discovery (LBD)
    approach, 81
Drug repurposing, 78–81, 79t
Drug revival approaches
  intrinsic properties modulation, 52–53, 53f
    chemical modulation, 53
    use of adjuvant (chemical or botanical),
      53, 55t
  repurposing for another indications, 56
  target modulation, 53
    multitarget modulation, 54
Drugs and biotech parks, 399–403
Drug–target network, 140f, 142f
DTDP-4-dehydrorhamnose 3,5-epimerase
  RmlC, 152–153
Dujieqing Oral Liquid (DJQ), 261

E

Echniacea purpurea, 337
EGb761, 250
EGFR-BRD4 inhibitors, 84
Electrospray ionization (ESI), 275
Eli Lilly-PD2/TD2 Initiatives, 69–70
Elongation factor 2 (EEF2), 284–285
Enantiomers, 14
Enbrel, 16–17
Enhanced green fluorescent protein (EGFP)
  mRNA, 241
Enoyl-acyl carrier protein reductase (ENR),
  154
Epigallocatechin 3-gallate, 154
Epigenomics/epigenetics, 235, 254–255,
  261–262
  mechanisms
    DNA methylation, 255
    histone modifications, 255–256
  methodologies, 256–261

modifications
  in cancer, 259–260
  in degenerative diseases, 259
  in infectious diseases, 257–258
  in lifestyle diseases, 258
  as therapeutic target, 260–261
ESA Biosciences, 353–354
Escherichia coli, 317–318
Esomeprazole (Nexium), 15
Ethnopharmacology, 3–5, 16, 261–262
  based natural product, 5
Ethyl carbamate, 23–25
Etoricoxib, 41–42
Evaporative Light Scattering Detection
  (ELSD), 353–354
Evodiamine/Vorinostat (HDAC inhibitor),
  83–84
Extensive metabolizers (EM), 197–198

F

Farnesyl pyrophosphate, 27–28
Fatty acid amide hydrolase (FAAH), 84
FDA review, 184
Fibrinogen like-2 (FGL2), 279
"Fire and forget" approach of modern
  medicine, 368–369
Fluorescent in situ sequencing (FISSEQ),
  245–248
Fluvastatin, 25–26
Formulation discovery, 18–19
Forward and reverse genetics/pharmacology
  approaches, 66f, 68–69
Forward chemical genetics, 189–190
Fragment based drug discovery (FBDD),
  71–72
Framingham Heart Study, 371
Fufang Xueshuantong (FXST) capsule,
  139–141
Functional pharmaceutical SEZs, India, 400

G

GAK (cyclin-G associated kinase), 279
Galen, 2
4,6-*O*-(S,S)-Gallagyl-alpha/beta-D-
  glucopyranose, 152–153
3-Galloylgallic acid, 153–154
Gallussaeure, 153–154
Gas Chromatography (GC) analysis, 354
Gasteiger–Marsili electrostatics, 176–177
Ge-Gen-Qin-Lian decoction, 139–141
Gemfibrozil, 26–27

Gene expression profiling, 273
Genenentech, 16–17
Genezyme, 16–17
Genome wide association studies (GWAS),
　73–74
Genomics-driven drug discovery process, 273
　academic research as a driver of innovation,
　　166–167
　clinical development, 182–183
　clinical research phase studies, 183–184
　　FDA review, 184
　　life cycle management, 184
　designing clinical trials, 183
　development of drug candidates, 182
　historical perspective, 165–166
　Investigational New Drug Process (IND), 182
　　for marketed drugs, 184
　lead identification, 172–175
　　assay development, 173
　　execution of confirmatory (on-target)
　　　assays and counter-screens (offtarget),
　　　174–175
　　generalized screening protocol, 173–174
　　promoter–reporter constructs, 172–173
　lead optimization strategies, 175–179
　　molecular modeling studies, 176–177
　　NMR structure-based ligand affinity
　　　screening, 178–179
　　probe prioritization, guidelines for,
　　　175–176
　　target-specific chemical probe
　　　optimization, 177
　　tasks of the Medicinal Chemistry team,
　　　177–178
　　using chemoinformatics, 175
　　X-ray crystallography study, 179
　preclinical studies, 179–181
　　evaluation of lead compound efficacy
　　　in vivo, 180–181
　　primary-tumor xenograft model, 180
　target identification, 170–172
　timeline and Go/No Go decision points, 186*f*
Gephi, 146
Geranyl-geranyl pyrophosphate, 27–28
Gglitazones. *See* Thiazolidinediones (THZs)
Ginkgo biloba, 250
Ginseng polysaccharides, 337
Ginsenoids, 4–5, 335
Gleevec, 16–17
Gln27Glu, 212–213
Glutathione peroxidase (GPx), 28
Glutathione S-transferases (GST), 207, 209

Gly16/Gly16, 212–213
Glycrrhiza glabra, 337
GPCR-focused drug discovery, 110–112
Gueriguian, Dr. John L., 34
Guggulsterone (GS), 4–5, 285
Gymnema sylvestre, 111

H

Haemophilus influenzae type b (Hib),
　315–316
Health care crisis, 387–389
Heat shock protein beta-1 (HSP27), 284–285
Hepatitis B vaccine, 328–329
HepG2 hepatic cells, 28
Heptares Therapeutics StaR(R) technology,
　110–111
Herbal medicines, 5
Herbal remedies, 4, 90
Herb–drug interactions, 287–288, 361
Herceptin, 16–17
High-performance capillary electrophoresis
　(HPCE), 256–257
High-performance liquid chromatography
　(HPLC), 256–257, 352–353, 355
High-Speed Counter-Current Chromatography
　(HSCCC), 353–354
High throughput screening (HTS)
　of druggable targets, 69–71
High throughput screening (HTS)
　technologies, 2, 235–236, 298
Hill, Sir Bradford, 90, 99
Histone acetylases (HAT), 255–256
Histone methyltransferases (HMTs), 255–256
HIV/AIDS death rate, 1
HIV/AIDS vaccine, 320–321
　clinical studies, 321–324
　current approaches for, 324
　　scientific paradigms for development,
　　　324–325
　major successes and failures of, 322*t*
Holarrhena alkaloids, 4–5
Holistic drug targeting, 75–78
Holistic targeting, 2
Hub proteins, 74
Human Genome Project (HGP), 16–17
Human protein atlas (HPA) database, 144
Hydralazine, 260
Hydroxylated CPT derivatives, 109–110, 110*f*
Hydroxypropyl cellulose, 43–44
Hypercholesteromia, 12–13
Hyperglycemia, 12–13

I

Ibuprofen, 41−42
Immunex, 16−17
Immunomodulators, 332−333
Indian Council of Medical Research (ICMR),
    398−399
Indomethacin, 41−42
Indoprofen, 23−25
Informatics, 295
Information Gain, 170−171
Innovation in drug discovery, 411
    irreproducible studies, 414−417
        application of statistics, 421−424, 422*f*
        clustering dilemma, 420*f*, 421
        cognitive bias, 417−421, 419*f*
        resources and conclusions, 424−425
        scientific misconduct, 415−416
    reducing risks, 412−414
Integrilin, 16−17
Intellectual property, protection of,
    403−404
Intermediate metabolizers (IM), 197−198
Investigational new drug (IND), 7−8
    process, 182
    for marketed drugs, 184
Irinotecan-induced myelosuppression, 216
Isoprenoids depletion, 27−29
    impacts
        on coenzyme Q10 synthesis, 27−28
        interference with posttranslational
            modifications, 28−29
        on selenoprotein synthesis, 28
        skeletal muscle weakness, 28−29, 30*f*
        on statin-induced apoptosis, 28−29
Isoprenylation, 27−29

J

JAK2/FLT3 kinase inhibitors, 84
Japanese (Kampo) medicine, 225
Jawaharlal Nehru Pharma City, 400

K

Kabat-Zinn, Dr Jon, 380−381
Keytruda, 1, 185
Kinase/bromodomain inhibitor, 84
Kolomogorov−Smirnov test, 171
Korean (Sasang constitution medicine), 225
Ku-Di-Dan, 355−356
Kyoto Encyclopedia of Genes and Genomes
    (KEGG), 142−144

L

Laborit, Henri, 78
Lactose, 43−44
Lead optimization, 251−252, 310
    genomics and, 175−179
        molecular modeling studies, 176−177
        NMR structure-based ligand affinity
            screening, 178−179
        probe prioritization, guidelines for,
            175−176
        target-specific chemical probe
            optimization, 177
        tasks of the Medicinal Chemistry team,
            177−178
        using chemoinformatics, 175
        X-ray crystallography study, 179
    proteomics and, 281
        hit/lead molecules properties, 281
Lifestyle diseases, 367−368
Ligation Independent Cloning (LIC) system,
    172−173
Light emitting diodes (LED), 351
Lilly's Phenotypic Drug Discovery Initiative,
    394−395
Linear ion trap (LIT) mass spectrometer, 275
Lipinski's rule of five, 69−70
Listeria monocytogenes, 242
Liu-Wei-Di-Huang pill, 139−141
LMMA (literature mining and microarray
    analysis), 129
Lovastatin, 25−26, 29−30
Lumiracoxib, 84
Lysine-specific demethylase 1 (LSD1),
    255−256

M

Magnesium stearate, 43−44
Malaria vaccine, 325
    challenges to developing, 327
    first successful, 326
MAP Kinase signaling pathways, 251
Matrix-assisted laser desorption/ionization
    (MALDI), 275
Meditation, 378−382
Meloxicam, 41−42
Metabolomics, 273
Metformin, 130−131
Methaqualone, 23−25
Methotrexate (MTX), 212
Methylated DNA immunoprecipitation
    (methyl-DIP), 256−257

Methylenetetrahydrofolate reductase (MTHFR) pathway, 212
Mevalonate, 27−28
MF59, 319−320
MG98, 260
Micellar Electrokinetic Capillary Chromatography, 353−354
Microarray technologies, 245
Microcrystalline cellulose, 43−44
Micro-RNAs (miRNAs), 172, 237−238, 258, 262
    genetic variants of, 242
Miller syndrome, 251
Mind−body therapies, 375, 378
Mindfulness-based, stress-reduction program, 380−381
Mindfulness medicine, 380−381
MiRNA−based biomarkers, 131
Modern pharmacology and drug discovery, 91−94
Molecular legos, 104−105
Morphine, 2
Mucunapruriens, 4−5
Multidrug toxin extrusion proteins (MATES), 209
Multitarget drug discovery approach (MTDD), 65−66, 77*f*, 83−85

N

N-acetyltransferases (NAT), 207−209
Nanopore sequencing, 247
Naproxen, 11, 41−42, 46
Natural products, 3−5
    based drug discovery, 4, 128
    based screens, 72
Natural products-based new chemical entities, 102−108
    background, 102−105
    isolation from plant species, 105−106
        design and synthesis of natural product analogs, 106−108
        fractionation, 106
        sample collection, 106
Nature-affiliated repository for data sets, 415, 417, 425
Neisseria meningitidis, 317−318
Network biology, 129−131
    accumulated-data integration, 129−130
    LMMA (literature mining and microarray analysis), 129
Network construction, 144−146
    nodes, 144−145

Network ethnopharmacology, 131−138
    Ayurveda and, 146
    knowledge bases for, 142−144
    traditional medicine inspired, 138−141
    of triphala, 146−147
Network pharmacology (NP), 16, 128−129
    applications, 154, 155*t*
    construction of networks, 141
    limitations and solutions, 154−156
    miRNA−based biomarkers, development of, 131
    network biology to, 129−131
    TCM formulations using, 134*t*
        synergistic effects of bioactives of, study of, 141
Network−recovery index (NRI), 141
Network target−based Identification of Multicomponent Synergy (NIMS), 139
Neuro-endocrine-immune (NEI) network, 132
New chemical entities (NCEs), 3, 90−91. *See also* Natural products-based new chemical entities
New Millennium Indian Technology Leadership Initiative (NMITLI), 396
    herbal drug project, 396−397
New-onset diabetes (NOD), 31*f*
Next generation of high-throughput sequencing (NGS) technologies, 245−248
    nanopore sequencing, 247
    polony sequencing, 246−247
    RNA-seq technology, 248
    sequencing by ligation, 247
    sequencing by synthesis (SBS), 246
    single molecule DNA sequencing, 247
Nicotinate-nucleotidepyrophosphorylase, 284−285
Noncommunicable diseases (NCD), 367−368
    lifestyle and behavioral interventions, 369−373
        clinical trials, 373−375
        effectiveness of, 372
        exercise and diet, 371−372
        mind−body therapies, 375
        research literature on, 371*t*
        stress management and resiliency training (SMART) program, 375
        walking, 372, 373*t*
Nonsteroidal antiinflammatory drug (NSAID), 41−42, 84
    mechanism of action, 42−43

Novel drug approvals, 9–10
Nrf2-Keap1, 251
Nyctanthes arbor-tristis, 98

O

O6-methylguanine-DNA methyltransferase (MGMT) gene, 261
Observational therapeutics, 97–98
Oligopeptide transporters, 209
Omeprazole, 15
On-target and off-target effects of withdrawal drug, 53
   multitarget modulation, 54
Opdivo, 1, 185
Open Source Drug Discovery (OSDD), 397
Oral hypoglycemic agents (OHAs), 31–32
Organic anion transporters (OATs and OATPs), 209–211
Organic cation transporters (OCTs), 209–211
Organogenesis, 16–17
Otanically-derived polysaccharides, 335–337

P

Paeonia tenufolia, 334
PAINS filters, 69–70
Panax ginseng, 337
Panax notoginseng saponin, 335
Parkinson's disease (PD), 101
Particle Swarm Optimization, 170–171
PASS tool, 302
Pelargonium grandiflorum, 335
Penicillium citrinum, 25–26
Peroxisome proliferator-activated receptor-g (PPARg), 32–33
Personalized medicine in traditional Indian medical system. *See* Ayurveda
Pert, Dr. Candace, 381–382
p glycoprotein (p-gp), 287
p-hacking, 423
PhaEZ Park, 400
Phage display, 190
Pharmaceutical products, retail sales of, 4
Pharmacodynamics (PD), 195
Pharmacogenomics, 195, 359–360
   clinical implementation of, 216–220
      clinically valuable tests for drug response, 218t
   in drug development, 220
   in drug response, 198
   of drug targets, 212–214
   of drug transporters, 209–211
   of phase I drug metabolites, 198–206
   of phase II drug metabolites, 207–209
Pharmacognosy, 72–73, 310–312
Pharmacokinetics (PD), 195
Pharma courting academia, 400–401
Pharmacovigilance, 360
Pharmacovigilance Program of India (PvPI), 360
Phospho-HSP27, 284–285
Phosphoproteomics, 281
Phosphostathmin, 284–285
Phyllanthins, 4–5
Phyllanthus emblica (amla) fruit, 356–357
Phyto-equivalence studies, 355
Picorrihiza kurroa, 337
Pioglitazone, 31–32
Piperidines, 4–5
Pirlindol, 81
Piroxicam, 41–42
Pitavastatin, 25–26, 29–30
PLK1 kinase inhibitors, 84
Poisons, 91–92
   mechanisms of actions, 92t
Polony sequencing, 246–247
Polycystic ovary syndrome (PCOS), 374
Polygala tenuifolia, 334
Polymerase chain reaction (PCR), 5
Polypharmacology, 83, 129–131, 236
Poor metabolizers (PM), 197–198
Pravastatin, 25–26, 29–30
Preclinical drug development, 73
Predictive toxicology (PredTox), 283–284
Preerythrocytic vaccine, 325
Prescription event monitoring (PEM), 360
Primary-tumor xenograft model, 180
Procainamide, 260
Procaine, 260
Prophylactic vaccine, 387–388
Prostaglandin inhibitors, 12–13
Prostate specific antigen (PSA) for prostate cancer, 278
Protein E6 of human papillomavirus 16 (HPV16), 153–154
Protein microarray technology, 276
Protein–protein interaction (PPI) network, 139f
Proteome-chip based microarrays, 190
Proteomics, 273
   advancement in technologies, 274–275
      electrospray ionization (ESI), 275
      linear ion trap (LIT) mass spectrometer, 275

Proteomics (*Continued*)
matrix-assisted laser desorption/
ionization (MALDI), 275
protein microarray technology, 276
surface-enhanced laser desorption/
ionization (SELDI) technology,
275–276
two-dimensional gel electrophoresis (2-
DE), 274–275
application in drug discovery, 276–277,
280*f*
biomarker discovery and identification of
potential therapeutic targets, 278–279
in ethnopharmacology research, 284–286
investigation of botanical medicine,
284–286
for evaluating drug toxicity, 282–284
in lead optimization, 281
limitations and future prospective, 288–289
MS-based, 284
in predicting herb–drug interactions,
287–288
in quality control and standardization of
herbal drugs, 286–287
quantitative, 280–281
in toxicokinetics, 287–288
understanding disease mechanisms,
279–281
vaccines and, 318
Psammaplin A, 260
Psoralens, 4–5
p-statistics, 424
PubChem (The PubChem Compound
Database), 176–177, 300
PU-H71, 280
Punicalins, 152–153
Pyrosequencing sequencing, 245–248
Pyruvate dehydrogenase, 282–283

Q
Qing-Luo-Yin pill, 139
QiShenYiQi formulation, 141
Quality control of botanical products
conventional approaches of, 352
new approaches of
DNA-based molecular markers, 355–358
hyphenated techniques, 352–355
phyto-equivalence studies, 355
Quantitative structure-activity relationship
(QSAR) methodology, 299–301,
303–304

Quercetin, 154, 284–285
Quillaja saponaria 21 (QS21), 326
Quinghaosu, 4–5
Quinine reductase-2, 279

R
Radix glycyrrhizae polysaccharides (GPS),
336
Random Aplified Polymeric DNA (RAPD)-
based molecular markers, 355–357,
357*f*
Rational drug design, 71–72
Rauwolfia alkaloids, 4–5
Rauwolfia serpentina, 93–94
Recombinant DNA technology, 5
Repurposed drugs, 79*t*
Restriction landmark genomic scanning
(RLGS), 256–257
Resveratrol (RVT), 284–285
Reversed-Phase (RP) columns, 352–353
Reverse engineering of vaccines, 318–319
Reverse pharmacology (RP), 89
approach to GPCR-focused drug discovery,
110–112
Ayurveda-inspired hits, 100–102, 103*t*
background of, 90–91
challenges and opportunities in, 117–118
clinical study designs and para-clinical
models in, 98–99
definition and origin, 94–95
experiential studies, 98
experimental and final clinical stage, 99
exploratory studies, 98–99
future direction and scope of differentiation
in, 118–120
ingenuity of, 90–91
new domains and, 108–110
novel biodynamic actions and, 111–112
opportunities for RP correlates, 119*t*
organization for academic development of,
115–117
Fellowship Program in RP and Drug
Development (FRPDD), 116
multisystem-multidisciplinary and
integrative nature of training program,
116
structural and functional elements for,
116*t*
scope of, 94–95
starting points of, 95*t*
transdisciplinary nature of, 119–120

Reverse vaccinology, 318–319, 320*f*
Rezulin. *See* Troglitazone
RG108 (N-Phthaloyl-L-tryptophan)/RG108
     analogs, 260
RICK (Rip-like interacting kinase), 279
Ring-closing metathesis (RCM), 107–108
Ritonavir, 252
RNAi screening, 9
RNAi silencing approaches, 167–168
RNA-mediated interference (RNAi),
     237–238, 416
  advantages of, 244
  application in diseases
     cardiac disorders, 242–244
     central nervous system disorders, 241
     pulmonary disorders, 242
  limitations, 244
  LVs, 241
  therapeutic application of, 238–240
     designing particle size, 239
     endosomal escape, 239
     in identification and validation of drug
        targets, 240–242, 240*f*
     internalization of pathways, 239
     mathematical models, 239–240
     off-target silencing, 238–239
     stability and targeting, 238
RNA-seq technology, 248
Rofecoxib, 14, 23–25. *See also* Vioxx
     (Rofecoxib)
R-omeprazole, 15
Rosiglitazone, 31–32
Rosuvastatin, 25–26, 29–30
RRx-001, 260

S

Safety of botanicals, 358–361
  herb–drug interactions, 361
  pharmacogenomics approach, 359–360
  pharmacovigilance, 360
  prescription event monitoring (PEM), 360
Salicin, 42
Salicylic acid, 42
Salvia miltiorrhiza, 261
Sanger sequencing, 251
Saponins, 334–335
Sarpagandha (*Rauwalfia serpentina*), 100
SB202190, 280
Science hubs, 394
Scientometrics, 370
Seeding Drug Discovery Initiative (SDDI),
     400–401

Selenocysteine-tRNA, isoprenalytion of, 28
Selenoproteins, 28
Sepbox concept, 105–106
Sequence Characterized Amplified Region
     (SCAR), 355–356
Sequencing by ligation, 247
Sequencing by synthesis (SBS) technology,
     246
Sequencing technologies, 245–248
Serial analysis of chromatin occupancy
     (SACO), 257
Serial analysis of gene expression (SAGE),
     244–245, 394–395
Serotonin (5-hydroxytryptamine, 5-HT), 359
Serturner, Frederik, 2
Serum Proteomic Pattern Diagnostics, 283
SGI-110, 260
SGI-1027, 260
Short hairpin RNAs (shRNAs), 240, 251–252
ShRNA gene screening, 167–168
Simvastatin, 25–26, 29–30
Single molecule DNA sequencing, 247
Single nucleotide polymorphisms (SNPs),
     197–198, 199*t*, 212–213
Single target specificity approach, 67
Sipuleucel-T, 319
Siwu decoction, 285–286
Size-Exclusion Chromatography (SEC),
     353–354
Small Business Innovation Research Initiative
     (SBIRI) scheme, 398
Small interfering RNA (siRNA), 237–238,
     240, 251–252
Small-molecule immunodrugs, 333
Society of Behavioral Medicine, 370
Soluble scavenger receptor cysteine-rich
     domain-containing protein (SSC5D),
     279
S-omeprazole, 15
Stability of proteins from rates of oxidation
     (SPROX), 190
Statin-induced diabetes, 29–31
  new-onset diabetes (NOD), 31*f*
  troglitazone, case of, 31–41
  type 2 diabetes, 26–27, 31–32
Statins
  adverse reactions, 26–27
     alteration of muscle cell membrane
        function, 26–27
     apoptosis, necrosis, and atrophy, 28–29
     cancers, 26–27
     depression, 26–27

Statins (*Continued*)
  hemorrhagic stroke, 26–27
  liver enzyme elevation, 26–27
  myopathy, 26–27
  myotoxicity, 28
  rhabdomyolysis, 26–27
  type 2 diabetes associated with, 26–27.
    See also Statin-induced diabetes
  compactin, 25–27
  discovery and development of, 25–29
  history of, 26*f*
  mevinolin, 25–26
Stem cell therapy, 1
STITCH database, 301
Stress management and resiliency training
    (SMART) program, 375, 377
Strong Anion-Exchange HPLC (SAX-HPLC),
    353–354
Structural vaccinology, 318
Structure-activity relationships (SARs),
    176–177, 295–296
Suberanilo-hydroxamic acid (SAHA)
    (vorinostat), 260–261
Sulphacarbamide, 23–25
SuperNatural database, 142–144
Supported oligonucleotide detection system
    (SOLiD), 245–248
Surface-enhanced laser desorption/ionization
    (SELDI) technology, 275–276
SYBYL program, 176–177
Synthetic biology, 318
Synthetic drugs, 3, 6
Systems-based approaches to vaccinology,
    327–328, 329*f*
  examples, 328–329
Systems biology, 326

T
Tai chi chuan (TCC), 381
Tamoxifen, 205
TANK-binding kinase-1, 279
Target–based drug discovery, 127
Target identification and validation, 67–68,
    156, 170–172
  chemical informatics and, 302–303
Taxol, 4, 334
TCMGeneDIT, 132–133
TCMSP database, 142–144
TCM@Taiwan database, 142–144
Terflavin B, 4-*O*-(S)-flavogallonyl-6-*O*-
    galloylbeta-D-glucopyranose, 152–153

Terminalia chebula, 361
Tetrahydrouridine (THU), 260
TG-101348, 84
Thalidomide, 49–51, 78
  adverse effects
    antiangiogenic actions, 50
    damage to embryos, 50
    gene expression profile changes, 50
    induced embryopathy (Phecomelia), 51*f*
  antiangiogenic, antiinflammatory, and
      antimyeloma roles, 51
  diseases associated with, 52*f*
  linked rings, 49–50
  teratogenic effects of S-enantiomer of,
      49–50
Therapeutic Targets Database (TTD), 144
Thiazolidinediones (THZs), 31–32, 37.
    See also Troglitazone (Rezulin)
  mechanism, 32–34, 34*f*
Thin layer chromatography (TLC), 352
Thiobutabarbital, 23–25
Thiopurine methyltransferase or thiopurine S-
    methyltransferase (TPMT), 207
TianMai Xiaoke tablet, 261
Toxicogenomics, 252–253
  limitations and scope, 253–254
  in risk assessment, 253
    cross-species extrapolations, 253
    developmental exposures, 253
    dose-response relationships, 253
    exposure assessment, 253
    hazard screening, 253
    variability in susceptibility, 253
Toxicoproteomics, 284
Traditional Chinese medicine (TCM),
    131–133, 225, 236, 261–262,
    285–286, 337, 347, 353
  addition and subtraction theory of,
      139–141
  network ethnopharmacological exploration
      of, 133
  plants, 90
Traditional Knowledge Digital Library
    (TKDL), 146
Traditional nonsteroidal antiinflammatory
    drug (tNSAIDs), 11, 43, 45–46
Traditional systems of medicine (TSM), 90
Transcendental Meditation (TM), 380
Transcriptomics, 235–248, 273
  application in drug discovery, 248–254, 249*f*
    herbal drugs, 249–250
    lead optimization, 251–252

for avoiding toxicity pathways, 252
interrogation of the transcriptome, 237
key aim of, 237
technologies
microarray, 245
sequencing, 245−248
serial analysis of gene expression
(SAGE), 244−245
in toxicogenomics, 252−253
Transmission-blocking vaccine, 325
Trichostatin, 280−281
Triphala. *See also* Ayurveda
antibacterial and wound healing activity of,
152
antimicrobial activity of, 152
bioactives of, 147, 152
network, 148*f*
in commercial antimicrobial agents, 152
human proteome and diseasome targeting
network of, 147−151, 149*f*, 150*f*
cancers, 149−150
cardiovascular diseases, 151
metabolic disorders, 151
nervous system disorders, 151
methanolic extract of, 151−152
microbial proteome targeting network of,
151−154, 153*f*
network ethnopharmacology of, 146−147
on *Plasmodium falciparum*, 154
protein targets of, 147−149
targets, 149−150
Triterpygium, 337
Troglitazone (Rezulin), 31−41, 283
cytotoxic response of, 38−39
induced acute liver failure, 37
mitochondrial injury, 38−39
hepatotoxicity of, 34−36, 40*f*
alanine aminotransferase (ALT)
elevations, 36, 38−39
formation of electrophilic reactive
intermediates, 41
host related factors, 41
inhibition of bile salt export pump
(BSEP), 39−41
insulin resistance, 35−36
targets of, 35*f*
timeline of events related to, 38*t*
withdrawals, 37
TTK protein kinase (TTK), 279
Turmeric (Curcuma longa), 343
Two-dimensional gel electrophoresis (2-DE),
274−275

Type 2 diabetes mellitus (T2DM), 345, 374
statin-induced, 26−27, 31−32
Tyrosine kinase receptor, 279

U
U0126, 280
Ubiquinone (coenzyme Q10), 27−28
Ubiquitin proteasome system (UPS), 252
UDP-glucuronosyltransferases (UGTs),
207−208
UGT1A1 enzyme, 216
Ultra High Pressure Liquid Chromatography
(UHPLC), 353
Ultra-rapid metabolizers (UM), 197−198
UNC0638, 280−281
Uncaria tomentosa, 337
UNITY fingerprints, 176−177
Universal Natural Products Database (UNPD),
142−144
US pharmaceutical market, 6

V
Vaccines
adjuvants, 329−330
botanically-derived polysaccharides as,
335−337
botanicals for, 334
discovery approaches, 337−338
immune response to a vaccine antigen,
330−332
immune targets for adjuvant discovery,
330−332
saponins, 334−335
small-molecule immunodrugs, 333
trends in, 332−333
Bacille Calmette−Guerin (BCG), 328
against complex pathogens, 320
discovery approaches for
empirical-based, 316−317
genomic approaches for discovery of
antigens, 317−320
proteomics-based, 318
rational-based, 317
structural vaccinology, 318
synthetic biology, 318
genome-wide association studies in,
328−329
HIV/AIDS vaccine, 320−321
malaria, 325
reverse engineering of, 318−319

Vaccines (*Continued*)
  systems-based approaches to vaccinology,
    327–328, 329*f*
    examples, 328–329
  yellow fever vaccine, 328
Vaidya, Dr. Rama, 96–97
Valdecoxib, 41–42
Valproate, 260–261
Van der Waals interactions, 306–308, 307*f*
Vane, Sir John, 99
VaxGen, 321
Vidaza (5-azacytidine), 260
Vioxx Gastrointestinal Outcomes Research
    (VIGOR), 11, 46
Vioxx (Rofecoxib), 11, 41–49
  absorption of, 44–46
  active ingredient in, 43–44
  adverse gastrointestinal effects, 45–46
  cardiovascular toxicity and, 48–49
  development of, 42–46
  forms, 43–44
  inhibition of COX (COX-1 and COX-2), 48
  molecular mechanism of, 49*f*
  preclinical and clinical studies, 44–46
  studies postapproval, 46–47
  targets, 45*f*
  withdrawal of, 47
Vipassana, 381
Virtual HTS (vHTS), 71–72
Visual network pharmacology (VNP), 145–146
Vitamin K epoxide reductase complex 1
    (VKORC1), 213

W
Warfarin, 213
Withania somnifera (Ashwagandha), 225, 285,
    337, 361
Withanolides, 4–5
World Health Organization declaration, 367

X
Ximelagatran, 11

Y
Yellow ferric oxide, 43–44
Yellow fever vaccine, 328
Yoga, 377
  breathing techniques, 379
  effects on, 377
  meditation, 378–382
  "Sun Salutation" exercise, 379–380

Z
Zebularine, 260
ZHENG, concept of, 131–132
  COLD, 132, 139
  HOT, 132, 139
Zhi-Zi-Da-Huang decoction, 139
Zingiber cassumunar, 357
Zingiber zerumbet, 357

Printed in the United States
By Bookmasters